Second National Report on Biochemical Indicators of Diet and Nutrition in the U.S. Population

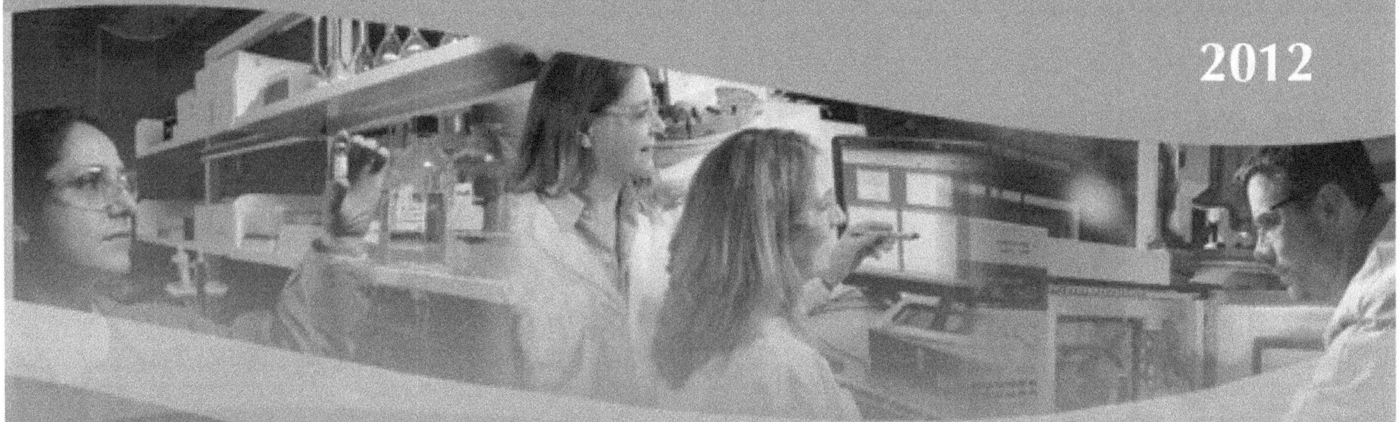

2012

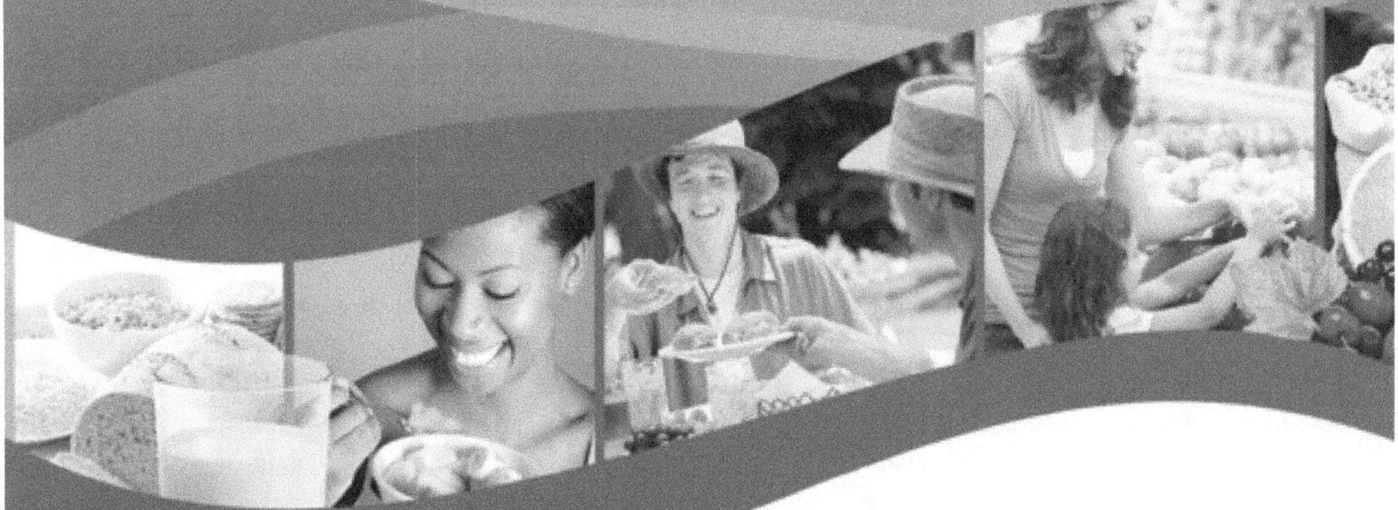

National Center for Environmental Health
Division of Laboratory Sciences

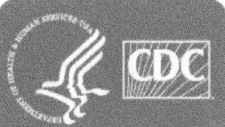

TABLE OF CONTENTS

* crea corr, creatinine corrected

** ODMA, O-desmethylangolensin

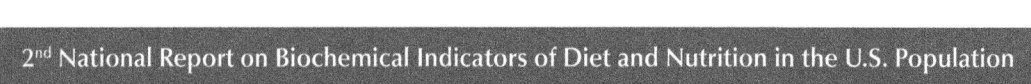

Introduction

- Background
- Addressing Data Needs
- Public Health Uses
- Data Presented for Each Biochemical Indicator
- Interpreting the Data
- Useful Sources of Information about Using Nutrition Monitoring to Interpret Data
- The National Health and Nutrition Examination Survey (NHANES)
- Data Analysis
- References

Introduction

Background

The National Report on Biochemical Indicators of Diet and Nutrition in the U.S. Population is a series of publications that provide ongoing assessment of the U.S. population's nutritional status by measuring blood or urine concentrations of diet-and-nutrition biochemical indicators. The Centers for Disease Control and Prevention's (CDC) Division of Laboratory Sciences at the National Center for Environmental Health (NCEH/DLS) conducted the laboratory analyses for 58 biochemical indicators presented in this 2012 report, which is the second in this series. CDC measured these indicators in specimens from a representative sample of the U.S. population during all or part of the four-year period from 2003 through 2006. Where available, data are also presented on changes of biochemical indicator concentrations over time since 1999. Similarly, data are also presented on the prevalence of low or high biochemical indicator concentrations during 2003–2006, and on changes in the prevalence over time since 1999. The first report of this series was published in July 2008 and contains information on 27 biochemical indicators from all or part of the four-year period from 1999 through 2002. Both reports can be accessed online: http://www.cdc.gov/nutritionreport.

Characteristic	First report, 2008	Second report, 2012
Years of NHANES covered	1999–2002	2003–2006
Number of indicators covered	27	58
Concentrations by race/ethnic group	Yes	Yes
Central 95% reference intervals	No	Yes
Graphic representation of age patterns	No	Yes
Concentrations over time	No	Yes (1999-2006)
Prevalence estimates	No	Yes
Prevalence estimates over time	No	Yes (1999-2006)

CDC's National Health and Nutrition Examination Survey (NHANES), conducted by the National Center for Health Statistics (NCHS), collected the specimens for this report. NHANES is a series of surveys designed to collect data on the health and nutritional status of the U.S. population. This report covers biochemical measurements—one important facet in the assessment of the U.S. population's nutritional status. Other nutrition-related aspects from NHANES, such as dietary intake, supplement usage, hematologic measurements, and anthropometric body measurements are not covered.

In this report, a biochemical indicator means a nutrient (e.g., vitamin, fatty acid, trace element), a metabolite (e.g., homocysteine, methylmalonic acid), or a dietary indicator with potential health relevance (e.g., isoflavone, lignan) measured in blood or urine. Although most biochemical indicators presented in this report enter the human body from foods or supplements, the body itself produces some indicators in response to dietary intake or environmental exposure. Blood and urine concentrations reflect the amount of nutrients and dietary compounds actually in the body or passing through the body from all these sources.

The biochemical indicator sections and new biochemical indicators covered in this report are:

Biochemical indicator sections	New biochemical indicators
• Water-soluble vitamins	• Vitamin B6
• Fat-soluble vitamins and nutrients	• Vitamin C
• Trace elements (iron indicators and iodine)	• Fatty acids
• Isoflavones and lignans	• Iron status: Transferrin receptor and body iron
• Acrylamide hemoglobin adducts	• Acrylamide hemoglobin adducts

Addressing Data Needs

This report is the second CDC product containing reference information on NCEH/DLS measurement data for a wide range of biochemical indicators of diet and nutrition from the most recent continuous NHANES survey, starting in 1999. In this comprehensive report, information on changes in concentrations of a large number of biochemical indicators during 1999–2006 is presented for the first time. Prevalence information on low or high biochemical indicator concentrations is also presented for the first time.

NCHS has historically released or commissioned a variety of products presenting NHANES results. Among these are Data Briefs, Data Tables, Advance Data, Series Reports, and Reports through the Life Sciences Research Office (LSRO). NHANES Series Reports (mainly Series 11) and LSRO Reports from surveys prior to the continuous NHANES have been of particular value to the nutrition community (see Appendix A). The NHANES Web site provides current information on results and products from this survey: http://www.cdc.gov/nchs/about/major/nhanes/survey_results_and_products.htm.

Public Health Uses

This report's primary objective is to inform public health scientists and policy makers about the concentrations of biochemical indicators of diet and nutrition in the general U.S. population and in selected subpopulations. These data will help physicians, scientists, and public health offcials assess inadequate or excess intake and will inform analyses on the relation between biochemical indicators and health outcomes. Other objectives and potential public health uses of the information include

- Establishing and improving on existing population reference levels that can be used to determine whether an individual or a group has an unusually high or low concentration of a diet-and-nutrition biochemical indicator.

- Determining whether the nutritional status of special population groups, such as minorities, children, women of childbearing age, or the elderly, is different from that of other groups, or whether such nutritional status needs improvement.

- Tracking trends over time in the population's biochemical indicator concentrations.

- Assessing the effectiveness of public health efforts to improve the diet and nutritional status of the U.S. population.

- Guide research to perform more in-depth analyses of the NHANES data and to generate hypotheses for future nutrition and human health studies.

Data Presented for Each Biochemical Indicator

This report contains tables and figures of descriptive statistics on the distribution of blood and urine concentrations during all or part of the four-year period from 2003 through 2006 for each diet-and-nutrition biochemical indicator. Statistics include unadjusted geometric means and selected percentiles with confidence intervals. For some biochemical indicators, additional information is included, as available, in the form of

- Tables and figures describing biochemical indicator concentrations across survey cycles during all or part of the eight-year period from 1999 through 2006. Statistics include unadjusted geometric means and selected percentiles with confidence intervals.

- Tables describing the prevalence of low or high concentrations of selected biochemical indicators during all or part of the four-year period from 2003 through 2006 and tables describing the prevalence across survey cycles during all or part of the eight-year period from 1999 through 2006. Statistics include unadjusted percentages with confidence intervals and estimated total number of persons affected.

See **Appendix B** for an overview of the type of information presented for each biochemical indicator. The data are grouped by age, gender, and race/ethnicity. The majority of the biochemical indicators reviewed in this report, with the exception of vitamin C and body iron, have a long upper tail (skewed right). For these biochemical indicators, a geometric mean provides a better estimate of central tendency because it is less influenced by high values than is the arithmetic mean. However, the arithmetic mean is presented for vitamin C and body iron as the distributions for these biochemical indicators were reasonably symmetric. Scientists can use the presented percentile levels to determine those serum, blood, or urine indicator concentrations common to people in the U.S. population and those that are unusual. Frequently, the central 95% reference interval (2.5th to 97.5th percentile) is used to describe normal concentrations in a population. Concentrations outside the reference interval are considered unusual. For urine measurements, data are shown for both the concentration and for the concentration corrected for the urinary creatinine level.

We present the following information for each biochemical indicator during all or part of 2003–2006:

- A table that presents the geometric mean and selected percentile (2.5th–97.5th, so called central 95% reference interval) concentrations by age, gender, or race/ethnicity (1-level stratified).

- A figure that presents the geometric mean concentrations by age and gender or by age and race/ethnicity (2-level stratified).

- Four detailed tables that present the geometric mean and selected percentile (5th or 10th, 50th, 90th or 95th) concentrations by age, gender, and race/ethnicity (3-level stratified). The first table is for the overall U.S. population stratified by age and gender, while the next three tables present data for each racial/ethnic group (Mexican American, non-Hispanic black, and non-Hispanic white) stratified by age and gender.

If data are available for multiple two-year survey cycles from 1999–2006, we present tables with geometric mean and selected percentile (5th–95th) concentrations by age, gender, or race/ethnicity for each available two-year survey cycle, as well as corresponding figures for selected percentiles (1-level stratified).

For biochemical indicators that have accepted cutoff values for low or high concentrations or for both (e.g., folate, vitamins A, B6, B12, C, D, E, ferritin, iodine)—suggesting deficiency or excess of certain micronutrients—we present tables with prevalence estimates by age, gender, or race/ethnicity during all or part of 2003–2006 (1-level stratified). We also present tables with prevalence estimates by age, gender, or race/ethnicity for each available two-year survey cycle from 1999–2006 to allow evaluation of changes in prevalence estimates over time (1-level stratified). See **Appendix C** for a complete listing of the cutoff values and populations described in this report.

Background text provides general information for each indicator to aid with interpreting the data.

To address sources of these nutrients, biochemical pathways in the body, and known health effects, the text contains a brief overview about each indicator.

Each chapter contains highlights followed by detailed observations that are derived from this report's data tables and figures.

The *highlights* are presented directly after the background text. They summarize important observations and discuss them in a public health context. For example, we present figures highlighting prevalence information by demographic subgroups. Where long-term trending information beyond the continuous NHANES is available and of public health interest, we present figures showing changes in biochemical indicator concentrations from NHANES III (1988–1994) to NHANES 1999–2002 and NHANES 2003–2006. The *detailed observations* describe selected categorical differences between demographic subgroups derived from the data tables and figures that follow next. Each chapter is concluded by a list of pertinent references.

Interpreting the Data

Blood or urine concentrations of biochemical indicators can help in assessing the adequacy of intake for the U.S. population. These measurements indicate cumulative intakes from foods, some fortified with micronutrients (e.g., iron, thiamin, riboflavin, niacin, folate, vitamin A, vitamin D), and from dietary supplements that contain vitamins, minerals, or both. However, blood or urine concentrations of biochemical indicators can also be influenced by factors other than diet, such as various diseases or exposures. For those nutrients without defined adequate intakes (e.g., carotenoids, isoflavones), biochemical indicators are useful for assessing intake without regard to adequacy.

Dietary deficiencies are well documented, and they have characteristic signs and symptoms. In addition, recent findings have determined that less than optimal biochemical concentrations (representing suboptimal status) have been associated with risks of adverse health effects. These health effects include cardiovascular disease, stroke, impaired cognitive function, cancer, eye diseases, poor bone health, and other conditions. Adverse health effects, including toxicity, are also possible from consuming excess amounts of certain nutrients and data to assist in the assessment of excessive intake is a feature of this report. Determining the concentrations of a biochemical indicator that may indicate risk for disease and the concentrations that are of negligible health concern requires future research studies that are separate from this report. In collaboration with other agencies and institutions, CDC encourages, and itself conducts research on the relationship between biochemical indicators and health effects.

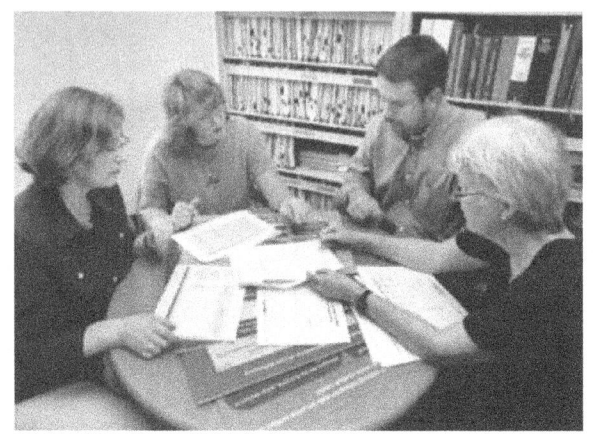

This report contains unadjusted geometric means, selected percentiles, and prevalence estimates of low or high concentrations of diet-and-nutrition biochemical indicators for the civilian, noninstitutionalized U.S. population. A limited interpretation of relative differences between population groups is possible by identifying groups with nonoverlapping confidence intervals. However, one should be careful about interpreting the observed differences as causal. The intent is to describe the characteristics of the population and of selected subgroups, not to explain why the groups display certain characteristics or why they differ from each other. Furthermore, differences in biochemical indicator concentrations of selected subgroups do not necessarily imply health status problems. And for several reasons, one should use caution when drawing temporal conclusions from comparisons of serial cross-sectional NHANES survey cycles. One of these reasons is that different or improved methods of measurement may be employed across the NHANES survey cycles. Another reason is that there are demographic changes to the U.S. population over time. Finally, sampling differences could explain some of the observed changes from one cycle to the next. More in-depth statistical analyses, such as developing models to adjust simultaneously for many covariates and taking into consideration interactions between two or more variables, are beyond the scope of this report. Nonetheless, unadjusted geometric means, selected percentiles, and prevalence estimates provided in this report are useful to summarize reference information for blood or urine concentrations of diet-and-nutrition biochemical indicators for the civilian, noninstitutionalized population in the United States and selected subgroups. We hope that the report will stimulate scientists to examine the data further through analyzing the raw data available at: http://www.cdc.gov/nchs/nhanes.htm.

Laboratories may use different methods for measuring the indicators reported here. However, different methods may result in different method-specific reference intervals. Consequently, to apply these results, health science professionals should check with their particular laboratory to be sure that their methods compare closely to those used in this report (see Appendix D).

Sources of Information on Nutrition Monitoring to Help Interpret the Data

Information about dietary intake is critical to research examining the reasons for nutritional inadequacies. Such information is also critical to programs seeking to improve diet and nutritional status. Selected NCHS Advance Data Reports provide useful overviews (see Appendix A). Also of value are the U.S. Department of Agriculture's (USDA) databases on food surveys and food composition:

What We Eat in America (WWEIA) is the dietary intake interview section of NHANES (http://www.ars.usda.gov/foodsurvey).

The Food and Nutrient Database for Dietary Studies (FNDDS) (http://www.ars.usda.gov/Services/docs.htm?docid=12089) is a database of foods, their nutrient values, and weights for typical food portions. This database is used to generate data for the WWEIA survey through application of the nutrient values from the National Nutrient Database for Standard Reference (http://www.ars.usda.gov/Services/docs.htm?docid=8964).

The National Health and Nutrition Examination Survey (NHANES)

CDC laboratory scientists used biological specimens obtained from NHANES participants to measure biochemical indicators of diet and nutrition for this publication. NHANES is a series of NCHS-conducted surveys designed to collect data on the health and nutritional status of the U.S. population. This is the only national survey that collects biological samples. The NHANES surveys began in 1960 with the first Health Examination Survey (HES 1). The nutritional component was added in the early 1970s in NHANES I. In 1999, NHANES became a continuous survey, sampling the U.S. population annually and releasing the data in two-year cycles.

NHANES collects information on a wide range of health-related behaviors, conducts physical examinations, and collects samples for laboratory tests. Because of physical examination and biological measures, NHANES is unique in its ability to examine public health issues in the U.S. population, such as risk factors for cardiovascular disease. To select a representative sample of the civilian, noninstitutionalized population in the United States, the survey sampling plan follows a complex, stratified, multistage, probability-cluster design. The civilian, noninstitutionalized population consists of persons who are neither in the military nor institutionalized (e.g., they are not residents of nursing homes, college dormitories, or prisons).

The NHANES protocol includes a home interview followed by a standardized physical examination at a mobile examination center. As part of the examination, for participants aged 1 year and older, blood is obtained by venipuncture. Urine specimens are collected from participants aged 6 years and older. By design, approximately half of the participants are evaluated after an overnight fast; for the other half of the participants, there is approximately an equal distribution between those who fasted less than 3 hours and those who fasted between 3 and 8 hours before providing a biological sample. Because weather can adversely affect the mobile examination centers, data are collected in northern latitudes in summer and in southern latitudes in winter. This seasonal-latitude structure might indirectly affect biochemical indicators.

Additional detailed information about the design and conduct of the NHANES survey is available at http://www.cdc.gov/nchs/nhanes.htm. Information about how biological specimens are collected is available at (http://www.cdc.gov/nchs/data/nhanes/blood.pdf) and included in the Laboratory Procedures Manual at http://www.cdc.gov/nchs/data/nhanes/lab1-6.pdf and at http://www.cdc.gov/nchs/data/nhanes/lab7-11.pdf.

Data Analysis

NCHS has developed a comprehensive Web-based tutorial (http://www.cdc.gov/nchs/tutorials/Nhanes/index.htm) to help users better understand the complex survey design and to help them analyze NHANES data.

Because the NHANES sample design is a complex, multistage probability sample, officials use sample weights when estimating the mean or other descriptive metrics. These weights are post-stratified to the U.S. Census Bureau estimates of the U.S. population to adjust for the unequal probability of selection into the survey and possible bias resulting from nonresponse. Demographic data files released by NCHS for each NHANES two-year survey cycle include a two-year interview weight and a medical examination weight. All estimates in this report use the appropriate medical examination weight. The selected medical examination weight depends on whether the specimens tested constitute a random subsample of all the eligible participants and how many survey cycles are combined to produce the estimate.

Combining data over multiple survey cycles can produce estimates with increased statistical reliability. In cases of combined estimates, new weights were constructed. For example, a four-year estimate for the years 2003–2006 was based on a four-year weight, which was created by assigning half the two-year weight for 2003–2004 or half the two-year weight for 2005–2006, depending when the person was sampled.

Results are shown for the total population and by age group, gender, and race/ethnicity, as defined in NHANES. For these analyses, race/ethnicity is presented as Mexican American, non-Hispanic black, and non-Hispanic white. Other racial or ethnic groups are sampled, but the proportion of the total population represented by these other groups is not large enough to produce valid estimates. Thus, this report does not include separate estimates for other racial subcategories. The other racial/ethnic groups, however, are included in the overall estimates.

Data were analyzed by use of the statistical software package Statistical Analysis System (SAS, Version 9.2) and SUDAAN (Release 10.0). SUDAAN uses sample weights and calculates variance estimates that account for the complex survey design. Guidelines for the analysis of NHANES data are provided by NCHS at: http://www.cdc.gov/nchs/nhanes/nhanes2003-2004/analytical_guidelines.htm.

Standard error estimates were calculated by use of the Taylor series (linearization) method within SUDAAN. The degrees of freedom for variance estimation are generated by subtracting the number of strata from the number of primary sampling units (PSUs).

Geometric means were calculated by taking the log of each concentration, calculating the mean of those log values, then taking the antilog of that mean (the calculation can be done by use of any log base, such as 10 or e). The confidence interval uses the standard error and mean on the log scale and the appropriate critical value from the t-distribution to calculate upper and lower confidence limits on the log scale. The confidence intervals of geometric means in this report are based on taking the antilog of those upper and lower confidence intervals.

Percentile estimates were calculated by use of linear interpolation. Confidence intervals for percentiles were calculated by the Woodruff method (1952). This method uses the standard error of the empirical distribution function at the selected percentile and constructs a 95% confidence interval, followed by back-transforming by use of the inverse of the empirical distribution (see **Appendix E** for more details). We used the unweighted sample size and assumed an average design effect of 1.4 as the criteria to estimate percentiles of sufficient precision (U.S. Centers for Disease for Control and Prevention 1996; Table 1 in Appendix B). In order for percentiles to be considered reliable, at least 112 persons had to be represented to allow estimation of the 10th and 90th percentiles, 224 persons for the 5th and 95th percentiles, and 448 persons for the 2.5th and 97.5th percentiles. We flagged and footnoted percentiles where these requirements were not met.

Prevalence estimates for low or high concentrations of biochemical indicators are the weighted percentage of persons who fall below or above a predefined cutoff value (see **Appendix C**). The confidence intervals for prevalence estimates are based on a logit transformation that ensures the confidence interval limits cannot fall outside of 0 and 1. We used the relative standard error (RSE) as a criterion for prevalence estimates of sufficient precision. The RSE is calculated as a percentage by dividing the standard error of the estimate by the estimate value and multiplying by 100. Prevalence estimates associated with a RSE between 30% and less than 40% are flagged and footnoted in this report. Estimates are not provided if they are associated with an RSE equal to or greater than 40%.

Estimates of the total number of persons who met the definition of having low or high concentrations of biochemical indicators were generated by multiplying the weighted prevalence estimate by the population size of interest, derived from the current population survey (CPS) at the midpoint of the available two-year cycle. Confidence intervals for the estimated total, while not presented, are calculated by multiplying the population size of interest by the upper and lower limits of the 95% confidence interval for the weighted prevalence. CPS-based population tables for NHANES by age, gender, and race/ethnicity are on the NHANES Web page for a given survey cycle, available at http://www.cdc.gov/nchs/nhanes/response_rates_CPS.htm. When estimates of the total count are based on combined survey cycles (2003–2006), the 2003–2004 CPS-based population table at the above link was used.

Figures in the highlight section that present age-adjusted geometric mean concentrations from NHANES III (1988–1994), NHANES 1999–2002, and NHANES 2003–2006 or age-adjusted prevalence estimates by demographic subgroups have been generated in SUDAAN by use of age-standardizing proportions from the 2000 U.S. Census population (using direct standardization). Statistically significant differences between age-adjusted geometric means and age-adjusted prevalences were assessed through pairwise comparisons. A reader should take care when interpreting these age-adjusted figures in isolation. The magnitude of an age-adjusted geometric mean or age-adjusted prevalence is completely arbitrary, and it depends upon the chosen standard population. Additionally, age-adjusted geometric means or age-adjusted prevalences can mask important information about trends if age-specific rates do not have a consistent relationship. It is worth noting that while NHANES 1999–2004 provided a race/ethnicity variable that was an analytic link to the NHANES III race/ethnicity variable called RIDRETH2, this variable is not included in the NHANES 2005–2006 demographics file. Therefore, the codes of the race/ethnicity variable called RIDRETH1 were used in displaying age-adjusted geometric means by race/ethnicity for NHANES 1999–2002 and NHANES 2003–2006. RIDRETH1 includes all multi-racial responses in the Other category; whereas, RIDRETH2 includes multi-racial responses for Non-Hispanics with primary race White or Black in the Non-Hispanic White or Non-Hispanic Black categories. This means that there are slightly fewer people coded as non-Hispanic white and non-Hispanic black through RIDRETH1 than for RIDRETH2; however, this difference does not affect the Mexican American category.

The limit of detection (LOD) is the level at which the measurement has a 95% probability of being greater than zero (Taylor 1987). For calculation of geometric means, concentrations less than the LOD were assigned a value equal to the LOD divided by the square root of 2. If the proportion of results less than the LOD (< LOD) was greater than 40%, geometric means were not calculated. Percentile estimates less than the LOD were reported as "< LOD". Most of the indicators had very few results below the LOD value, so that the choice of statistical analysis to handle these results makes little practical difference. There were a few exceptions, however (e.g., serum *cis-beta*-carotene, retinyl palmitate and retinyl stearate; urinary O-desmethylangolensin and equol), where a larger proportion of results were < LOD. **Appendix F** contains a table of LOD values for each biochemical indicator, as well as the unweighted percent of data values that were < LOD for each survey cycle. LOD values may change over the time period of the report as a result of changes in analytical methods. We used the higher of the two LOD values for the analysis of the combined four-year data for 2003–2006.

Due to changes to analytical methods for plasma total homocysteine, serum 25-hydroxyvitamin D, and serum ferritin, an adjustment equation was applied to the data, as described in the NHANES documentation:

- http://www.cdc.gov/nchs/nhanes/nhanes1999-2000/LAB06.htm#Component_Description
- http://www.cdc.gov/nchs/nhanes/nhanes2003-2004/L06VID_C.htm
- http://www.cdc.gov/nchs/nhanes/nhanes2003-2004/L06TFR_C.htm#Analytic_Notes.

For biochemical indicators measured in urine, we present separate tables for the concentration of the indicator expressed as "per volume of urine" (uncorrected table) and the concentration of the indicator expressed as "per gram of creatinine" (creatinine-corrected table). Comparison of an individual participant's result to population data in the tables requires correction for urinary dilution; thus, an individual creatinine-corrected result is needed and should be compared to the creatinine-corrected data tables. Otherwise, health scientists may compare means and percentiles from other studies to the tables having either of the corresponding units. We used the uncorrected tables to compare urine concentrations across groups. Because instrument responses are measured in units of weight per volume, LOD calculations were performed by use of the concentration of the indicator expressed as per volume of urine. For this reason, LOD results for urine measurements in **Appendix F** are in weight per volume of urine. In the creatinine-corrected tables, a result for a geometric mean or a percentile was reported as < LOD if the corresponding geometric mean or percentile was < LOD in the uncorrected table. Thus, for example, if the 5th percentile for males was < LOD in the uncorrected table, it would also be < LOD in the creatinine-corrected table.

References

Taylor JK. Quality assurance of chemical measurements. Chelsea (MI): Lewis Publishing; 1987.

U.S. Centers for Disease Control and Prevention. NHANES analytic guidelines, the Third National Health and Nutrition Examination Survey, NHANES III (1988–94). Hyattsville (MD): National Center for Health Statistics; October 1996 [cited 2011]. Available at: http://www.cdc.gov/nchs/data/nhanes/nhanes3/nh3gui.pdf.

Woodruff RS. Confidence intervals for medians and other position measures. J Am Stat Assoc. 1952;57:622–627.

1. Water-Soluble Vitamins

B Vitamins and Related Biochemical Compounds

- Folate (serum and red blood cell)
- Vitamin B6
  - » Pyridoxal-5'-phosphate
  - » 4-Pyridoxic acid
- Vitamin B12
- Homocysteine
- Methylmalonic acid

Vitamin C (Ascorbic Acid)

B Vitamins and Related Biochemical Compounds

Background Information

Sources and Physiological Functions. Folate, vitamins B6, and B12 belong to the group of water-soluble B vitamins that occur naturally in food. Leafy green vegetables (such as spinach and turnip greens), fruits (such as citrus fruits and juices), and dried beans and peas are all natural sources of folate. Folic acid is the synthetic form of folate found in supplements and added to fortified foods. Because of wide consumption of fortified foods in the United States, these products have become an important contributor of folic acid to the U.S. diet. Folate functions as a coenzyme in single-carbon transfers in the metabolism of nucleic and amino acids. It is therefore especially important during periods of rapid cell division and growth, such as occurs during pregnancy and infancy.

The most abundant dietary sources of vitamin B6 are meats, whole grains (with the highest concentrations of B6 in the germ and aleuronic layer), vegetables, and nuts. Vitamin B6 is used as a cofactor for nearly 200 biochemical reactions in the human body, mostly related to amino acid metabolism. Its three major forms are pyridoxine (the major form in plants) and pyridoxal and pyridoxamine (the two most abundant forms in humans and animals); pyridoxal-5'-phosphate (PLP) is the most biologically active coenzyme form. 4-Pyridoxic acid (4PA) is the end product of vitamin B6 catabolism.

Vitamin B12 (cobalamin) is found naturally in animal foods, including fish, meat, poultry, eggs, milk, and milk products. For vegetarians, fortified breakfast cereals are a particularly valuable source of vitamin B12. The current Dietary Guidelines for Americans list vitamin B12 as a nutrient of concern for specific population groups. The guidelines recommend that persons 50 years and older consume foods fortified with vitamin B12 or dietary supplements (U.S. Department of Agriculture and U.S. Department of Health and Human Services 2010). Vitamin B12 functions as a coenzyme for a critical methyl transfer reaction that converts homocysteine to methionine and for a separate reaction that converts L-methylmalonyl-coenzyme A to succinyl-coenzyme A.

Homocysteine (Hcy) is an amino acid naturally found in the blood. Plasma Hcy concentrations are strongly influenced by diet as well as by genetic factors. Elevated concentrations of total Hcy (tHcy; the sum of free, protein-bound, and disulfides) are found in people whose folate, vitamin B12, or vitamin B6 status is suboptimal (Selhub 1993) and in people with impaired renal function (Wollensen 1999).

Methylmalonic acid (MMA) is a dicarboxylic acid naturally found in the blood. Plasma MMA concentrations are elevated when serum vitamin B12 concentrations are low or intermediate; such concentrations are therefore a useful diagnostic test for confirming vitamin B12 deficiency (Baik 1999). As with plasma tHcy, MMA concentrations are also elevated in people with impaired renal function (Rasmussen 1990).

Health Effects. A chronic dietary deficiency of either folate or vitamin B12 causes macrocytic anemia, although strict dietary deficiencies are rare. Due to the wide abundance of vitamin B6 in foods, dietary deficiencies of vitamin B6 are also rare. Signs of vitamin B6 deficiency include dermatitis, glossitis (inflammation of the tongue), depression, confusion, convulsions, and anemia. Symptoms do not appear immediately, however, for ~80% of the vitamin B6 in the body is stored in muscle tissue and will remain stable until intake has been low for several weeks (Coburn 1990). Certain drugs (e.g., alcohol, methotrexate, anticonvulsants, sulfa drugs) may interfere with the absorption or utilization of folate, and disorders of the small bowel that limit absorption (e.g., Crohn's disease, jejunal bypass surgery) can cause folate deficiency (Halsted 1990). Drugs that react with carbonyl groups have the potential to interact with PLP. Isoniazid—used in the treatment of tuberculosis—and L-DOPA have been shown to reduce plasma PLP concentrations, and a small decrease in vitamin B6 status has been seen in women taking high-dose oral contraceptives (Institute of Medicine 1998). Most people who develop a vitamin B12 deficiency have an underlying stomach or intestinal disorder that limits the absorption of vitamin B12. Subtly reduced cognitive function resulting from early vitamin B12 deficiency is sometimes the only symptom of these intestinal disorders. Severe vitamin B12 deficiency can cause permanent nerve damage and dementia. Hematologic signs, however, are not always present in vitamin B12 deficiency, and hematologic signs and neurologic abnormalities can be inversely correlated (Baik 1999).

Clinical trials have shown that folic acid supplementation effectively reduces the number of neural tube birth defects (NTDs) (Czeizel 1992; MRC Vitamin Study Research Group 1991). Thus, the U.S. Public Health Service recommended that every woman who could become pregnant consume at least 400 micrograms (μg) of folic acid each day (U.S. Centers for Disease Control and Prevention 1992). This recommendation has also been incorporated into the current Dietary Guidelines for Americans, which list folate as a nutrient of concern for specific population groups (U.S. Department of Agriculture 2010). Since 1998, the U.S. Food and Drug Administration (FDA) has required the addition of folic acid to enriched breads, cereals, flours, corn meals, pastas, rice, and other grain products (U.S. Food and Drug Administration 1996). After the introduction of fortification, NTD rates have decreased by 36% (U.S. Centers for Disease Control and Prevention 2010); nevertheless, in the era of folic acid fortification, NTD rates are still highest among Hispanic women (Williams 2005). The higher prevalence in Hispanics could be due to their lower consumption of total folic acid, which is specifically true for less acculturated populations (Hamner 2011). This suggests that there may be factors in addition to folate status, such as genetic or environmental factors, that modulate NTD prevalence and possibly lead to higher folate requirements for some population groups. Recent observational studies have also suggested other potential benefits of the U.S. folic acid fortification, such as decreased prevalence of inadequate serum and RBC folate concentrations (Pfeiffer 2007), and declines in the incidence of stroke (Yang 2006) and neuroblastoma (French 2003). Potential roles of B vitamins in modulating the risk for diseases (e.g., heart disease, cancer, and cognitive impairment) are currently being studied. Two national health objectives that relate to folate and maternal, infant, and child health are part of the objectives for Healthy People 2020: Objective MICH HP2020-14 (increase the proportion of women of childbearing potential with intake of at least 400 μg of folic acid from fortified foods or dietary supplements) and Objective MICH HP2020-15 (reduce the proportion of women of childbearing potential who have low red blood cell folate concentrations) (http://www.healthypeople.gov/HP2020/).

Intake Recommendations. The recommended dietary allowance (RDA) for both men and women is 400 μg per day of dietary folate equivalents (DFEs). DFEs adjust for the nearly 50% lower bioavailability of dietary folate compared to the bioavailability of folic acid: 1 mg of dietary folate equivalent equals 0.6 mg of folic acid from fortified food or from a supplement taken on an empty stomach (Institute of Medicine 1998). The RDA for vitamin B6 is 1.3 mg for both men and women (19–50 years), 1.7 mg for men and 1.5 mg for women aged 51 years and older, and 1.9 mg for pregnant women (2.0 mg if lactating) (Institute of Medicine 1998). The RDA for vitamin B12 for adults is 2.4 μg per day. Because as many as 10 to 30% of older people may be unable to absorb naturally occurring vitamin B12, it is advisable for people older than 50 years to meet their RDA mainly by consuming foods fortified with vitamin B12 or by taking a supplement containing vitamin B12. People with vitamin B12 deficiency caused by a lack of intrinsic factor or intestinal malabsorption require parenteral B12 treatment (Institute of Medicine 1998).

Prolonged consumption of very high daily intakes of folic acid has the potential to delay the diagnosis of anemia among adults with vitamin B12 deficiency. This may result in increased risk of progressive, unrecognized neurological damage from untreated vitamin B12 deficiency. Consequently, the Institute of Medicine (1998) set the Tolerable Upper Intake Level (UL) for folic acid intake for adults (aged 19 years and older) at 1000 µg per day. The UL is defined as the "maximum daily intake levels at which no risk of adverse health effects is expected for almost all individuals in the general population—including sensitive individuals—when the nutrient is consumed over long periods of time" (Institute of Medicine 2000). Because no data were available for children, the Institute of Medicine used the UL for adults adjusted by weight: 300–800 µg

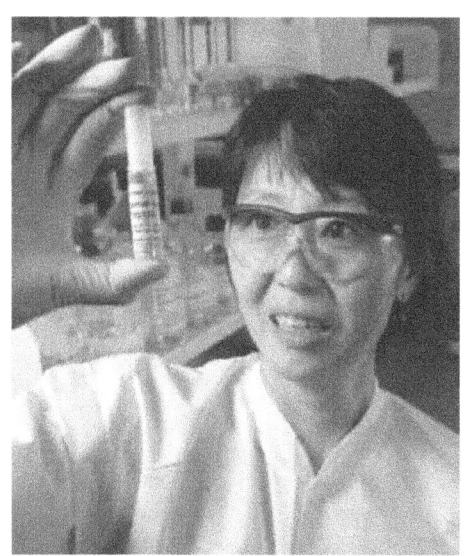

per day, depending on the age group. Folate intake from food is not associated with any health risk. The UL for vitamin B6 for adults is 100 mg per day (Institute of Medicine 1998). If more is ingested through supplements, sensory neuropathy, dermatological lesions, and reversible nerve damage to the arms and legs can occur. No adverse effects have been seen, however, from getting large amounts of vitamin B6 through food sources (Institute of Medicine 1998). No adverse effects have been associated with excess vitamin B12 intake from food or supplements in healthy individuals, and no UL has been set (Institute of Medicine 1998).

Biochemical Indicators and Methods. Folate status can be assessed by measuring serum or plasma folate, which provides information on recent intake, and red blood cell (RBC) folate, indicative of body folate stores and long-term nutritional status. Vitamin B6 status is typically assessed by measuring the level of one or more of the B6 vitamers in serum or plasma. Serum PLP is generally viewed as the best single indicator of status. Serum or urinary 4PA, the end product of vitamin B6 catabolism, is an indicator of recent intake. Vitamin B12 status can be assessed by measuring serum or plasma total cobalamins or serum holo-transcobalamin II, the transport protein of absorbed cobalamin. Urinary or serum MMA is a specific functional indicator of vitamin B12 status. Plasma tHcy is a functional indicator of folate, vitamin B6, and/or B12 status, but it is not specific for either vitamin. As B vitamin concentrations decrease, plasma tHcy concentrations increase.

Clinical laboratories typically use conventional units for measuring concentrations of folate (nanograms per milliliter [ng/mL]) and vitamin B12 (picograms [pg]/mL) and international system (SI) units for vitamin B6 (nanomole per liter [nmol/L]), tHcy (micromole [µmol]/L), and MMA (nmol/L). Conversion factors to SI units are as follows: 1 ng/mL = 2.266 nmol/L for folate and 1 pg/mL = 0.738 picomol (pmol)/L for vitamin B12.

Traditionally, folate has been measured by microbiologic assay; however, in clinical settings, radioprotein-binding assays or commercial non-radio-protein-binding assays on automated clinical analyzers offering high throughput are used (Shane 2011). In research settings, chromatography-based methods, nowadays coupled to tandem mass spectrometry (LC-MS/MS), are often used to measure individual forms of folate in serum or whole blood (Pfeiffer 2010). International reference materials for serum folate from the U.S. National Institute of Standards and Technology (NIST) and the United Kingdom National Institute for Biological Standards and Control (NIBSC), with certified or reference values by higher-order reference methods (LC-MS/MS), have been available only for the last few years: NIST SRM 1955 and 1950, and NIBSC 03/178. A reference material for whole blood folate has been available from the NIBSC (95/528) for several years; however, the value assignment for this material was by consensus of various protein-binding and microbiological assays. Because of observed method differences in measuring folate concentrations (Gunter 1996, Pfeiffer 2010), caution should be used in comparing other datasets to the tables in this report. Method-specific cutoff values and reference intervals for use in medical diagnostics have been suggested previously (Life Sciences Research Office 1994, Gunter 1996) and may be required until clinical assays have been standardized.

Vitamin B6 forms in serum are most commonly measured by high performance liquid chromatography (HPLC) with fluorometric detection; chemical derivatization (sample, online, or post-column) is almost always used to enhance PLP fluorescence (Rybak 2004). Enzymatic (radioactive or nonradioactive) and microbiological methods have also been employed (Coburn 2000). LC-MS/MS methods are emerging (Midttun 2005). The comparability of methods could be improved (Rybak 2005); such improvement is expected to occur in the future due to the new availability of NIST SRM 1950 and 3950 (certified concentrations for serum PLP by LC-MS/MS).

Serum vitamin B12 is commonly measured by competitive protein-binding assay (Carmel 2011). Research methods for tHcy determination are HPLC with fluorescence detection or coupled to tandem mass spectrometry; clinical methods are based on immunoassay or enzymatic principle (Refsum 2004). MMA is measured by gas chromatography coupled to mass spectrometry (GC-MS) or by LC-MS/MS (Pedersen 2011). The comparability among methods for serum vitamin B12, plasma Hcy, and MMA is superior to that for folate. The following international reference materials are available: NIBSC 03/178 for serum vitamin B12 (consensus value); and NIST SRM 1955 and 1950 for plasma tHcy (certified concentration by LC-MS/MS or GC-MS).

Data in NHANES. Folate and vitamin B12 data presented in this report were generated by use of the commercial BioRad Quantaphase II radio-protein-binding assay kit. This is the same method used during the first four years of the continuous NHANES survey (1999-2002) and during NHANES III (1988-1994) (Yetley 2011). The BioRad assay measures approximately 35% lower than the traditional microbiologic assay (Life Sciences Research Office 1994). As a result, the conventional cutoff values of less than 3 ng/mL for low serum folate concentrations, representing a negative folate balance at the time the blood sample was drawn, and less than 140 ng/mL for low RBC folate concentrations (Life Sciences Research Office 1984) should be adjusted to less than 2 ng/mL and less than 95 ng/mL, respectively (Wright 1998). A 2005 WHO Technical Consultation on folate and vitamin B12 deficiencies estimated blood folate and vitamin B12 concentrations below which plasma metabolite concentrations (tHcy for folate and MMA for vitamin B12) became elevated. It arrived at the following consensus cutoff values: 4 ng/mL (10 nmol/L) for serum folate, 151 ng/mL (340 nmol/L) for RBC folate, and 203 pg/mL (150 pmol/L) for serum vitamin B12 (de Benoist 2008). Because the folate data used to derive these cutoff values were generated with the microbiologic assay, the cutoff values are not directly applicable to data generated with the BioRad radio-protein-binding assay. For this report, we used cutoff values of 2 ng/mL and 95 ng/mL, respectively, to estimate the prevalence of low serum and RBC folate concentrations. To estimate the prevalence of low serum vitamin B12 concentrations, we used a cutoff value of 200 pg/mL. This cutoff value is very close to the WHO consensus cutoff value and has been widely used in previous studies (Carmel 2011).

Vitamin B6 data presented in this report include serum PLP and 4PA. They were generated by use of HPLC with post-column derivatization and fluorometric detection (Rybak 2004; Rybak 2009). We used a cutoff value of 20 nmol/L to indicate low serum PLP concentrations. This cutoff value was used by the Institute of Medicine as the basis for the Estimated Average Requirement (EAR) (1998); it may overestimate the vitamin B6 requirement for health maintenance of more than half the group.

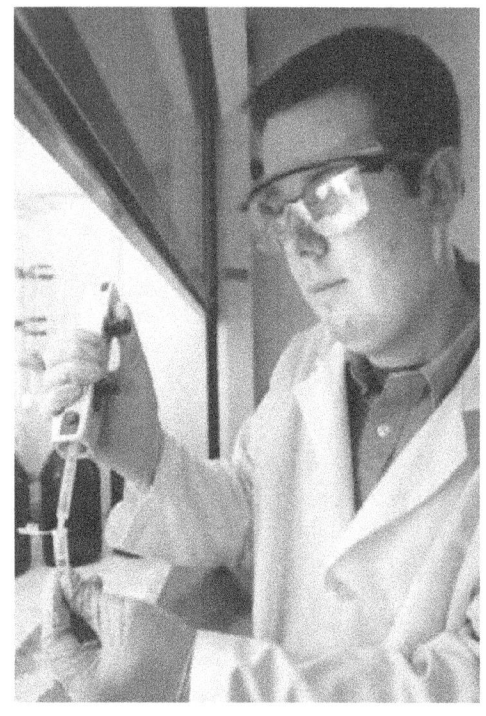

tHcy data presented in this report were generated by use of the commercial Abbott fluorescence polarization immunoassay kit. MMA data were generated through a GC-MS method. Frequently used cutoff values for elevated concentrations of plasma tHcy and MMA are 13 µmol/L (Jacques 1999) and 271 nmol/L (Allen 1990), respectively.

Monitoring the folate status of the U.S. population over time has been a priority (Yetley 2011). It has been so first because serum and RBC folate results from NHANES II (1976–1980) (Senti 1985) and NHANES III (1988–1994) (Wright 1998) suggested that the folate status of some population groups might be of public health concern; a second reason was to assess the impact of folic acid fortification (Pfeiffer 2007). Vitamin B12 status of the U.S. population has been monitored during the second phase of NHANES III (1991–1994) (Wright 1998) and during eight years of the continuous survey (1999–2006). Plasma metabolite concentrations have also been monitored during several years of the continuous survey (tHcy 1999–2006; MMA 1999–2004).

Pfeiffer et al. (2007) showed that the introduction of folic acid fortification has substantially increased serum and RBC folate concentrations in each age group. Serum vitamin B12 concentrations, however, did not change appreciably. Circulating tHcy concentrations from prefortification to postfortification decreased by approximately 10% in a national sample of the U.S. population (Pfeiffer 2008).

For more information on B vitamins and related biochemical indicators, see the Institute of Medicine's Dietary Reference Intake reports (Institute of Medicine 1998) and fact sheets from the National Institutes of Health (NIH), Office of Dietary Supplements (http://ods.od.nih.gov/Health_Information/Information_About_Individual_Dietary_Supplements.aspx).

Highlights

Blood concentrations of water-soluble B vitamins (folate, vitamins B6 and B12) in the U.S. population showed the following demographic patterns and characteristics:

- The highest concentrations were generally found in the youngest age group, except for RBC folate and the vitamin B6 catabolite 4-pyridoxic acid where the highest concentrations were found in the oldest age group.

- No consistent pattern was observed with regard to gender.

- A specific race/ethnic pattern was observed: non-Hispanic blacks had the lowest folate and the highest vitamin B12 status, non-Hispanic whites had the highest folate and the lowest vitamin B12 status, and Mexican Americans had intermediate folate and vitamin B12 status.

- In the era of folic acid fortification, the prevalence of folate deficiency was very low throughout the population.

- The likelihood of being vitamin B6 and B12 deficient was higher in persons 40 years and older compared to younger persons.

Monitoring the continued effect of the U.S. folic acid fortification program of enriched grains and cereal products on serum and RBC folate concentrations is of great public health interest. Serum folate concentrations more than doubled and RBC folate concentrations increased by approximately 50% after the introduction of fortification in 1998. Regardless of gender or race/ethnicity, we observed small decreases (< 10%) in serum and RBC folate concentrations from the earlier (1999–2002) to the later (2003–2006) post-fortification period (Figures H.1.a and H.1.b). However, during the first eight years post-fortification covered in this report (1999–2006), the prevalence of low serum (< 2 ng/mL) and RBC folate (< 95 ng/mL) concentrations was less than 1% in the U.S. population, including women of childbearing age, regardless of race/ethnicity (data not shown). Folate deficiency was virtually non-existent in the general population, and it may be limited to persons with malabsorption, alcohol abusers, or consumers of certain drugs.

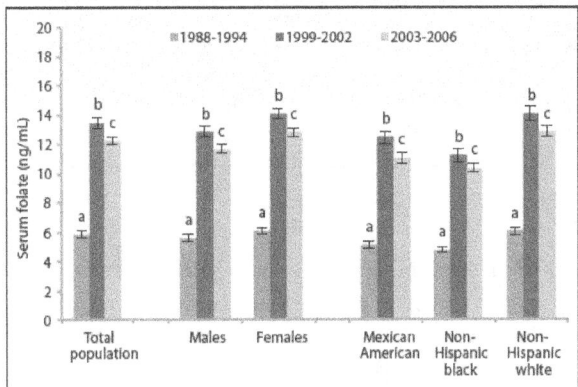 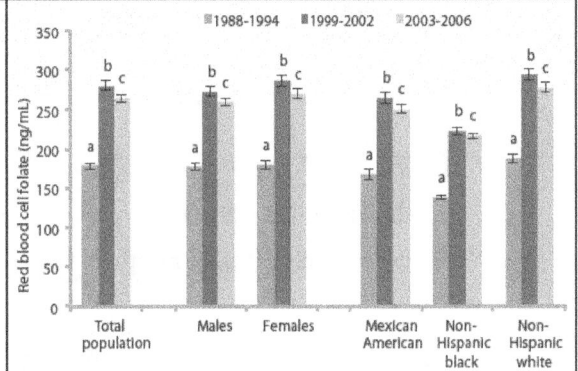

Figure H.1.a. *Age-adjusted geometric mean concentrations of serum folate in the U.S. population aged 4 years and older by gender or race/ethnicity, National Health and Nutrition Examination Survey, 1988–2006.*

Error bars represent 95% confidence intervals. Within a demographic group, bars not sharing a common letter differ (p < 0.05). Age adjustment was done using direct standardization.

Figure H.1.b. *Age-adjusted geometric mean concentrations of RBC folate in the U.S. population aged 4 years and older by gender or race/ethnicity, National Health and Nutrition Examination Survey, 1988–2006.*

Error bars represent 95% confidence intervals. Within a demographic group, bars not sharing a common letter differ (p < 0.05). Age-adjustment was done using direct standardization.

Because of the close relationship of folate and vitamin B12 in one-carbon metabolism, it is of interest to see whether serum vitamin B12 concentrations changed since the introduction of folic acid fortification and whether there are differences among race/ethnic groups. We observed a small increase in serum vitamin B12 concentrations from pre- (1991–1994) to post-fortification (1999–2002). We then found similar concentrations during 2003–2006 for the total population and for males and females (Figure H.1.c). The increase from pre- to post-fortification was observed for non-Hispanic whites, but not for non-Hispanic blacks and Mexican Americans; the latter two groups had higher serum vitamin B12 concentrations than non-Hispanic whites during both pre- and post-fortification.

Assessing the extent of inadequate vitamin B12 status in the older U.S. population is challenging because serum vitamin B12 is not sensitive enough, plasma tHcy is not specific, and both plasma MMA and tHcy are artificially elevated when renal function is impaired, which is common in older persons. As expected, we found a higher prevalence of elevated plasma MMA (17%) or tHcy (19%) concentrations, potentially indicating suboptimal vitamin B12 status, than we found in the prevalence of low serum vitamin B12 concentrations (4%) in older persons (Figure H.1.d). Defining better cutoff values for vitamin B12 status biomarkers remains a continued area of research (Bailey 2011).

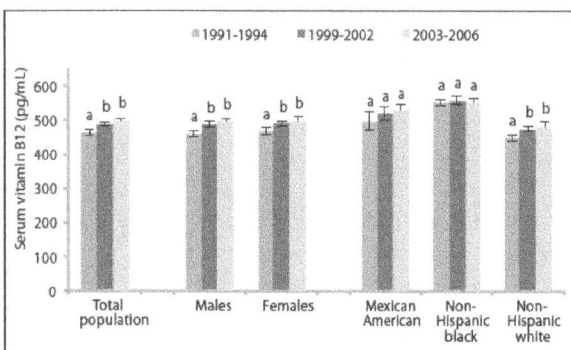

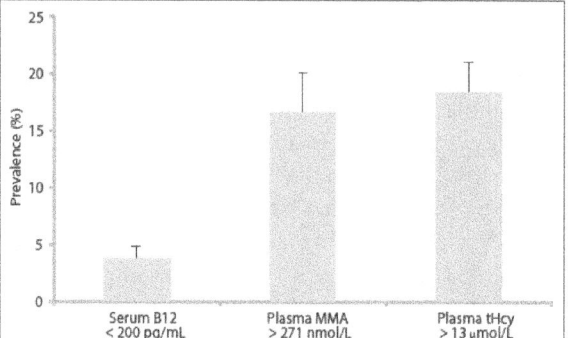

Figure H.1.c. *Age-adjusted geometric mean concentrations of serum vitamin B12 in the U.S. population aged 4 years and older by gender or race/ethnicity, National Health and Nutrition Examination Survey, 1991–2006.*

Error bars represent 95% confidence intervals. Within a demographic group, bars not sharing a common letter differ (p < 0.05). Age adjustment was done using direct standardization.

Figure H.1.d. *Prevalence estimates of low serum vitamin B12 (B12), high plasma methylmalonic acid (MMA), and high plasma total homocysteine (tHcy) concentrations in U.S. persons 60 years and older, National Health and Nutrition Examination Survey, 2003–2006.*

Data shown for plasma MMA are from NHANES 2003–2004 only. Error bars represent 95% confidence intervals.

Detailed Observations

The selected observations mentioned below are derived from the tables and figures presented next. Statements about categorical differences between demographic groups noted below are based on non-overlapping confidence limits from univariate analysis without adjusting for demographic variables (e.g., age, gender, race/ethnicity) or other blood concentration determinants (e.g., dietary intake, supplement usage, smoking, BMI). A multivariate analysis may alter the size and statistical significance of these categorical differences. Furthermore, additional significant differences of smaller magnitude may be present despite their lack of mention here (e.g., if confidence limits slightly overlap or if differences are not statistically significant before covariate adjustment has occurred). For a selection of citations of descriptive NHANES papers related to these biochemical indicators of diet and nutrition, see **Appendix G**.

Geometric mean concentrations (NHANES 2003–2006):

- Serum and RBC folate concentrations followed a U-shaped age pattern, with the lowest concentrations seen in adolescents and young adults, respectively (Tables 1.1.a.1 and 1.2.a.1; Figures 1.1.a and 1.2.a).

- Serum PLP concentrations declined from childhood to adolescence, then stabilized in older age groups (Table 1.3.a.1 and Figure 1.3.a). Serum 4PA concentrations were lowest in adolescence and increased steadily through the oldest age group (Table 1.4.a.1 and Figure 1.4.a).

- Serum vitamin B12 concentrations declined from childhood to adolescence and then stabilized in older age groups (Table 1.5.a.1), while plasma MMA concentrations were relatively stable through young adulthood, and then increased with age (Table 1.7.a.1 and Figure 1.7.a).

- Plasma tHcy concentrations in adults increased with age (Table 1.6.a.1 and Figure 1.6.a).

- Females had higher serum and RBC folate concentrations than males (Tables 1.1.a.1 and 1.2.a.1); males had higher serum PLP and plasma tHcy concentrations than females (Tables 1.3.a.1 and 1.6.a.1); males and females had similar serum 4PA (Table 1.4.a.1), vitamin B12 (Table 1.5.a.1) and plasma MMA (Table 1.7.a.1) concentrations.

- Non-Hispanic whites had the highest concentrations of serum and RBC folate (Tables 1.1.a.1 and 1.2.a.1), serum 4PA (Table 1.4.a.1), and plasma MMA (Table 1.7.a.1). They also had the lowest concentrations of serum vitamin B12 (Table 1.5.a.1). Non-Hispanic blacks had the lowest concentrations of RBC folate (Table 1.2.a.1) and serum PLP (Table 1.3.a.1). Mexican Americans had the lowest concentrations of plasma tHcy (Table 1.6.a.1).

Changes in geometric mean concentrations across survey cycles:

- Serum folate concentrations decreased slightly (< 10%) between the 1999–2000 and 2001–2002 survey cycles; however, concentrations stabilized over the next two survey cycles (Table 1.1.b).

- RBC folate concentrations were similar across all survey cycles except for a < 10% decrease between the 2001–2002 and 2003–2004 survey cycles (Table 1.2.b).

- We observed no changes in serum vitamin B12 (Table 1.5.b), plasma tHcy (Table 1.6.b), or plasma MMA (Table 1.7.b) concentrations over time.

Prevalence estimates of low or high biochemical indicator concentrations:

- In 2003–2006, less than 1% of the population aged 1 year and older had RBC folate concentrations < 95 ng/mL (Table 1.2.c). Similarly, less than 1% of the population had low serum folate concentrations < 2 ng/mL; however, the estimates had large variances and we do not present a prevalence table for this indicator.

- Of the population aged 1 year and older, approximately 11% had serum PLP concentrations < 20 nmol/L in 2005–2006 (Table 1.3.c). Compared to the prevalence of low PLP concentrations in persons 20–39 years of age, the prevalence of low PLP concentrations was lower in all younger age groups and higher in all older age groups.

- Approximately 2% of the population aged 1 year and older and 4% of persons 60 years and older had serum vitamin B12 concentrations < 200 pg/mL in 2003-2006 (Table 1.5.c).

- We found elevated plasma tHcy concentrations (> 13 μmol/L) in 2003–2006 in approximately 8% of the population aged 20 years and older and in 19% of persons 60 years and older (Table 1.6.c).

- Approximately 7% of the population aged 3 years and older and 17% of persons 60 years and older had plasma MMA concentrations > 271 nmol/L in 2003-2004 (Table 1.7.c).

- Between 1999 and 2006 (2004 for MMA), we did not observe any change in the prevalence of low RBC folate (Table 1.2.d), low serum vitamin B12 (Table 1.5.d), high plasma tHcy (Table 1.6.d), and high plasma MMA (Table 1.7.d) concentrations.

Table 1.1.a.1. Serum folate: Concentrations

Geometric mean and selected percentiles of serum concentrations (in ng/mL) for the total U.S. population aged 1 year and older, National Health and Nutrition Examination Survey, 2003–2006.

	Geometric mean (95% conf. interval)	Selected percentiles (95% conf. interval)					Sample size
		2.5th	5th	50th	95th	97.5th	
Total, 1 year and older	12.3 (12.0 – 12.6)	4.51 (4.36 – 4.61)	5.46 (5.26 – 5.66)	12.2 (11.9 – 12.5)	28.5 (27.5 – 29.5)	34.0 (32.5 – 36.0)	16,411
Age group							
1–5 years	16.2 (15.5 – 16.9)	6.29 (5.51 – 6.93)	7.61 (6.92 – 8.24)	16.0 (15.5 – 16.5)	36.0 (32.0 – 41.9)	50.8 (37.7 – 77.7)	1,690
6–11 years	16.1 (15.6 – 16.6)	8.21 (7.82 – 8.58)	9.04 (8.63 – 9.58)	15.7 (15.3 – 16.2)	29.9 (27.5 – 35.0)	35.9 (32.3 – 46.3)	1,749
12–19 years	11.2 (11.0 – 11.5)	4.86 (4.57 – 5.11)	5.62 (5.45 – 5.83)	11.3 (10.9 – 11.6)	20.9 (19.9 – 21.8)	24.6 (23.4 – 25.8)	4,028
20–39 years	10.4 (10.1 – 10.7)	4.24 (4.08 – 4.46)	4.93 (4.75 – 5.09)	10.5 (10.1 – 10.9)	20.5 (19.5 – 22.9)	26.1 (23.1 – 29.9)	3,242
40–59 years	11.6 (11.2 – 12.0)	4.23 (3.70 – 4.40)	5.09 (4.57 – 5.42)	11.6 (11.3 – 11.9)	25.2 (24.1 – 28.1)	32.8 (29.2 – 37.1)	2,649
60 years and older	15.6 (15.0 – 16.1)	5.31 (4.83 – 5.57)	6.32 (5.95 – 6.61)	15.8 (15.2 – 16.3)	35.7 (34.2 – 37.7)	45.7 (42.1 – 49.6)	3,053
Gender							
Males	11.7 (11.4 – 12.0)	4.39 (4.29 – 4.60)	5.32 (5.00 – 5.55)	11.6 (11.3 – 11.9)	26.4 (25.6 – 27.8)	32.2 (30.6 – 34.8)	8,050
Females	12.9 (12.5 – 13.3)	4.56 (4.41 – 4.81)	5.61 (5.33 – 5.91)	12.9 (12.5 – 13.2)	29.7 (28.8 – 31.2)	35.6 (33.6 – 37.8)	8,361
Race/ethnicity							
Mexican Americans	11.1 (10.7 – 11.4)	4.67 (4.52 – 4.92)	5.49 (5.17 – 5.68)	11.1 (10.8 – 11.4)	22.2 (20.8 – 23.4)	25.9 (24.3 – 28.8)	4,212
Non-Hispanic Blacks	10.4 (10.1 – 10.7)	4.19 (4.01 – 4.36)	4.83 (4.56 – 5.07)	10.3 (9.94 – 10.8)	22.6 (21.4 – 23.5)	27.0 (25.6 – 29.3)	4,297
Non-Hispanic Whites	13.0 (12.5 – 13.4)	4.58 (4.40 – 4.81)	5.72 (5.36 – 5.98)	12.9 (12.5 – 13.3)	30.1 (29.2 – 31.5)	36.0 (34.2 – 38.5)	6,633

Figure 1.1.a. Serum folate: Concentrations by age group

Geometric mean (95% confidence interval), National Health and Nutrition Examination Survey, 2003–2006

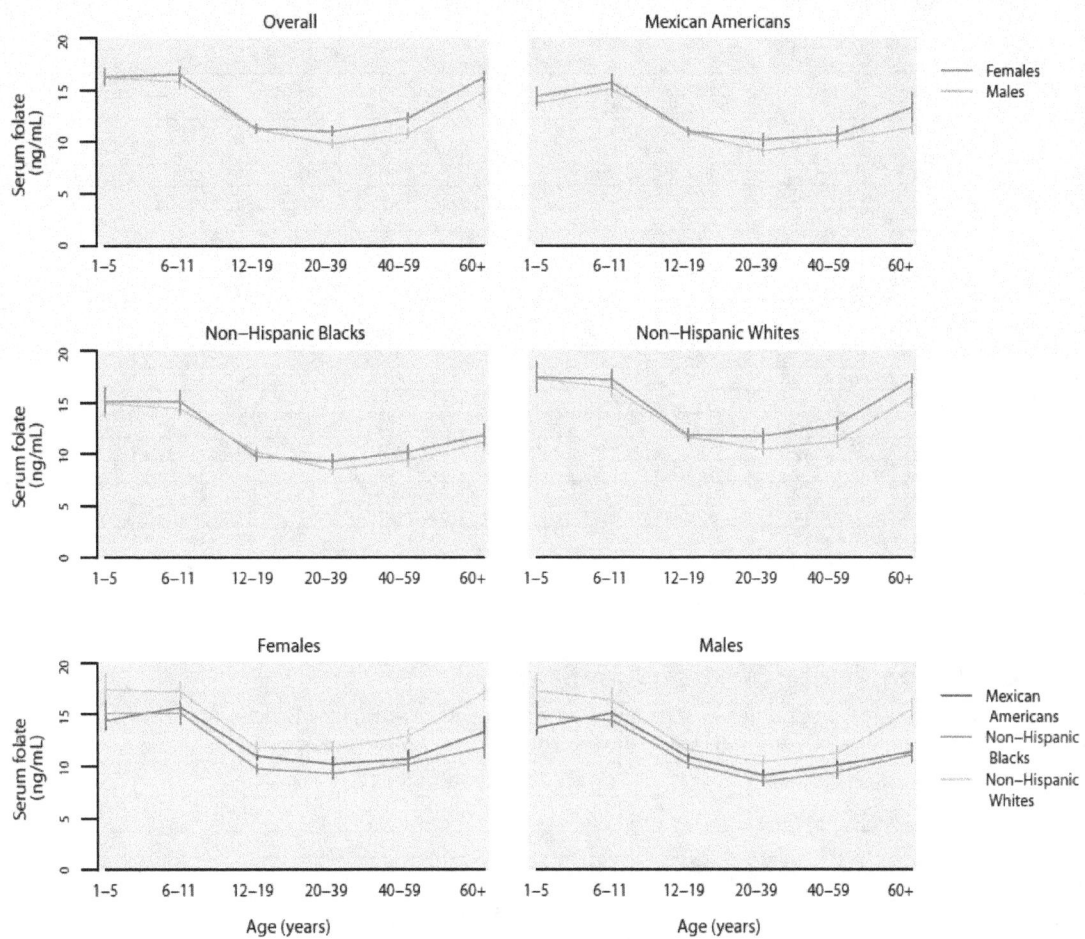

Table 1.1.a.2. Serum folate: Total population

Geometric mean and selected percentiles of serum concentrations (in ng/mL) for the total U.S. population aged 1 year and older, National Health and Nutrition Examination Survey, 2003–2006.

	Geometric mean (95% conf. interval)	Selected percentiles (95% conf. interval)						Sample size
		5th		50th		95th		
Males and Females								
Total, 1 year and older	12.3	(12.0 – 12.6)	5.46	(5.26 – 5.66)	12.2	(11.9 – 12.5)	28.5	(27.5 – 29.5)	16,411
1–5 years	16.2	(15.5 – 16.9)	7.61	(6.92 – 8.24)	16.0	(15.5 – 16.5)	36.0	(32.0 – 41.9)	1,690
6–11 years	16.1	(15.6 – 16.6)	9.04	(8.63 – 9.58)	15.7	(15.3 – 16.2)	29.9	(27.5 – 35.0)	1,749
12–19 years	11.2	(11.0 – 11.5)	5.62	(5.45 – 5.83)	11.3	(10.9 – 11.6)	20.9	(19.9 – 21.8)	4,028
20–39 years	10.4	(10.1 – 10.7)	4.93	(4.75 – 5.09)	10.5	(10.1 – 10.9)	20.5	(19.5 – 22.9)	3,242
40–59 years	11.6	(11.2 – 12.0)	5.09	(4.57 – 5.42)	11.6	(11.3 – 11.9)	25.2	(24.1 – 28.1)	2,649
60 years and older	15.6	(15.0 – 16.1)	6.32	(5.95 – 6.61)	15.8	(15.2 – 16.3)	35.7	(34.2 – 37.7)	3,053
Males								
Total, 1 year and older	11.7	(11.4 – 12.0)	5.32	(5.00 – 5.55)	11.6	(11.3 – 11.9)	26.4	(25.6 – 27.8)	8,050
1–5 years	16.2	(15.3 – 17.1)	7.56	(6.40 – 8.53)	15.8	(15.2 – 16.3)	36.2	(32.0 – 46.5)	854
6–11 years	15.8	(15.2 – 16.4)	9.10	(8.37 – 9.77)	15.3	(14.8 – 16.0)	29.1	(26.2 – 34.9)	854
12–19 years	11.2	(10.9 – 11.5)	5.45	(4.94 – 5.82)	11.3	(10.9 – 11.6)	20.5	(19.8 – 21.9)	2,041
20–39 years	9.83	(9.51 – 10.2)	4.84	(4.66 – 5.03)	9.89	(9.53 – 10.3)	18.3	(17.6 – 20.0)	1,462
40–59 years	10.8	(10.4 – 11.3)	4.84	(4.39 – 5.26)	11.0	(10.4 – 11.4)	22.7	(20.5 – 25.8)	1,305
60 years and older	14.7	(14.0 – 15.6)	6.12	(5.81 – 6.42)	14.7	(13.7 – 15.7)	34.9	(32.5 – 41.9)	1,534
Females								
Total, 1 year and older	12.9	(12.5 – 13.3)	5.61	(5.33 – 5.91)	12.9	(12.5 – 13.2)	29.7	(28.8 – 31.2)	8,361
1–5 years	16.3	(15.6 – 17.0)	7.65	(6.80 – 8.30)	16.3	(15.8 – 17.0)	34.6	(30.2 – 46.5)	836
6–11 years	16.5	(15.8 – 17.2)	9.01	(8.62 – 9.59)	16.2	(15.5 – 16.9)	30.8	(28.2 – 36.6)	895
12–19 years	11.3	(10.9 – 11.7)	5.76	(5.57 – 6.04)	11.2	(10.9 – 11.6)	21.3	(19.6 – 23.4)	1,987
20–39 years	11.0	(10.6 – 11.5)	5.05	(4.63 – 5.27)	11.1	(10.7 – 11.6)	23.1	(21.1 – 26.1)	1,780
40–59 years	12.3	(11.9 – 12.8)	5.37	(4.56 – 5.96)	12.4	(11.9 – 12.9)	27.6	(25.2 – 32.1)	1,344
60 years and older	16.2	(15.7 – 16.8)	6.57	(6.05 – 6.92)	16.5	(15.9 – 17.2)	36.1	(34.4 – 38.5)	1,519

Table 1.1.a.3. Serum folate: Mexican Americans

Geometric mean and selected percentiles of serum concentrations (in ng/mL) for Mexican Americans in the U.S. population aged 1 year and older, National Health and Nutrition Examination Survey, 2003–2006.

	Geometric mean (95% conf. interval)	Selected percentiles (95% conf. interval)						Sample size
		5th		50th		95th		
Males and Females								
Total, 1 year and older	11.1	(10.7 – 11.4)	5.49	(5.17 – 5.68)	11.1	(10.8 – 11.4)	22.2	(20.8 – 23.4)	4,212
1–5 years	14.1	(13.4 – 14.7)	7.56	(6.85 – 8.17)	14.0	(13.3 – 14.8)	26.2	(23.8 – 29.4)	542
6–11 years	15.4	(14.7 – 16.2)	9.03	(8.32 – 9.67)	15.2	(14.2 – 16.0)	28.2	(26.2 – 32.2)	586
12–19 years	10.9	(10.6 – 11.2)	5.89	(5.43 – 6.28)	11.1	(10.8 – 11.5)	19.1	(18.2 – 19.8)	1,281
20–39 years	9.60	(9.24 – 9.96)	5.04	(4.70 – 5.19)	9.62	(9.07 – 10.2)	18.1	(16.8 – 19.6)	781
40–59 years	10.4	(9.76 – 11.1)	5.13	(4.59 – 5.67)	10.1	(9.51 – 11.0)	21.0	(18.7 – 23.7)	469
60 years and older	12.4	(11.6 – 13.2)	5.36	(4.61 – 6.41)	12.1	(11.6 – 12.6)	27.1	(24.6 – 37.1)	553
Males								
Total, 1 year and older	10.6	(10.3 – 11.0)	5.35	(4.99 – 5.65)	10.7	(10.3 – 11.0)	20.2	(19.5 – 22.4)	2,042
1–5 years	13.7	(13.1 – 14.5)	8.03	(6.22 – 8.33)	13.5	(12.7 – 14.5)	23.9	(21.2 – 31.4)	263
6–11 years	15.1	(14.3 – 16.0)	8.68	(7.46 – 9.86)	14.9	(13.7 – 16.0)	28.3	(25.4 – 32.3)	285
12–19 years	10.9	(10.5 – 11.3)	5.62	(4.99 – 5.94)	11.1	(10.6 – 11.4)	19.1	(17.7 – 20.6)	638
20–39 years	9.11	(8.67 – 9.57)	4.90	(4.47 – 5.37)	9.09	(8.68 – 9.70)	15.6	(14.7 – 18.7)	347
40–59 years	10.1	(9.43 – 10.8)	5.11	(4.48 – 5.91)	10.0	(9.19 – 10.7)	19.1	(18.1 – 22.5)	237
60 years and older	11.4	(10.7 – 12.1)	5.27	(4.61 – 6.23)	10.5	(9.85 – 12.1)	26.0	(22.9 – 36.9)	272
Females								
Total, 1 year and older	11.5	(11.1 – 12.0)	5.64	(5.15 – 5.87)	11.6	(11.3 – 11.8)	23.3	(21.8 – 25.6)	2,170
1–5 years	14.4	(13.6 – 15.2)	7.34	(6.41 – 8.10)	14.4	(13.7 – 15.9)	26.5	(24.5 – 31.9)	279
6–11 years	15.7	(14.9 – 16.5)	9.13	(8.01 – 10.2)	15.5	(14.8 – 16.3)	27.8	(25.9 – 34.2)	301
12–19 years	11.0	(10.7 – 11.3)	6.23	(5.78 – 6.54)	11.2	(10.8 – 11.6)	19.0	(18.2 – 21.0)	643
20–39 years	10.2	(9.62 – 10.8)	5.11	(4.74 – 5.38)	10.4	(9.53 – 11.0)	19.3	(18.1 – 21.8)	434
40–59 years	10.7	(10.0 – 11.5)	5.16	(3.80 – 5.85)	10.4	(9.57 – 11.4)	22.4	(19.1 – 40.0)	232
60 years and older	13.3	(12.0 – 14.7)	5.62	(4.00 – 6.65)	13.0	(12.1 – 13.7)	29.7	(25.3 – 64.8)	281

Table 1.1.a.4. Serum folate: Non-Hispanic blacks

Geometric mean and selected percentiles of serum concentrations (in ng/mL) for non-Hispanic blacks in the U.S.population aged 1 year and older, National Health and Nutrition Examination Survey, 2003–2006.

	Geometric mean (95% conf. interval)	Selected percentiles (95% conf. interval) 5th	Selected percentiles (95% conf. interval) 50th	Selected percentiles (95% conf. interval) 95th	Sample size
Males and Females					
Total, 1 year and older	10.4 (10.1 – 10.7)	4.83 (4.56 – 5.07)	10.3 (9.94 – 10.8)	22.6 (21.4 – 23.5)	4,297
1–5 years	15.0 (14.0 – 16.0)	7.08 (5.99 – 7.80)	14.9 (14.3 – 15.6)	32.9 (28.0 – 40.7)	481
6–11 years	14.8 (14.2 – 15.3)	8.62 (7.91 – 9.03)	14.6 (14.0 – 15.2)	25.3 (23.9 – 29.4)	554
12–19 years	9.98 (9.63 – 10.4)	5.19 (4.98 – 5.39)	9.91 (9.59 – 10.3)	18.3 (17.7 – 19.1)	1,417
20–39 years	8.92 (8.56 – 9.29)	4.56 (4.26 – 4.81)	8.73 (8.34 – 9.23)	17.7 (16.7 – 19.1)	711
40–59 years	9.81 (9.28 – 10.4)	4.34 (3.93 – 4.99)	9.75 (9.04 – 10.3)	20.0 (18.8 – 26.0)	621
60 years and older	11.5 (10.8 – 12.3)	4.88 (4.48 – 5.29)	11.3 (10.7 – 11.9)	27.2 (24.5 – 36.0)	513
Males					
Total, 1 year and older	10.1 (9.84 – 10.4)	4.67 (4.34 – 4.94)	10.1 (9.76 – 10.5)	21.1 (19.7 – 23.2)	2,141
1–5 years	14.9 (13.7 – 16.2)	6.69 (5.91 – 7.81)	14.7 (13.9 – 15.5)	36.5 (29.0 – 51.9)	238
6–11 years	14.4 (13.8 – 15.1)	8.87 (8.20 – 9.55)	14.3 (13.6 – 14.9)	24.3 (21.2 – 30.8)	273
12–19 years	10.2 (9.85 – 10.6)	5.02 (4.75 – 5.19)	10.3 (9.82 – 10.8)	19.0 (17.9 – 19.8)	742
20–39 years	8.48 (8.07 – 8.91)	4.33 (4.01 – 4.81)	8.35 (7.82 – 8.89)	15.4 (14.5 – 17.7)	339
40–59 years	9.41 (8.82 – 10.0)	4.11 (3.42 – 4.99)	9.38 (8.49 – 10.1)	18.7 (17.3 – 32.9)	291
60 years and older	11.1 (10.4 – 11.8)	4.73 (3.87 – 5.82)	10.7 (9.77 – 11.3)	29.0 (23.9 – 32.7)	258
Females					
Total, 1 year and older	10.6 (10.2 – 11.0)	5.00 (4.62 – 5.23)	10.5 (10.0 – 11.1)	23.3 (22.0 – 24.9)	2,156
1–5 years	15.1 (14.0 – 16.4)	7.33 (5.00 – 8.42)	15.1 (14.2 – 16.3)	28.8 (26.7 – 40.8)	243
6–11 years	15.1 (14.1 – 16.1)	8.03 (7.24 – 8.98)	14.9 (14.0 – 15.9)	26.0 (24.3 – 33.6)	281
12–19 years	9.76 (9.35 – 10.2)	5.42 (4.98 – 5.57)	9.67 (9.21 – 10.0)	17.7 (16.9 – 18.4)	675
20–39 years	9.30 (8.78 – 9.86)	4.68 (4.44 – 5.01)	9.00 (8.52 – 9.59)	19.1 (17.8 – 20.8)	372
40–59 years	10.2 (9.56 – 10.8)	4.48 (4.07 – 5.18)	10.1 (9.24 – 10.7)	22.1 (19.2 – 27.7)	330
60 years and older	11.8 (10.8 – 12.9)	4.95 (4.26 – 5.65)	11.6 (11.0 – 12.8)	26.8 (23.9 – 45.8)	255

Table 1.1.a.5. Serum folate: Non-Hispanic whites

Geometric mean and selected percentiles of serum concentrations (in ng/mL) for non-Hispanic whites in the U.S.population aged 1 year and older, National Health and Nutrition Examination Survey, 2003–2006.

	Geometric mean (95% conf. interval)	Selected percentiles (95% conf. interval) 5th	Selected percentiles (95% conf. interval) 50th	Selected percentiles (95% conf. interval) 95th	Sample size
Males and Females					
Total, 1 year and older	13.0 (12.5 – 13.4)	5.72 (5.36 – 5.98)	12.9 (12.5 – 13.3)	30.1 (29.2 – 31.5)	6,633
1–5 years	17.4 (16.2 – 18.6)	7.94 (6.77 – 8.99)	17.0 (16.0 – 17.8)	37.9 (34.7 – 56.0)	478
6–11 years	16.8 (16.1 – 17.5)	9.54 (8.59 – 10.0)	16.5 (15.9 – 17.2)	31.7 (28.0 – 37.6)	449
12–19 years	11.7 (11.3 – 12.1)	5.83 (5.57 – 6.19)	11.6 (11.3 – 12.2)	22.1 (21.2 – 23.4)	1,048
20–39 years	11.0 (10.6 – 11.5)	5.22 (4.82 – 5.54)	11.1 (10.7 – 11.5)	22.9 (20.6 – 26.2)	1,453
40–59 years	12.0 (11.5 – 12.6)	5.14 (4.55 – 5.61)	12.1 (11.7 – 12.6)	26.1 (24.3 – 31.7)	1,357
60 years and older	16.3 (15.7 – 17.0)	6.55 (6.19 – 6.92)	16.7 (16.1 – 17.2)	36.8 (34.9 – 39.4)	1,848
Males					
Total, 1 year and older	12.3 (11.8 – 12.7)	5.56 (5.04 – 5.93)	12.1 (11.7 – 12.6)	28.0 (26.4 – 29.8)	3,268
1–5 years	17.3 (16.0 – 18.8)	8.02 (5.84 – 9.82)	16.5 (15.7 – 17.9)	36.3 (32.6 – 55.8)	259
6–11 years	16.4 (15.5 – 17.5)	8.91† (7.81 – 10.0)	16.2 (15.1 – 16.9)	30.4† (26.1 – 52.6)	216
12–19 years	11.6 (11.2 – 12.0)	5.58 (4.93 – 6.17)	11.6 (11.2 – 12.1)	21.8 (20.4 – 23.3)	528
20–39 years	10.4 (9.94 – 10.9)	5.30 (4.75 – 5.82)	10.5 (9.93 – 11.0)	19.5 (18.1 – 22.9)	638
40–59 years	11.2 (10.6 – 11.9)	4.95 (4.36 – 5.35)	11.5 (10.9 – 12.1)	22.9 (20.9 – 26.8)	689
60 years and older	15.5 (14.5 – 16.5)	6.35 (5.91 – 6.72)	15.6 (14.5 – 16.6)	37.0 (32.7 – 45.3)	938
Females					
Total, 1 year and older	13.7 (13.2 – 14.1)	5.88 (5.45 – 6.20)	13.7 (13.2 – 14.2)	31.6 (30.3 – 32.9)	3,365
1–5 years	17.4 (16.0 – 18.9)	7.79† (6.32 – 8.79)	17.1 (15.9 – 18.0)	42.7† (30.9 – 73.2)	219
6–11 years	17.2 (16.4 – 18.1)	9.71 (8.72 – 10.2)	17.0 (15.9 – 17.7)	31.7 (28.3 – 38.2)	233
12–19 years	11.8 (11.3 – 12.4)	5.90 (5.64 – 6.67)	11.8 (11.1 – 12.5)	22.2 (20.5 – 25.1)	520
20–39 years	11.7 (11.1 – 12.4)	5.19 (4.54 – 5.60)	11.8 (11.1 – 12.5)	25.7 (22.8 – 30.7)	815
40–59 years	12.9 (12.3 – 13.5)	5.40 (4.54 – 6.22)	13.1 (12.3 – 13.7)	30.9 (25.5 – 34.0)	668
60 years and older	17.1 (16.5 – 17.7)	6.85 (6.21 – 7.22)	17.6 (16.8 – 18.4)	36.6 (34.9 – 39.7)	910

† Estimate is subject to greater uncertainty due to small cell size.

Table 1.1.b. Serum folate: Concentrations by survey cycle

Geometric mean and selected percentiles of serum concentrations (in ng/mL) for the U.S. population, National Health and Nutrition Examination Survey, 1999–2006.

	Geometric mean (95% conf. interval)	Selected percentiles (95% conf. interval) 5th	Selected percentiles (95% conf. interval) 50th	Selected percentiles (95% conf. interval) 95th	Sample size
Total, 3 years and older					
1999–2000	14.0 (13.4 – 14.8)	5.74 (5.35 – 6.10)	14.2 (13.4 – 15.0)	33.1 (31.6 – 34.9)	7,526
2001–2002	12.9 (12.5 – 13.3)	5.73 (5.36 – 6.05)	13.0 (12.7 – 13.4)	27.2 (26.4 – 28.5)	8,386
2003–2004	12.1 (11.7 – 12.6)	5.40 (5.12 – 5.69)	11.9 (11.5 – 12.4)	28.2 (27.1 – 29.7)	7,836
2005–2006	12.4 (11.9 – 12.9)	5.47 (5.10 – 5.80)	12.3 (11.9 – 12.7)	28.5 (26.5 – 30.2)	7,774
Age group					
3–5 years					
1999–2000	20.1 (18.8 – 21.4)	10.5 (7.89 – 12.2)	19.1 (17.9 – 21.6)	38.2 (34.0 – 45.1)	361
2001–2002	17.3 (16.3 – 18.4)	9.44 (7.08 – 10.6)	17.1 (16.1 – 18.3)	31.9 (29.5 – 38.5)	438
2003–2004	16.6 (15.1 – 18.2)	8.59 (5.22 – 9.61)	16.2 (15.2 – 17.0)	34.5 (29.4 – 57.9)	448
2005–2006	17.6 (16.5 – 18.8)	9.56 (8.34 – 10.3)	16.7 (16.1 – 17.9)	37.6 (31.3 – 77.2)	441
6–11 years					
1999–2000	19.3 (18.4 – 20.3)	11.0 (10.6 – 11.4)	19.3 (18.4 – 19.9)	33.4 (31.6 – 36.3)	885
2001–2002	17.2 (16.6 – 17.9)	9.31 (8.75 – 9.78)	17.1 (16.3 – 17.8)	32.7 (29.9 – 37.9)	1,023
2003–2004	15.6 (14.9 – 16.3)	9.39 (8.66 – 9.85)	15.2 (14.7 – 16.0)	27.4 (24.4 – 34.0)	843
2005–2006	16.7 (15.9 – 17.5)	8.77 (8.26 – 9.60)	16.3 (15.5 – 17.1)	32.4 (29.5 – 36.9)	906
12–19 years					
1999–2000	13.3 (12.6 – 14.0)	6.26 (5.72 – 6.61)	13.3 (12.7 – 14.0)	27.6 (25.6 – 31.3)	2,124
2001–2002	12.2 (11.6 – 12.8)	5.91 (5.29 – 6.28)	12.5 (11.9 – 13.3)	22.1 (21.2 – 23.4)	2,208
2003–2004	11.0 (10.5 – 11.5)	5.56 (5.20 – 6.02)	11.0 (10.5 – 11.4)	19.7 (19.1 – 22.1)	2,058
2005–2006	11.5 (11.2 – 11.8)	5.65 (5.39 – 5.90)	11.6 (11.1 – 12.1)	21.8 (21.1 – 22.6)	1,970
20–39 years					
1999–2000	11.8 (11.0 – 12.7)	5.15 (4.40 – 5.55)	11.6 (10.6 – 12.8)	28.6 (25.6 – 30.8)	1,470
2001–2002	11.1 (10.6 – 11.6)	5.27 (4.78 – 5.59)	11.1 (10.6 – 11.6)	22.6 (20.6 – 24.3)	1,714
2003–2004	10.2 (9.78 – 10.6)	4.83 (4.62 – 5.01)	10.2 (9.59 – 10.8)	20.0 (19.1 – 22.9)	1,555
2005–2006	10.6 (10.2 – 11.1)	5.07 (4.76 – 5.33)	10.8 (10.3 – 11.2)	21.1 (19.2 – 25.9)	1,687
40–59 years					
1999–2000	13.6 (12.7 – 14.5)	5.37 (4.37 – 6.08)	13.6 (12.7 – 14.7)	31.6 (30.0 – 35.4)	1,199
2001–2002	12.2 (11.7 – 12.7)	5.63 (4.86 – 6.06)	12.5 (11.9 – 13.1)	24.0 (22.4 – 25.3)	1,475
2003–2004	11.6 (11.0 – 12.3)	5.20 (4.57 – 5.60)	11.6 (11.1 – 11.9)	26.0 (23.8 – 32.8)	1,276
2005–2006	11.6 (11.0 – 12.2)	4.85 (4.39 – 5.57)	11.7 (11.1 – 12.1)	24.4 (22.8 – 29.0)	1,373
60 years and older					
1999–2000	17.4 (16.7 – 18.1)	7.09 (6.48 – 7.51)	17.4 (16.5 – 18.2)	42.3 (39.2 – 44.8)	1,487
2001–2002	16.1 (15.4 – 16.8)	6.50 (5.75 – 7.09)	16.6 (15.4 – 17.5)	37.3 (34.2 – 40.7)	1,528
2003–2004	15.7 (15.1 – 16.4)	6.53 (6.13 – 7.00)	15.6 (14.8 – 16.4)	34.9 (32.9 – 37.7)	1,656
2005–2006	15.4 (14.5 – 16.4)	6.06 (5.40 – 6.58)	15.8 (15.0 – 16.8)	36.4 (34.4 – 41.9)	1,397
Gender					
Males					
1999–2000	13.3 (12.7 – 14.0)	5.53 (4.73 – 6.13)	13.4 (12.7 – 14.2)	30.6 (29.0 – 32.2)	3,684
2001–2002	12.3 (11.8 – 12.8)	5.64 (5.17 – 6.00)	12.5 (12.1 – 13.0)	25.0 (23.7 – 27.0)	4,063
2003–2004	11.6 (11.1 – 12.1)	5.31 (4.93 – 5.69)	11.5 (11.1 – 11.9)	26.2 (24.7 – 28.1)	3,871
2005–2006	11.7 (11.2 – 12.1)	5.24 (4.74 – 5.59)	11.6 (11.2 – 12.0)	26.2 (25.2 – 28.5)	3,780
Females					
1999–2000	14.8 (14.0 – 15.6)	5.94 (5.60 – 6.18)	14.8 (14.1 – 16.0)	35.3 (33.7 – 37.5)	3,842
2001–2002	13.5 (13.1 – 13.9)	5.80 (5.39 – 6.35)	13.6 (13.2 – 14.0)	29.3 (27.3 – 31.6)	4,323
2003–2004	12.6 (12.1 – 13.1)	5.51 (5.12 – 5.84)	12.5 (12.0 – 13.0)	29.5 (28.3 – 31.6)	3,965
2005–2006	13.1 (12.5 – 13.7)	5.66 (5.25 – 6.14)	13.2 (12.6 – 13.8)	29.9 (28.2 – 32.2)	3,994
Race/ethnicity					
Mexican Americans					
1999–2000	13.2 (12.8 – 13.7)	6.10 (5.49 – 6.51)	13.5 (12.9 – 14.0)	28.4 (27.1 – 30.2)	2,571
2001–2002	11.6 (10.9 – 12.4)	5.48 (4.66 – 6.08)	11.8 (11.1 – 12.5)	22.5 (20.0 – 26.1)	2,124
2003–2004	10.9 (10.4 – 11.5)	5.20 (5.09 – 5.50)	11.1 (10.7 – 11.6)	20.9 (19.2 – 23.4)	1,919
2005–2006	11.1 (10.7 – 11.5)	5.56 (5.18 – 5.79)	11.0 (10.6 – 11.5)	23.1 (21.6 – 25.0)	2,012
Non-Hispanic Blacks					
1999–2000	11.7 (11.1 – 12.4)	5.15 (4.67 – 5.42)	11.6 (10.9 – 12.4)	27.3 (24.9 – 31.5)	1,712
2001–2002	10.9 (10.2 – 11.6)	5.06 (4.47 – 5.39)	10.7 (10.1 – 11.4)	23.6 (21.7 – 25.2)	2,004
2003–2004	10.1 (9.66 – 10.6)	4.65 (4.28 – 5.11)	10.1 (9.37 – 10.8)	21.9 (19.9 – 23.7)	2,057
2005–2006	10.6 (10.1 – 11.1)	4.95 (4.68 – 5.15)	10.5 (9.92 – 11.2)	22.9 (21.4 – 24.0)	2,040
Non-Hispanic Whites					
1999–2000	14.8 (13.8 – 15.8)	6.11 (5.52 – 6.55)	15.0 (13.9 – 16.2)	34.2 (32.6 – 36.0)	2,557
2001–2002	13.4 (13.0 – 13.9)	5.90 (5.62 – 6.21)	13.6 (13.2 – 14.1)	28.4 (27.2 – 29.9)	3,590
2003–2004	12.9 (12.2 – 13.5)	5.76 (5.31 – 6.08)	12.7 (12.1 – 13.3)	30.0 (28.5 – 32.1)	3,272
2005–2006	13.0 (12.4 – 13.6)	5.62 (4.96 – 6.04)	12.9 (12.4 – 13.5)	29.9 (28.3 – 32.2)	3,120

Figure 1.1.b. Serum folate: Concentrations by survey cycle

Selected percentiles in ng/mL (95% confidence intervals), National Health and Nutrition Examination Survey, 1999–2006

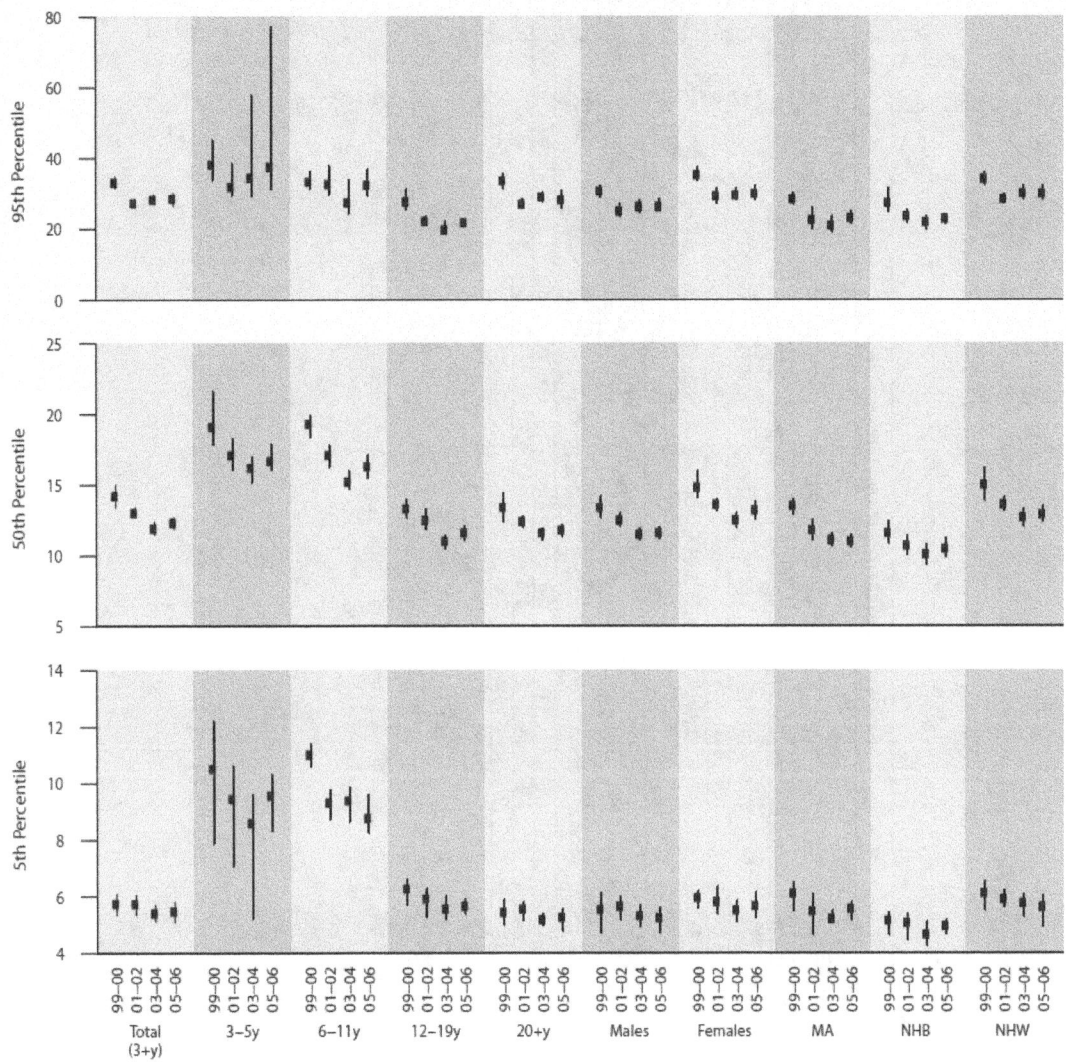

Table 1.2.a.1. Red blood cell folate: Concentrations

Geometric mean and selected percentiles of red blood cell concentrations (in ng/mL) for the total U.S. population aged 1 year and older, National Health and Nutrition Examination Survey, 2003–2006.

	Geometric mean (95% conf. interval)	Selected percentiles (95% conf. interval)						Sample size
		2.5th	5th	50th	95th	97.5th	
Total, 1 year and older	265 (261 – 270)	133 (129 – 136)	149 (146 – 152)	261 (256 – 265)	501 (487 – 515)	581 (566 – 604)	16,670
Age group							
1–5 years	272 (265 – 279)	152 (149 – 160)	174 (169 – 178)	266 (261 – 272)	483 (436 – 531)	560 (521 – 668)	1,861
6–11 years	263 (258 – 268)	164 (152 – 171)	180 (172 – 184)	259 (254 – 264)	430 (400 – 456)	470 (457 – 511)	1,779
12–19 years	229 (225 – 234)	126 (123 – 130)	140 (134 – 146)	229 (224 – 233)	370 (355 – 390)	436 (398 – 471)	4,050
20–39 years	244 (238 – 250)	126 (119 – 131)	140 (136 – 144)	241 (235 – 247)	449 (421 – 480)	512 (483 – 547)	3,262
40–59 years	270 (264 – 276)	132 (126 – 137)	149 (143 – 154)	273 (266 – 279)	481 (461 – 510)	554 (519 – 605)	2,649
60 years and older	324 (317 – 332)	147 (140 – 151)	161 (157 – 166)	327 (315 – 338)	656 (622 – 705)	768 (724 – 860)	3,069
Gender							
Males	259 (253 – 264)	133 (128 – 138)	149 (144 – 153)	255 (250 – 259)	469 (453 – 489)	551 (529 – 588)	8,172
Females	272 (267 – 277)	132 (127 – 136)	149 (146 – 153)	268 (262 – 273)	522 (508 – 535)	604 (576 – 642)	8,498
Race/ethnicity							
Mexican Americans	247 (242 – 252)	133 (125 – 138)	149 (138 – 155)	241 (237 – 246)	452 (434 – 465)	529 (506 – 558)	4,304
Non-Hispanic Blacks	214 (210 – 218)	112 (107 – 116)	125 (120 – 130)	213 (210 – 216)	382 (367 – 398)	428 (419 – 449)	4,404
Non-Hispanic Whites	281 (274 – 288)	144 (137 – 149)	160 (154 – 165)	276 (269 – 282)	529 (510 – 537)	617 (594 – 653)	6,675

Figure 1.2.a. Red blood cell folate: Concentrations by age group

Geometric mean (95% confidence interval), National Health and Nutrition Examination Survey, 2003–2006

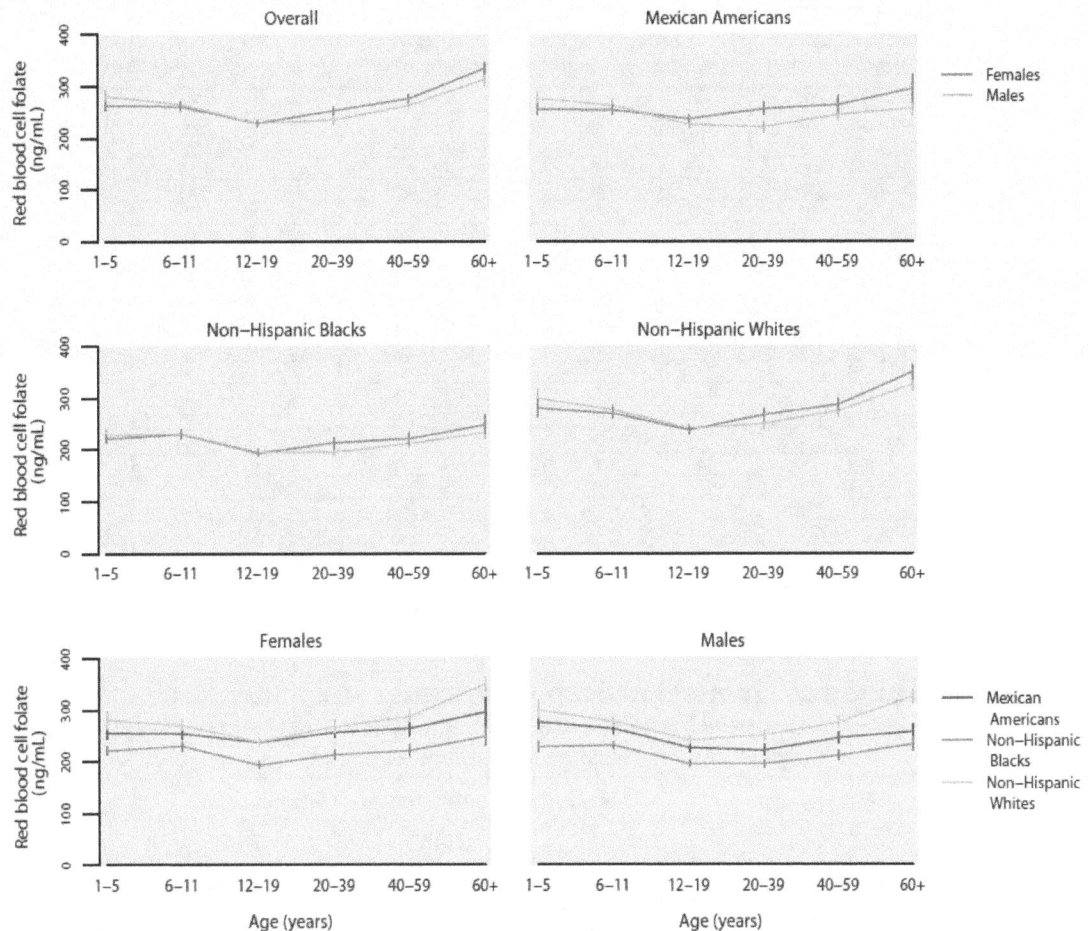

Table 1.2.a.2. Red blood cell folate: Total population

Geometric mean and selected percentiles of red blood cell concentrations (in ng/mL) for the total U.S. population aged 1 year and older, National Health and Nutrition Examination Survey, 2003–2006.

	Geometric mean (95% conf. interval)	Selected percentiles (95% conf. interval)						Sample size
		5th		50th		95th		
Males and Females								
Total, 1 year and older	265 (261 – 270)	149	(146 – 152)	261	(256 – 265)	501	(487 – 515)	16,670
1–5 years	272 (265 – 279)	174	(169 – 178)	266	(261 – 272)	483	(436 – 531)	1,861
6–11 years	263 (258 – 268)	180	(172 – 184)	259	(254 – 264)	430	(400 – 456)	1,779
12–19 years	229 (225 – 234)	140	(134 – 146)	229	(224 – 233)	370	(355 – 390)	4,050
20–39 years	244 (238 – 250)	140	(136 – 144)	241	(235 – 247)	449	(421 – 480)	3,262
40–59 years	270 (264 – 276)	149	(143 – 154)	273	(266 – 279)	481	(461 – 510)	2,649
60 years and older	324 (317 – 332)	161	(157 – 166)	327	(315 – 338)	656	(622 – 705)	3,069
Males								
Total, 1 year and older	259 (253 – 264)	149	(144 – 153)	255	(250 – 259)	469	(453 – 489)	8,172
1–5 years	281 (271 – 290)	176	(170 – 185)	271	(264 – 281)	507	(460 – 560)	941
6–11 years	265 (259 – 271)	182	(173 – 188)	257	(251 – 264)	439	(414 – 468)	867
12–19 years	229 (225 – 234)	142	(135 – 148)	229	(223 – 233)	361	(353 – 385)	2,051
20–39 years	235 (228 – 242)	140	(131 – 148)	235	(226 – 244)	397	(379 – 429)	1,467
40–59 years	263 (256 – 271)	149	(140 – 154)	265	(256 – 275)	463	(431 – 513)	1,309
60 years and older	313 (302 – 324)	159	(154 – 163)	311	(297 – 328)	651	(595 – 709)	1,537
Females								
Total, 1 year and older	272 (267 – 277)	149	(146 – 153)	268	(262 – 273)	522	(508 – 535)	8,498
1–5 years	263 (255 – 270)	173	(161 – 177)	262	(254 – 267)	436	(395 – 531)	920
6–11 years	261 (254 – 269)	176	(162 – 183)	260	(253 – 267)	402	(379 – 459)	912
12–19 years	229 (223 – 234)	138	(130 – 146)	229	(223 – 234)	373	(354 – 398)	1,999
20–39 years	253 (246 – 261)	139	(134 – 145)	248	(239 – 258)	486	(461 – 529)	1,795
40–59 years	276 (269 – 284)	149	(139 – 157)	278	(271 – 288)	501	(467 – 536)	1,340
60 years and older	334 (324 – 344)	162	(157 – 172)	338	(325 – 352)	661	(616 – 744)	1,532

Table 1.2.a.3. Red blood cell folate: Mexican Americans

Geometric mean and selected percentiles of red blood cell concentrations (in ng/mL) for Mexican Americans in the U.S. population aged 1 year and older, National Health and Nutrition Examination Survey, 2003–2006.

	Geometric mean (95% conf. interval)	Selected percentiles (95% conf. interval)						Sample size
		5th		50th		95th		
Males and Females								
Total, 1 year and older	247 (242 – 252)	149	(138 – 155)	241	(237 – 246)	452	(434 – 465)	4,304
1–5 years	266 (257 – 275)	170	(152 – 177)	258	(249 – 266)	477	(441 – 507)	610
6–11 years	259 (252 – 266)	170	(156 – 183)	256	(249 – 262)	443	(396 – 483)	595
12–19 years	231 (225 – 237)	144	(136 – 154)	225	(221 – 232)	402	(386 – 423)	1,288
20–39 years	237 (228 – 246)	139	(125 – 154)	232	(223 – 241)	437	(402 – 463)	787
40–59 years	254 (245 – 264)	149	(132 – 157)	249	(235 – 264)	451	(415 – 520)	471
60 years and older	277 (263 – 292)	147	(130 – 156)	271	(258 – 290)	565	(483 – 646)	553
Males								
Total, 1 year and older	238 (231 – 245)	146	(133 – 153)	234	(230 – 239)	413	(388 – 445)	2,087
1–5 years	276 (263 – 289)	171	(151 – 189)	267	(260 – 275)	481	(445 – 553)	298
6–11 years	263 (253 – 274)	171	(151 – 189)	258	(249 – 265)	466	(422 – 523)	289
12–19 years	226 (219 – 233)	139	(134 – 147)	223	(214 – 230)	378	(340 – 455)	639
20–39 years	221 (211 – 231)	136	(106 – 153)	220	(211 – 231)	367	(333 – 406)	350
40–59 years	245 (235 – 255)	149	(122 – 158)	234	(226 – 250)	429	(373 – 538)	238
60 years and older	257 (243 – 271)	146	(121 – 150)	248	(234 – 268)	478	(438 – 542)	273
Females								
Total, 1 year and older	257 (252 – 263)	154	(140 – 161)	250	(246 – 256)	477	(460 – 505)	2,217
1–5 years	255 (245 – 265)	165	(139 – 177)	248	(240 – 258)	445	(398 – 506)	312
6–11 years	254 (245 – 263)	170	(153 – 180)	253	(246 – 261)	405	(358 – 477)	306
12–19 years	237 (230 – 243)	153	(135 – 158)	230	(224 – 237)	420	(398 – 450)	649
20–39 years	256 (247 – 267)	149	(135 – 161)	250	(236 – 267)	490	(458 – 587)	437
40–59 years	264 (249 – 281)	144	(110 – 159)	263	(244 – 287)	486	(424 – 746)	233
60 years and older	295 (269 – 322)	148	(91.6 – 168)	306	(267 – 329)	587	(550 – 682)	280

Table 1.2.a.4. Red blood cell folate: Non–Hispanic blacks

Geometric mean and selected percentiles of red blood cell concentrations (in ng/mL) for non–Hispanic blacks in the U.S. population aged 1 year and older, National Health and Nutrition Examination Survey, 2003–2006.

	Geometric mean (95% conf. interval)		Selected percentiles (95% conf. interval)						Sample size
			5th		50th		95th		
Males and Females									
Total, 1 year and older	214	(210 – 218)	125	(120 – 130)	213	(210 – 216)	382	(367 – 398)	4,404
1–5 years	225	(218 – 232)	143	(132 – 152)	226	(221 – 231)	350	(330 – 371)	525
6–11 years	230	(225 – 235)	156	(146 – 165)	231	(224 – 238)	336	(321 – 370)	572
12–19 years	194	(190 – 199)	118	(111 – 124)	195	(191 – 200)	312	(299 – 319)	1,432
20–39 years	204	(199 – 210)	119	(115 – 122)	203	(193 – 209)	370	(350 – 406)	717
40–59 years	216	(208 – 225)	124	(107 – 132)	215	(209 – 221)	386	(359 – 436)	630
60 years and older	242	(231 – 254)	131	(125 – 137)	237	(221 – 252)	449	(423 – 508)	528
Males									
Total, 1 year and older	209	(205 – 213)	122	(119 – 129)	208	(204 – 213)	355	(344 – 375)	2,189
1–5 years	228	(219 – 238)	143	(122 – 152)	227	(220 – 235)	359	(333 – 418)	259
6–11 years	231	(225 – 237)	164	(146 – 170)	231	(222 – 239)	337	(319 – 386)	282
12–19 years	195	(190 – 201)	123	(110 – 131)	198	(190 – 204)	305	(289 – 320)	750
20–39 years	195	(188 – 201)	116	(113 – 121)	192	(184 – 204)	309	(298 – 337)	339
40–59 years	211	(202 – 220)	120	(95.7 – 133)	209	(201 – 218)	375	(355 – 435)	295
60 years and older	233	(222 – 245)	128	(123 – 134)	224	(211 – 240)	461	(413 – 541)	264
Females									
Total, 1 year and older	219	(214 – 224)	127	(119 – 131)	216	(212 – 221)	397	(374 – 416)	2,215
1–5 years	221	(214 – 228)	146	(124 – 158)	224	(218 – 232)	334	(301 – 361)	266
6–11 years	230	(221 – 239)	149	(142 – 161)	230	(219 – 242)	334	(314 – 388)	290
12–19 years	193	(188 – 200)	113	(109 – 119)	194	(190 – 200)	314	(299 – 341)	682
20–39 years	213	(204 – 221)	121	(108 – 132)	210	(199 – 219)	406	(371 – 428)	378
40–59 years	221	(210 – 233)	128	(99.8 – 133)	219	(211 – 232)	389	(353 – 494)	335
60 years and older	248	(232 – 267)	135	(104 – 150)	245	(220 – 275)	445	(421 – 521)	264

Table 1.2.a.5. Red blood cell folate: Non–Hispanic whites

Geometric mean and selected percentiles of red blood cell concentrations (in ng/mL) for non–Hispanic whites in the U.S. population aged 1 year and older, National Health and Nutrition Examination Survey, 2003–2006.

	Geometric mean (95% conf. interval)		Selected percentiles (95% conf. interval)						Sample size
			5th		50th		95th		
Males and Females									
Total, 1 year and older	281	(274 – 288)	160	(154 – 165)	276	(269 – 282)	529	(510 – 537)	6,675
1–5 years	290	(277 – 304)	191	(179 – 201)	278	(267 – 293)	528	(484 – 598)	523
6–11 years	274	(267 – 281)	191	(187 – 197)	268	(261 – 275)	439	(411 – 464)	454
12–19 years	239	(233 – 246)	152	(145 – 158)	238	(231 – 246)	376	(356 – 407)	1,046
20–39 years	258	(250 – 267)	152	(143 – 159)	254	(246 – 262)	464	(435 – 504)	1,460
40–59 years	281	(273 – 290)	159	(150 – 165)	285	(275 – 293)	494	(466 – 532)	1,346
60 years and older	339	(330 – 348)	173	(162 – 183)	340	(328 – 350)	673	(645 – 732)	1,846
Males									
Total, 1 year and older	274	(267 – 281)	161	(153 – 167)	269	(262 – 278)	493	(473 – 524)	3,294
1–5 years	299	(284 – 316)	200	(173 – 208)	283	(268 – 312)	537	(498 – 659)	286
6–11 years	277	(268 – 286)	193†	(188 – 202)	269	(258 – 278)	447†	(425 – 517)	218
12–19 years	241	(234 – 248)	152	(139 – 158)	238	(231 – 249)	374	(355 – 437)	527
20–39 years	250	(240 – 260)	154	(141 – 165)	248	(238 – 258)	414	(395 – 447)	641
40–59 years	275	(265 – 286)	160	(148 – 165)	280	(266 – 292)	474	(433 – 534)	688
60 years and older	326	(314 – 338)	170	(161 – 184)	322	(306 – 340)	660	(609 – 716)	934
Females									
Total, 1 year and older	288	(280 – 296)	158	(153 – 164)	282	(273 – 290)	546	(531 – 569)	3,381
1–5 years	280	(264 – 296)	183	(152 – 196)	272	(263 – 286)	486	(428 – 584)	237
6–11 years	270	(261 – 280)	188	(170 – 198)	267	(259 – 276)	390	(373 – 456)	236
12–19 years	238	(231 – 245)	149	(136 – 160)	237	(230 – 244)	381	(350 – 447)	519
20–39 years	267	(257 – 278)	149	(139 – 155)	263	(251 – 272)	502	(473 – 557)	819
40–59 years	287	(277 – 298)	158	(148 – 167)	289	(276 – 302)	506	(477 – 545)	658
60 years and older	350	(337 – 362)	177	(158 – 186)	352	(338 – 370)	689	(630 – 796)	912

† Estimate is subject to greater uncertainty due to small cell size.

Table 1.2.b. Red blood cell folate: Concentrations by survey cycle

Geometric mean and selected percentiles of red blood cell concentrations (in ng/mL) for the U.S. population, National Health and Nutrition Examination Survey, 1999–2006.

	Geometric mean (95% conf. interval)	Selected percentiles (95% conf. interval) 5th	50th	95th	Sample size
Total, 3 years and older					
1999–2000	281 (269 – 293)	153 (144 – 162)	277 (266 – 288)	522 (499 – 556)	7,614
2001–2002	277 (269 – 285)	155 (148 – 160)	274 (265 – 282)	519 (500 – 540)	8,488
2003–2004	258 (251 – 266)	146 (139 – 151)	254 (246 – 262)	483 (464 – 506)	7,849
2005–2006	272 (267 – 277)	152 (148 – 155)	267 (263 – 270)	517 (497 – 534)	7,906
Age group					
3–5 years					
1999–2000	293 (282 – 306)	198 (182 – 206)	290 (283 – 301)	446 (397 – 608)	380
2001–2002	284 (273 – 296)	188 (163 – 201)	283 (270 – 296)	468 (394 – 522)	460
2003–2004	263 (253 – 273)	181 (172 – 187)	258 (245 – 268)	385 (364 – 583)	453
2005–2006	282 (269 – 295)	191 (181 – 197)	271 (265 – 281)	463 (432 – 598)	493
6–11 years					
1999–2000	284 (275 – 293)	190 (177 – 202)	282 (274 – 292)	423 (389 – 502)	898
2001–2002	276 (266 – 287)	183 (171 – 189)	272 (260 – 283)	444 (422 – 512)	1,040
2003–2004	258 (251 – 265)	176 (170 – 183)	255 (246 – 264)	414 (372 – 447)	849
2005–2006	269 (260 – 277)	182 (173 – 189)	263 (257 – 271)	434 (396 – 494)	930
12–19 years					
1999–2000	247 (237 – 256)	152 (146 – 158)	244 (238 – 255)	415 (391 – 456)	2,136
2001–2002	242 (231 – 253)	148 (138 – 157)	238 (228 – 249)	406 (381 – 446)	2,226
2003–2004	223 (217 – 230)	137 (129 – 145)	223 (215 – 230)	356 (338 – 386)	2,063
2005–2006	235 (229 – 241)	145 (133 – 151)	234 (228 – 240)	380 (358 – 414)	1,987
20–39 years					
1999–2000	256 (244 – 268)	141 (130 – 150)	254 (237 – 270)	460 (439 – 515)	1,474
2001–2002	254 (246 – 263)	144 (134 – 152)	251 (240 – 262)	448 (432 – 471)	1,721
2003–2004	236 (228 – 245)	138 (131 – 143)	234 (221 – 245)	426 (403 – 461)	1,555
2005–2006	252 (244 – 261)	143 (138 – 150)	249 (242 – 256)	462 (428 – 525)	1,707
40–59 years					
1999–2000	294 (279 – 311)	156 (144 – 167)	292 (274 – 309)	538 (502 – 613)	1,213
2001–2002	289 (280 – 298)	163 (155 – 170)	287 (281 – 295)	526 (484 – 585)	1,496
2003–2004	264 (253 – 275)	148 (137 – 156)	270 (258 – 279)	465 (430 – 514)	1,273
2005–2006	276 (270 – 282)	150 (145 – 155)	277 (270 – 284)	495 (465 – 544)	1,376
60 years and older					
1999–2000	340 (328 – 352)	169 (154 – 182)	343 (323 – 363)	667 (629 – 701)	1,513
2001–2002	334 (323 – 345)	167 (158 – 178)	336 (325 – 349)	654 (608 – 721)	1,545
2003–2004	320 (310 – 329)	162 (154 – 171)	321 (310 – 337)	642 (589 – 725)	1,656
2005–2006	329 (316 – 342)	161 (155 – 168)	332 (312 – 347)	662 (618 – 733)	1,413
Gender					
Males					
1999–2000	274 (262 – 286)	153 (144 – 161)	270 (259 – 280)	499 (478 – 526)	3,721
2001–2002	269 (259 – 278)	155 (147 – 160)	265 (254 – 276)	485 (465 – 520)	4,106
2003–2004	252 (244 – 260)	147 (138 – 153)	248 (239 – 257)	452 (431 – 485)	3,874
2005–2006	264 (257 – 271)	151 (144 – 157)	259 (255 – 264)	481 (459 – 508)	3,845
Females					
1999–2000	288 (275 – 301)	154 (142 – 164)	286 (272 – 298)	549 (515 – 590)	3,893
2001–2002	285 (276 – 294)	155 (148 – 159)	282 (274 – 291)	540 (518 – 575)	4,382
2003–2004	264 (256 – 273)	146 (138 – 151)	261 (251 – 271)	502 (483 – 530)	3,975
2005–2006	280 (273 – 287)	153 (148 – 157)	274 (267 – 282)	538 (528 – 557)	4,061
Race/ethnicity					
Mexican Americans					
1999–2000	261 (253 – 268)	159 (151 – 166)	256 (251 – 262)	452 (429 – 465)	2,592
2001–2002	256 (244 – 268)	146 (132 – 161)	252 (241 – 265)	458 (434 – 497)	2,134
2003–2004	242 (234 – 251)	149 (136 – 157)	236 (231 – 244)	414 (398 – 462)	1,919
2005–2006	250 (244 – 256)	148 (129 – 158)	244 (239 – 249)	461 (452 – 482)	2,057
Non-Hispanic Blacks					
1999–2000	225 (218 – 233)	125 (113 – 135)	226 (221 – 234)	386 (366 – 427)	1,738
2001–2002	216 (210 – 222)	122 (119 – 124)	214 (208 – 220)	376 (355 – 412)	2,045
2003–2004	209 (203 – 214)	119 (114 – 127)	209 (204 – 214)	366 (349 – 389)	2,091
2005–2006	220 (215 – 224)	131 (124 – 136)	217 (212 – 221)	402 (376 – 422)	2,084
Non-Hispanic Whites					
1999–2000	298 (281 – 315)	165 (147 – 175)	293 (275 – 309)	555 (527 – 592)	2,585
2001–2002	293 (286 – 300)	166 (160 – 172)	289 (283 – 295)	542 (524 – 566)	3,625
2003–2004	273 (262 – 285)	158 (146 – 166)	269 (258 – 280)	504 (485 – 531)	3,256
2005–2006	288 (281 – 295)	162 (155 – 167)	282 (276 – 289)	539 (527 – 567)	3,149

Figure 1.2.b. Red blood cell folate: Concentrations by survey cycle

Selected percentiles in ng/mL (95% confidence intervals), National Health and Nutrition Examination Survey, 1999–2006

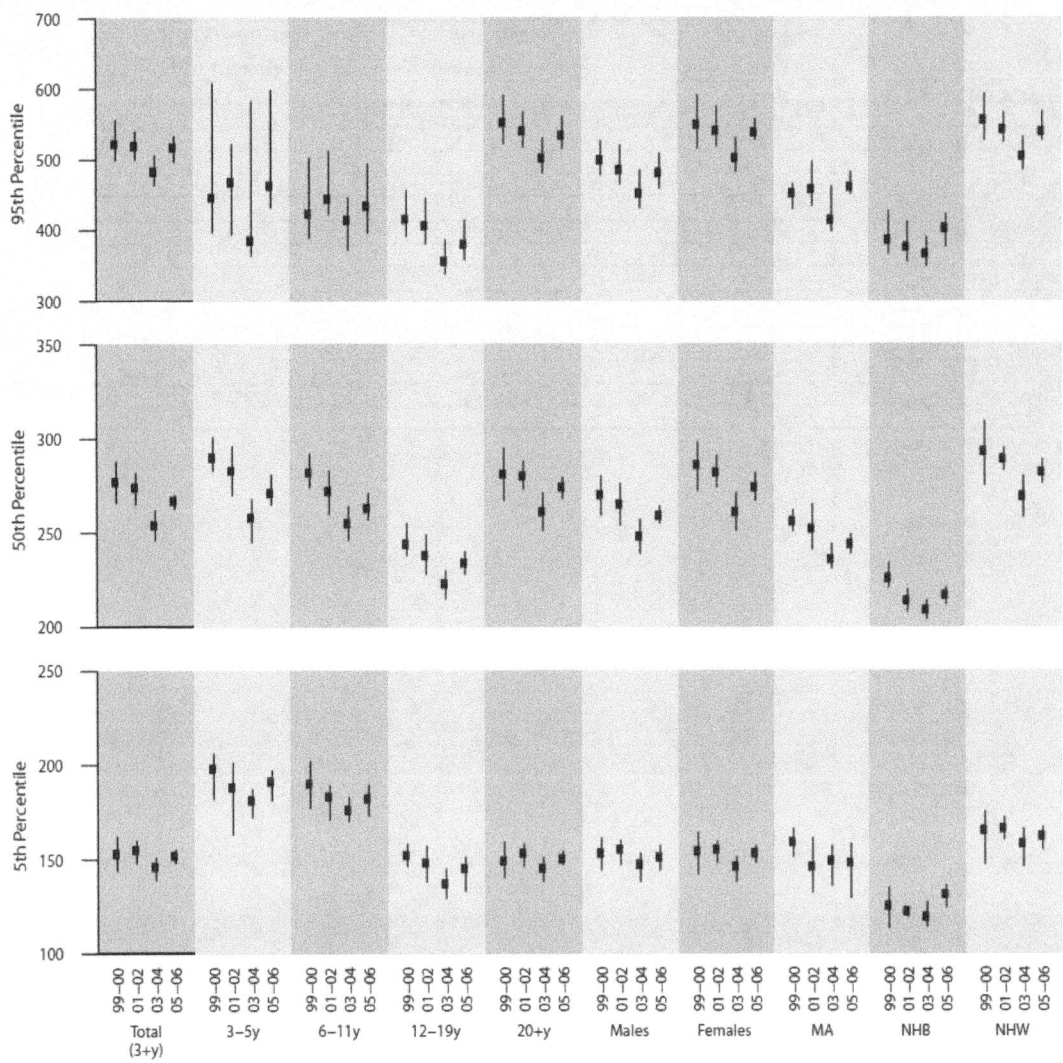

Table 1.2.c. Red blood cell folate: Prevalence

Prevalence (in percent) of low red blood cell folate concentration (< 95 ng/mL) for the U.S. population aged 1 year and older, National Health and Nutrition Examination Survey, 2003–2006.

	Sample size	Prevalence (95% conf. interval)	Estimated total number of persons
Total, 1 year and older	16,670	0.2 (0.2 – 0.4)	704,000
Age group			
1–5 years	1,861	§	§
6–11 years	1,779	§	§
12–19 years	4,050	0.2 (0.1 – 0.4)	76,000
20–39 years	3,262	§	§
40–59 years	2,649	0.4 (0.2 – 0.7)	331,000
60 years and older	3,069	§	§
Gender			
Males	8,172	0.2 (0.1 – 0.4)	301,000
Females	8,498	0.3 (0.2 – 0.5)	404,000
Race/ethnicity			
Mexican Americans	4,304	0.3‡ (0.1 – 0.6)	72,000‡
Non-Hispanic Blacks	4,404	0.9 (0.6 – 1.5)	313,000
Non-Hispanic Whites	6,675	§	§

‡ Estimate flagged: 30% ≤ RSE < 40% for the prevalence estimate.
§ Estimate suppressed: RSE ≥ 40% for the prevalence estimate.

Table 1.2.d. Red blood cell folate: Prevalence by survey cycle

Prevalence (in percent) of low red blood cell folate concentration (< 95 ng/mL) for the U.S. population, National Health and Nutrition Examination Survey, 1999–2006.

	Sample size	Prevalence (95% conf. interval)		Estimated total number of persons
Total, 3 years and older				
1999–2000	7,614	§		§
2001–2002	8,488	0.2‡	(0.1 – 0.4)	562,000‡
2003–2004	7,849	0.3	(0.2 – 0.6)	947,000
2005–2006	7,906	0.2	(0.1 – 0.3)	434,000
Age group				
3–5 years				
1999–2000	380	§		§
2001–2002	460	§		§
2003–2004	453	§		§
2005–2006	493	§		§
6–11 years				
1999–2000	898	§		§
2001–2002	1,040	§		§
2003–2004	849	§		§
2005–2006	930	§		§
12–19 years				
1999–2000	2,136	§		§
2001–2002	2,226	§		§
2003–2004	2,063	0.3‡	(0.1 – 0.5)	88,000‡
2005–2006	1,987	0.2‡	(0.1 – 0.4)	64,000‡
20–39 years				
1999–2000	1,474	§		§
2001–2002	1,721	§		§
2003–2004	1,555	§		§
2005–2006	1,707	§		§
40–59 years				
1999–2000	1,213	§		§
2001–2002	1,496	§		§
2003–2004	1,273	0.7‡	(0.3 – 1.5)	555,000‡
2005–2006	1,376	0.1‡	(0.1 – 0.3)	118,000‡
60 years and older				
1999–2000	1,513	§		§
2001–2002	1,545	0.3‡	(0.1 – 0.7)	147,000‡
2003–2004	1,656	§		§
2005–2006	1,413	§		§
Gender				
Males				
1999–2000	3,721	0.2‡	(0.1 – 0.4)	217,000‡
2001–2002	4,106	§		§
2003–2004	3,874	0.3‡	(0.1 – 0.6)	378,000‡
2005–2006	3,845	0.1	(0.1 – 0.2)	201,000
Females				
1999–2000	3,893	§		§
2001–2002	4,382	0.1‡	(0.1 – 0.3)	161,000‡
2003–2004	3,975	0.4‡	(0.2 – 0.9)	570,000‡
2005–2006	4,061	§		§
Race/ethnicity				
Mexican Americans				
1999–2000	2,592	§		§
2001–2002	2,134	§		§
2003–2004	1,919	§		§
2005–2006	2,057	§		§
Non-Hispanic Blacks				
1999–2000	1,738	1.0	(0.5 – 1.7)	318,000
2001–2002	2,045	0.7‡	(0.3 – 1.5)	238,000‡
2003–2004	2,091	1.0	(0.5 – 1.9)	333,000
2005–2006	2,084	0.8‡	(0.3 – 1.8)	261,000‡
Non-Hispanic Whites				
1999–2000	2,585	§		§
2001–2002	3,625	§		§
2003–2004	3,256	§		§
2005–2006	3,149	0.0	(0.0 – 0.1)	85,000

‡ Estimate flagged: 30% ≤ RSE < 40% for the prevalence estimate.
§ Estimate suppressed: RSE ≥ 40% for the prevalence estimate.

Table 1.3.a.1. Serum pyridoxal-5'-phosphate: Concentrations

Geometric mean and selected percentiles of serum concentrations (in nmol/L) for the total U.S. population aged 1 year and older, National Health and Nutrition Examination Survey, 2005–2006.

	Geometric mean (95% conf. interval)	Selected percentiles (95% conf. interval)						Sample size
		2.5th	5th	50th	95th	97.5th	
Total, 1 year and older	51.4 (49.1 – 53.8)	11.3 (10.0 – 12.5)	14.3 (13.3 – 15.3)	49.3 (46.9 – 51.2)	214 (199 – 245)	302 (279 – 330)	8,311
Age group							
1–5 years	65.0 (61.2 – 69.0)	20.7 (18.2 – 23.6)	25.4 (21.3 – 29.9)	66.1 (63.1 – 70.4)	160 (148 – 182)	185 (176 – 202)	915
6–11 years	60.5 (56.9 – 64.4)	22.9 (20.0 – 24.1)	25.5 (23.3 – 28.2)	60.0 (55.3 – 65.5)	157 (137 – 185)	188 (169 – 223)	922
12–19 years	49.4 (46.7 – 52.3)	17.4 (16.4 – 18.4)	20.7 (19.2 – 21.6)	47.8 (44.9 – 51.0)	127 (118 – 150)	174 (140 – 206)	1,985
20–39 years	51.0 (47.7 – 54.6)	11.8 (10.3 – 13.7)	15.6 (13.6 – 17.0)	47.3 (43.9 – 50.5)	219 (194 – 273)	322 (279 – 379)	1,699
40–59 years	49.0 (45.1 – 53.3)	9.84 (8.61 – 11.3)	12.8 (11.2 – 13.8)	45.6 (41.5 – 50.3)	262 (212 – 302)	342 (297 – 399)	1,381
60 years and older	50.4 (46.7 – 54.5)	9.13 (8.70 – 9.95)	11.6 (9.96 – 12.9)	46.9 (41.9 – 53.5)	262 (217 – 311)	324 (281 – 385)	1,409
Gender							
Males	56.0 (53.6 – 58.5)	13.3 (11.7 – 14.5)	17.1 (15.2 – 18.9)	53.9 (52.0 – 56.0)	209 (191 – 254)	320 (282 – 352)	4,055
Females	47.4 (44.7 – 50.3)	10.2 (9.46 – 11.2)	12.9 (11.7 – 13.9)	44.1 (40.8 – 47.0)	222 (210 – 249)	291 (266 – 323)	4,256
Race/ethnicity							
Mexican Americans	49.3 (47.2 – 51.4)	12.9 (10.8 – 14.7)	17.5 (14.5 – 19.5)	46.4 (44.9 – 48.3)	157 (147 – 174)	212 (190 – 262)	2,212
Non-Hispanic Blacks	40.5 (37.4 – 44.0)	9.41 (8.45 – 10.5)	12.7 (11.3 – 13.2)	39.0 (35.9 – 41.7)	155 (129 – 212)	238 (183 – 302)	2,157
Non-Hispanic Whites	53.8 (50.8 – 57.0)	11.3 (9.84 – 12.8)	14.1 (12.9 – 15.3)	51.7 (49.5 – 54.6)	234 (212 – 269)	319 (289 – 344)	3,285

Figure 1.3.a. Serum pyridoxal–5'–phosphate: Concentrations by age group

Geometric mean (95% confidence interval), National Health and Nutrition Examination Survey, 2005–2006

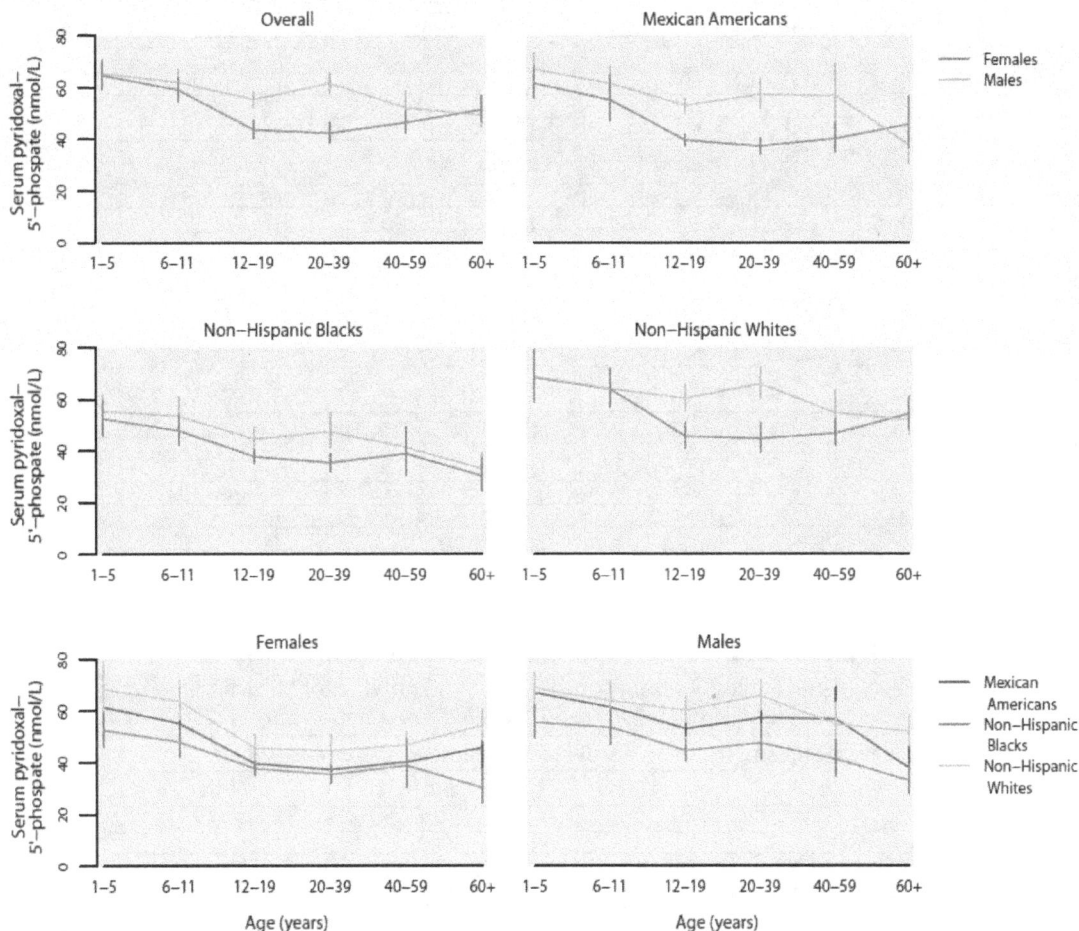

Table 1.3.a.2. Serum pyridoxal-5'-phosphate: Total population

Geometric mean and selected percentiles of serum concentrations (in nmol/L) for the total U.S. population aged 1 year and older, National Health and Nutrition Examination Survey, 2005–2006.

	Geometric mean (95% conf. interval)	Selected percentiles (95% conf. interval)						Sample size
		10th		50th		90th		
Males and Females								
Total, 1 year and older	51.4 (49.1 – 53.8)	19.5	(18.2 – 20.6)	49.3	(46.9 – 51.2)	154	(139 – 162)	8,311
1–5 years	65.0 (61.2 – 69.0)	31.7	(29.2 – 35.0)	66.1	(63.1 – 70.4)	126	(116 – 140)	915
6–11 years	60.5 (56.9 – 64.4)	30.7	(28.0 – 33.5)	60.0	(55.3 – 65.5)	126	(110 – 138)	922
12–19 years	49.4 (46.7 – 52.3)	24.8	(23.3 – 26.3)	47.8	(44.9 – 51.0)	105	(92.9 – 114)	1,985
20–39 years	51.0 (47.7 – 54.6)	20.0	(18.0 – 21.6)	47.3	(43.9 – 50.5)	153	(130 – 183)	1,699
40–59 years	49.0 (45.1 – 53.3)	16.5	(14.3 – 19.0)	45.6	(41.5 – 50.3)	166	(147 – 192)	1,381
60 years and older	50.4 (46.7 – 54.5)	15.1	(13.0 – 17.5)	46.9	(41.9 – 53.5)	187	(173 – 209)	1,409
Males								
Total, 1 year and older	56.0 (53.6 – 58.5)	22.6	(20.3 – 24.6)	53.9	(52.0 – 56.0)	149	(136 – 162)	4,055
1–5 years	65.3 (61.2 – 69.6)	31.6	(26.3 – 35.2)	66.8	(63.2 – 71.9)	127	(117 – 135)	455
6–11 years	62.0 (57.4 – 66.9)	31.6	(30.5 – 33.4)	60.8	(54.8 – 68.4)	130	(113 – 143)	454
12–19 years	55.4 (52.4 – 58.6)	28.9	(27.0 – 30.6)	54.8	(51.3 – 57.9)	110	(101 – 122)	991
20–39 years	61.6 (58.0 – 65.4)	26.8	(24.8 – 28.8)	55.3	(52.7 – 58.3)	165	(139 – 202)	741
40–59 years	52.1 (46.4 – 58.5)	19.1	(14.8 – 22.6)	51.0	(43.7 – 56.9)	158	(125 – 188)	680
60 years and older	49.3 (44.7 – 54.3)	16.1	(13.5 – 19.3)	45.9	(40.0 – 54.4)	171	(156 – 196)	734
Females								
Total, 1 year and older	47.4 (44.7 – 50.3)	17.2	(15.2 – 18.8)	44.1	(40.8 – 47.0)	156	(141 – 165)	4,256
1–5 years	64.6 (59.3 – 70.5)	32.1	(28.5 – 36.1)	65.2	(60.9 – 71.1)	124	(106 – 156)	460
6–11 years	59.1 (54.9 – 63.6)	29.7	(25.3 – 33.6)	58.3	(52.0 – 64.0)	118	(104 – 156)	468
12–19 years	43.7 (40.5 – 47.2)	21.8	(21.0 – 22.8)	41.4	(39.0 – 45.1)	90.6	(78.4 – 111)	994
20–39 years	42.4 (38.8 – 46.3)	16.5	(14.6 – 18.4)	37.6	(35.1 – 41.8)	132	(111 – 166)	958
40–59 years	46.4 (42.5 – 50.6)	14.4	(13.0 – 17.6)	41.6	(36.3 – 46.6)	172	(161 – 207)	701
60 years and older	51.4 (46.6 – 56.7)	14.1	(12.7 – 16.2)	47.6	(39.8 – 57.1)	206	(176 – 246)	675

Table 1.3.a.3. Serum pyridoxal-5'-phosphate: Mexican Americans

Geometric mean and selected percentiles of serum concentrations (in nmol/L) for Mexican Americans in the U.S. population aged 1 year and older, National Health and Nutrition Examination Survey, 2005–2006.

	Geometric mean (95% conf. interval)	Selected percentiles (95% conf. interval)						Sample size
		10th		50th		90th		
Males and Females								
Total, 1 year and older	49.3 (47.2 – 51.4)	22.3	(19.8 – 23.9)	46.4	(44.9 – 48.3)	121	(105 – 136)	2,212
1–5 years	64.2 (60.1 – 68.7)	32.4	(28.0 – 34.2)	65.0	(59.0 – 71.1)	126	(115 – 142)	322
6–11 years	58.3 (52.5 – 64.6)	30.3	(24.0 – 34.9)	56.4	(50.8 – 65.8)	116	(98.9 – 137)	321
12–19 years	46.0 (44.4 – 47.6)	24.7	(23.0 – 26.6)	44.4	(42.5 – 47.6)	91.1	(83.7 – 100)	657
20–39 years	47.1 (44.1 – 50.4)	20.4	(15.7 – 24.8)	42.9	(40.1 – 45.6)	127	(97.0 – 143)	453
40–59 years	47.9 (42.4 – 54.1)	20.2	(14.5 – 23.3)	42.2	(38.5 – 49.4)	141	(115 – 170)	249
60 years and older	42.0 (34.9 – 50.5)	15.0	(13.1 – 17.2)	38.6	(30.2 – 50.1)	142	(101 – 184)	210
Males								
Total, 1 year and older	56.4 (53.7 – 59.1)	27.9	(23.5 – 30.6)	53.7	(51.2 – 55.8)	124	(108 – 140)	1,056
1–5 years	67.0 (61.3 – 73.3)	30.4	(22.2 – 38.5)	67.7	(60.0 – 76.3)	129	(108 – 180)	153
6–11 years	61.4 (55.5 – 67.9)	32.0	(27.9 – 35.2)	57.5	(52.4 – 65.7)	126	(97.0 – 151)	157
12–19 years	53.0 (50.2 – 55.9)	28.2	(26.7 – 32.3)	51.6	(47.7 – 55.8)	104	(87.7 – 113)	318
20–39 years	57.2 (51.9 – 63.1)	29.4	(22.0 – 32.5)	51.9	(46.1 – 60.9)	135	(108 – 152)	200
40–59 years	56.7 (46.6 – 68.9)	24.0	(16.0 – 34.1)	53.3	(45.1 – 59.2)	122	(91.1 – 478)	123
60 years and older	37.8 (30.0 – 47.6)	14.7†	(10.7 – 18.6)	35.6	(26.8 – 50.9)	95.5†	(71.3 – 209)	105
Females								
Total, 1 year and older	42.6 (40.8 – 44.6)	19.1	(16.4 – 20.8)	39.4	(38.2 – 40.3)	111	(96.5 – 130)	1,156
1–5 years	61.5 (55.9 – 67.7)	33.2	(28.9 – 34.9)	61.2	(55.2 – 68.8)	120	(97.3 – 176)	169
6–11 years	55.1 (47.2 – 64.3)	27.6	(17.6 – 34.7)	54.3	(44.6 – 68.7)	105	(87.9 – 133)	164
12–19 years	39.6 (37.6 – 41.7)	20.7	(19.0 – 22.6)	38.8	(37.2 – 39.7)	76.8	(69.9 – 87.9)	339
20–39 years	37.3 (34.3 – 40.4)	17.7	(11.8 – 19.6)	34.1	(31.7 – 36.1)	89.7	(71.6 – 134)	253
40–59 years	40.2 (35.0 – 46.3)	14.9	(10.3 – 18.9)	33.2	(29.7 – 39.1)	155	(110 – 199)	126
60 years and older	45.7 (36.9 – 56.6)	16.6†	(12.6 – 19.8)	39.3	(30.7 – 53.3)	160†	(106 – 212)	105

† Estimate is subject to greater uncertainty due to small cell size.

Table 1.3.a.4. Serum pyridoxal-5′-phosphate: Non-Hispanic blacks

Geometric mean and selected percentiles of serum concentrations (in nmol/L) for non-Hispanic blacks in the U.S. population aged 1 year and older, National Health and Nutrition Examination Survey, 2005–2006.

	Geometric mean (95% conf. interval)	Selected percentiles (95% conf. interval)			Sample size
		10th	50th	90th	
Males and Females					
Total, 1 year and older	40.5 (37.4 – 44.0)	16.3 (15.4 – 17.2)	39.0 (35.9 – 41.7)	104 (90.5 – 132)	2,157
1–5 years	54.0 (49.4 – 58.9)	25.2 (22.3 – 29.5)	51.2 (46.4 – 58.8)	115 (99.1 – 138)	226
6–11 years	50.6 (45.4 – 56.4)	27.2 (25.0 – 29.8)	46.4 (41.9 – 55.9)	97.1 (90.0 – 123)	254
12–19 years	41.0 (38.1 – 44.1)	21.6 (19.8 – 22.7)	39.5 (37.1 – 43.2)	82.8 (73.6 – 90.9)	676
20–39 years	40.5 (36.8 – 44.5)	16.3 (13.2 – 18.1)	38.5 (35.3 – 43.5)	105 (94.0 – 142)	371
40–59 years	39.9 (33.5 – 47.5)	14.9 (13.2 – 17.4)	36.3 (31.1 – 41.7)	132 (82.8 – 204)	339
60 years and older	31.3 (26.8 – 36.6)	10.7 (8.73 – 12.6)	29.1 (24.5 – 35.7)	104 (79.0 – 152)	291
Males					
Total, 1 year and older	44.3 (40.5 – 48.6)	19.0 (17.3 – 20.1)	43.7 (39.3 – 47.3)	104 (92.0 – 137)	1,071
1–5 years	55.4 (49.5 – 61.9)	24.6† (19.3 – 32.2)	53.6 (46.6 – 60.4)	120† (103 – 147)	109
6–11 years	53.5 (47.2 – 60.7)	29.6 (26.0 – 31.8)	52.5 (41.9 – 61.7)	100 (92.0 – 124)	133
12–19 years	44.6 (40.6 – 48.9)	22.9 (21.1 – 25.1)	44.5 (38.8 – 49.5)	89.2 (74.9 – 103)	348
20–39 years	47.5 (41.2 – 54.8)	19.7 (14.5 – 23.5)	45.2 (37.7 – 53.5)	130 (95.2 – 185)	170
40–59 years	41.2 (34.9 – 48.7)	16.0 (9.17 – 20.7)	40.7 (31.6 – 46.6)	102 (79.6 – 203)	157
60 years and older	33.0 (27.9 – 39.1)	12.4 (10.2 – 13.4)	27.9 (24.1 – 38.1)	103 (79.1 – 194)	154
Females					
Total, 1 year and older	37.5 (34.2 – 41.1)	14.8 (13.4 – 16.1)	35.6 (32.3 – 39.2)	103 (85.9 – 128)	1,086
1–5 years	52.5 (46.3 – 59.4)	26.0 (11.1 – 30.5)	51.1 (42.8 – 59.8)	109 (88.7 – 149)	117
6–11 years	47.9 (42.4 – 54.2)	25.0 (22.9 – 29.8)	42.9 (38.0 – 52.0)	93.0 (84.6 – 128)	121
12–19 years	37.7 (35.2 – 40.3)	20.7 (18.7 – 21.6)	36.8 (33.7 – 39.1)	73.6 (68.9 – 85.6)	328
20–39 years	35.4 (32.2 – 38.9)	14.4 (9.31 – 16.8)	33.8 (28.4 – 37.9)	99.7 (80.0 – 141)	201
40–59 years	38.8 (30.8 – 48.9)	14.4 (13.0 – 16.1)	33.8 (26.5 – 41.0)	145 (81.3 – 261)	182
60 years and older	30.2 (24.5 – 37.2)	9.48 (8.20 – 11.2)	29.9 (22.4 – 37.0)	95.0 (74.2 – 157)	137

† Estimate is subject to greater uncertainty due to small cell size

Table 1.3.a.5. Serum pyridoxal-5′-phosphate: Non-Hispanic whites

Geometric mean and selected percentiles of serum concentrations (in nmol/L) for non-Hispanic whites in the U.S. population aged 1 year and older, National Health and Nutrition Examination Survey, 2005–2006.

	Geometric mean (95% conf. interval)	Selected percentiles (95% conf. interval)			Sample size
		10th	50th	90th	
Males and Females					
Total, 1 year and older	53.8 (50.8 – 57.0)	19.2 (17.7 – 20.7)	51.7 (49.5 – 54.6)	167 (156 – 181)	3,285
1–5 years	68.5 (63.0 – 74.4)	34.0 (30.5 – 37.3)	68.4 (63.3 – 77.5)	130 (114 – 157)	263
6–11 years	63.9 (58.7 – 69.5)	31.6 (29.2 – 34.2)	63.3 (54.9 – 72.7)	133 (117 – 170)	251
12–19 years	52.7 (48.7 – 57.1)	25.7 (23.8 – 27.2)	51.5 (47.4 – 56.8)	109 (96.0 – 127)	505
20–39 years	54.3 (48.9 – 60.3)	20.9 (17.7 – 22.7)	50.6 (44.9 – 55.8)	168 (133 – 211)	718
40–59 years	50.6 (45.6 – 56.1)	16.2 (13.7 – 19.0)	47.9 (42.7 – 52.8)	173 (153 – 199)	691
60 years and older	53.2 (49.0 – 57.9)	15.7 (13.3 – 18.2)	50.6 (44.0 – 57.5)	196 (177 – 215)	857
Males					
Total, 1 year and older	58.8 (55.1 – 62.7)	22.8 (20.2 – 25.5)	57.4 (53.8 – 60.6)	166 (147 – 183)	1,636
1–5 years	68.7 (62.9 – 74.9)	34.9 (30.2 – 37.2)	70.8 (65.3 – 78.3)	126 (115 – 137)	146
6–11 years	63.9 (57.3 – 71.4)	31.6 (29.3 – 33.7)	64.7 (50.1 – 75.8)	135 (106 – 190)	121
12–19 years	60.3 (55.5 – 65.5)	29.5 (27.3 – 33.8)	59.7 (54.7 – 65.2)	117 (105 – 148)	255
20–39 years	65.9 (60.4 – 72.0)	27.9 (25.3 – 30.8)	58.4 (53.9 – 66.8)	183 (152 – 228)	310
40–59 years	54.7 (47.4 – 63.2)	19.1 (14.6 – 22.8)	53.1 (43.6 – 61.7)	173 (140 – 194)	356
60 years and older	52.0 (46.4 – 58.2)	16.7 (13.7 – 20.5)	50.4 (42.2 – 59.3)	174 (157 – 204)	448
Females					
Total, 1 year and older	49.4 (45.8 – 53.2)	16.4 (14.4 – 18.7)	46.4 (42.5 – 50.4)	170 (161 – 182)	1,649
1–5 years	68.3 (59.0 – 79.0)	32.6 (26.5 – 40.3)	66.6 (59.0 – 79.5)	141 (105 – 183)	117
6–11 years	63.8 (56.8 – 71.8)	31.3 (23.7 – 35.9)	62.7 (51.7 – 74.6)	126 (108 – 175)	130
12–19 years	45.6 (41.0 – 50.8)	21.8 (19.7 – 23.9)	42.1 (39.0 – 47.8)	94.0 (80.0 – 126)	250
20–39 years	44.6 (39.3 – 50.7)	16.5 (14.4 – 18.8)	38.4 (34.5 – 45.7)	156 (112 – 216)	408
40–59 years	46.8 (42.2 – 52.0)	13.9 (12.6 – 16.4)	44.4 (35.8 – 48.3)	174 (155 – 221)	335
60 years and older	54.3 (48.6 – 60.6)	14.6 (12.5 – 17.0)	50.6 (41.6 – 62.5)	213 (184 – 254)	409

Table 1.3.c. Serum pyridoxal-5'-phosphate: Prevalence

Prevalence (in percent) of low serum pyridoxal-5'-phosphate concentration (< 20 nmol/L) for the U.S. population aged 1 year and older, National Health and Nutrition Examination Survey, 2005–2006.

	Sample size	Prevalence (95% conf. interval)	Estimated total number of persons
Total, 1 year and older	8,311	10.5 (9.1 – 12.0)	30,146,000
Age group			
1–5 years	915	2.1‡ (1.1 – 4.2)	435,000‡
6–11 years	922	1.2‡ (0.5 – 2.7)	280,000‡
12–19 years	1,985	4.6 (3.6 – 5.7)	1,529,000
20–39 years	1,699	9.9 (7.7 – 12.6)	7,877,000
40–59 years	1,381	13.9 (11.2 – 17.1)	11,371,000
60 years and older	1,409	16.0 (13.1 – 19.5)	7,741,000
Gender			
Males	4,055	7.3 (5.7 – 9.4)	10,305,000
Females	4,256	13.5 (11.7 – 15.5)	19,830,000
Race/ethnicity			
Mexican Americans	2,212	7.5 (5.3 – 10.4)	2,031,000
Non-Hispanic Blacks	2,157	15.7 (13.6 – 18.0)	5,459,000
Non-Hispanic Whites	3,285	10.7 (9.1 – 12.5)	20,588,000

‡ Estimate flagged: 30% ≤ RSE < 40% for the prevalence estimate.

Table 1.4.a.1. Serum 4-pyridoxic acid: Concentrations

Geometric mean and selected percentiles of serum concentrations (in nmol/L) for the total U.S. population aged 1 year and older, National Health and Nutrition Examination Survey, 2005–2006.

| | Geometric mean (95% conf. interval) | Selected percentiles (95% conf. interval) | | | | | Sample size |
		2.5th	5th	50th	95th	97.5th	
Total, 1 year and older	31.9 (30.3 – 33.7)	8.73 (8.19 – 9.06)	9.87 (9.53 – 10.2)	25.5 (24.6 – 26.5)	194 (174 – 223)	385 (329 – 505)	8,312
Age group							
1-5 years	25.9 (23.8 – 28.2)	8.90 (8.00 – 9.22)	10.5 (9.07 – 11.3)	24.2 (22.2 – 25.8)	96.9 (75.6 – 125)	130 (104 – 214)	917
6-11 years	23.5 (21.8 – 25.5)	8.11 (7.12 – 8.98)	9.46 (8.57 – 10.2)	21.6 (19.8 – 23.9)	85.6 (64.3 – 115)	111 (92.4 – 133)	922
12-19 years	20.9 (19.9 – 22.0)	7.74 (7.17 – 8.22)	8.85 (8.28 – 9.47)	19.0 (18.2 – 20.1)	70.5 (59.8 – 84.4)	94.5 (79.4 – 131)	1,985
20-39 years	26.8 (24.3 – 29.5)	8.02 (7.49 – 8.47)	9.16 (8.78 – 9.53)	22.2 (20.4 – 23.9)	160 (125 – 198)	271 (184 – 447)	1,698
40-59 years	34.7 (31.9 – 37.7)	9.36 (8.56 – 10.0)	10.7 (9.90 – 11.4)	27.3 (25.8 – 29.1)	212 (162 – 344)	705 (278 – 2,150)	1,381
60 years and older	58.6 (54.7 – 62.9)	11.6 (10.2 – 12.4)	13.1 (12.3 – 14.1)	47.6 (45.0 – 52.3)	464 (355 – 611)	873 (557 – 1,700)	1,409
Gender							
Males	32.1 (30.0 – 34.2)	9.24 (8.43 – 9.77)	10.6 (9.91 – 11.2)	26.0 (24.9 – 27.4)	171 (146 – 212)	334 (271 – 427)	4,055
Females	31.8 (30.2 – 33.5)	8.21 (7.89 – 8.65)	9.50 (9.15 – 9.76)	24.7 (23.4 – 26.1)	214 (188 – 255)	465 (349 – 712)	4,257
Race/ethnicity							
Mexican Americans	22.5 (21.0 – 24.1)	7.90 (7.09 – 8.46)	9.13 (8.66 – 9.55)	19.0 (18.1 – 20.1)	90.9 (74.7 – 136)	169 (127 – 355)	2,213
Non-Hispanic Blacks	21.6 (19.4 – 24.0)	7.21 (6.78 – 7.57)	8.04 (7.72 – 8.44)	17.8 (16.3 – 19.3)	119 (89.8 – 196)	232 (159 – 493)	2,157
Non-Hispanic Whites	37.1 (35.1 – 39.1)	9.65 (9.04 – 10.1)	11.1 (10.6 – 11.5)	29.3 (27.8 – 30.6)	224 (203 – 265)	498 (370 – 717)	3,285

Figure 1.4.a. Serum 4–pyridoxic acid: Concentrations by age group
Geometric mean (95% confidence interval), National Health and Nutrition Examination Survey, 2005–2006

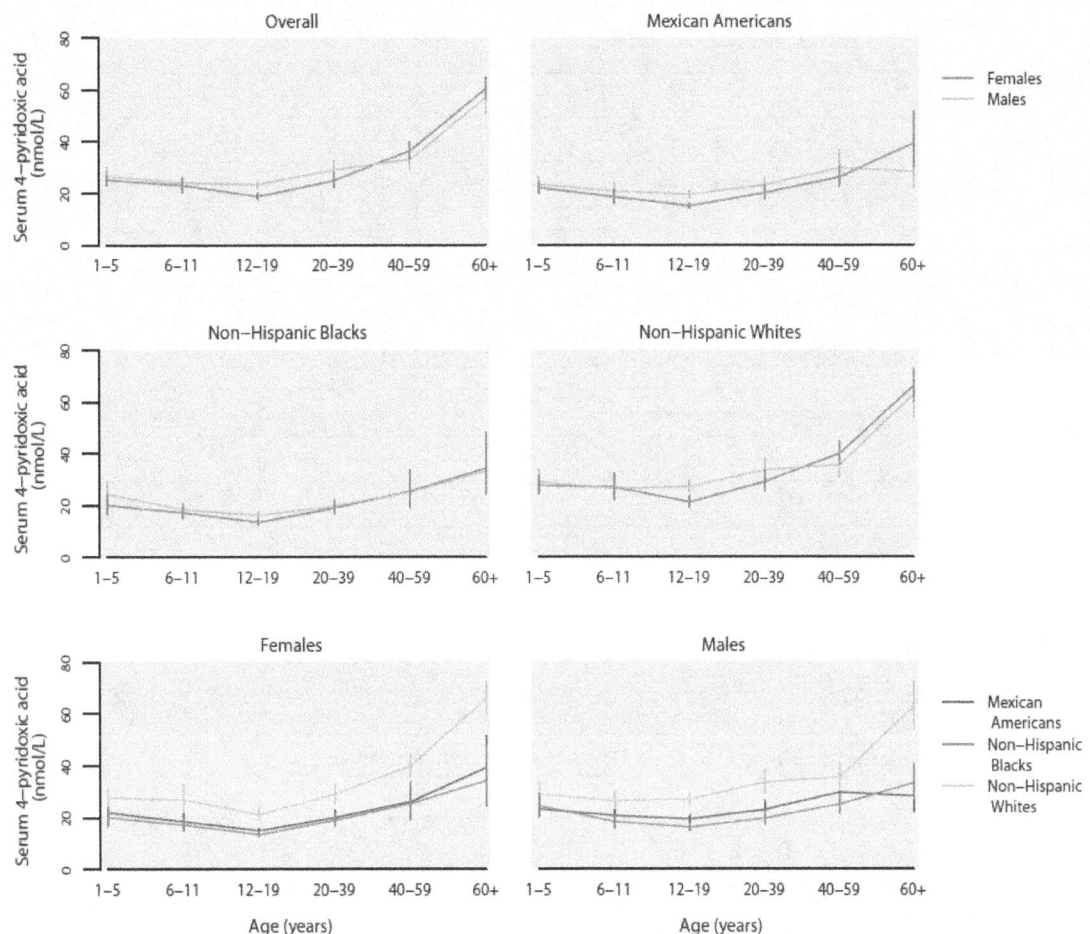

Table 1.4.a.2. Serum 4-pyridoxic acid: Total population

Geometric mean and selected percentiles of serum concentrations (in nmol/L) for the total U.S. population aged 1 year and older, National Health and Nutrition Examination Survey, 2005–2006.

	Geometric mean (95% conf. interval)	Selected percentiles (95% conf. interval)						Sample size
		10th		50th		90th		
Males and Females								
Total, 1 year and older	31.9 (30.3 – 33.7)	11.7	(11.4 – 12.2)	25.5	(24.6 – 26.5)	116	(105 – 128)	8,312
1–5 years	25.9 (23.8 – 28.2)	12.5	(11.4 – 13.3)	24.2	(22.2 – 25.8)	59.8	(49.8 – 79.6)	917
6–11 years	23.5 (21.8 – 25.5)	11.2	(10.2 – 12.0)	21.6	(19.8 – 23.9)	56.7	(48.4 – 71.5)	922
12–19 years	20.9 (19.9 – 22.0)	10.2	(9.88 – 10.6)	19.0	(18.2 – 20.1)	48.1	(44.1 – 54.5)	1,985
20–39 years	26.8 (24.3 – 29.5)	10.7	(10.0 – 11.1)	22.2	(20.4 – 23.9)	90.9	(73.2 – 115)	1,698
40–59 years	34.7 (31.9 – 37.7)	12.6	(11.8 – 13.6)	27.3	(25.8 – 29.1)	117	(105 – 138)	1,381
60 years and older	58.6 (54.7 – 62.9)	16.4	(14.9 – 18.3)	47.6	(45.0 – 52.3)	248	(208 – 321)	1,409
Males								
Total, 1 year and older	32.1 (30.0 – 34.2)	12.9	(12.1 – 13.6)	26.0	(24.9 – 27.4)	103	(92.2 – 118)	4,055
1–5 years	26.7 (23.7 – 30.0)	11.9	(10.5 – 14.1)	25.2	(22.8 – 27.0)	63.6	(48.5 – 111)	456
6–11 years	24.0 (22.1 – 26.1)	11.6	(9.92 – 12.4)	21.9	(20.2 – 24.1)	56.4	(46.0 – 83.0)	454
12–19 years	23.3 (21.9 – 24.7)	11.9	(10.9 – 12.6)	20.8	(19.7 – 21.9)	55.0	(46.8 – 67.0)	991
20–39 years	29.0 (26.1 – 32.2)	12.0	(10.9 – 13.2)	24.3	(22.5 – 26.0)	89.5	(65.9 – 124)	740
40–59 years	33.0 (29.3 – 37.2)	13.8	(11.8 – 15.2)	26.5	(24.4 – 30.2)	101	(76.3 – 124)	680
60 years and older	56.7 (50.7 – 63.5)	17.2	(15.1 – 18.9)	46.8	(41.8 – 53.3)	220	(178 – 292)	734
Females								
Total, 1 year and older	31.8 (30.2 – 33.5)	11.1	(10.9 – 11.3)	24.7	(23.4 – 26.1)	133	(116 – 151)	4,257
1–5 years	25.1 (23.3 – 27.1)	12.6	(11.9 – 13.0)	22.7	(20.8 – 25.4)	59.2	(48.3 – 76.4)	461
6–11 years	23.0 (20.5 – 25.8)	10.7	(9.57 – 11.5)	20.8	(18.6 – 24.2)	54.9	(44.7 – 90.5)	468
12–19 years	18.7 (17.7 – 19.8)	9.59	(9.31 – 9.88)	17.1	(16.3 – 18.0)	42.9	(35.5 – 52.2)	994
20–39 years	24.8 (22.3 – 27.5)	9.74	(9.31 – 10.4)	19.2	(17.3 – 22.1)	92.5	(77.5 – 118)	958
40–59 years	36.4 (33.3 – 39.8)	12.1	(11.3 – 12.7)	28.1	(25.2 – 31.1)	145	(116 – 192)	701
60 years and older	60.2 (56.1 – 64.8)	15.6	(14.0 – 17.9)	48.7	(43.5 – 56.9)	257	(219 – 328)	675

Table 1.4.a.3. Serum 4-pyridoxic acid: Mexican Americans

Geometric mean and selected percentiles of serum concentrations (in nmol/L) for Mexican Americans in the U.S. population aged 1 year and older, National Health and Nutrition Examination Survey, 2005–2006.

	Geometric mean (95% conf. interval)	Selected percentiles (95% conf. interval)						Sample size
		10th		50th		90th		
Males and Females								
Total, 1 year and older	22.5 (21.0 – 24.1)	10.7	(10.0 – 11.2)	19.0	(18.1 – 20.1)	57.9	(48.0 – 66.1)	2,213
1–5 years	22.7 (20.7 – 24.8)	11.9	(10.7 – 12.8)	20.3	(19.1 – 22.2)	52.3	(41.3 – 62.3)	324
6–11 years	19.6 (17.7 – 21.7)	9.67	(8.75 – 10.7)	18.5	(16.0 – 20.3)	44.2	(36.3 – 58.1)	321
12–19 years	17.1 (16.4 – 17.8)	9.29	(8.70 – 9.81)	15.8	(14.8 – 16.8)	34.6	(31.5 – 42.8)	657
20–39 years	21.6 (19.3 – 24.1)	10.7	(9.33 – 11.4)	18.3	(16.8 – 19.9)	53.3	(43.8 – 76.4)	452
40–59 years	27.9 (24.6 – 31.6)	11.7	(10.1 – 12.7)	22.4	(20.5 – 24.6)	71.1	(60.0 – 114)	249
60 years and older	33.8 (27.9 – 41.0)	12.5	(11.0 – 14.7)	27.3	(23.6 – 31.2)	117	(75.3 – 311)	210
Males								
Total, 1 year and older	23.6 (21.9 – 25.6)	11.5	(10.8 – 12.0)	20.7	(19.4 – 21.7)	58.1	(45.6 – 68.9)	1,057
1–5 years	23.3 (20.4 – 26.5)	11.8	(10.7 – 13.7)	20.9	(18.9 – 22.9)	48.8	(38.0 – 78.1)	155
6–11 years	20.7 (18.2 – 23.6)	10.3	(8.64 – 11.4)	18.9	(16.5 – 20.9)	47.4	(39.5 – 59.3)	157
12–19 years	19.4 (18.2 – 20.6)	10.3	(9.71 – 10.8)	17.3	(16.8 – 18.4)	41.6	(34.1 – 59.2)	318
20–39 years	23.0 (20.1 – 26.2)	11.2	(9.36 – 12.7)	19.5	(17.6 – 22.2)	55.0	(42.2 – 85.5)	199
40–59 years	29.7 (24.2 – 36.4)	12.9	(12.5 – 13.9)	24.2	(21.2 – 28.4)	65.1	(45.1 – 230)	123
60 years and older	28.2 (22.0 – 36.1)	11.6†	(5.00 – 14.6)	26.0	(19.9 – 33.3)	72.5†	(50.8 – 193)	105
Females								
Total, 1 year and older	21.4 (20.1 – 22.7)	9.91	(9.35 – 10.6)	17.3	(16.4 – 18.3)	57.0	(49.5 – 70.1)	1,156
1–5 years	22.0 (19.9 – 24.4)	11.9	(9.70 – 12.5)	20.2	(17.5 – 22.6)	52.3	(38.6 – 64.8)	169
6–11 years	18.5 (16.3 – 21.1)	9.60	(7.35 – 10.7)	17.3	(15.1 – 20.4)	41.2	(31.1 – 53.4)	164
12–19 years	15.0 (14.3 – 15.8)	8.55	(7.66 – 9.16)	14.1	(13.2 – 15.1)	28.2	(25.2 – 33.6)	339
20–39 years	20.0 (17.6 – 22.8)	9.73	(7.90 – 11.1)	16.3	(14.7 – 18.6)	49.5	(41.4 – 81.1)	253
40–59 years	26.1 (22.4 – 30.3)	10.9	(9.79 – 11.6)	19.1	(14.7 – 25.2)	90.5	(54.6 – 289)	126
60 years and older	39.2 (30.0 – 51.4)	13.9†	(11.1 – 15.7)	28.0	(23.3 – 35.2)	162†	(78.4 – 3,380)	105

† Estimate is subject to greater uncertainty due to small cell size.

Table 1.4.a.4. Serum 4-pyridoxic acid: Non-Hispanic blacks

Geometric mean and selected percentiles of serum concentrations (in nmol/L) for non-Hispanic blacks in the U.S. population aged 1 year and older, National Health and Nutrition Examination Survey, 2005–2006.

	Geometric mean (95% conf. interval)	Selected percentiles (95% conf. interval)			Sample size
		10th	50th	90th	
Males and Females					
Total, 1 year and older	21.6 (19.4 – 24.0)	9.28 (8.85 – 9.59)	17.8 (16.3 – 19.3)	60.5 (51.3 – 81.9)	2,157
1–5 years	22.2 (19.2 – 25.8)	10.1 (8.17 – 11.2)	19.5 (17.6 – 22.5)	61.7 (44.0 – 96.8)	226
6–11 years	17.8 (16.0 – 19.8)	9.03 (8.25 – 9.53)	15.3 (14.3 – 17.4)	43.9 (32.5 – 67.1)	254
12–19 years	14.8 (14.0 – 15.7)	8.28 (7.64 – 8.65)	13.9 (13.1 – 14.6)	28.9 (25.7 – 34.0)	676
20–39 years	19.3 (18.1 – 20.7)	8.89 (8.39 – 9.47)	15.4 (14.2 – 17.6)	51.4 (45.3 – 60.6)	371
40–59 years	25.3 (21.3 – 30.0)	9.62 (8.24 – 10.8)	19.2 (17.6 – 21.2)	103 (57.1 – 164)	339
60 years and older	33.8 (26.3 – 43.4)	12.2 (9.71 – 14.1)	27.4 (23.1 – 30.6)	113 (81.9 – 246)	291
Males					
Total, 1 year and older	21.8 (19.7 – 24.3)	9.68 (9.16 – 10.3)	18.5 (17.3 – 20.0)	55.7 (44.4 – 82.8)	1,070
1–5 years	24.5 (20.6 – 29.1)	10.3† (6.27 – 12.2)	20.9 (17.7 – 24.4)	83.7† (48.8 – 152)	108
6–11 years	18.4 (16.2 – 21.0)	9.50 (8.53 – 10.3)	15.9 (14.5 – 18.5)	44.1 (33.3 – 66.5)	133
12–19 years	16.2 (15.0 – 17.5)	9.11 (8.59 – 9.35)	15.5 (14.1 – 16.5)	30.9 (26.8 – 39.1)	348
20–39 years	19.7 (17.6 – 22.2)	9.68 (8.96 – 10.9)	17.4 (14.3 – 20.4)	44.3 (32.7 – 68.2)	170
40–59 years	25.1 (21.7 – 29.0)	9.58 (7.97 – 10.6)	19.3 (17.7 – 20.8)	71.2 (52.9 – 134)	157
60 years and older	33.2 (27.1 – 40.7)	12.5 (11.8 – 13.4)	24.3 (22.7 – 30.2)	109 (80.8 – 246)	154
Females					
Total, 1 year and older	21.3 (18.7 – 24.3)	8.88 (8.38 – 9.44)	17.1 (15.0 – 19.1)	64.9 (52.5 – 94.0)	1,087
1–5 years	20.1 (16.7 – 24.2)	8.59 (7.62 – 11.1)	19.0 (16.1 – 22.5)	42.6 (34.5 – 65.2)	118
6–11 years	17.2 (15.1 – 19.7)	8.50 (7.72 – 9.43)	14.8 (13.1 – 17.4)	40.6 (31.1 – 86.4)	121
12–19 years	13.5 (12.6 – 14.4)	7.56 (6.46 – 8.33)	12.7 (11.8 – 13.4)	25.6 (22.0 – 32.8)	328
20–39 years	19.0 (16.9 – 21.5)	8.42 (7.62 – 8.98)	14.3 (12.7 – 16.9)	57.7 (45.3 – 85.7)	201
40–59 years	25.4 (19.2 – 33.7)	9.64 (7.95 – 11.0)	18.8 (15.5 – 25.8)	107 (53.1 – 217)	182
60 years and older	34.2 (24.3 – 48.1)	11.6 (8.02 – 15.3)	28.0 (21.9 – 33.8)	116 (75.1 – 431)	137

† Estimate is subject to greater uncertainty due to small cell size.

Table 1.4.a.5. Serum 4-pyridoxic acid: Non-Hispanic whites

Geometric mean and selected percentiles of serum concentrations (in nmol/L) for non-Hispanic whites in the U.S. population aged 1 year and older, National Health and Nutrition Examination Survey, 2005–2006.

	Geometric mean (95% conf. interval)	Selected percentiles (95% conf. interval)			Sample size
		10th	50th	90th	
Males and Females					
Total, 1 year and older	37.1 (35.1 – 39.1)	13.2 (12.6 – 13.8)	29.3 (27.8 – 30.6)	138 (120 – 154)	3,285
1–5 years	28.4 (25.2 – 31.8)	13.6 (11.9 – 15.1)	26.7 (24.2 – 29.2)	59.9 (49.8 – 104)	263
6–11 years	26.7 (24.1 – 29.5)	12.6 (11.8 – 13.3)	24.5 (22.4 – 26.0)	63.5 (50.7 – 96.3)	251
12–19 years	24.1 (22.4 – 26.0)	11.5 (10.6 – 12.8)	21.5 (21.0 – 22.2)	55.9 (47.7 – 74.7)	505
20–39 years	31.2 (27.5 – 35.4)	11.5 (10.7 – 12.6)	25.2 (22.6 – 28.1)	113 (89.1 – 155)	718
40–59 years	37.7 (34.1 – 41.6)	13.7 (12.5 – 14.8)	30.2 (27.9 – 32.2)	130 (111 – 148)	691
60 years and older	64.4 (58.5 – 70.9)	18.2 (15.3 – 20.2)	53.7 (48.7 – 57.9)	257 (220 – 328)	857
Males					
Total, 1 year and older	36.8 (34.1 – 39.6)	14.9 (13.7 – 15.7)	29.5 (27.7 – 31.3)	116 (105 – 136)	1,636
1–5 years	29.0 (24.9 – 33.7)	14.0 (9.91 – 16.0)	27.2 (24.5 – 31.1)	59.8 (47.3 – 130)	146
6–11 years	26.4 (23.7 – 29.5)	12.5 (11.7 – 13.9)	24.9 (21.6 – 26.0)	66.7 (45.2 – 92.9)	121
12–19 years	27.1 (25.0 – 29.4)	14.2 (13.4 – 15.5)	23.5 (21.4 – 26.1)	64.0 (54.7 – 80.3)	255
20–39 years	33.6 (29.4 – 38.4)	14.4 (12.0 – 15.6)	26.9 (24.2 – 29.4)	105 (71.2 – 187)	310
40–59 years	35.5 (30.7 – 41.1)	14.9 (12.5 – 17.5)	29.3 (26.0 – 33.1)	102 (81.5 – 141)	356
60 years and older	62.6 (54.1 – 72.5)	18.8 (15.9 – 21.2)	52.3 (44.8 – 60.1)	232 (195 – 344)	448
Females					
Total, 1 year and older	37.3 (35.4 – 39.4)	12.4 (11.6 – 12.7)	29.2 (26.8 – 31.4)	155 (136 – 176)	1,649
1–5 years	27.7 (24.5 – 31.3)	13.1 (11.1 – 15.1)	25.4 (20.8 – 29.9)	59.9 (49.8 – 99.2)	117
6–11 years	26.9 (22.4 – 32.3)	12.5 (10.7 – 13.7)	24.3 (20.7 – 29.2)	62.1 (47.7 – 189)	130
12–19 years	21.2 (19.2 – 23.5)	10.2 (9.58 – 11.0)	19.8 (18.0 – 21.1)	47.3 (40.3 – 69.4)	250
20–39 years	29.0 (25.5 – 33.0)	10.6 (9.87 – 11.0)	23.1 (19.3 – 26.9)	117 (90.2 – 161)	408
40–59 years	39.9 (35.9 – 44.5)	12.8 (12.1 – 13.6)	30.5 (26.6 – 34.8)	155 (128 – 223)	335
60 years and older	65.9 (60.1 – 72.4)	17.6 (14.1 – 20.4)	54.9 (47.4 – 63.8)	270 (242 – 343)	409

Table 1.5.a.1. Serum vitamin B12: Concentrations

Geometric mean and selected percentiles of serum concentrations (in pg/mL) for the total U.S. population aged 1 year and older, National Health and Nutrition Examination Survey, 2003–2006.

	Geometric mean (95% conf. interval)	Selected percentiles (95% conf. interval)					Sample size
		2.5th	5th	50th	95th	97.5th	
Total, 1 year and older	500 (489 – 511)	206 (201 – 212)	236 (227 – 244)	495 (483 – 505)	1,090 (1,050 – 1,110)	1,300 (1,250 – 1,340)	16,316
Age group							
1–5 years	804 (776 – 833)	327 (280 – 368)	397 (344 – 432)	814 (783 – 858)	1,520 (1,470 – 1,630)	1,710 (1,600 – 1,810)	1,678
6–11 years	728 (713 – 743)	354 (342 – 363)	396 (367 – 431)	724 (707 – 747)	1,280 (1,240 – 1,350)	1,440 (1,360 – 1,570)	1,747
12–19 years	510 (499 – 521)	238 (224 – 250)	271 (264 – 277)	509 (495 – 526)	938 (901 – 975)	1,050 (1,020 – 1,140)	4,013
20–39 years	454 (443 – 465)	210 (201 – 214)	231 (223 – 243)	451 (441 – 462)	884 (859 – 904)	1,010 (962 – 1,060)	3,214
40–59 years	466 (451 – 482)	197 (177 – 210)	226 (214 – 237)	460 (446 – 475)	1,020 (934 – 1,100)	1,180 (1,110 – 1,350)	2,629
60 years and older	482 (468 – 496)	166 (151 – 179)	210 (202 – 217)	481 (466 – 499)	1,070 (1,020 – 1,190)	1,380 (1,280 – 1,570)	3,035
Gender							
Males	500 (490 – 509)	216 (210 – 222)	249 (238 – 259)	494 (484 – 505)	1,030 (994 – 1,060)	1,200 (1,150 – 1,240)	7,999
Females	500 (487 – 514)	200 (189 – 206)	227 (216 – 236)	495 (480 – 508)	1,140 (1,100 – 1,180)	1,370 (1,330 – 1,410)	8,317
Race/ethnicity							
Mexican Americans	549 (530 – 569)	224 (212 – 241)	260 (248 – 274)	527 (513 – 547)	1,170 (1,110 – 1,240)	1,600 (1,370 – 1,950)	4,205
Non-Hispanic Blacks	565 (550 – 580)	223 (210 – 233)	266 (258 – 276)	556 (537 – 576)	1,240 (1,200 – 1,320)	1,430 (1,370 – 1,540)	4,285
Non-Hispanic Whites	482 (470 – 495)	201 (194 – 209)	229 (222 – 239)	478 (465 – 491)	1,040 (999 – 1,080)	1,230 (1,170 – 1,310)	6,571

Figure 1.5.a. Serum vitamin B12: Concentrations by age group

Geometric mean (95% condence interval), National Health and Nutrition Examination Survey, 2003–2006

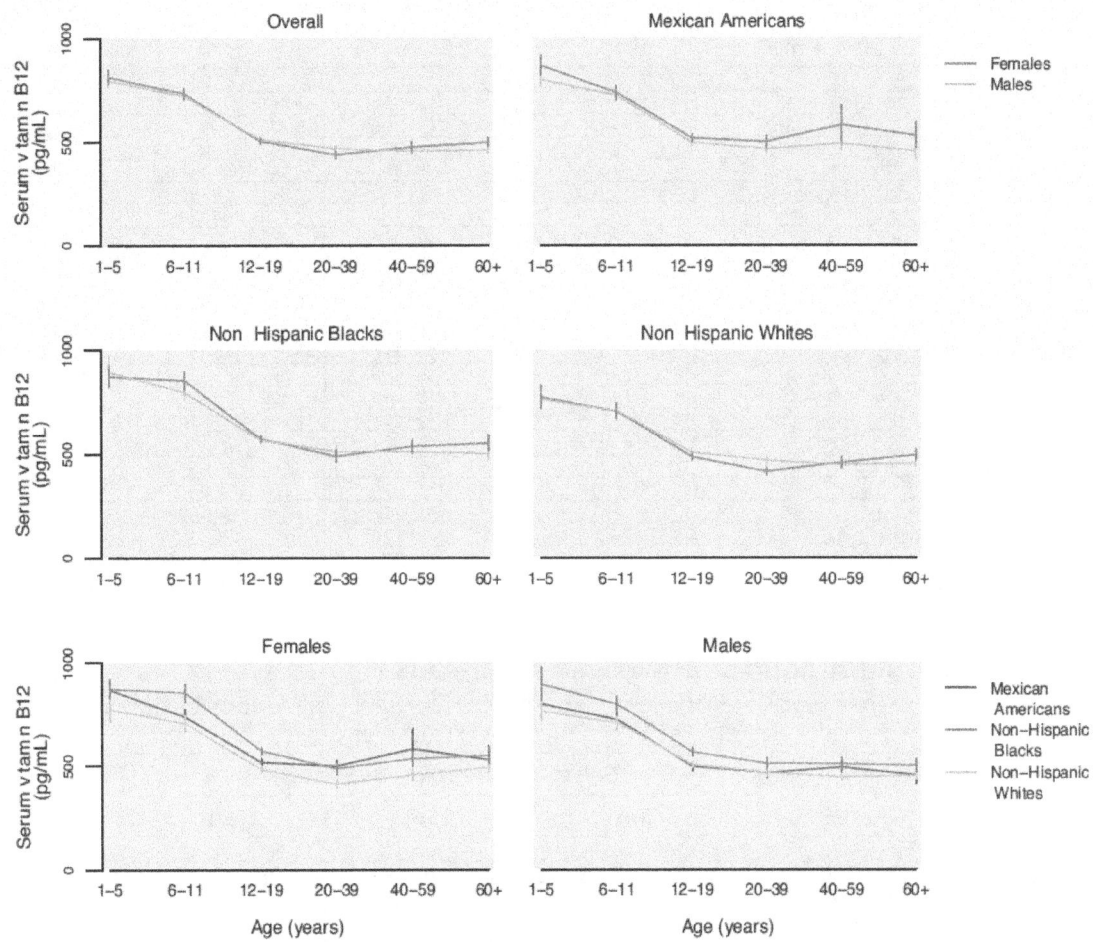

Table 1.5.a.2. Serum vitamin B12: Total population

Geometric mean and selected percentiles of serum concentrations (in pg/mL) for the total U.S. population aged 1 year and older, National Health and Nutrition Examination Survey, 2003–2006.

	Geometric mean (95% conf. interval)		Selected percentiles (95% conf. interval)						Sample size
			5th		50th		95th		
Males and Females									
Total, 1 year and older	500	(489 – 511)	236	(227 – 244)	495	(483 – 505)	1,090	(1,050 – 1,110)	16,316
1–5 years	804	(776 – 833)	397	(344 – 432)	814	(783 – 858)	1,520	(1,470 – 1,630)	1,678
6–11 years	728	(713 – 743)	396	(367 – 431)	724	(707 – 747)	1,280	(1,240 – 1,350)	1,747
12–19 years	510	(499 – 521)	271	(264 – 277)	509	(495 – 526)	938	(901 – 975)	4,013
20–39 years	454	(443 – 465)	231	(223 – 243)	451	(441 – 462)	884	(859 – 904)	3,214
40–59 years	466	(451 – 482)	226	(214 – 237)	460	(446 – 475)	1,020	(934 – 1,100)	2,629
60 years and older	482	(468 – 496)	210	(202 – 217)	481	(466 – 499)	1,070	(1,020 – 1,190)	3,035
Males									
Total, 1 year and older	500	(490 – 509)	249	(238 – 259)	494	(484 – 505)	1,030	(994 – 1,060)	7,999
1–5 years	796	(761 – 832)	379	(302 – 423)	816	(775 – 862)	1,470	(1,430 – 1,520)	844
6–11 years	722	(701 – 744)	411	(363 – 439)	735	(713 – 761)	1,220	(1,140 – 1,270)	853
12–19 years	513	(500 – 526)	292	(272 – 309)	510	(494 – 534)	904	(866 – 951)	2,031
20–39 years	469	(456 – 483)	258	(242 – 270)	469	(454 – 485)	856	(820 – 893)	1,451
40–59 years	456	(440 – 472)	226	(212 – 246)	456	(442 – 469)	896	(825 – 985)	1,296
60 years and older	461	(447 – 475)	210	(193 – 223)	458	(442 – 480)	990	(937 – 1,100)	1,524
Females									
Total, 1 year and older	500	(487 – 514)	227	(216 – 236)	495	(480 – 508)	1,140	(1,100 – 1,180)	8,317
1–5 years	813	(781 – 847)	401	(343 – 444)	810	(772 – 863)	1,560	(1,470 – 1,740)	834
6–11 years	734	(710 – 758)	393	(362 – 421)	714	(687 – 748)	1,360	(1,290 – 1,460)	894
12–19 years	506	(492 – 520)	254	(243 – 266)	507	(487 – 526)	973	(928 – 1,050)	1,982
20–39 years	439	(425 – 453)	217	(206 – 227)	431	(420 – 446)	909	(868 – 980)	1,763
40–59 years	476	(455 – 499)	223	(200 – 241)	467	(444 – 489)	1,090	(1,020 – 1,160)	1,333
60 years and older	499	(479 – 521)	210	(200 – 218)	504	(477 – 530)	1,140	(1,050 – 1,310)	1,511

Table 1.5.a.3. Serum vitamin B12: Mexican Americans

Geometric mean and selected percentiles of serum concentrations (in pg/mL) for Mexican Americans in the U.S. population aged 1 year and older, National Health and Nutrition Examination Survey, 2003–2006.

	Geometric mean (95% conf. interval)		Selected percentiles (95% conf. interval)						Sample size
			5th		50th		95th		
Males and Females									
Total, 1 year and older	549	(530 – 569)	260	(248 – 274)	527	(513 – 547)	1,170	(1,110 – 1,240)	4,205
1–5 years	833	(802 – 866)	450	(417 – 468)	842	(811 – 880)	1,480	(1,390 – 1,670)	540
6–11 years	730	(708 – 753)	409	(367 – 441)	729	(704 – 762)	1,210	(1,150 – 1,290)	587
12–19 years	508	(493 – 524)	270	(250 – 295)	505	(486 – 525)	909	(873 – 951)	1,280
20–39 years	483	(463 – 503)	249	(225 – 260)	467	(449 – 493)	955	(883 – 1,150)	778
40–59 years	535	(491 – 582)	248	(207 – 274)	483	(457 – 515)	1,310	(996 – 3,160)	468
60 years and older	496	(465 – 528)	220	(193 – 239)	458	(435 – 489)	1,240	(1,070 – 2,490)	552
Males									
Total, 1 year and older	526	(510 – 543)	258	(251 – 267)	513	(492 – 533)	1,060	(1,010 – 1,110)	2,036
1–5 years	801	(766 – 838)	423	(364 – 467)	805	(776 – 844)	1,450	(1,330 – 1,630)	261
6–11 years	724	(696 – 752)	386	(345 – 462)	735	(705 – 771)	1,150	(1,080 – 1,250)	285
12–19 years	498	(478 – 519)	271	(239 – 305)	494	(476 – 516)	866	(810 – 920)	637
20–39 years	467	(443 – 492)	252	(217 – 264)	459	(431 – 494)	855	(794 – 978)	345
40–59 years	493	(460 – 529)	249	(191 – 263)	463	(446 – 494)	1,050	(915 – 2,230)	236
60 years and older	456	(412 – 505)	224	(195 – 237)	404	(376 – 448)	1,210	(929 – 5,710)	272
Females									
Total, 1 year and older	574	(548 – 602)	263	(241 – 288)	550	(522 – 573)	1,290	(1,180 – 1,630)	2,169
1–5 years	869	(824 – 916)	456	(420 – 500)	887	(834 – 910)	1,590	(1,400 – 1,890)	279
6–11 years	738	(704 – 772)	413	(370 – 441)	716	(690 – 762)	1,280	(1,160 – 1,620)	302
12–19 years	519	(502 – 536)	269	(255 – 291)	518	(495 – 549)	951	(892 – 1,060)	643
20–39 years	501	(476 – 528)	248	(220 – 271)	476	(452 – 509)	1,190	(984 – 2,080)	433
40–59 years	582	(500 – 678)	243	(182 – 306)	520	(464 – 574)	1,950	(1,010 – 6,830)	232
60 years and older	531	(475 – 594)	210	(169 – 258)	494	(459 – 537)	1,370	(1,110 – 2,950)	280

Table 1.5.a.4. Serum vitamin B12: Non-Hispanic blacks

Geometric mean and selected percentiles of serum concentrations (in pg/mL) for non-Hispanic blacks in the U.S. population aged 1 year and older, National Health and Nutrition Examination Survey, 2003–2006.

	Geometric mean (95% conf. interval)		Selected percentiles (95% conf. interval)						Sample size
			5th		50th		95th		
Males and Females									
Total, 1 year and older	565	(550 – 580)	266	(258 – 276)	556	(537 – 576)	1,240	(1,200 – 1,320)	4,285
1–5 years	885	(835 – 938)	431	(340 – 479)	899	(827 – 965)	1,770	(1,550 – 2,020)	476
6–11 years	827	(800 – 854)	448	(398 – 470)	817	(800 – 842)	1,560	(1,440 – 1,670)	553
12–19 years	570	(557 – 584)	284	(270 – 297)	571	(551 – 585)	1,110	(1,050 – 1,160)	1,415
20–39 years	499	(483 – 516)	259	(227 – 277)	497	(480 – 512)	941	(894 – 1,050)	706
40–59 years	524	(506 – 543)	264	(220 – 286)	515	(494 – 544)	1,120	(1,070 – 1,200)	622
60 years and older	530	(504 – 558)	225	(199 – 252)	531	(505 – 565)	1,240	(1,100 – 1,510)	513
Males									
Total, 1 year and older	564	(549 – 580)	267	(257 – 282)	546	(533 – 571)	1,230	(1,140 – 1,320)	2,136
1–5 years	896	(821 – 977)	418	(293 – 494)	910	(822 – 1,010)	1,800	(1,570 – 2,150)	236
6–11 years	799	(762 – 837)	428	(350 – 466)	811	(743 – 840)	1,540	(1,370 – 1,780)	272
12–19 years	567	(550 – 585)	294	(268 – 322)	567	(541 – 585)	1,040	(993 – 1,140)	742
20–39 years	512	(488 – 536)	277	(256 – 290)	507	(482 – 527)	950	(872 – 1,160)	337
40–59 years	510	(482 – 539)	241	(204 – 269)	509	(488 – 541)	988	(863 – 1,250)	292
60 years and older	502	(472 – 533)	211	(142 – 241)	494	(459 – 521)	1,220	(998 – 1,770)	257
Females									
Total, 1 year and older	565	(545 – 587)	265	(233 – 282)	563	(531 – 597)	1,250	(1,200 – 1,340)	2,149
1–5 years	874	(829 – 922)	431	(257 – 489)	880	(798 – 957)	1,650	(1,470 – 2,050)	240
6–11 years	856	(815 – 899)	468	(383 – 501)	834	(801 – 887)	1,570	(1,430 – 1,710)	281
12–19 years	574	(558 – 590)	272	(259 – 288)	576	(551 – 595)	1,160	(1,110 – 1,210)	673
20–39 years	489	(464 – 515)	231	(207 – 271)	487	(460 – 518)	938	(880 – 1,080)	369
40–59 years	536	(507 – 566)	273	(219 – 295)	527	(492 – 568)	1,170	(1,100 – 1,400)	330
60 years and older	551	(514 – 590)	232	(187 – 265)	576	(524 – 613)	1,280	(1,110 – 1,620)	256

Table 1.5.a.5. Serum vitamin B12: Non-Hispanic whites

Geometric mean and selected percentiles of serum concentrations (in pg/mL) for non-Hispanic whites in the U.S. population aged 1 year and older, National Health and Nutrition Examination Survey, 2003–2006.

	Geometric mean (95% conf. interval)		Selected percentiles (95% conf. interval)						Sample size
			5th		50th		95th		
Males and Females									
Total, 1 year and older	482	(470 – 495)	229	(222 – 239)	478	(465 – 491)	1,040	(999 – 1,080)	6,571
1–5 years	769	(730 – 810)	375	(298 – 411)	777	(730 – 830)	1,470	(1,410 – 1,560)	476
6–11 years	707	(686 – 729)	392	(345 – 435)	703	(674 – 734)	1,230	(1,170 – 1,350)	448
12–19 years	496	(484 – 509)	269	(253 – 276)	498	(481 – 517)	887	(833 – 952)	1,042
20–39 years	440	(426 – 455)	226	(215 – 238)	438	(424 – 452)	853	(814 – 889)	1,434
40–59 years	453	(435 – 471)	225	(208 – 236)	448	(434 – 465)	980	(867 – 1,090)	1,340
60 years and older	476	(461 – 492)	209	(200 – 217)	477	(460 – 499)	1,050	(990 – 1,170)	1,831
Males									
Total, 1 year and older	487	(475 – 498)	244	(228 – 256)	483	(471 – 496)	981	(946 – 1,030)	3,235
1–5 years	764	(720 – 811)	353	(261 – 416)	799	(739 – 861)	1,380	(1,320 – 1,500)	254
6–11 years	708	(678 – 740)	405†	(343 – 441)	715	(680 – 753)	1,160†	(1,080 – 1,250)	216
12–19 years	507	(492 – 522)	293	(271 – 316)	505	(486 – 535)	847	(803 – 941)	523
20–39 years	468	(448 – 488)	263	(230 – 275)	469	(448 – 493)	826	(786 – 900)	631
40–59 years	447	(430 – 465)	226	(199 – 248)	448	(435 – 464)	879	(781 – 984)	682
60 years and older	454	(439 – 469)	208	(181 – 221)	455	(434 – 481)	952	(887 – 1,050)	929
Females									
Total, 1 year and older	478	(462 – 494)	220	(210 – 230)	471	(454 – 488)	1,080	(1,040 – 1,140)	3,336
1–5 years	774	(721 – 831)	381†	(325 – 431)	763	(700 – 835)	1,530†	(1,450 – 1,760)	222
6–11 years	706	(671 – 743)	377	(316 – 421)	679	(648 – 742)	1,340	(1,180 – 1,490)	232
12–19 years	485	(470 – 501)	246	(226 – 259)	486	(468 – 508)	913	(842 – 1,030)	519
20–39 years	414	(398 – 431)	211	(197 – 223)	405	(387 – 427)	874	(797 – 936)	803
40–59 years	458	(432 – 485)	220	(199 – 236)	447	(419 – 483)	1,040	(900 – 1,180)	658
60 years and older	494	(471 – 519)	210	(199 – 217)	500	(470 – 523)	1,090	(1,030 – 1,320)	902

† Estimate is subject to greater uncertainty due to small cell size.

Table 1.5.b. Serum vitamin B12: Concentrations by survey cycle

Geometric mean and selected percentiles of serum concentrations (in pg/mL) for the U.S. population, National Health and Nutrition Examination Survey, 1999–2006.

	Geometric mean (95% conf. interval)	Selected percentiles (95% conf. interval) 5th	Selected percentiles (95% conf. interval) 50th	Selected percentiles (95% conf. interval) 95th	Sample size
Total, 3 years and older					
1999–2000	487 (481 – 494)	240 (234 – 245)	483 (474 – 494)	993 (970 – 1,040)	7,524
2001–2002	488 (479 – 497)	236 (232 – 241)	485 (474 – 494)	1,000 (971 – 1,040)	8,390
2003–2004	489 (472 – 507)	238 (225 – 252)	486 (467 – 500)	1,020 (979 – 1,080)	7,837
2005–2006	502 (489 – 516)	231 (221 – 242)	497 (482 – 511)	1,100 (1,060 – 1,130)	7,694
Age group					
3–5 years					
1999–2000	757 (682 – 839)	441 (321 – 459)	735 (663 – 827)	1,380 (1,300 – 1,730)	361
2001–2002	804 (773 – 837)	471 (426 – 518)	815 (783 – 836)	1,380 (1,250 – 1,560)	439
2003–2004	768 (716 – 824)	393 (285 – 422)	775 (716 – 852)	1,550 (1,310 – 1,800)	449
2005–2006	877 (841 – 913)	482 (437 – 507)	894 (826 – 950)	1,470 (1,430 – 1,660)	444
6–11 years					
1999–2000	695 (659 – 733)	362 (330 – 401)	704 (676 – 738)	1,250 (1,170 – 1,340)	885
2001–2002	691 (669 – 714)	386 (340 – 412)	696 (672 – 724)	1,270 (1,190 – 1,330)	1,022
2003–2004	711 (689 – 733)	375 (344 – 419)	714 (679 – 736)	1,240 (1,190 – 1,360)	843
2005–2006	745 (721 – 769)	418 (381 – 442)	741 (710 – 768)	1,290 (1,230 – 1,370)	904
12–19 years					
1999–2000	501 (491 – 511)	263 (235 – 280)	506 (494 – 518)	954 (905 – 1,010)	2,123
2001–2002	511 (495 – 528)	269 (256 – 289)	516 (496 – 536)	934 (899 – 983)	2,208
2003–2004	500 (483 – 518)	267 (255 – 282)	504 (481 – 528)	911 (871 – 949)	2,059
2005–2006	519 (505 – 534)	273 (269 – 281)	519 (496 – 544)	966 (907 – 1,040)	1,954
20–39 years					
1999–2000	445 (438 – 451)	234 (219 – 240)	448 (432 – 459)	807 (791 – 824)	1,470
2001–2002	445 (432 – 458)	230 (217 – 239)	445 (432 – 457)	822 (776 – 893)	1,715
2003–2004	451 (434 – 468)	240 (225 – 253)	449 (431 – 465)	826 (787 – 888)	1,555
2005–2006	457 (443 – 472)	227 (214 – 239)	452 (440 – 468)	913 (889 – 964)	1,659
40–59 years					
1999–2000	460 (447 – 474)	234 (208 – 256)	447 (432 – 466)	909 (861 – 952)	1,198
2001–2002	460 (450 – 471)	232 (221 – 238)	456 (443 – 465)	942 (879 – 1,020)	1,478
2003–2004	460 (435 – 486)	226 (215 – 243)	456 (438 – 479)	957 (833 – 1,110)	1,276
2005–2006	472 (452 – 493)	223 (195 – 244)	464 (444 – 485)	1,060 (984 – 1,130)	1,353
60 years and older					
1999–2000	482 (467 – 496)	228 (212 – 243)	470 (460 – 483)	1,030 (950 – 1,130)	1,487
2001–2002	473 (455 – 491)	220 (204 – 231)	479 (465 – 493)	1,000 (962 – 1,030)	1,528
2003–2004	477 (459 – 496)	208 (198 – 221)	477 (454 – 494)	1,060 (967 – 1,310)	1,655
2005–2006	487 (466 – 508)	211 (197 – 219)	495 (464 – 511)	1,070 (1,030 – 1,220)	1,380
Gender					
Males					
1999–2000	487 (479 – 495)	255 (235 – 264)	488 (478 – 498)	956 (901 – 1,020)	3,682
2001–2002	490 (476 – 505)	247 (235 – 257)	485 (468 – 497)	963 (919 – 1,010)	4,059
2003–2004	490 (476 – 505)	250 (229 – 266)	486 (469 – 499)	971 (944 – 1,020)	3,871
2005–2006	500 (487 – 514)	247 (226 – 259)	497 (482 – 512)	1,040 (987 – 1,110)	3,740
Females					
1999–2000	488 (481 – 495)	233 (222 – 241)	478 (465 – 495)	1,030 (981 – 1,090)	3,842
2001–2002	486 (476 – 496)	230 (219 – 237)	485 (474 – 495)	1,040 (998 – 1,090)	4,331
2003–2004	488 (467 – 509)	228 (212 – 245)	486 (463 – 504)	1,080 (1,010 – 1,160)	3,966
2005–2006	504 (486 – 523)	224 (208 – 236)	497 (476 – 516)	1,150 (1,110 – 1,190)	3,954
Race/ethnicity					
Mexican Americans					
1999–2000	551 (523 – 581)	268 (259 – 281)	527 (509 – 542)	1,200 (1,140 – 1,310)	2,571
2001–2002	516 (491 – 543)	249 (227 – 271)	496 (468 – 535)	1,050 (1,010 – 1,120)	2,124
2003–2004	543 (513 – 575)	285 (264 – 304)	520 (504 – 538)	1,080 (994 – 1,210)	1,919
2005–2006	536 (512 – 561)	245 (223 – 257)	515 (487 – 554)	1,180 (1,110 – 1,280)	2,009
Non-Hispanic Blacks					
1999–2000	582 (565 – 599)	286 (261 – 304)	583 (569 – 603)	1,220 (1,150 – 1,270)	1,712
2001–2002	556 (542 – 570)	269 (250 – 282)	554 (544 – 568)	1,160 (1,100 – 1,220)	2,000
2003–2004	561 (538 – 585)	281 (262 – 294)	553 (523 – 584)	1,150 (1,090 – 1,310)	2,058
2005–2006	559 (540 – 579)	256 (231 – 270)	546 (528 – 575)	1,250 (1,200 – 1,340)	2,032
Non-Hispanic Whites					
1999–2000	468 (460 – 476)	235 (231 – 240)	467 (454 – 478)	916 (890 – 951)	2,556
2001–2002	474 (462 – 485)	233 (227 – 237)	473 (460 – 486)	959 (899 – 1,020)	3,594
2003–2004	470 (452 – 489)	228 (216 – 244)	469 (449 – 488)	966 (920 – 1,050)	3,272
2005–2006	487 (470 – 504)	228 (217 – 239)	482 (462 – 502)	1,050 (1,010 – 1,100)	3,062

Figure 1.5.b. Serum vitamin B12: Concentrations by survey cycle

Selected percentiles in pg/mL (95% conence intervals), National Health and
Nutrition Examination Survey, 1999–2006

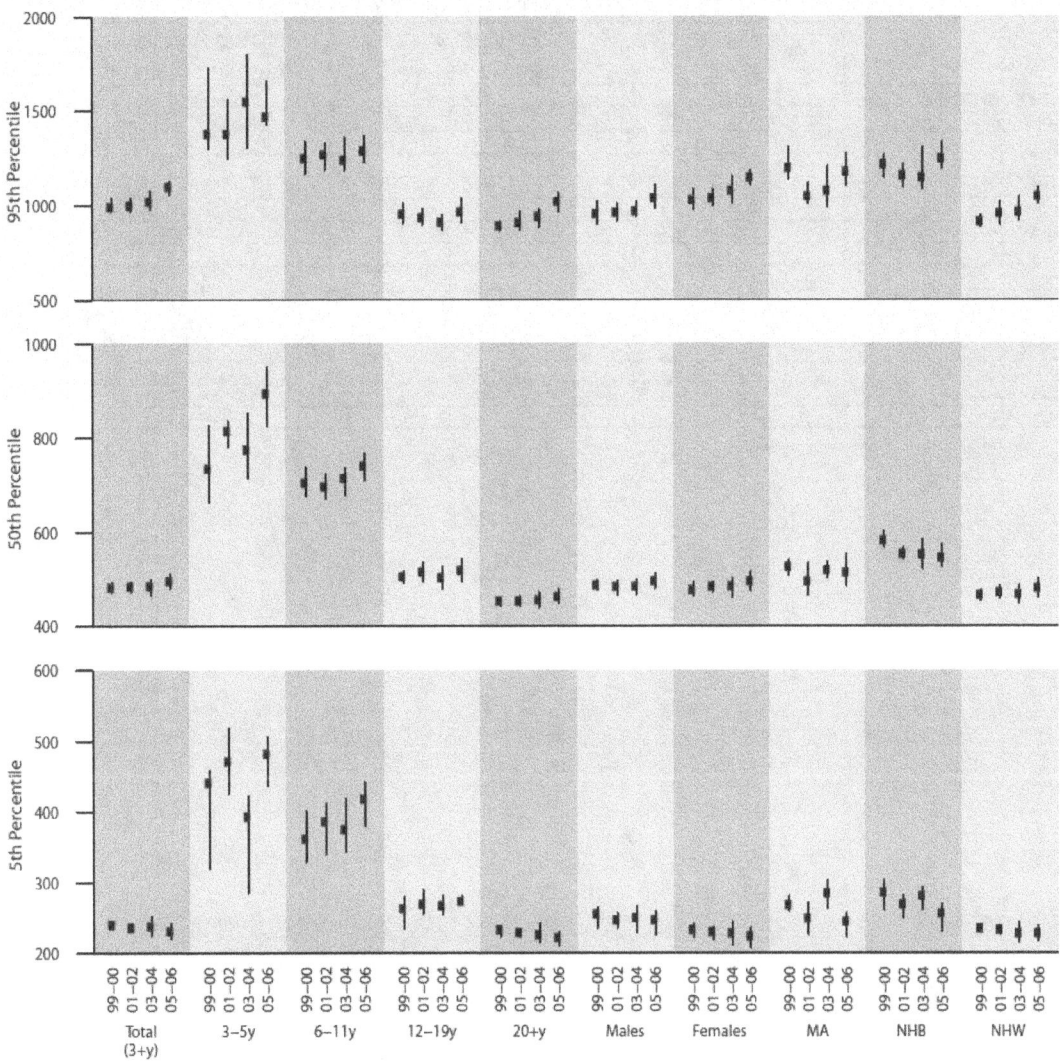

Table 1.5.c. Serum vitamin B12: Prevalence

Prevalence (in percent) of low serum vitamin B12 concentration (< 200 pg/mL) for the U.S. population aged 1 year and older, National Health and Nutrition Examination Survey, 2003–2006.

	Sample size	Prevalence (95% conf. interval)	Estimated total number of persons
Total, 1 year and older	16,316	2.0 (1.6 – 2.4)	5,563,000
Age group			
1–5 years	1,678	§	§
6–11 years	1,747	§	§
12–19 years	4,013	0.6 (0.4 – 1.0)	210,000
20–39 years	3,214	1.5 (1.2 – 2.0)	1,211,000
40–59 years	2,629	2.6 (1.8 – 3.7)	2,057,000
60 years and older	3,035	3.9 (3.1 – 4.9)	1,815,000
Gender			
Males	7,999	1.6 (1.3 – 2.0)	2,165,000
Females	8,317	2.3 (1.9 – 2.9)	3,402,000
Race/ethnicity			
Mexican Americans	4,205	1.0 (0.7 – 1.5)	265,000
Non-Hispanic Blacks	4,285	1.2 (0.8 – 1.8)	398,000
Non-Hispanic Whites	6,571	2.2 (1.8 – 2.7)	4,289,000

§ Estimate suppressed: RSE ≥ 40% for the prevalence estimate.

Table 1.5.d. Serum vitamin B12: Prevalence by survey cycle

Prevalence (in percent) of low serum vitamin B12 concentration (< 200 pg/mL) for the U.S. population, National Health and Nutrition Examination Survey, 1999–2006.

	Sample size	Prevalence (95% conf. interval)	Estimated total number of persons
Total, 3 years and older			
1999–2000	7,524	1.9 (1.5 – 2.3)	4,933,000
2001–2002	8,390	1.8 (1.5 – 2.2)	4,762,000
2003–2004	7,837	1.6 (1.2 – 2.2)	4,506,000
2005–2006	7,694	2.4 (1.9 – 3.0)	6,642,000
Age group			
3–5 years			
1999–2000	361	§	§
2001–2002	439	§	§
2003–2004	449	§	§
2005–2006	444	§	§
6–11 years			
1999–2000	885	§	§
2001–2002	1,022	§	§
2003–2004	843	§	§
2005–2006	904	§	§
12–19 years			
1999–2000	2,123	0.8‡ (0.4 – 1.7)	251,000‡
2001–2002	2,208	0.9 (0.5 – 1.6)	276,000
2003–2004	2,059	0.6‡ (0.3 – 1.3)	214,000‡
2005–2006	1,954	0.6‡ (0.3 – 1.2)	209,000‡
20–39 years			
1999–2000	1,470	2.2 (1.4 – 3.3)	1,683,000
2001–2002	1,715	1.8 (1.2 – 2.8)	1,436,000
2003–2004	1,555	1.0‡ (0.5 – 2.0)	805,000‡
2005–2006	1,659	2.0 (1.6 – 2.7)	1,636,000
40–59 years			
1999–2000	1,198	2.4 (1.5 – 4.0)	1,708,000
2001–2002	1,478	1.8 (1.1 – 3.1)	1,399,000
2003–2004	1,276	1.9 (1.3 – 2.9)	1,508,000
2005–2006	1,353	3.3 (1.9 – 5.5)	2,695,000
60 years and older			
1999–2000	1,487	2.7 (1.9 – 3.8)	1,159,000
2001–2002	1,528	3.6 (2.7 – 4.6)	1,590,000
2003–2004	1,655	3.9 (2.9 – 5.3)	1,806,000
2005–2006	1,380	3.9 (2.8 – 5.5)	1,895,000
Gender			
Males			
1999–2000	3,682	1.7 (1.2 – 2.4)	2,113,000
2001–2002	4,059	1.3 (1.0 – 1.8)	1,699,000
2003–2004	3,871	1.3 (0.9 – 1.9)	1,727,000
2005–2006	3,740	1.9 (1.4 – 2.5)	2,615,000
Females			
1999–2000	3,842	2.1 (1.7 – 2.6)	2,824,000
2001–2002	4,331	2.2 (1.7 – 3.0)	3,063,000
2003–2004	3,966	2.0 (1.4 – 2.8)	2,787,000
2005–2006	3,954	2.8 (2.0 – 3.9)	4,024,000
Race/ethnicity			
Mexican Americans			
1999–2000	2,571	0.8‡ (0.4 – 1.5)	154,000‡
2001–2002	2,124	1.8 (1.0 – 3.3)	419,000
2003–2004	1,919	0.7‡ (0.3 – 1.4)	166,000‡
2005–2006	2,009	1.5 (0.8 – 2.5)	376,000
Non-Hispanic Blacks			
1999–2000	1,712	§	§
2001–2002	2,000	§	§
2003–2004	2,058	0.7‡ (0.3 – 1.6)	239,000‡
2005–2006	2,032	1.6 (1.0 – 2.6)	551,000
Non-Hispanic Whites			
1999–2000	2,556	2.1 (1.6 – 2.7)	3,858,000
2001–2002	3,594	2.0 (1.6 – 2.5)	3,733,000
2003–2004	3,272	1.9 (1.3 – 2.7)	3,572,000
2005–2006	3,062	2.6 (2.0 – 3.5)	4,978,000

‡ Estimate flagged: 30% ≤ RSE < 40% for the prevalence estimate.
§ Estimate suppressed: RSE ≥ 40% for the prevalence estimate.

Table 1.6.a.1. Plasma total homocysteine: Concentrations

Geometric mean and selected percentiles of plasma concentrations (in μmol/L) for the total U.S. population aged 20 years and older, National Health and Nutrition Examination Survey, 2003–2006.

	Geometric mean (95% conf. interval)	Selected percentiles (95% conf. interval)						Sample size
		2.5th	5th	50th	95th	97.5th		
Total, 20 years and older	8.21 (8.06 – 8.37)	4.48 (4.35 – 4.57)	5.00 (4.85 – 5.12)	8.04 (7.91 – 8.17)	14.3 (13.9 – 15.0)	17.2 (16.5 – 18.3)		8,999
Age group								
20–39 years	7.14 (7.04 – 7.24)	3.93 (3.77 – 4.05)	4.44 (4.30 – 4.52)	7.09 (6.99 – 7.22)	11.2 (10.9 – 11.6)	12.4 (12.1 – 13.0)		3,267
40–59 years	8.33 (8.17 – 8.50)	4.84 (4.61 – 5.02)	5.25 (5.15 – 5.36)	8.13 (8.02 – 8.29)	13.9 (13.3 – 14.5)	16.8 (15.8 – 18.3)		2,651
60 years and older	10.1 (9.85 – 10.4)	5.79 (5.56 – 5.99)	6.37 (6.07 – 6.50)	9.79 (9.57 – 10.1)	17.9 (17.1 – 18.9)	21.2 (20.1 – 22.7)		3,081
Gender								
Males	9.00 (8.83 – 9.18)	5.64 (5.48 – 5.73)	5.96 (5.86 – 6.08)	8.68 (8.56 – 8.84)	14.8 (14.2 – 15.6)	18.0 (16.6 – 19.7)		4,329
Females	7.55 (7.36 – 7.74)	4.12 (3.94 – 4.20)	4.52 (4.40 – 4.69)	7.30 (7.13 – 7.47)	13.8 (13.1 – 14.8)	16.8 (15.8 – 17.9)		4,670
Race/ethnicity								
Mexican Americans	7.09 (6.95 – 7.23)	3.91 (3.76 – 4.01)	4.35 (4.20 – 4.50)	7.02 (6.87 – 7.18)	11.7 (11.2 – 12.2)	12.9 (12.3 – 13.9)		1,814
Non-Hispanic Blacks	8.22 (8.03 – 8.42)	4.42 (4.20 – 4.58)	4.89 (4.61 – 5.05)	8.00 (7.82 – 8.22)	14.8 (14.4 – 15.7)	18.2 (17.0 – 20.0)		1,871
Non-Hispanic Whites	8.39 (8.22 – 8.57)	4.65 (4.43 – 4.85)	5.18 (5.03 – 5.34)	8.21 (8.07 – 8.37)	14.5 (14.0 – 15.2)	17.0 (16.4 – 18.1)		4,670

Figure 1.6.a. Plasma total homocysteine: Concentrations by age group
Geometric mean (95% confidence interval), National Health and Nutrition Examination Survey, 2003–2006

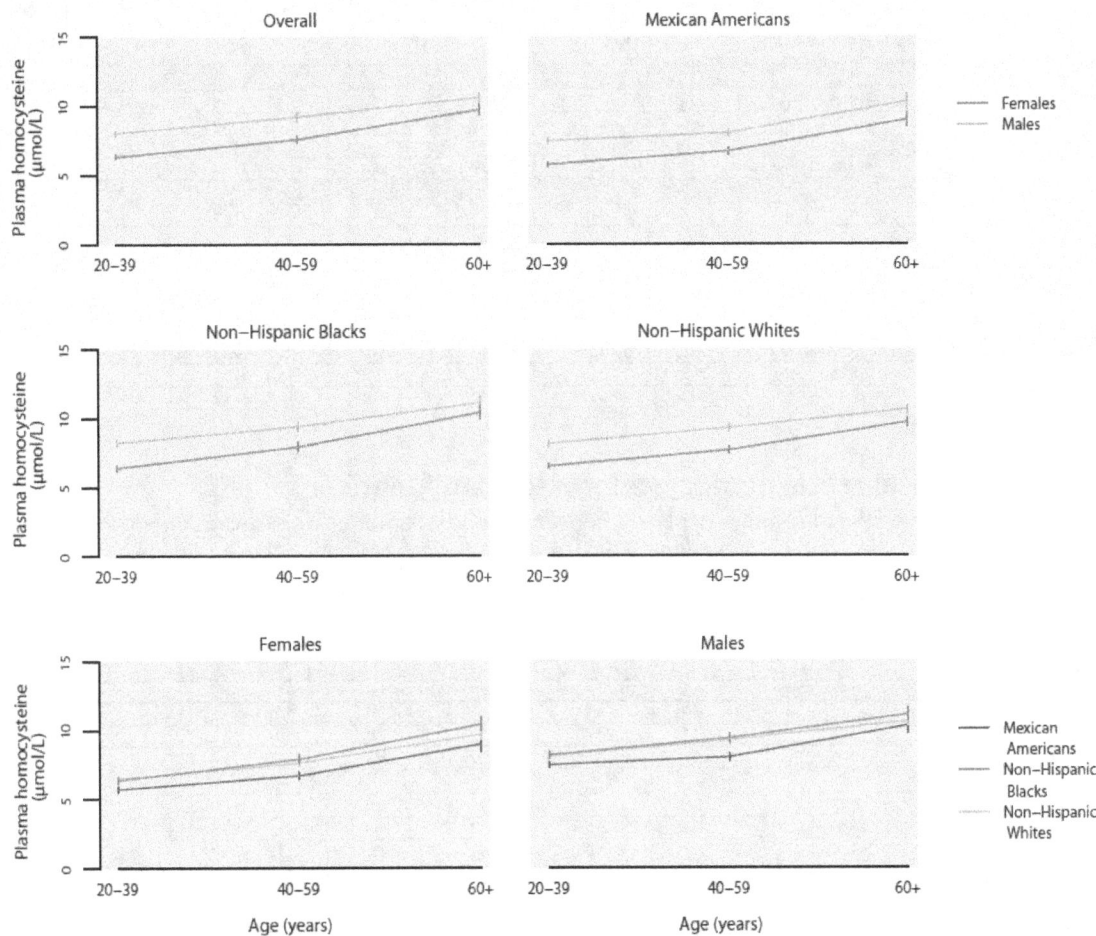

Table 1.6.a.2. Plasma total homocysteine: Total population

Geometric mean and selected percentiles of plasma concentrations (in μmol/L) for the total U.S. population aged 20 years and older, National Health and Nutrition Examination Survey, 2003–2006.

	Geometric mean (95% conf. interval)		Selected percentiles (95% conf. interval)						Sample size
			5th		50th		95th		
Males and Females									
Total, 20 years and older	8.21	(8.06 – 8.37)	5.00	(4.85 – 5.12)	8.04	(7.91 – 8.17)	14.3	(13.9 – 15.0)	8,999
20–39 years	7.14	(7.04 – 7.24)	4.44	(4.30 – 4.52)	7.09	(6.99 – 7.22)	11.2	(10.9 – 11.6)	3,267
40–59 years	8.33	(8.17 – 8.50)	5.25	(5.15 – 5.36)	8.13	(8.02 – 8.29)	13.9	(13.3 – 14.5)	2,651
60 years and older	10.1	(9.85 – 10.4)	6.37	(6.07 – 6.50)	9.79	(9.57 – 10.1)	17.9	(17.1 – 18.9)	3,081
Males									
Total, 20 years and older	9.00	(8.83 – 9.18)	5.96	(5.86 – 6.08)	8.68	(8.56 – 8.84)	14.8	(14.2 – 15.6)	4,329
20–39 years	8.05	(7.90 – 8.20)	5.65	(5.47 – 5.76)	7.94	(7.80 – 8.05)	11.9	(11.5 – 12.5)	1,473
40–59 years	9.21	(8.96 – 9.47)	6.28	(6.15 – 6.43)	8.86	(8.61 – 9.08)	14.3	(13.6 – 15.9)	1,306
60 years and older	10.6	(10.3 – 10.9)	6.89	(6.52 – 7.10)	10.4	(10.0 – 10.8)	18.0	(16.9 – 19.0)	1,550
Females									
Total, 20 years and older	7.55	(7.36 – 7.74)	4.52	(4.40 – 4.69)	7.30	(7.13 – 7.47)	13.8	(13.1 – 14.8)	4,670
20–39 years	6.33	(6.21 – 6.46)	3.96	(3.79 – 4.11)	6.31	(6.17 – 6.46)	9.87	(9.47 – 10.5)	1,794
40–59 years	7.58	(7.38 – 7.78)	4.90	(4.67 – 5.07)	7.30	(7.11 – 7.53)	13.0	(12.1 – 15.1)	1,345
60 years and older	9.72	(9.40 – 10.1)	6.02	(5.75 – 6.27)	9.43	(9.05 – 9.69)	17.8	(16.7 – 19.2)	1,531

Table 1.6.a.3. Plasma total homocysteine: Mexican Americans

Geometric mean and selected percentiles of plasma concentrations (in μmol/L) for Mexican Americans in the U.S. population aged 20 years and older, National Health and Nutrition Examination Survey, 2003–2006.

	Geometric mean (95% conf. interval)		Selected percentiles (95% conf. interval)						Sample size
			5th		50th		95th		
Males and Females									
Total, 20 years and older	7.09	(6.95 – 7.23)	4.35	(4.20 – 4.50)	7.02	(6.87 – 7.18)	11.7	(11.2 – 12.2)	1,814
20–39 years	6.61	(6.48 – 6.74)	4.05	(3.88 – 4.31)	6.61	(6.47 – 6.73)	10.6	(9.97 – 11.1)	789
40–59 years	7.36	(7.21 – 7.52)	4.77	(4.38 – 4.92)	7.33	(7.20 – 7.47)	10.9	(10.5 – 12.3)	470
60 years and older	9.55	(9.14 – 9.98)	6.07	(5.48 – 6.41)	9.32	(8.82 – 9.88)	16.0	(15.2 – 18.0)	555
Males									
Total, 20 years and older	7.85	(7.70 – 8.01)	5.50	(5.33 – 5.69)	7.74	(7.56 – 7.90)	12.2	(11.6 – 12.6)	866
20–39 years	7.47	(7.30 – 7.64)	5.38	(5.05 – 5.59)	7.38	(7.15 – 7.68)	11.3	(10.9 – 11.9)	353
40–59 years	8.03	(7.80 – 8.26)	5.71	(4.81 – 6.08)	7.91	(7.67 – 8.25)	11.8	(10.7 – 13.4)	239
60 years and older	10.3	(9.78 – 10.8)	6.79	(5.75 – 7.27)	10.0	(9.44 – 10.5)	16.0	(15.1 – 18.4)	274
Females									
Total, 20 years and older	6.34	(6.17 – 6.51)	3.91	(3.76 – 4.02)	6.28	(6.10 – 6.50)	10.6	(10.1 – 11.5)	948
20–39 years	5.73	(5.57 – 5.91)	3.67	(3.41 – 3.82)	5.77	(5.57 – 5.99)	8.52	(8.11 – 9.49)	436
40–59 years	6.71	(6.49 – 6.94)	4.39	(3.91 – 4.78)	6.68	(6.36 – 6.86)	10.1	(9.32 – 12.2)	231
60 years and older	8.98	(8.49 – 9.49)	5.67	(4.83 – 6.08)	8.50	(8.07 – 9.07)	15.9	(14.2 – 19.8)	281

Table 1.6.a.4. Plasma total homocysteine: Non-Hispanic blacks

Geometric mean and selected percentiles of plasma concentrations (in µmol/L) for non-Hispanic blacks in the U.S. population aged 20 years and older, National Health and Nutrition Examination Survey, 2003–2006.

	Geometric mean (95% conf. interval)	Selected percentiles (95% conf. interval)						Sample size
		5th		50th		95th		
Males and Females								
Total, 20 years and older	8.22	(8.03 – 8.42)	4.89	(4.61 – 5.05)	8.00	(7.82 – 8.22)	14.8	(14.4 – 15.7)	1,871
20–39 years	7.14	(6.95 – 7.34)	4.46	(4.20 – 4.61)	7.14	(6.98 – 7.36)	11.2	(10.8 – 11.8)	720
40–59 years	8.55	(8.31 – 8.79)	5.28	(5.10 – 5.39)	8.42	(8.14 – 8.70)	14.7	(13.9 – 17.1)	626
60 years and older	10.7	(10.4 – 11.0)	6.45	(6.00 – 6.95)	10.3	(10.1 – 10.7)	20.7	(18.8 – 23.6)	525
Males								
Total, 20 years and older	9.09	(8.91 – 9.27)	5.93	(5.73 – 6.16)	8.78	(8.58 – 8.96)	15.3	(14.5 – 16.4)	896
20–39 years	8.19	(7.95 – 8.44)	5.72	(5.42 – 5.88)	8.04	(7.80 – 8.25)	12.1	(11.6 – 13.1)	340
40–59 years	9.40	(9.12 – 9.70)	6.17	(5.70 – 6.41)	9.11	(8.82 – 9.41)	15.3	(14.2 – 18.2)	292
60 years and older	11.1	(10.7 – 11.6)	6.76	(6.39 – 7.30)	10.9	(10.3 – 11.3)	21.1	(17.5 – 24.9)	264
Females								
Total, 20 years and older	7.59	(7.34 – 7.85)	4.52	(4.23 – 4.74)	7.23	(7.07 – 7.53)	14.7	(13.5 – 15.9)	975
20–39 years	6.38	(6.19 – 6.58)	4.19	(3.80 – 4.38)	6.43	(6.25 – 6.72)	9.79	(9.22 – 10.6)	380
40–59 years	7.90	(7.56 – 8.25)	4.98	(4.46 – 5.23)	7.73	(7.22 – 8.08)	13.7	(11.9 – 16.1)	334
60 years and older	10.4	(9.98 – 10.9)	6.15	(5.74 – 6.83)	9.93	(9.50 – 10.5)	20.7	(18.7 – 24.7)	261

Table 1.6.a.5. Plasma total homocysteine: Non-Hispanic whites

Geometric mean and selected percentiles of plasma concentrations (in µmol/L) for non-Hispanic whites in the U.S. population aged 20 years and older, National Health and Nutrition Examination Survey, 2003–2006.

	Geometric mean (95% conf. interval)	Selected percentiles (95% conf. interval)						Sample size
		5th		50th		95th		
Males and Females								
Total, 20 years and older	8.39	(8.22 – 8.57)	5.18	(5.03 – 5.34)	8.21	(8.07 – 8.37)	14.5	(14.0 – 15.2)	4,670
20–39 years	7.26	(7.13 – 7.40)	4.51	(4.33 – 4.79)	7.26	(7.07 – 7.39)	11.2	(10.9 – 11.9)	1,458
40–59 years	8.40	(8.21 – 8.60)	5.36	(5.19 – 5.51)	8.24	(8.09 – 8.44)	13.6	(13.1 – 14.9)	1,353
60 years and older	10.1	(9.82 – 10.4)	6.38	(6.09 – 6.59)	9.82	(9.57 – 10.1)	17.6	(16.7 – 18.4)	1,859
Males								
Total, 20 years and older	9.15	(8.94 – 9.36)	6.13	(5.95 – 6.24)	8.80	(8.61 – 8.99)	14.9	(14.2 – 16.0)	2,274
20–39 years	8.11	(7.91 – 8.32)	5.69	(5.47 – 5.85)	8.00	(7.85 – 8.14)	11.8	(11.2 – 12.7)	641
40–59 years	9.28	(8.98 – 9.59)	6.35	(6.21 – 6.55)	8.89	(8.61 – 9.16)	14.2	(13.4 – 16.0)	687
60 years and older	10.6	(10.3 – 10.9)	6.95	(6.65 – 7.15)	10.4	(10.0 – 10.8)	17.8	(16.6 – 19.0)	946
Females								
Total, 20 years and older	7.75	(7.54 – 7.96)	4.72	(4.49 – 4.93)	7.53	(7.34 – 7.70)	14.0	(13.3 – 15.2)	2,396
20–39 years	6.50	(6.35 – 6.65)	3.98	(3.77 – 4.13)	6.46	(6.29 – 6.59)	10.2	(9.55 – 11.0)	817
40–59 years	7.63	(7.40 – 7.87)	4.99	(4.70 – 5.18)	7.38	(7.16 – 7.62)	13.0	(11.8 – 15.8)	666
60 years and older	9.69	(9.34 – 10.0)	6.03	(5.71 – 6.28)	9.48	(9.05 – 9.73)	17.1	(16.3 – 18.7)	913

Table 1.6.b. Plasma total homocysteine: Concentrations by survey cycle

Geometric mean and selected percentiles of plasma concentrations (in µmol/L) for the U.S. population, National Health and Nutrition Examination Survey, 1999–2006.

	Geometric mean (95% conf. interval)	Selected percentiles (95% conf. interval) 5th	50th	95th	Sample size
Total, 20 years and older					
1999–2000	8.07 (7.95 – 8.18)	4.82 (4.65 – 5.02)	7.94 (7.82 – 8.04)	14.3 (13.5 – 15.0)	4,192
2001–2002	8.21 (8.04 – 8.38)	5.01 (4.86 – 5.15)	8.01 (7.84 – 8.17)	14.4 (13.9 – 15.1)	4,759
2003–2004	8.56 (8.32 – 8.81)	5.31 (5.15 – 5.40)	8.33 (8.14 – 8.55)	14.9 (14.2 – 15.9)	4,509
2005–2006	7.88 (7.73 – 8.04)	4.78 (4.60 – 4.94)	7.76 (7.60 – 7.90)	13.7 (13.1 – 14.5)	4,490
Age group					
3–5 years					
1999–2000	4.21 (4.05 – 4.39)	2.81 (2.56 – 2.98)	4.19 (4.02 – 4.42)	6.31 (5.75 – 7.70)	376
2001–2002	4.31 (4.16 – 4.46)	2.95 (2.65 – 3.21)	4.28 (4.20 – 4.44)	6.15 (5.89 – 6.50)	454
2003–2004	4.36 (4.18 – 4.55)	3.10 (2.87 – 3.19)	4.42 (4.14 – 4.65)	6.28 (5.72 – 6.66)	454
6–11 years					
1999–2000	4.35 (4.18 – 4.54)	2.91 (2.55 – 3.09)	4.36 (4.20 – 4.50)	6.49 (6.21 – 6.78)	899
2001–2002	4.67 (4.58 – 4.77)	3.27 (3.04 – 3.44)	4.61 (4.53 – 4.73)	6.94 (6.60 – 7.21)	1,034
2003–2004	4.65 (4.53 – 4.78)	3.22 (2.99 – 3.37)	4.68 (4.51 – 4.82)	6.62 (6.44 – 6.77)	852
12–19 years					
1999–2000	5.87 (5.70 – 6.05)	3.65 (3.37 – 3.81)	5.83 (5.70 – 6.01)	9.58 (9.23 – 10.6)	2,132
2001–2002	6.03 (5.88 – 6.19)	3.96 (3.64 – 4.14)	5.90 (5.73 – 6.11)	9.48 (9.30 – 10.1)	2,225
2003–2004	6.30 (6.14 – 6.47)	4.26 (4.08 – 4.36)	6.21 (6.02 – 6.43)	10.0 (9.43 – 10.7)	2,073
20–39 years					
1999–2000	7.19 (7.04 – 7.35)	4.23 (4.06 – 4.42)	7.26 (7.03 – 7.43)	11.9 (11.3 – 12.5)	1,474
2001–2002	7.27 (7.12 – 7.42)	4.42 (4.21 – 4.67)	7.16 (7.08 – 7.25)	12.0 (11.6 – 12.8)	1,720
2003–2004	7.47 (7.33 – 7.62)	4.71 (4.47 – 4.99)	7.42 (7.30 – 7.58)	11.3 (11.0 – 12.0)	1,561
2005–2006	6.81 (6.67 – 6.95)	4.21 (3.99 – 4.42)	6.72 (6.61 – 6.84)	11.0 (10.4 – 11.5)	1,706
40–59 years					
1999–2000	8.27 (8.07 – 8.48)	5.18 (5.05 – 5.27)	8.08 (7.94 – 8.26)	13.5 (12.4 – 15.6)	1,209
2001–2002	8.30 (8.17 – 8.43)	5.35 (5.16 – 5.48)	8.17 (8.02 – 8.31)	13.4 (12.7 – 14.1)	1,494
2003–2004	8.67 (8.42 – 8.93)	5.60 (5.33 – 5.74)	8.44 (8.20 – 8.61)	14.4 (13.6 – 16.2)	1,280
2005–2006	8.01 (7.84 – 8.18)	5.13 (4.82 – 5.25)	7.90 (7.70 – 8.07)	12.8 (12.5 – 14.1)	1,371
60 years and older					
1999–2000	9.78 (9.53 – 10.0)	6.10 (6.03 – 6.17)	9.45 (9.23 – 9.75)	17.6 (16.9 – 18.7)	1,509
2001–2002	10.2 (9.76 – 10.6)	6.36 (6.12 – 6.64)	9.79 (9.33 – 10.2)	18.6 (17.7 – 19.6)	1,545
2003–2004	10.6 (10.2 – 10.9)	6.62 (6.33 – 6.99)	10.3 (9.93 – 10.6)	19.0 (17.6 – 20.2)	1,668
2005–2006	9.69 (9.36 – 10.0)	6.01 (5.75 – 6.29)	9.40 (9.05 – 9.75)	17.5 (16.2 – 18.5)	1,413
Gender					
(20 years and older)					
Males					
1999–2000	8.90 (8.69 – 9.11)	5.77 (5.57 – 5.92)	8.65 (8.42 – 8.92)	15.0 (14.2 – 16.6)	1,959
2001–2002	9.06 (8.89 – 9.23)	6.08 (5.86 – 6.24)	8.74 (8.53 – 8.96)	14.9 (14.3 – 15.8)	2,255
2003–2004	9.35 (9.06 – 9.65)	6.28 (6.09 – 6.42)	8.92 (8.67 – 9.17)	15.3 (14.5 – 16.7)	2,177
2005–2006	8.67 (8.49 – 8.84)	5.82 (5.70 – 5.92)	8.42 (8.25 – 8.59)	14.2 (13.2 – 15.2)	2,152
Females					
1999–2000	7.37 (7.23 – 7.52)	4.31 (4.07 – 4.53)	7.30 (7.14 – 7.42)	13.1 (12.7 – 14.3)	2,233
2001–2002	7.50 (7.32 – 7.68)	4.53 (4.32 – 4.73)	7.23 (7.06 – 7.36)	13.6 (12.9 – 14.8)	2,504
2003–2004	7.89 (7.61 – 8.18)	4.86 (4.51 – 5.03)	7.60 (7.39 – 7.87)	14.3 (13.4 – 15.8)	2,332
2005–2006	7.22 (7.00 – 7.45)	4.40 (4.19 – 4.51)	6.98 (6.80 – 7.15)	13.1 (12.1 – 14.9)	2,338
Race/ethnicity					
(20 years and older)					
Mexican Americans					
1999–2000	7.28 (7.06 – 7.50)	4.22 (3.96 – 4.58)	7.08 (6.88 – 7.36)	12.5 (11.8 – 13.9)	1,146
2001–2002	7.18 (6.85 – 7.53)	4.27 (4.00 – 4.47)	7.10 (6.80 – 7.34)	12.4 (11.8 – 13.7)	1,009
2003–2004	7.30 (7.11 – 7.49)	4.49 (4.25 – 4.57)	7.31 (7.17 – 7.42)	11.9 (11.3 – 12.7)	904
2005–2006	6.90 (6.74 – 7.05)	4.31 (3.99 – 4.44)	6.75 (6.62 – 6.94)	11.2 (10.8 – 12.2)	910
Non-Hispanic Blacks					
1999–2000	8.14 (7.87 – 8.41)	4.71 (4.25 – 4.87)	7.91 (7.51 – 8.34)	15.3 (14.7 – 16.6)	773
2001–2002	8.29 (8.03 – 8.55)	4.64 (4.40 – 5.08)	7.93 (7.72 – 8.17)	15.4 (14.4 – 17.9)	872
2003–2004	8.53 (8.24 – 8.83)	5.04 (4.84 – 5.24)	8.29 (7.99 – 8.59)	14.9 (14.4 – 16.6)	869
2005–2006	7.94 (7.72 – 8.17)	4.73 (4.50 – 4.90)	7.74 (7.50 – 7.95)	14.7 (14.0 – 15.5)	1,002
Non-Hispanic Whites					
1999–2000	8.19 (8.07 – 8.30)	5.09 (4.82 – 5.19)	8.03 (7.93 – 8.22)	14.3 (13.5 – 14.8)	1,874
2001–2002	8.37 (8.21 – 8.54)	5.18 (5.04 – 5.26)	8.14 (7.98 – 8.28)	14.6 (14.0 – 15.7)	2,514
2003–2004	8.74 (8.50 – 8.99)	5.46 (5.37 – 5.57)	8.53 (8.29 – 8.72)	15.1 (14.2 – 16.1)	2,406
2005–2006	8.06 (7.89 – 8.24)	4.97 (4.70 – 5.15)	7.94 (7.83 – 8.04)	13.9 (13.2 – 14.8)	2,264

Figure 1.6.b. Plasma total homocysteine: Concentrations by survey cycle

Selected percentiles in µmol/L (95% con dence intervals), National Health and Nutrition Examination Survey, 1999–2006

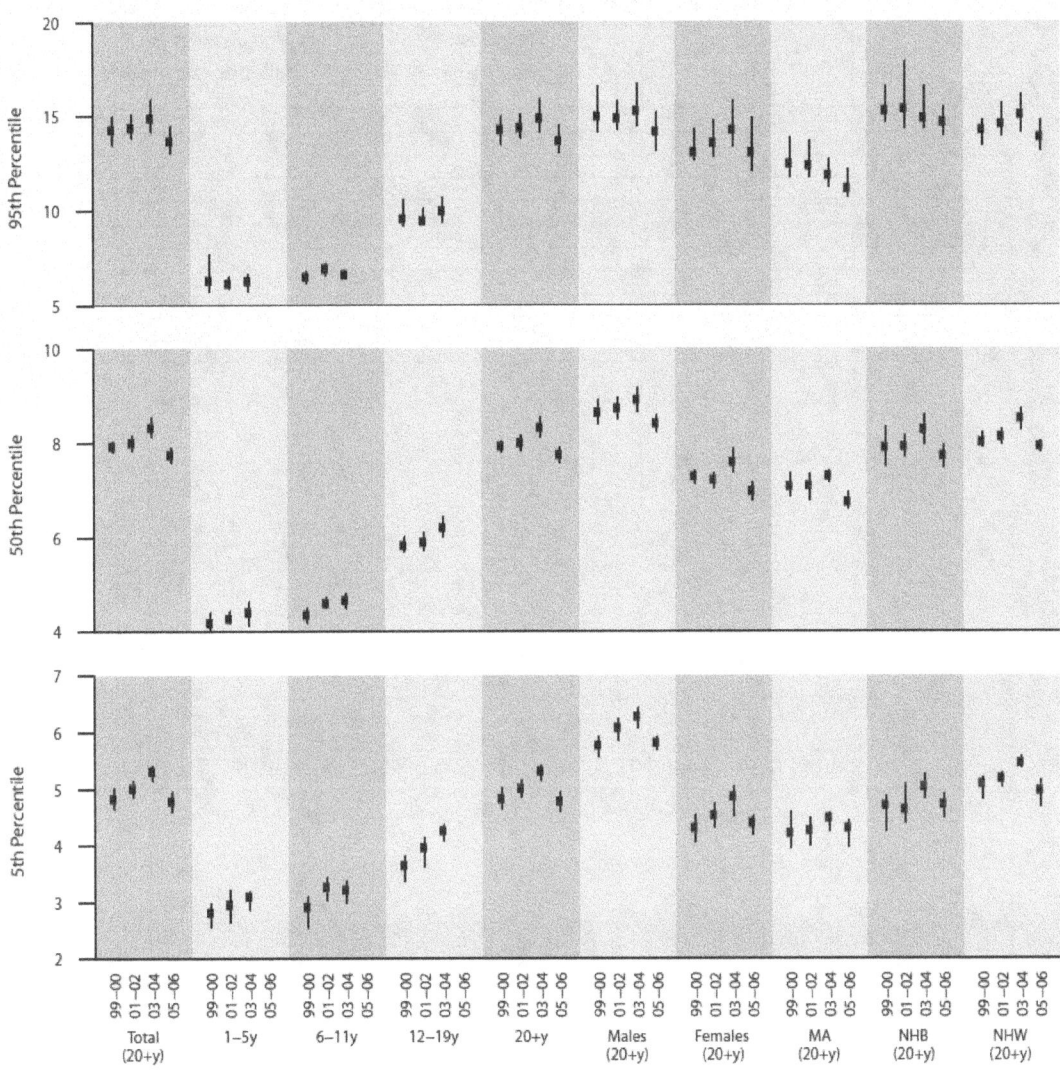

Table 1.6.c. Plasma total homocysteine: Prevalence

Prevalence (in percent) of high Plasma total homocysteine concentration (> 13 µmol/L) for the U.S. population aged 20 years and older, National Health and Nutrition Examination Survey, 2003–2006.

	Sample size	Prevalence (95% conf. interval)	Estimated total number of persons
Total, 20 years and older	8,999	7.7 (6.8 – 8.8)	15,825,000
Age group			
20–39 years	3,267	1.9 (1.4 – 2.4)	1,482,000
40–59 years	2,651	7.0 (5.6 – 8.7)	5,553,000
60 years and older	3,081	18.5 (16.3 – 21.0)	8,620,000
Gender			
Males	4,329	9.2 (7.9 – 10.6)	9,021,000
Females	4,670	6.4 (5.2 – 7.7)	6,796,000
Race/ethnicity			
Mexican Americans	1,814	2.1 (1.5 – 2.9)	336,000
Non-Hispanic Blacks	1,871	8.9 (7.7 – 10.2)	2,005,000
Non-Hispanic Whites	4,670	8.3 (7.1 – 9.6)	12,066,000

Table 1.6.d. Plasma total homocysteine: Prevalence by survey cycle

Prevalence (in percent) of high Plasma total homocysteine concentration (> 13 μmol/L) for the U.S. population, National Health and Nutrition Examination Survey, 1999–2006.

	Sample size	Prevalence (95% conf. interval)	Estimated total number of persons
Total, 20 years and older			
1999–2000	4,192	6.9 (6.0 – 8.1)	13,319,000
2001–2002	4,759	7.8 (6.5 – 9.2)	15,479,000
2003–2004	4,509	9.5 (7.9 – 11.3)	19,421,000
2005–2006	4,490	6.0 (5.1 – 6.9)	12,553,000
Age group			
3–5 years			
1999–2000	376	§	§
2001–2002	454	§	§
2003–2004	454	§	§
6–11 years			
1999–2000	899	§	§
2001–2002	1,034	§	§
2003–2004	852	§	§
12–19 years			
1999–2000	2,132	1.5‡ (0.8 – 2.8)	466,000‡
2001–2002	2,225	0.9 (0.5 – 1.6)	294,000
2003–2004	2,073	1.1‡ (0.5 – 2.1)	358,000‡
20–39 years			
1999–2000	1,474	2.6 (1.6 – 4.3)	2,058,000
2001–2002	1,720	3.2 (2.2 – 4.6)	2,505,000
2003–2004	1,561	2.4 (1.7 – 3.4)	1,923,000
2005–2006	1,706	1.3 (0.8 – 2.2)	1,034,000
40–59 years			
1999–2000	1,209	5.9 (4.3 – 8.1)	4,188,000
2001–2002	1,494	5.8 (4.4 – 7.5)	4,378,000
2003–2004	1,280	9.4 (7.0 – 12.4)	7,396,000
2005–2006	1,371	4.7 (3.6 – 6.2)	3,894,000
60 years and older			
1999–2000	1,509	17.3 (14.8 – 20.3)	7,441,000
2001–2002	1,545	20.5 (17.1 – 24.5)	9,180,000
2003–2004	1,668	21.6 (19.2 – 24.2)	10,039,000
2005–2006	1,413	15.6 (12.3 – 19.5)	7,527,000
Gender			
(20 years and older)			
Males			
1999–2000	1,959	8.6 (7.0 – 10.4)	7,854,000
2001–2002	2,255	9.6 (7.8 – 11.7)	9,136,000
2003–2004	2,177	11.4 (9.4 – 13.7)	11,197,000
2005–2006	2,152	7.0 (5.6 – 8.7)	7,036,000
Females			
1999–2000	2,233	5.4 (4.5 – 6.6)	5,459,000
2001–2002	2,504	6.1 (4.9 – 7.5)	6,342,000
2003–2004	2,332	7.7 (6.0 – 9.8)	8,202,000
2005–2006	2,338	5.1 (3.8 – 6.8)	5,525,000
Race/ethnicity			
(20 years and older)			
Mexican Americans			
1999–2000	1,146	4.4 (3.3 – 5.9)	542,000
2001–2002	1,009	3.8 (2.5 – 5.5)	542,000
2003–2004	904	2.7 (1.8 – 4.0)	426,000
2005–2006	910	1.6 (1.0 – 2.5)	263,000
Non-Hispanic Blacks			
1999–2000	773	8.6 (6.7 – 10.8)	1,872,000
2001–2002	872	9.6 (7.8 – 11.8)	2,120,000
2003–2004	869	10.8 (8.7 – 13.2)	2,435,000
2005–2006	1,002	7.0 (6.0 – 8.2)	1,640,000
Non-Hispanic Whites			
1999–2000	1,874	7.0 (6.0 – 8.1)	9,938,000
2001–2002	2,514	8.4 (6.9 – 10.3)	12,142,000
2003–2004	2,406	10.1 (8.3 – 12.2)	14,718,000
2005–2006	2,264	6.5 (5.4 – 7.7)	9,541,000

‡ Estimate flagged: 30% ≤ RSE < 40% for the prevalence estimate.
§ Estimate suppressed: RSE ≥ 40% for the prevalence estimate.

Table 1.7.a.1. Plasma methylmalonic acid: Concentrations

Geometric mean and selected percentiles of plasma concentrations (in nmol/L) for the total U.S. population aged 3 years and older, National Health and Nutrition Examination Survey, 2003–2004.

	Geometric mean (95% conf. interval)	Selected percentiles (95% conf. interval)					Sample size
		2.5th	5th	50th	95th	97.5th	
Total, 3 years and older	134 (128 – 140)	63.2 (60.5 – 65.6)	70.0 (67.3 – 72.8)	127 (122 – 132)	293 (277 – 320)	387 (359 – 428)	7,544
Age group							
3–5 years	120 (110 – 130)	61.1† (54.6 – 63.4)	65.2 (56.6 – 72.1)	117 (109 – 124)	269 (235 – 307)	299† (271 – 516)	421
6–11 years	117 (111 – 123)	60.6 (56.9 – 64.4)	67.5 (61.0 – 72.6)	113 (109 – 118)	228 (204 – 253)	258 (229 – 461)	806
12–19 years	118 (115 – 122)	62.4 (56.8 – 64.4)	67.3 (64.8 – 70.0)	115 (110 – 118)	222 (210 – 263)	280 (247 – 326)	1,979
20–39 years	122 (116 – 127)	61.4 (57.0 – 64.4)	67.3 (64.2 – 69.6)	116 (110 – 123)	246 (231 – 275)	303 (279 – 368)	1,496
40–59 years	137 (129 – 144)	62.9 (59.2 – 67.8)	70.9 (66.6 – 75.0)	130 (124 – 138)	275 (252 – 338)	387 (324 – 572)	1,230
60 years and older	177 (169 – 186)	79.7 (73.5 – 83.6)	89.9 (83.6 – 94.5)	163 (156 – 170)	429 (392 – 482)	628 (536 – 822)	1,612
Gender							
Males	136 (130 – 142)	65.0 (63.0 – 67.9)	72.4 (69.4 – 75.4)	127 (123 – 132)	299 (277 – 339)	406 (364 – 526)	3,719
Females	131 (125 – 138)	61.3 (58.2 – 63.9)	68.1 (65.2 – 71.3)	126 (120 – 132)	287 (272 – 315)	362 (328 – 403)	3,825
Race/ethnicity							
Mexican Americans	111 (108 – 114)	56.2 (53.3 – 58.0)	61.9 (58.6 – 64.4)	106 (100 – 112)	230 (209 – 254)	300 (248 – 387)	1,834
Non-Hispanic Blacks	109 (104 – 114)	55.3 (52.3 – 57.9)	61.1 (57.7 – 64.1)	105 (99.3 – 111)	224 (206 – 246)	270 (249 – 298)	1,993
Non-Hispanic Whites	143 (136 – 150)	69.4 (65.1 – 72.9)	76.9 (73.1 – 79.9)	135 (129 – 141)	308 (283 – 340)	393 (360 – 480)	3,152

† Estimate is subject to greater uncertainty due to small cell size.

Figure 1.7.a. Plasma methylmalonic acid: Concentrations by age group

Geometric mean (95% confidence interval), National Health and Nutrition Examination Survey, 2003–2004

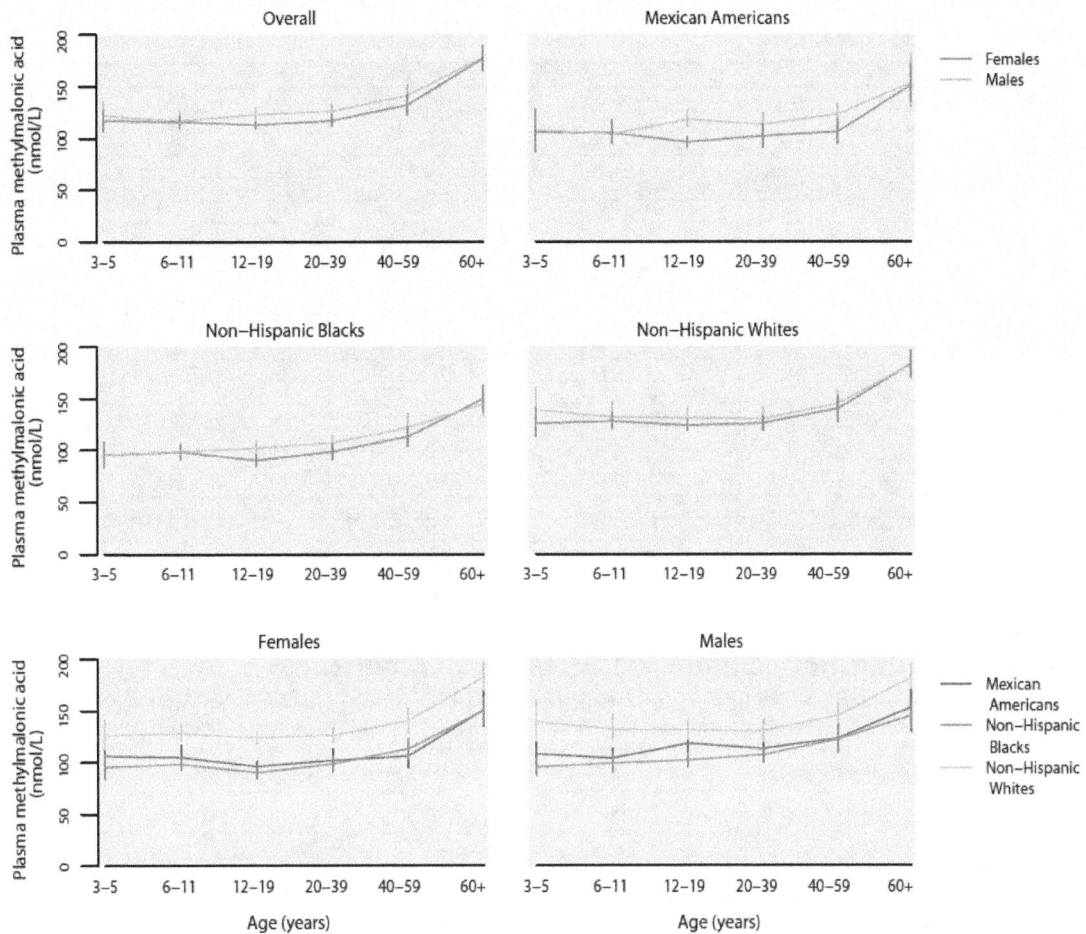

Table 1.7.a.2. Plasma methylmalonic acid: Total population

Geometric mean and selected percentiles of plasma concentrations (in nmol/L) for the total U.S. population aged 3 years and older, National Health and Nutrition Examination Survey, 2003–2004.

	Geometric mean (95% conf. interval)	Selected percentiles (95% conf. interval)					Sample size
		10th		50th		90th	
Males and Females							
Total, 3 years and older	134 (128 – 140)	79.6	(76.4 – 82.4)	127	(122 – 132)	231 (218 – 249)	7,544
3–5 years	120 (110 – 130)	74.5	(67.8 – 79.0)	117	(109 – 124)	198 (169 – 269)	421
6–11 years	117 (111 – 123)	77.6	(72.5 – 79.9)	113	(109 – 118)	184 (168 – 205)	806
12–19 years	118 (115 – 122)	75.1	(72.5 – 78.2)	115	(110 – 118)	189 (179 – 201)	1,979
20–39 years	122 (116 – 127)	75.5	(71.7 – 79.2)	116	(110 – 123)	201 (188 – 219)	1,496
40–59 years	137 (129 – 144)	82.3	(77.2 – 86.3)	130	(124 – 138)	223 (209 – 238)	1,230
60 years and older	177 (169 – 186)	102	(96.8 – 106)	163	(156 – 170)	328 (312 – 358)	1,612
Males							
Total, 3 years and older	136 (130 – 142)	82.8	(79.4 – 85.3)	127	(123 – 132)	231 (217 – 253)	3,719
3–5 years	122 (110 – 135)	71.6	(65.1 – 78.7)	118	(103 – 129)	239 (180 – 272)	223
6–11 years	117 (109 – 126)	75.9	(69.5 – 79.4)	112	(107 – 119)	191 (167 – 223)	385
12–19 years	123 (118 – 129)	79.2	(76.7 – 81.4)	119	(112 – 125)	197 (179 – 210)	1,016
20–39 years	126 (120 – 133)	78.7	(72.6 – 85.9)	119	(111 – 125)	209 (194 – 223)	705
40–59 years	141 (132 – 151)	86.2	(79.9 – 93.2)	134	(128 – 141)	224 (206 – 266)	608
60 years and older	178 (168 – 189)	99.0	(93.0 – 103)	162	(155 – 174)	351 (328 – 373)	782
Females							
Total, 3 years and older	131 (125 – 138)	77.5	(73.7 – 81.0)	126	(120 – 132)	231 (217 – 250)	3,825
3–5 years	117 (107 – 127)	75.5	(65.7 – 79.7)	117	(109 – 122)	169 (155 – 276)	198
6–11 years	116 (111 – 122)	78.7	(73.9 – 81.4)	115	(109 – 119)	177 (164 – 207)	421
12–19 years	113 (110 – 116)	71.4	(67.8 – 74.1)	109	(106 – 113)	181 (171 – 203)	963
20–39 years	117 (112 – 123)	73.0	(68.4 – 76.5)	113	(106 – 120)	197 (180 – 218)	791
40–59 years	132 (123 – 142)	79.0	(71.2 – 85.3)	126	(119 – 136)	222 (208 – 236)	622
60 years and older	177 (165 – 189)	106	(97.3 – 111)	164	(155 – 170)	315 (291 – 357)	830

Table 1.7.a.3. Plasma methylmalonic acid: Mexican Americans

Geometric mean and selected percentiles of plasma concentrations (in nmol/L) for Mexican Americans in the U.S. population aged 3 years and older, National Health and Nutrition Examination Survey, 2003–2004.

	Geometric mean (95% conf. interval)	Selected percentiles (95% conf. interval)					Sample size
		10th		50th		90th	
Males and Females							
Total, 3 years and older	111 (108 – 114)	69.4	(67.1 – 72.4)	106	(100 – 112)	186 (174 – 201)	1,834
3–5 years	107 (94.2 – 122)	74.1†	(65.1 – 76.9)	106	(87.8 – 118)	150† (133 – 279)	111
6–11 years	105 (96.7 – 113)	70.8	(61.5 – 77.1)	101	(92.6 – 112)	152 (142 – 192)	258
12–19 years	107 (102 – 112)	65.8	(62.4 – 69.8)	104	(98.3 – 109)	167 (160 – 184)	599
20–39 years	108 (99.2 – 117)	67.7	(65.0 – 70.6)	103	(92.6 – 116)	181 (156 – 242)	322
40–59 years	115 (110 – 119)	71.7	(65.4 – 75.8)	108	(102 – 115)	201 (178 – 220)	216
60 years and older	152 (138 – 168)	87.6	(81.1 – 92.8)	138	(125 – 159)	272 (245 – 368)	328
Males							
Total, 3 years and older	116 (114 – 119)	74.3	(69.8 – 77.3)	109	(106 – 114)	199 (185 – 217)	911
3–5 years	108 (93.9 – 124)	72.6†	(57.0 – 81.5)	105	(87.6 – 119)	145† (131 – 307)	59
6–11 years	104 (96.1 – 113)	70.2	(50.9 – 79.4)	105	(90.5 – 113)	148 (138 – 232)	124
12–19 years	118 (111 – 126)	72.9	(67.6 – 78.7)	111	(104 – 119)	198 (171 – 242)	306
20–39 years	113 (104 – 124)	75.6	(64.0 – 81.1)	106	(99.5 – 113)	189 (157 – 363)	149
40–59 years	123 (114 – 133)	73.4	(65.2 – 76.6)	116	(103 – 131)	218 (173 – 330)	113
60 years and older	153 (130 – 181)	89.1	(80.1 – 95.3)	137	(119 – 158)	268 (234 – 411)	160
Females							
Total, 3 years and older	105 (99.3 – 112)	67.0	(61.7 – 68.7)	102	(92.6 – 110)	176 (157 – 201)	923
3–5 years	106 (87.6 – 128)	74.1†	(57.0 – 81.0)	105	(80.4 – 127)	152† (124 – 228)	52
6–11 years	105 (94.3 – 117)	72.4	(58.9 – 77.7)	99.7	(89.6 – 115)	160 (145 – 218)	134
12–19 years	96.2 (91.3 – 101)	61.6	(55.1 – 66.5)	95.5	(90.0 – 102)	150 (142 – 156)	293
20–39 years	102 (91.2 – 113)	65.4	(56.5 – 68.0)	99.5	(81.5 – 119)	170 (147 – 208)	173
40–59 years	106 (95.2 – 117)	69.8†	(58.0 – 75.4)	101	(95.6 – 109)	181† (137 – 247)	103
60 years and older	151 (135 – 170)	83.4	(77.3 – 96.5)	140	(120 – 171)	279 (243 – 333)	168

† Estimate is subject to greater uncertainty due to small cell size.

Table 1.7.a.4. Plasma methylmalonic acid: Non-Hispanic blacks

Geometric mean and selected percentiles of plasma concentrations (in nmol/L) for non-Hispanic blacks in the U.S. population aged 3 years and older, National Health and Nutrition Examination Survey, 2003–2004.

	Geometric mean (95% conf. interval)	Selected percentiles (95% conf. interval)			Sample size
		10th	50th	90th	
Males and Females					
Total, 3 years and older	109 (104 – 114)	68.4 (65.1 – 71.0)	105 (99.3 – 111)	177 (167 – 188)	1,993
3–5 years	95.4 (87.4 – 104)	62.7 (54.6 – 72.2)	99.4 (86.5 – 106)	139 (125 – 159)	146
6–11 years	98.7 (92.9 – 105)	65.9 (56.1 – 71.0)	96.6 (92.1 – 103)	147 (139 – 159)	290
12–19 years	96.0 (90.6 – 102)	63.9 (60.0 – 66.4)	93.2 (89.7 – 97.7)	147 (135 – 160)	721
20–39 years	102 (96.5 – 108)	66.7 (56.2 – 70.0)	99.3 (91.3 – 107)	161 (151 – 177)	328
40–59 years	117 (108 – 126)	74.1 (63.5 – 78.1)	114 (99.8 – 122)	193 (161 – 246)	275
60 years and older	148 (137 – 159)	91.8 (76.6 – 105)	142 (131 – 147)	245 (217 – 299)	233
Males					
Total, 3 years and older	112 (107 – 117)	69.6 (67.8 – 72.6)	108 (101 – 113)	184 (171 – 199)	992
3–5 years	95.4 (87.4 – 104)	65.2† (< LOD – 73.4)	101 (87.6 – 107)	125† (121 – 140)	76
6–11 years	99.0 (90.5 – 108)	64.3 (50.7 – 69.3)	97.4 (86.2 – 109)	150 (138 – 177)	135
12–19 years	102 (95.5 – 109)	69.5 (64.4 – 72.8)	97.9 (92.3 – 103)	154 (143 – 179)	381
20–39 years	107 (99.9 – 114)	69.3 (64.1 – 72.9)	102 (97.0 – 114)	157 (149 – 182)	161
40–59 years	122 (110 – 136)	71.5 (61.4 – 77.4)	117 (104 – 124)	226 (179 – 280)	130
60 years and older	145 (133 – 158)	85.0† (77.2 – 98.7)	138 (125 – 150)	237† (212 – 322)	109
Females					
Total, 3 years and older	107 (100 – 114)	66.9 (62.2 – 70.8)	104 (95.7 – 110)	172 (161 – 187)	1,001
3–5 years	95.4 (84.0 – 108)	59.3† (< LOD – 71.8)	95.6 (80.0 – 108)	141† (126 – 268)	70
6–11 years	98.4 (92.6 – 105)	68.7 (57.1 – 74.3)	95.9 (89.5 – 105)	145 (135 – 155)	155
12–19 years	90.3 (84.7 – 96.2)	59.4 (56.1 – 64.1)	89.6 (85.8 – 94.5)	139 (128 – 151)	340
20–39 years	98.5 (91.3 – 106)	64.5 (52.6 – 68.2)	92.9 (85.7 – 101)	162 (142 – 197)	167
40–59 years	113 (104 – 123)	75.0 (62.0 – 82.2)	110 (97.7 – 120)	169 (151 – 211)	145
60 years and older	150 (137 – 163)	96.5 (72.9 – 107)	143 (129 – 152)	247 (216 – 334)	124

< LOD means less than the limit of detection, which may vary for some compounds by year. See Appendix D for LOD.
† Estimate is subject to greater uncertainty due to small cell size.

Table 1.7.a.5. Plasma methylmalonic acid: Non-Hispanic whites

Geometric mean and selected percentiles of plasma concentrations (in nmol/L) for non-Hispanic whites in the U.S. population aged 3 years and older, National Health and Nutrition Examination Survey, 2003–2004.

	Geometric mean (95% conf. interval)	Selected percentiles (95% conf. interval)			Sample size
		10th	50th	90th	
Males and Females					
Total, 3 years and older	143 (136 – 150)	86.7 (82.8 – 89.9)	135 (129 – 141)	242 (229 – 266)	3,152
3–5 years	133 (123 – 145)	80.5 (64.1 – 94.6)	128 (119 – 140)	246 (200 – 274)	115
6–11 years	130 (122 – 139)	87.3 (77.5 – 95.7)	122 (114 – 135)	213 (189 – 232)	196
12–19 years	128 (122 – 133)	79.9 (77.7 – 83.3)	122 (119 – 127)	203 (188 – 217)	525
20–39 years	128 (121 – 136)	82.7 (76.3 – 87.1)	123 (115 – 132)	204 (194 – 228)	708
40–59 years	142 (134 – 152)	86.6 (80.6 – 92.9)	136 (128 – 145)	227 (210 – 258)	642
60 years and older	182 (173 – 192)	105 (99.1 – 109)	167 (161 – 176)	341 (316 – 365)	966
Males					
Total, 3 years and older	144 (137 – 152)	91.0 (85.8 – 94.2)	134 (127 – 142)	240 (224 – 274)	1,535
3–5 years	139 (121 – 160)	73.7† (63.0 – 99.4)	130 (118 – 155)	267† (242 – 279)	62
6–11 years	132 (120 – 146)	91.6† (72.1 – 101)	120 (111 – 141)	207† (184 – 266)	91
12–19 years	131 (122 – 141)	83.4 (78.2 – 89.6)	125 (119 – 133)	204 (179 – 256)	266
20–39 years	130 (120 – 141)	88.1 (69.7 – 93.3)	123 (113 – 137)	205 (186 – 231)	319
40–59 years	145 (135 – 157)	95.7 (82.6 – 99.6)	138 (130 – 145)	224 (203 – 275)	321
60 years and older	182 (171 – 195)	101 (95.8 – 104)	168 (159 – 187)	364 (330 – 390)	476
Females					
Total, 3 years and older	141 (135 – 148)	84.1 (79.2 – 88.1)	135 (129 – 141)	246 (231 – 261)	1,617
3–5 years	126 (113 – 141)	80.7† (54.0 – 103)	122 (113 – 140)	168† (151 – 311)	53
6–11 years	128 (121 – 136)	86.5† (71.3 – 92.4)	122 (116 – 129)	209† (170 – 251)	105
12–19 years	124 (119 – 129)	77.6 (73.9 – 80.2)	119 (115 – 127)	202 (179 – 231)	259
20–39 years	126 (119 – 133)	80.0 (75.3 – 84.5)	121 (114 – 132)	203 (187 – 239)	389
40–59 years	140 (128 – 152)	82.8 (71.4 – 90.2)	135 (122 – 147)	231 (219 – 259)	321
60 years and older	183 (170 – 196)	109 (103 – 116)	166 (161 – 175)	318 (299 – 360)	490

† Estimate is subject to greater uncertainty due to small cell size.

Table 1.7.b. Plasma methylmalonic acid: Concentrations by survey cycle

Geometric mean and selected percentiles of plasma concentrations (in nmol/L) for the U.S. population, National Health and Nutrition Examination Survey, 1999–2004.

	Geometric mean (95% conf. interval)	Selected percentiles (95% conf. interval)			Sample size
		5th	50th	95th	
Total, 3 years and older					
1999–2000	132 (129 – 136)	64.9 (62.8 – 67.0)	123 (119 – 126)	280 (266 – 298)	7,597
2001–2002	130 (126 – 133)	63.8 (61.3 – 66.4)	119 (116 – 123)	276 (263 – 293)	8,451
2003–2004	134 (128 – 140)	70.0 (67.3 – 72.8)	127 (122 – 132)	293 (277 – 320)	7,544
Age group					
3–5 years					
1999–2000	124 (118 – 131)	67.4 (61.8 – 71.6)	116 (111 – 122)	237 (197 – 332)	376
2001–2002	116 (112 – 121)	63.9 (61.8 – 66.0)	108 (104 – 113)	219 (195 – 244)	453
2003–2004	120 (110 – 130)	65.2 (56.6 – 72.1)	117 (109 – 124)	269 (235 – 307)	421
6–11 years					
1999–2000	125 (117 – 134)	66.9 (63.5 – 70.3)	117 (107 – 130)	210 (191 – 319)	898
2001–2002	118 (114 – 122)	62.6 (57.7 – 66.8)	113 (109 – 118)	200 (187 – 224)	1,031
2003–2004	117 (111 – 123)	67.5 (61.0 – 72.6)	113 (109 – 118)	228 (204 – 253)	806
12–19 years					
1999–2000	118 (112 – 125)	60.2 (55.1 – 63.5)	109 (103 – 117)	231 (206 – 291)	2,132
2001–2002	115 (112 – 119)	56.9 (54.6 – 59.1)	107 (104 – 110)	228 (216 – 264)	2,220
2003–2004	118 (115 – 122)	67.3 (64.8 – 70.0)	115 (110 – 118)	222 (210 – 263)	1,979
20–39 years					
1999–2000	124 (119 – 129)	62.4 (59.7 – 64.9)	116 (110 – 121)	259 (235 – 295)	1,474
2001–2002	121 (116 – 125)	59.5 (55.9 – 61.8)	112 (107 – 117)	239 (226 – 268)	1,715
2003–2004	122 (116 – 127)	67.3 (64.2 – 69.6)	116 (110 – 123)	246 (231 – 275)	1,496
40–59 years					
1999–2000	133 (130 – 137)	65.4 (62.6 – 68.1)	124 (122 – 127)	251 (239 – 277)	1,210
2001–2002	131 (127 – 135)	71.2 (66.4 – 73.4)	120 (117 – 124)	264 (231 – 302)	1,491
2003–2004	137 (129 – 144)	70.9 (66.6 – 75.0)	130 (124 – 138)	275 (252 – 338)	1,230
60 years and older					
1999–2000	168 (163 – 174)	80.3 (67.7 – 89.1)	149 (145 – 155)	423 (392 – 458)	1,507
2001–2002	172 (164 – 180)	76.9 (74.1 – 79.8)	156 (150 – 162)	487 (413 – 604)	1,541
2003–2004	177 (169 – 186)	89.9 (83.6 – 94.5)	163 (156 – 170)	429 (392 – 482)	1,612
Gender					
Males					
1999–2000	136 (132 – 141)	67.2 (64.5 – 70.0)	127 (123 – 131)	288 (265 – 309)	3,708
2001–2002	133 (129 – 138)	66.4 (62.7 – 70.1)	123 (120 – 127)	273 (258 – 294)	4,091
2003–2004	136 (130 – 142)	72.4 (69.4 – 75.4)	127 (123 – 132)	299 (277 – 339)	3,719
Females					
1999–2000	128 (124 – 132)	63.3 (61.1 – 65.5)	118 (114 – 122)	276 (262 – 294)	3,889
2001–2002	126 (123 – 130)	62.3 (59.9 – 64.7)	115 (111 – 119)	277 (261 – 301)	4,360
2003–2004	131 (125 – 138)	68.1 (65.2 – 71.3)	126 (120 – 132)	287 (272 – 315)	3,825
Race/ethnicity					
Mexican Americans					
1999–2000	110 (106 – 114)	56.2 (54.9 – 57.5)	100 (97.3 – 103)	225 (198 – 270)	2,595
2001–2002	111 (107 – 115)	53.7 (51.0 – 56.5)	103 (99.0 – 108)	225 (218 – 235)	2,131
2003–2004	111 (108 – 114)	61.9 (58.6 – 64.4)	106 (100 – 112)	230 (209 – 254)	1,834
Non-Hispanic Blacks					
1999–2000	108 (103 – 113)	57.5 (52.6 – 60.7)	98.3 (91.5 – 105)	217 (192 – 250)	1,732
2001–2002	112 (108 – 116)	55.6 (53.0 – 58.2)	102 (98.3 – 107)	220 (200 – 258)	2,036
2003–2004	109 (104 – 114)	61.1 (57.7 – 64.1)	105 (99.3 – 111)	224 (206 – 246)	1,993
Non-Hispanic Whites					
1999–2000	140 (136 – 144)	72.0 (69.8 – 74.2)	131 (126 – 135)	290 (272 – 311)	2,573
2001–2002	137 (133 – 141)	70.6 (66.8 – 72.7)	126 (122 – 130)	288 (272 – 304)	3,605
2003–2004	143 (136 – 150)	76.9 (73.1 – 79.9)	135 (129 – 141)	308 (283 – 340)	3,152

Figure 1.7.b. Plasma methylmalonic acid: Concentrations by survey cycle

Selected percentiles in nmol/L (95% condence intervals), National Health and Nutrition Examination Survey, 1999–2004

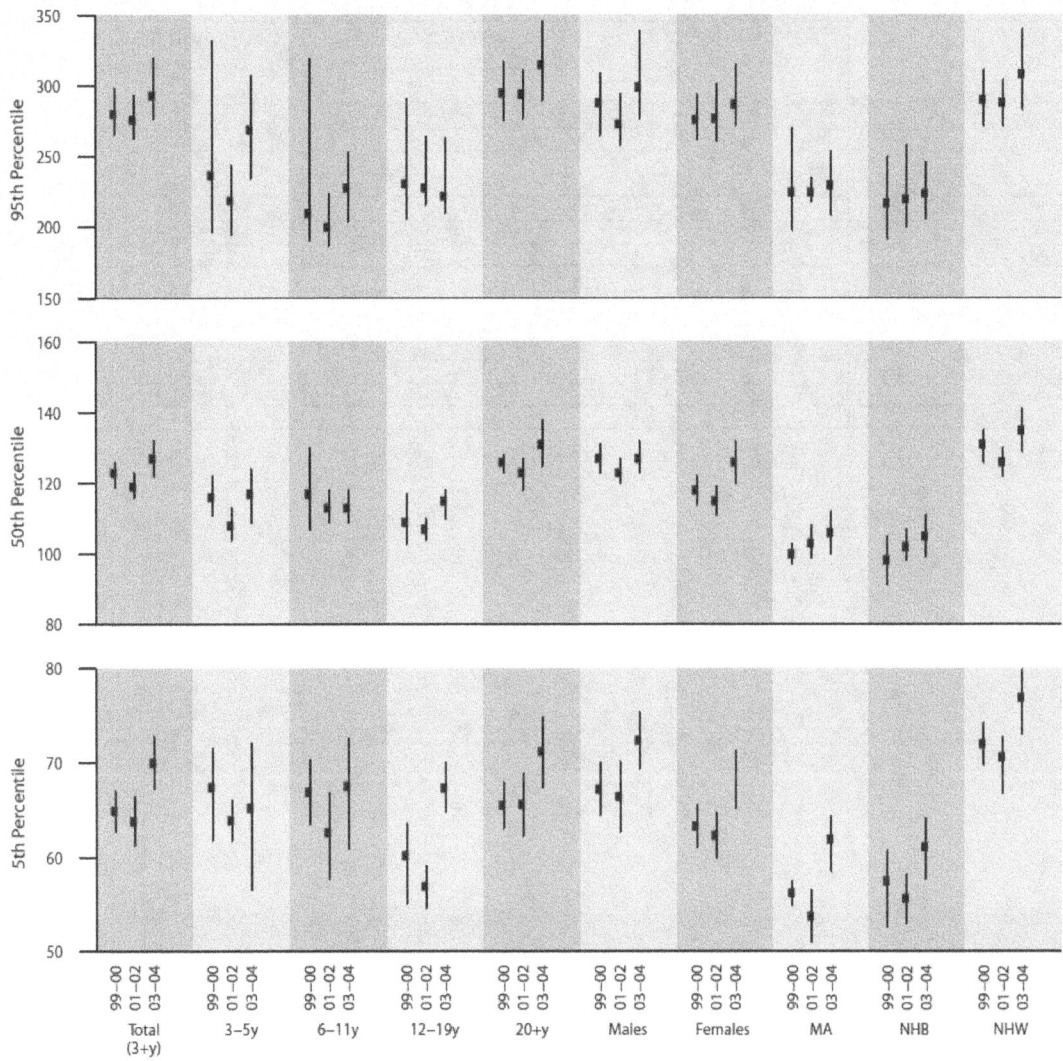

Table 1.7.c. Plasma methylmalonic acid: Prevalence

Prevalence (in percent) of high plasma methylmalonic acid concentration (> 271 nmol/L) for the U.S. population aged 3 years and older, National Health and Nutrition Examination Survey, 2003–2004.

	Sample size	Prevalence (95% conf. interval)	Estimated total number of persons
Total, 3 years and older	7,544	6.5 (5.3 – 7.9)	18,411,000
Age group			
3–5 years	421	4.5‡ (2.0 – 9.7)	916,000‡
6–11 years	806	§	§
12–19 years	1,979	3.2 (2.2 – 4.6)	1,054,000
20–39 years	1,496	3.8 (2.9 – 5.1)	3,066,000
40–59 years	1,230	5.8 (4.1 – 8.1)	4,557,000
60 years and older	1,612	16.7 (13.7 – 20.1)	7,748,000
Gender			
Males	3,719	6.8 (5.4 – 8.6)	9,439,000
Females	3,825	6.2 (5.0 – 7.7)	8,965,000
Race/ethnicity			
Mexican Americans	1,834	2.8 (1.7 – 4.4)	722,000
Non-Hispanic Blacks	1,993	2.5 (1.8 – 3.4)	846,000
Non-Hispanic Whites	3,152	7.6 (6.1 – 9.4)	14,546,000

‡ Estimate flagged: 30% ≤ RSE < 40% for the prevalence estimate.
§ Estimate suppressed: RSE ≥ 40% for the prevalence estimate.

Table 1.7.d. Plasma methylmalonic acid: Prevalence by survey cycle

Prevalence (in percent) of high plasma methylmalonic acid concentration (> 271 nmol/L) for the U.S. population, National Health and Nutrition Examination Survey, 1999–2004.

	Sample size	Prevalence (95% conf. interval)	Estimated total number of persons
Total, 3 years and older			
1999–2000	7,597	5.5 (4.8 – 6.3)	14,367,000
2001–2002	8,451	5.3 (4.6 – 6.0)	14,218,000
2003–2004	7,544	6.5 (5.3 – 7.9)	17,887,000
Age group			
3–5 years			
1999–2000	376	§	§
2001–2002	453	§	§
2003–2004	421	4.5‡ (2.0 – 9.7)	553,000‡
6–11 years			
1999–2000	898	2.5‡ (1.1 – 5.6)	623,000‡
2001–2002	1,031	1.5‡ (0.7 – 3.0)	372,000‡
2003–2004	806	§	§
12–19 years			
1999–2000	2,132	3.3 (2.1 – 5.3)	1,061,000
2001–2002	2,220	3.3 (2.1 – 5.3)	1,079,000
2003–2004	1,979	3.2 (2.2 – 4.6)	1,054,000
20–39 years			
1999–2000	1,474	4.5 (3.2 – 6.1)	3,496,000
2001–2002	1,715	3.7 (2.6 – 5.0)	2,888,000
2003–2004	1,496	3.8 (2.9 – 5.1)	3,066,000
40–59 years			
1999–2000	1,210	4.0 (3.0 – 5.2)	2,803,000
2001–2002	1,491	4.7 (3.6 – 6.1)	3,557,000
2003–2004	1,230	5.8 (4.1 – 8.1)	4,557,000
60 years and older			
1999–2000	1,507	13.9 (11.7 – 16.6)	5,986,000
2001–2002	1,541	13.9 (12.0 – 16.1)	6,225,000
2003–2004	1,612	16.7 (13.7 – 20.1)	7,748,000
Gender			
Males			
1999–2000	3,708	5.7 (4.7 – 6.9)	7,231,000
2001–2002	4,091	5.1 (4.3 – 6.0)	6,671,000
2003–2004	3,719	6.8 (5.4 – 8.6)	9,157,000
Females			
1999–2000	3,889	5.3 (4.5 – 6.3)	7,133,000
2001–2002	4,360	5.5 (4.6 – 6.5)	7,546,000
2003–2004	3,825	6.2 (5.0 – 7.7)	8,723,000
Race/ethnicity			
Mexican Americans			
1999–2000	2,595	3.2 (2.0 – 5.0)	632,000
2001–2002	2,131	2.9 (2.2 – 3.8)	656,000
2003–2004	1,834	2.8 (1.7 – 4.4)	687,000
Non-Hispanic Blacks			
1999–2000	1,732	2.5 (1.6 – 3.7)	803,000
2001–2002	2,036	2.6 (1.7 – 3.9)	842,000
2003–2004	1,993	2.5 (1.8 – 3.4)	817,000
Non-Hispanic Whites			
1999–2000	2,573	6.1 (5.3 – 7.1)	11,346,000
2001–2002	3,605	5.9 (5.2 – 6.8)	11,036,000
2003–2004	3,152	7.6 (6.1 – 9.4)	14,198,000

‡ Estimate flagged: 30% ≤ RSE < 40% for the prevalence estimate.
§ Estimate suppressed: RSE ≥ 40% for the prevalence estimate.

References

Allen RH, Stabler SP, Savage DG, Lindenbaum J. Diagnosis of cobalamin deficiency I: Usefulness of serum methylmalonic acid and total homocysteine concentrations. Am J Hematol. 1990;34:90–98.

Baik HW, Russel RM. Vitamin B12 deficiency in the elderly. Annu Rev Nutr. 1999;19:357–377.

Bailey RL, Carmel R, Green R, Pfeiffer CM, Cogswell ME, Osterloh JD, et al. Monitoring of vitamin B-12 nutritional status in the United States by using plasma methylmalonic acid and serum vitamin B-12. Am J Clin Nutr. 2011;94:552-561.

Carmel R. Biomarkers of cobalamin (vitamin B-12) status in the epidemiologic setting: a critical overview of context, applications, and performance characteristics of cobalamin, methylmalonic acid, and holotranscobalamin II. Am J Clin Nutr. 2011;94:348S–358S.

Coburn SP. Location and turnover of vitamin B6 pools and vitamin B6 requirements of humans. Ann NY Acad Sci 1990;585:76–85.

Coburn SP. Vitamin B6. In: Song WO, Beecher GR, Eitenmiller RR, editors. Modern Analytical Methodologies in Fat- and Water-Soluble Vitamins. New York: John Wiley & Sons, Inc.; 2000. pp. 291–311.

Czeizel AE, Dudas I. Prevention of the first occurrence of neural-tube defects by periconceptional vitamin supplementation. N Engl J Med. 1992;327:1832–1835.

de Benoist B. Conclusions of a WHO technical consultation on folate and vitamin B12 deficiencies. Food Nutr Bull. 2008;29:S238–244.

French AE, Grant R, Weitzman S, Ray JG, Vermeulen MJ, Sung L, et al. Folic acid food fortification is associated with a decline in neuroblastoma. Clin Pharmacol Ther. 2003;74:288–294.

Gunter EW, Bowman BA, Caudill SP, Twite DB, Adams MJ, Sampson EJ. Results of an international round robin for serum folate and whole-blood folate. Clin Chem. 1996;42:1689–1694.

Halsted CH. Intestinal absorption of dietary folates. In: Picciano MF, Stokstad ELR, Gregory JF, editors. Folic acid metabolism in health and disease. New York: Wiley-Liss, Inc.; 1990. pp. 23–45.

Hamner HC, Cogswell ME, Johnson MA. Acculturation factors are associated with folate intakes among Mexican American women. J Nutr. 2011;141:1889–1897.

Institute of Medicine, Food and Nutrition Board. Dietary reference intakes: Thiamin, riboflavin, niacin, vitamin B6, folate, vitamin B12, pantothenic acid, biotin, and choline. Washington, D.C.: National Academy Press; 1998.

Institute of Medicine, Food and Nutrition Board. Applications in dietary assessment. Washington, D.C.: National Academy Press; 2000.

Jacques PF, Selhub J, Bostom AG, Wilson PF, Rosenberg IH. The effect of folic acid fortification on plasma folate and total homocysteine concentrations. N Engl J Med. 1999;340:1449–1454.

Life Sciences Research Office, Center for Food Safety and Applied Nutrition. Assessment of the folate nutritional status of the U.S. population based on data collected in the Second National Health and Nutrition Survey, 1976–1980. Washington, D.C.: U.S. Food and Drug Administration, Department of Health and Human Services; 1984.

Life Sciences Research Office, Center for Food Safety and Applied Nutrition. Assessment of folate methodology used in the Third National Health and Nutrition Survey (NHANES 1988–1994). Washington, D.C.: U.S. Food and Drug Administration, Department of Health and Human Services; 1994.

Midttun O, Hustad S, Solheim E, Schneeded J, Ueland PM. Multianalyte quantification of vitamin B6 and B2 species in the nanomolar range in human plasma by liquid chromatography-tandem mass spectrometry. Clin Chem. 2005;51:1206–1216.

MRC Vitamin Study Research Group. Prevention of neural tube defects: results of the Medical Research Council Vitamin Study. Lancet. 1991;338:131–137.

Pedersen TL, Keyes WR, Shahab-Ferdows S, Allen LH, Newman JW. Methylmalonic acid quantification in low serum volumes by UPLC–MS/MS. J Chrom B. 2011;879:1502–1506.

Pfeiffer CM, Johnson CL, Jain RB, Yetley EA, Picciano MF, Rader JI, et al. Trends in blood folate and vitamin B12 concentrations in the United States, 1988–2004. Am J Clin Nutr. 2007;86:718–727.

Pfeiffer CM, Osterloh JD, Kennedy-Stephenson J, Picciano MF, Yetley EA, Rader JI, et al. Trends in circulating concentrations of total homocysteine among US adolescents and adults: findings from the 1991–1994 and 1999–2004 National Health and Nutrition Examination Surveys. Clin Chem. 2008;54:801–813.

Pfeiffer CM, Fazili Z, Zhang M. Folate analytical methodology. In: Bailey LB, editor. Folate in Health and Disease. 2nd ed. Boca Raton: CRC Press, Taylor & Francis Group; 2010. pp. 517–574.

Rasmussen K, Vyberg B, Pedersen KO, Brochner-Mortensen J. Methylmalonic acid in renal insufficiency: Evidence of accumulation and implications for diagnosis of cobalamin deficiency. Clin Chem. 1990;36:1523–1524.

Refsum H, Smith AD, Ueland PM, Nexo E, Clarke R, McPartlin J, et al. Facts and recommendations about total homocysteine determinations: an expert opinion. Clin Chem. 2004;50:3–32.

Rybak ME, Pfeiffer CM. Clinical analysis of vitamin B6: Determination of pyridoxal 5'-phosphate and 4-pyridoxic acid in human serum by reversed-phase high-performance liquid chromatography with chlorite postcolumn derivatization. Anal Biochem. 2004;333:336–344.

Rybak ME, Jain RB, Pfeiffer CM. Clinical vitamin B_6 analysis: an inter-laboratory comparison of pyridoxal 5'-phosphate measurements in serum. Clin Chem. 2005;51:1223–1231.

Rybak ME, Pfeiffer CM. A simplified protein precipitation and filtration procedure for determining serum vitamin B6 by high-performance liquid chromatography. Anal Biochem. 2009;388:175–177.

Selhub J, Jacques PF, Wilson PWF, Rush D, Rosenberg IH. Vitamin status and intake as primary determinants of homocysteinemia in an elderly population. JAMA. 1993;270:2693–2698.

Senti FR, Pilch SM. Analysis of folate data from the Second National Health and Nutrition Examination Survey (NHANES II). J Nutr. 1985;115:1398–1402.

Shane B. Folate status assessment history: implications for measurement of biomarkers in NHANES. Am J Clin Nutr. 2011;94:337S–342S.

U.S. Centers for Disease Control and Prevention. Recommendations for the use of folic acid to reduce the number of cases of spina bifida and other neural tube defects. Morb Mort Wkly Rep. 1992;41(No. RR-14):001.

U.S. Centers for Disease Control and Prevention. CDC Grand Rounds: Additional opportunities to prevent neural tube defects with folic acid fortification. Morb Mort Wkly Rep. 2010;59:980-984.

U.S. Department of Agriculture and U.S. Department of Health and Human Services. Dietary Guidelines for Americans, 2010. 7th Edition, Washington, DC: U.S. Government Printing Office, December 2010. [cited 2011]. Available at: http://www.cnpp.usda.gov/DGAs2010-PolicyDocument.htm.

U.S. Food and Drug Administration. Food standards: amendment of standards of identity for enriched grain products to require addition of folic acid. Final rule. Fed Regist. 1996;61(44):8781–8797.

Williams LJ, Rasmussen SA, Flores A, Kirby RS, Edmonds LD. Decline in the prevalence of spina bifida and anencephaly by race/ethnicity: 1995–2002. Pediatrics. 2005;116:580–586.

Wollensen F, Brattstrom L, Refsum H, Ueland PM, Berglund L, Berne C. Plasma total homocysteine and cysteine in relation to glomerular filtration rate in diabetes mellitus. Kidney Int. 1999;55:1028–1035.

Wright JD, Bialostosky K, Gunter EW, Carroll MD, Najjar MF, Bowman BA, et al. Blood folate and vitamin B12: United States, 1988–1994. National Center for Health Statistics. Vital Health Stat Series No. 11(243), 1998.

Yang Q, Botto LD, Erickson JD, Berry RJ, Sambell C, Johansen H, et al. Improvement in stroke mortality in Canada and the United States, 1990 to 2002. Circulation. 2006;113:1335–1343.

Yetley EA and Johnson CL. Folate and vitamin B-12 biomarkers in NHANES: history of their measurement and use. Am J Clin Nutr. 2011;94:322S–331S.

Vitamin C (Ascorbic Acid)

Background Information

Sources and Physiological Functions. Vitamin C, a water-soluble vitamin, is a collective term used to refer to L-ascorbic acid (the functional form of the vitamin), dehydro-L-ascorbic acid (the oxidized form, DHA), and monodehydro-L-ascorbic acid (the free radical form). Greater than 95% of vitamin C in human plasma exists as ascorbic acid (Jacob 1990). The most abundant dietary sources of vitamin C are orange juice, grapefruit juice, peaches, sweet red peppers, and papayas, followed by a variety of other fruits, vegetables, and fortified cereals. Vitamin C is a powerful antioxidant and a cofactor in various reduction reactions; it is a known electron donor for at least eight human enzymes involved in the hydroxylation of collagen and the biosynthesis of carnitine, hormones, and amino acids. Humans and a few other mammals, such as monkeys and guinea pigs, are unable to biosynthesize vitamin C from glucose and must obtain the vitamin from outside sources.

Approximately 70–90% of the ascorbic acid consumed is absorbed by the human body at usual intakes of 30–180 milligrams per day (mg/d). Bioavailability of vitamin C from food or supplemental sources is equivalent. Vitamin C administered after the plasma has reached a point of saturation (approximately 70 μmol/L) will likely be excreted as unmetabolized ascorbic acid in the urine (Institute of Medicine 2000).

Health Effects. The clinical manifestation of vitamin C deficiency is scurvy. Scurvy can occur if intake is below 10 mg/d for many weeks. Important signs and symptoms of scurvy include coiled hairs, follicular hyperkeratosis, fatigue, bleeding gums, and delayed wound-healing (Institute of Medicine 2000). Too much vitamin C can cause gastrointestinal upset, but such upset is generally seen only at an intake exceeding 2 gram/d, and it usually disappears within one to two weeks of discontinuation. High intakes of vitamin C supplements have the potential to increase urinary oxalate excretion, which is a risk factor for the formation of calcium oxalate kidney stones, but evidence is conflicting.

Vitamin C, in combination with other supplements, including vitamin E, zinc, and *beta*-carotene, has been shown to slow the progression of age-related macular degeneration (AREDS Research Group 2001). There is conflicting evidence for the reduction of risk of cardiovascular disease mortality by vitamin C supplementation and its effect on cardiovascular health in general (Shekelle 2003). More research is also needed to determine the role vitamin C plays in cancer prevention and treatment.

Intake Recommendations. The recommended daily allowance (RDA) of vitamin C for adults is 120% of the EAR (estimated average requirement), which was determined by the maximally protective neutrophil vitamin C concentration. For men, this equates to 90 mg/d, with 75 mg being the appropriate daily amount for women (Institute of Medicine 2000). RDAs range from 15–25 mg/d for children one to eight years of age, 45–75 mg/d for boys aged nine to 18 years, and 45–65 mg/d for girls aged nine to 18 years. For infants aged 0 to 12 months, the RDA is set at the amount of vitamin C commonly received through regular breastfeeding and the additional amount obtained through solid foods during the seven to 12 month period (an average of 45 mg/d). A number of factors, such as bioavailability, interactions with other nutrients, smoking status, age, and gender, affect the amount of vitamin C required by humans. For example, people who smoke require an additional 35 mg/d of vitamin C due to the increased ascorbic acid needed to repair oxidant damage (Institute of Medicine 2000).

Biochemical Indicators and Methods.
Vitamin C status can be assessed by measuring total ascorbic acid (oxidized and reduced) in serum or plasma, buffy-coat, or leucocytes. Ascorbic acid in plasma is considered an index of the circulating vitamin available to tissues, and in leucocytes (particularly polymorphonuclear) it is believed to be a good indicator of tissue stores. Vitamin C deficiency is generally defined as plasma or serum concentrations less than 11.4 micromoles per liter (μmol/L), or the level at which signs and symptoms of scurvy may appear. Serum ascorbic acid concentrations between 11.4–23 μmol/L are considered low (Gibson 2005).

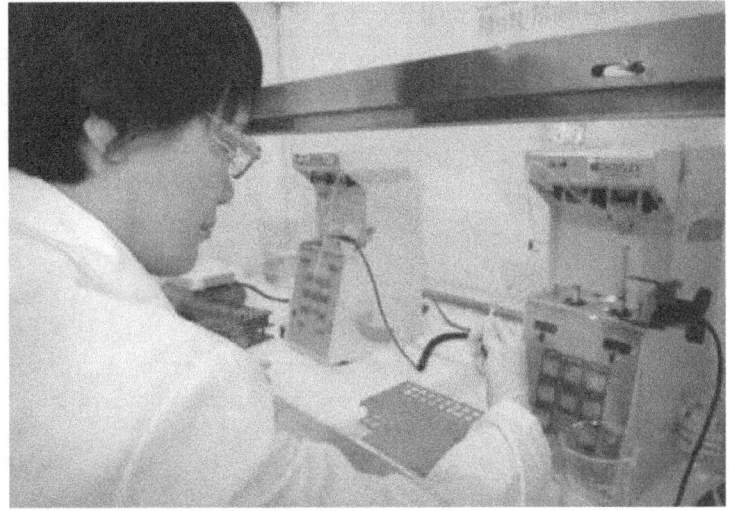

Clinical laboratories generally use international system (SI) units for vitamin C (μmol/L); however, some use conventional units (mg per deciliter [mg/dL]). The conversion factor to conventional units is: 1 μmol/L = 0.0176 mg/dL.

High-performance liquid chromatography (HPLC) methods with electrochemical detection, which provide necessary sensitivity and specificity, are generally used to quantitate serum vitamin C concentrations. Older spectrophotometric assays were susceptible to interferences from a number of substances, such as riboflavin and aspirin. A multi-level standard reference material (SRM 970) is available from the National Institute of Standards and Technology (NIST) for human serum with certified values for ascorbic acid. The Micronutrients Measurement Quality Assurance Program (MMQAP) sponsored by NIST hosts inter-laboratory comparison studies directed at assuring high quality measurements of serum vitamin C.

Data in NHANES. An HPLC method with electrochemical detection was used to determine serum vitamin C concentrations in NHANES 2003–2006 (McCoy 2005). Because of the incorporation of an internal standard, improved accuracy and precision was achieved with this method compared to the previous method used during NHANES III (1988–1994).

An analysis of NHANES 2003–2004 data showed that the highest serum concentrations of vitamin C were found in children and older persons. Mean concentrations among adult smokers were one-third lower than those of nonsmokers. In NHANES 2003–2004, the prevalence of vitamin C deficiency was significantly lower than that during NHANES III, but smokers and low-income persons were among those at increased risk of deficiency (Schleicher 2009).

For more information about vitamin C, see the Institute of Medicine's Dietary Reference Intake reports (Institute of Medicine, Food and Nutrition Board 2000) and fact sheets from the National Institutes of Health, Office of Dietary Supplements (http://ods.od.nih.gov/factsheets/VitaminC_pf.asp).

Highlights

Serum vitamin C concentrations in the U.S. population showed the following demographic patterns and characteristics:

- The highest concentrations were generally found in the youngest age group and higher concentrations were found in females compared to males.

- The likelihood of being vitamin C deficient or having low serum vitamin C concentrations varied by demographic subgroup.

Serum vitamin C concentrations less than 11.4 µmol/L may indicate vitamin C deficiency. Compared to non-Hispanic whites, Mexican Americans and non-Hispanic blacks had a lower risk of deficiency; compared to females, males had a higher risk of deficiency (Figure H.1.e). A number of important variables that impact vitamin C status are not addressed in this analysis, including smoking, overweight/obesity, socioeconomic status, and supplement use (Schleicher 2009). Considering that manifest vitamin C deficiency is rare in the United States (Olmedo 2006), persons categorized as vitamin C deficient may more likely experience latent scurvy, which is characterized by fatigue, irritability, vague, dull aching pains and weight loss (Prinzo 1999).

Serum vitamin C concentrations between 11.4–23 µmol/L are considered low. The prevalence of deficient (< 11.4 µmol/L) and of low (11.4–23 µmol/L) serum vitamin C concentrations was significantly lower in children than in persons 20 years and older (Figure H.1.f).

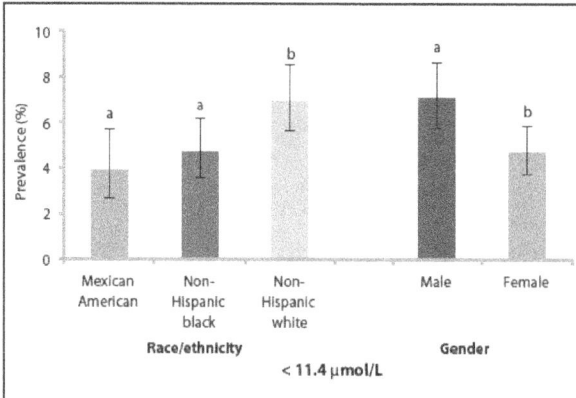

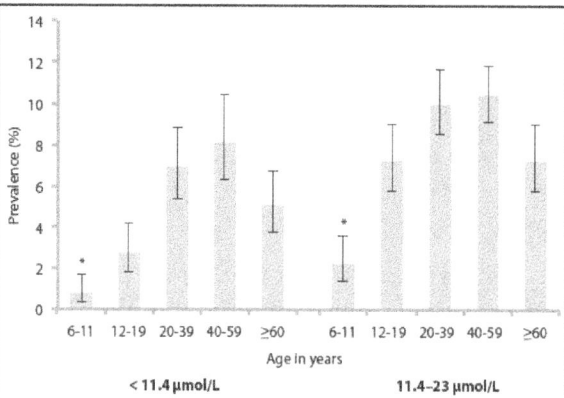

Figure H.1.e. Age-adjusted prevalence estimates of vitamin C deficiency (serum concentrations less than 11.4 µmol/L) in the U.S. population aged 6 years and older by race/ethnicity or gender, National Health and Nutrition Examination Survey, 2003–2006.

Error bars represent 95% confidence intervals. Bars not sharing a common letter differ by race/ethnicity or gender (p < 0.05). Age-adjustment was done using direct standardization.

Figure H.1.f. Prevalence estimates of vitamin C deficiency (serum concentrations less than 11.4 µmol/L) and of low vitamin C concentrations (11.4–23 µmol/L) in the U.S. population aged 6 years and older by age group, National Health and Nutrition Examination Survey, 2003–2006.

Error bars represent 95% confidence intervals. *Prevalence in children is significantly lower than prevalence in persons 20 years and older (p < 0.05).

Detailed Observations

The selected observations mentioned below are derived from the tables and figures presented next. Statements about categorical differences between demographic groups noted below are based on non-overlapping confidence limits from univariate analysis without adjusting for demographic variables (e.g., age, sex, race/ethnicity) or other blood concentration determinants (e.g., dietary intake, supplement usage, smoking, BMI). A multivariate analysis may alter the size and statistical significance of these categorical differences. Furthermore, additional significant differences of smaller magnitude may be present despite their lack of mention here (e.g., if confidence limits slightly overlap or if differences are not statistically significant before covariate adjustment has occurred). For a selection of citations of descriptive NHANES papers related to these biochemical indicators of diet and nutrition, see **Appendix G**.

Arithmetic mean concentrations (NHANES 2003–2006):

- The distribution of serum vitamin C concentrations was reasonably symmetric and for that reason we present arithmetic means.

- Serum vitamin C concentrations followed a U-shaped pattern, with the lowest concentrations seen in 20–59 year old persons (Table 1.8.a.1 and Figure 1.8.a).

- Females had higher serum vitamin C concentrations than males (Table 1.8.a.1).

- We observed no differences in serum vitamin C concentrations among race/ethnic groups (Table 1.8.a.1).

Changes in arithmetic mean concentrations across survey cycles:

- No changes in the serum vitamin C concentrations (Table 1.8.b) were observed between 2003–2004 and 2005–2006.

Prevalence estimates of low or high biochemical indicator concentrations:

- Six percent of the population aged 6 years and older had serum vitamin C concentrations < 11.4 μmol/L (Table 1.8.c).

- Children (<1%) and adolescents (3%) had a lower prevalence of low serum vitamin C concentrations than older age groups (5–8%).

- Non-Hispanic whites (7%) had a higher prevalence of low serum vitamin C concentrations than non-Hispanic blacks (4%) and Mexican Americans (3%).

Table 1.8.a.1. Serum vitamin C: Concentrations

Arithmetic mean and selected percentiles of serum concentrations (in μmol/L) for the total U.S. population aged 6 years and older, National Health and Nutrition Examination Survey, 2003–2006.

	Arithmetic mean (95% conf. interval)	Selected percentiles (95% conf. interval)						Sample size
		2.5th	5th	50th	95th	97.5th		
Total, 6 years and older	56.1 (54.6 – 57.6)	6.12 (5.47 – 6.91)	9.61 (8.17 – 10.9)	56.3 (54.9 – 57.6)	103 (101 – 105)	116 (113 – 120)		14,579
Age group								
6–11 years	75.1 (73.0 – 77.2)	21.3 (16.1 – 24.2)	29.0 (25.0 – 33.7)	74.5 (72.6 – 76.5)	123 (115 – 131)	138 (128 – 153)		1,703
12–19 years	58.0 (55.9 – 60.2)	10.2 (7.68 – 11.9)	15.2 (11.9 – 17.0)	58.6 (55.9 – 60.7)	98.9 (94.5 – 103)	109 (105 – 115)		3,984
20–39 years	51.0 (48.8 – 53.2)	6.01 (4.60 – 7.31)	9.00 (7.48 – 10.3)	51.4 (49.2 – 53.9)	92.9 (89.4 – 96.9)	102 (98.0 – 107)		3,233
40–59 years	51.6 (49.7 – 53.4)	4.92 (4.06 – 5.69)	7.41 (5.91 – 8.77)	52.4 (50.6 – 53.9)	97.2 (94.3 – 101)	111 (105 – 117)		2,635
60 years and older	63.0 (61.5 – 64.6)	6.91 (5.53 – 7.90)	10.7 (8.16 – 13.6)	62.5 (61.1 – 63.9)	117 (112 – 121)	131 (127 – 142)		3,024
Gender								
Males	52.4 (50.9 – 54.0)	5.80 (4.89 – 6.48)	8.38 (7.09 – 9.70)	52.6 (51.2 – 54.0)	98.9 (96.4 – 102)	110 (107 – 115)		7,155
Females	59.7 (57.9 – 61.4)	7.06 (5.74 – 8.15)	11.2 (9.61 – 12.9)	59.6 (58.1 – 61.2)	106 (103 – 111)	121 (117 – 128)		7,424
Race/ethnicity								
Mexican Americans	55.2 (52.7 – 57.7)	9.49 (7.64 – 12.1)	15.1 (11.6 – 18.7)	55.1 (52.8 – 57.7)	93.7 (90.7 – 96.0)	101 (97.6 – 107)		3,628
Non-Hispanic Blacks	54.3 (52.7 – 56.0)	7.38 (5.75 – 9.18)	11.9 (10.0 – 14.0)	54.0 (52.2 – 55.9)	95.2 (92.7 – 97.5)	104 (101 – 110)		3,784
Non-Hispanic Whites	56.5 (54.6 – 58.4)	5.75 (5.05 – 6.36)	8.56 (7.26 – 9.92)	56.9 (54.9 – 58.7)	105 (103 – 108)	120 (115 – 125)		6,089

Figure 1.8.a. Serum vitamin C: Concentrations by age group

Arithmetic mean (95% confidence interval), National Health and Nutrition Examination Survey, 2003–2006

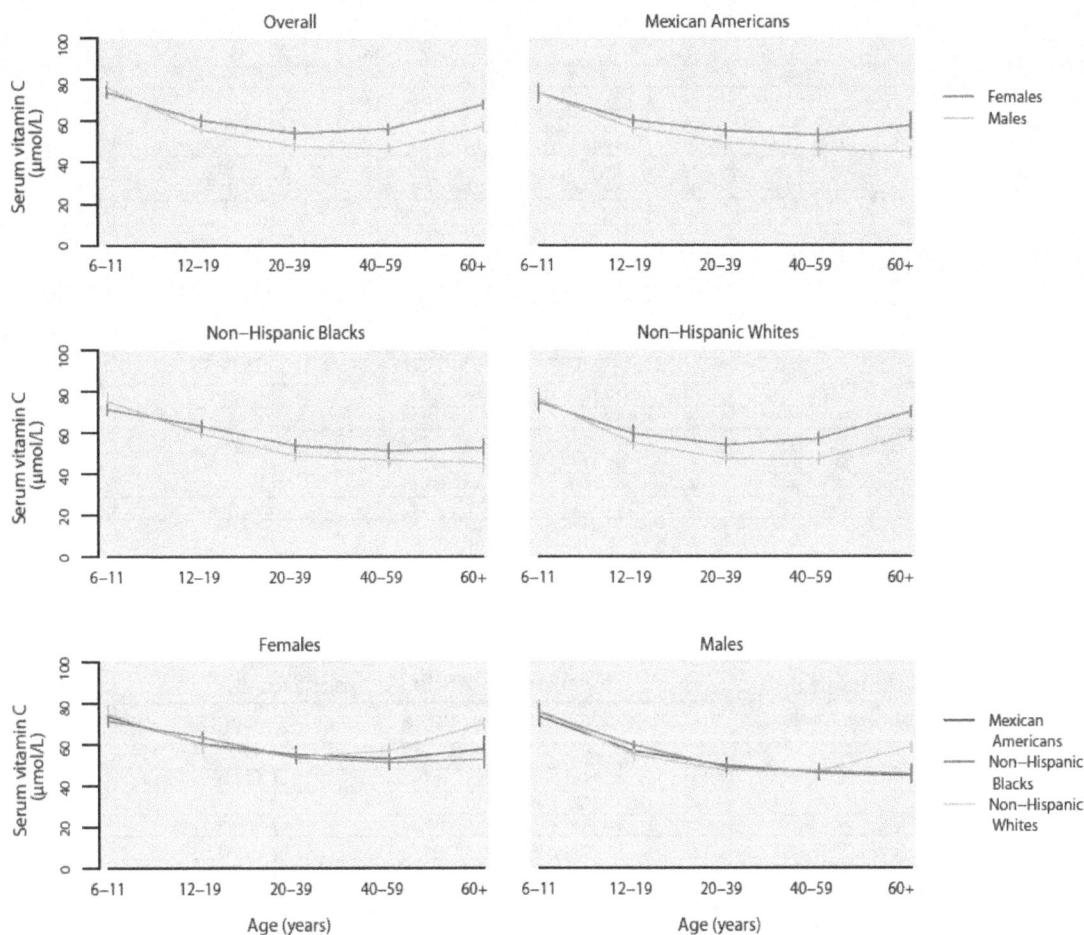

Table 1.8.a.2. Serum vitamin C: Total population

Arithmetic mean and selected percentiles of serum concentrations (in μmol/L) for the total U.S. population aged 6 years and older, National Health and Nutrition Examination Survey, 2003–2006.

	Arithmetic mean (95% conf. interval)	Selected percentiles (95% conf. interval)						Sample size
		5th		50th		95th		
Males and Females								
Total, 6 years and older	56.1 (54.6 – 57.6)	9.61	(8.17 – 10.9)	56.3	(54.9 – 57.6)	103	(101 – 105)	14,579
6–11 years	75.1 (73.0 – 77.2)	29.0	(25.0 – 33.7)	74.5	(72.6 – 76.5)	123	(115 – 131)	1,703
12–19 years	58.0 (55.9 – 60.2)	15.2	(11.9 – 17.0)	58.6	(55.9 – 60.7)	98.9	(94.5 – 103)	3,984
20–39 years	51.0 (48.8 – 53.2)	9.00	(7.48 – 10.3)	51.4	(49.2 – 53.9)	92.9	(89.4 – 96.9)	3,233
40–59 years	51.6 (49.7 – 53.4)	7.41	(5.91 – 8.77)	52.4	(50.6 – 53.9)	97.2	(94.3 – 101)	2,635
60 years and older	63.0 (61.5 – 64.6)	10.7	(8.16 – 13.6)	62.5	(61.1 – 63.9)	117	(112 – 121)	3,024
Males								
Total, 6 years and older	52.4 (50.9 – 54.0)	8.38	(7.09 – 9.70)	52.6	(51.2 – 54.0)	98.9	(96.4 – 102)	7,155
6–11 years	76.3 (73.1 – 79.5)	30.4	(21.7 – 37.7)	76.2	(72.5 – 78.7)	123	(113 – 138)	837
12–19 years	55.8 (53.6 – 58.1)	14.7	(11.2 – 16.5)	56.0	(53.4 – 58.5)	94.0	(91.2 – 100)	2,022
20–39 years	47.9 (45.3 – 50.4)	8.58	(6.68 – 9.87)	48.4	(45.2 – 50.8)	87.5	(82.8 – 95.4)	1,463
40–59 years	46.7 (44.5 – 48.9)	6.38	(4.89 – 7.94)	48.2	(46.1 – 50.2)	88.4	(84.8 – 96.3)	1,305
60 years and older	57.2 (54.9 – 59.4)	7.92	(6.72 – 10.1)	57.2	(54.7 – 59.4)	110	(105 – 118)	1,528
Females								
Total, 6 years and older	59.7 (57.9 – 61.4)	11.2	(9.61 – 12.9)	59.6	(58.1 – 61.2)	106	(103 – 111)	7,424
6–11 years	73.8 (71.1 – 76.6)	28.5	(20.3 – 35.9)	72.4	(69.2 – 75.9)	123	(115 – 131)	866
12–19 years	60.4 (57.8 – 62.9)	15.7	(11.0 – 18.8)	61.4	(58.6 – 63.9)	102	(98.2 – 110)	1,962
20–39 years	54.1 (51.5 – 56.7)	9.90	(7.73 – 11.5)	55.3	(51.9 – 58.6)	96.1	(91.9 – 101)	1,770
40–59 years	56.2 (53.7 – 58.7)	9.34	(6.29 – 12.0)	56.4	(53.6 – 58.2)	103	(97.4 – 110)	1,330
60 years and older	67.8 (65.9 – 69.7)	14.3	(10.9 – 16.4)	67.0	(65.1 – 69.0)	121	(116 – 129)	1,496

Table 1.8.a.3. Serum vitamin C: Mexican Americans

Arithmetic mean and selected percentiles of serum concentrations (in μmol/L) for Mexican Americans in the U.S. population aged 6 years and older, National Health and Nutrition Examination Survey, 2003–2006.

	Arithmetic mean (95% conf. interval)	Selected percentiles (95% conf. interval)						Sample size
		5th		50th		95th		
Males and Females								
Total, 6 years and older	55.2 (52.7 – 57.7)	15.1	(11.6 – 18.7)	55.1	(52.8 – 57.7)	93.7	(90.7 – 96.0)	3,628
6–11 years	73.4 (69.4 – 77.4)	28.3	(20.7 – 37.8)	74.2	(71.7 – 76.4)	113	(107 – 130)	563
12–19 years	58.5 (56.4 – 60.5)	20.3	(14.9 – 23.9)	59.0	(57.4 – 60.7)	92.7	(90.6 – 95.2)	1,266
20–39 years	52.2 (49.4 – 54.9)	15.9	(12.2 – 20.6)	52.4	(49.9 – 54.5)	85.7	(80.9 – 90.6)	782
40–59 years	49.5 (46.9 – 52.1)	9.55	(7.54 – 14.0)	51.0	(47.5 – 54.7)	83.6	(80.0 – 85.2)	470
60 years and older	51.8 (47.8 – 55.8)	9.48	(2.78 – 14.5)	50.5	(46.0 – 55.9)	93.6	(88.9 – 103)	547
Males								
Total, 6 years and older	52.7 (50.0 – 55.5)	13.6	(8.67 – 17.5)	53.3	(50.4 – 55.7)	90.8	(87.6 – 94.5)	1,762
6–11 years	73.4 (69.0 – 77.8)	28.2	(20.8 – 37.5)	74.6	(71.4 – 77.2)	113	(108 – 134)	275
12–19 years	56.7 (54.3 – 59.1)	18.9	(10.6 – 23.3)	57.4	(55.2 – 59.5)	90.1	(86.9 – 93.0)	628
20–39 years	49.6 (46.2 – 53.1)	14.2	(7.50 – 22.1)	50.8	(47.7 – 54.4)	79.5	(73.6 – 86.6)	351
40–59 years	46.2 (42.8 – 49.7)	8.27	(4.43 – 13.6)	46.3	(43.5 – 53.5)	76.5	(73.9 – 87.2)	239
60 years and older	44.8 (41.6 – 47.9)	7.27	(1.70 – 10.0)	44.0	(38.1 – 48.9)	86.3	(78.5 – 94.2)	269
Females								
Total, 6 years and older	58.0 (55.4 – 60.6)	18.6	(14.1 – 21.5)	58.1	(54.8 – 60.8)	95.1	(92.4 – 99.2)	1,866
6–11 years	73.4 (69.1 – 77.7)	26.5	(18.0 – 41.2)	73.3	(70.7 – 76.2)	113	(103 – 129)	288
12–19 years	60.3 (57.8 – 62.8)	22.4	(18.8 – 24.7)	60.7	(58.4 – 62.7)	95.1	(90.9 – 104)	638
20–39 years	55.1 (51.7 – 58.6)	18.5	(12.8 – 22.6)	54.0	(50.6 – 58.0)	90.0	(84.3 – 102)	431
40–59 years	53.1 (49.9 – 56.3)	10.6	(7.49 – 18.2)	54.5	(50.0 – 58.9)	85.2	(83.9 – 92.9)	231
60 years and older	57.7 (51.6 – 63.8)	14.3	(1.10 – 23.2)	58.7	(48.3 – 64.2)	97.9	(93.4 – 116)	278

Table 1.8.a.4. Serum vitamin C: Non-Hispanic blacks

Arithmetic mean and selected percentiles of serum concentrations (in µmol/L) for non-Hispanic blacks in the U.S. population aged 6 years and older, National Health and Nutrition Examination Survey, 2003–2006.

	Arithmetic mean (95% conf. interval)	Selected percentiles (95% conf. interval)			Sample size
		5th	50th	95th	
Males and Females					
Total, 6 years and older	54.3 (52.7 – 56.0)	11.9 (10.0 – 14.0)	54.0 (52.2 – 55.9)	95.2 (92.7 – 97.5)	3,784
6–11 years	73.4 (70.8 – 75.9)	39.7 (34.0 – 43.0)	72.8 (69.0 – 75.9)	107 (103 – 118)	544
12–19 years	61.5 (59.7 – 63.2)	28.1 (25.9 – 30.3)	61.3 (59.1 – 63.2)	95.0 (91.7 – 98.3)	1,400
20–39 years	51.5 (49.4 – 53.5)	14.7 (11.2 – 16.9)	50.4 (48.1 – 53.2)	87.3 (83.4 – 91.3)	711
40–59 years	49.2 (46.3 – 52.1)	8.58 (4.80 – 11.2)	48.9 (45.3 – 52.7)	93.1 (83.9 – 101)	619
60 years and older	49.8 (46.8 – 52.8)	6.69 (4.99 – 8.42)	50.8 (47.0 – 54.1)	95.9 (90.8 – 101)	510
Males					
Total, 6 years and older	52.6 (51.0 – 54.1)	10.2 (7.77 – 12.6)	52.1 (50.4 – 54.2)	92.8 (90.2 – 97.3)	1,895
6–11 years	75.3 (71.0 – 79.6)	42.4 (34.1 – 44.3)	75.8 (69.8 – 79.9)	108 (104 – 118)	272
12–19 years	59.6 (58.0 – 61.2)	28.6 (24.2 – 30.2)	58.8 (56.4 – 61.0)	91.6 (89.5 – 96.1)	735
20–39 years	48.7 (46.3 – 51.2)	12.4 (6.93 – 16.2)	48.0 (44.0 – 50.9)	81.5 (76.6 – 91.0)	337
40–59 years	46.7 (43.3 – 50.1)	7.24 (4.00 – 10.4)	46.6 (42.2 – 51.3)	82.8 (77.1 – 97.4)	291
60 years and older	45.6 (41.0 – 50.3)	5.02 (2.96 – 6.19)	45.6 (38.6 – 50.9)	93.0 (89.0 – 106)	260
Females					
Total, 6 years and older	55.8 (53.7 – 58.0)	13.5 (11.3 – 15.8)	55.8 (53.5 – 58.1)	95.9 (94.1 – 99.8)	1,889
6–11 years	71.3 (68.9 – 73.7)	36.8 (30.8 – 41.4)	68.8 (67.0 – 73.1)	106 (102 – 114)	272
12–19 years	63.4 (60.7 – 66.1)	27.6 (25.9 – 30.8)	63.8 (60.6 – 67.0)	96.0 (92.8 – 102)	665
20–39 years	53.7 (50.9 – 56.6)	15.7 (11.5 – 21.5)	52.7 (49.4 – 56.3)	90.5 (86.6 – 95.8)	374
40–59 years	51.3 (47.8 – 54.8)	9.84 (4.02 – 14.5)	50.4 (47.2 – 55.2)	95.9 (86.6 – 106)	328
60 years and older	52.7 (48.8 – 56.7)	9.64 (4.66 – 11.2)	54.0 (50.1 – 58.2)	96.5 (90.0 – 108)	250

Table 1.8.a.5. Serum vitamin C: Non-Hispanic whites

Arithmetic mean and selected percentiles of serum concentrations (in µmol/L) for non-Hispanic whites in the U.S. population aged 6 years and older, National Health and Nutrition Examination Survey, 2003–2006.

	Arithmetic mean (95% conf. interval)	Selected percentiles (95% conf. interval)			Sample size
		5th	50th	95th	
Males and Females					
Total, 6 years and older	56.5 (54.6 – 58.4)	8.56 (7.26 – 9.92)	56.9 (54.9 – 58.7)	105 (103 – 108)	6,089
6–11 years	75.6 (72.5 – 78.8)	25.7 (18.7 – 31.8)	74.8 (70.9 – 77.7)	128 (118 – 144)	436
12–19 years	57.2 (54.0 – 60.4)	12.3 (9.88 – 15.7)	58.0 (53.2 – 61.5)	101 (95.4 – 107)	1,037
20–39 years	50.6 (47.8 – 53.3)	7.99 (6.39 – 8.99)	51.2 (47.7 – 55.1)	96.2 (91.2 – 102)	1,442
40–59 years	52.0 (49.7 – 54.3)	6.80 (5.56 – 8.33)	52.8 (51.2 – 55.2)	99.8 (96.0 – 103)	1,346
60 years and older	64.8 (63.0 – 66.7)	11.7 (8.22 – 14.7)	63.9 (62.4 – 65.3)	118 (114 – 123)	1,828
Males					
Total, 6 years and older	52.3 (50.4 – 54.1)	7.71 (6.50 – 8.82)	52.4 (50.5 – 54.5)	101 (98.2 – 104)	2,990
6–11 years	76.5 (71.7 – 81.4)	25.4† (14.0 – 34.1)	75.8 (69.2 – 80.6)	127† (117 – 155)	210
12–19 years	54.9 (51.7 – 58.1)	12.6 (9.73 – 16.2)	54.8 (51.4 – 59.1)	94.4 (91.6 – 104)	524
20–39 years	47.2 (44.2 – 50.3)	7.92 (6.52 – 8.79)	47.5 (44.1 – 50.7)	93.8 (85.8 – 98.7)	636
40–59 years	47.0 (44.3 – 49.8)	6.19 (4.90 – 7.44)	48.5 (46.4 – 51.0)	90.2 (86.4 – 101)	687
60 years and older	58.5 (56.0 – 61.1)	8.15 (6.84 – 11.5)	58.4 (55.6 – 60.7)	112 (106 – 119)	933
Females					
Total, 6 years and older	60.5 (58.2 – 62.8)	9.92 (8.18 – 11.7)	60.7 (58.5 – 62.8)	110 (106 – 114)	3,099
6–11 years	74.7 (70.3 – 79.0)	25.2 (9.65 – 36.1)	72.8 (68.7 – 78.2)	129 (115 – 145)	226
12–19 years	59.6 (55.8 – 63.5)	12.0 (8.98 – 15.7)	61.1 (56.9 – 64.7)	104 (98.6 – 120)	513
20–39 years	53.9 (50.4 – 57.4)	8.06 (5.40 – 9.86)	56.0 (50.2 – 60.7)	99.0 (93.1 – 106)	806
40–59 years	57.0 (53.9 – 60.0)	8.63 (5.81 – 11.1)	57.4 (53.5 – 59.8)	105 (98.0 – 113)	659
60 years and older	70.0 (67.7 – 72.3)	15.0 (10.9 – 17.9)	69.1 (66.5 – 72.6)	123 (117 – 131)	895

† Estimate is subject to greater uncertainty due to small cell size.

Table 1.8.b. Serum vitamin C: Concentrations by survey cycle

Arithmetic mean and selected percentiles of serum concentrations (in μmol/L) for the U.S. population, National Health and Nutrition Examination Survey, 2003–2006.

	Arithmetic mean (95% conf. interval)	Selected percentiles (95% conf. interval)			Sample size
		5th	50th	95th	
Total, 6 years and older					
2003–2004	55.8 (53.1 – 58.5)	8.55 (6.57 – 10.2)	56.3 (53.4 – 58.8)	103 (101 – 108)	7,277
2005–2006	56.4 (54.8 – 58.0)	11.1 (9.22 – 12.4)	56.3 (55.0 – 57.6)	102 (99.2 – 105)	7,302
Age group					
6–11 years					
2003–2004	74.3 (70.9 – 77.8)	27.8 (16.6 – 35.5)	73.7 (70.8 – 76.8)	126 (112 – 139)	823
2005–2006	75.9 (73.1 – 78.7)	32.0 (26.2 – 36.6)	75.0 (72.4 – 78.1)	121 (114 – 130)	880
12–19 years					
2003–2004	56.3 (52.9 – 59.8)	13.6 (10.2 – 16.2)	56.2 (52.1 – 60.0)	98.4 (93.6 – 106)	2,016
2005–2006	59.7 (57.0 – 62.4)	17.0 (13.4 – 20.8)	60.3 (57.3 – 63.5)	99.3 (93.0 – 107)	1,968
20–39 years					
2003–2004	49.7 (46.0 – 53.5)	7.34 (5.42 – 9.22)	50.0 (45.7 – 54.1)	95.0 (87.9 – 102)	1,540
2005–2006	52.2 (49.7 – 54.8)	11.3 (9.71 – 12.5)	52.8 (49.7 – 55.7)	91.9 (87.8 – 97.1)	1,693
40–59 years					
2003–2004	52.6 (49.4 – 55.8)	6.71 (5.02 – 8.71)	53.5 (51.2 – 56.6)	100 (95.5 – 105)	1,266
2005–2006	50.6 (48.3 – 52.9)	7.92 (5.51 – 10.9)	51.3 (48.9 – 53.4)	94.4 (90.1 – 100)	1,369
60 years and older					
2003–2004	63.2 (60.8 – 65.6)	10.3 (7.88 – 13.3)	62.5 (60.2 – 64.7)	119 (114 – 124)	1,632
2005–2006	62.9 (60.7 – 65.1)	11.8 (6.99 – 15.1)	62.6 (60.7 – 64.5)	113 (108 – 119)	1,392
Gender					
Males					
2003–2004	52.2 (49.4 – 54.9)	7.32 (5.74 – 9.08)	52.7 (50.1 – 55.2)	100 (97.7 – 103)	3,590
2005–2006	52.7 (51.0 – 54.3)	9.74 (7.88 – 11.0)	52.4 (50.9 – 53.9)	97.3 (93.7 – 102)	3,565
Females					
2003–2004	59.3 (56.4 – 62.3)	9.76 (7.89 – 11.4)	59.8 (56.7 – 62.5)	108 (102 – 115)	3,687
2005–2006	60.0 (57.9 – 62.1)	13.1 (11.1 – 15.6)	59.4 (57.7 – 61.4)	105 (101 – 111)	3,737
Race/ethnicity					
Mexican Americans					
2003–2004	55.4 (50.6 – 60.2)	14.0 (7.30 – 20.1)	55.6 (51.7 – 60.0)	93.1 (89.3 – 97.1)	1,766
2005–2006	55.1 (52.8 – 57.5)	17.1 (10.8 – 20.6)	54.6 (51.7 – 57.5)	94.2 (90.8 – 97.3)	1,862
Non-Hispanic Blacks					
2003–2004	52.9 (50.3 – 55.4)	11.1 (7.65 – 13.5)	52.0 (49.7 – 55.5)	93.7 (90.5 – 99.1)	1,880
2005–2006	55.7 (53.6 – 57.9)	13.0 (9.49 – 16.8)	55.4 (53.5 – 57.6)	95.6 (94.0 – 99.2)	1,904
Non-Hispanic Whites					
2003–2004	56.7 (53.1 – 60.3)	7.82 (6.24 – 9.09)	57.4 (53.1 – 60.6)	108 (103 – 115)	3,103
2005–2006	56.3 (54.5 – 58.0)	10.0 (7.77 – 11.7)	56.4 (54.7 – 58.0)	103 (100 – 106)	2,986

Figure 1.8.b. Serum vitamin C: Concentrations by survey cycle
Selected percentiles in μmol/L (95% condence intervals), National Health and
Nutrition Examination Survey, 2003–2006

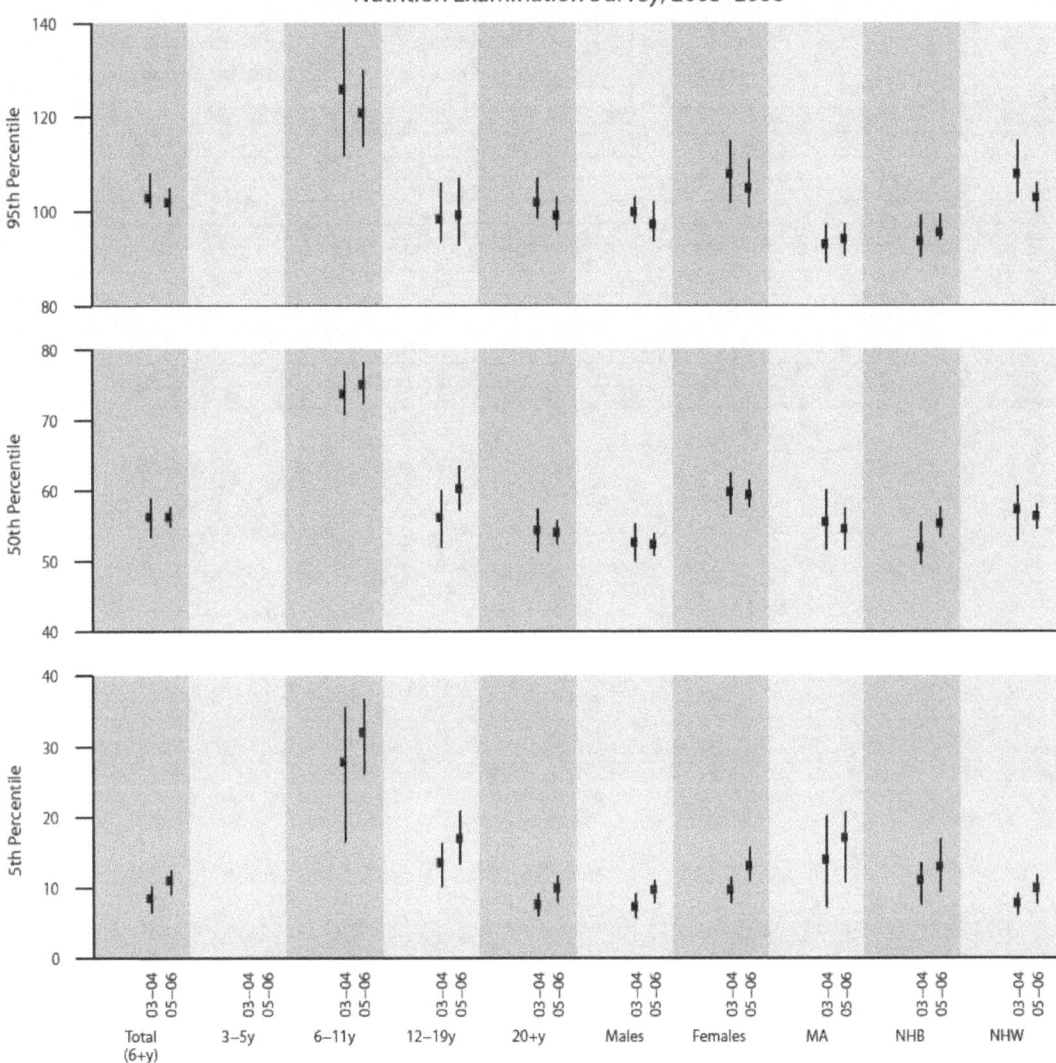

Table 1.8.c. Serum vitamin C: Prevalence

Prevalence (in percent) of low serum vitamin C concentration (< 11.4 µmol/L) for the U.S. population aged 6 years and older, National Health and Nutrition Examination Survey, 2003–2006.

	Sample size	Prevalence (95% conf. interval)	Estimated total number of persons
Total, 6 years and older	14,579	6.0 (4.9 – 7.3)	15,757,000
Age group			
6–11 years	1,703	0.8‡ (0.4 – 1.7)	191,000‡
12–19 years	3,984	2.8 (1.9 – 4.2)	931,000
20–39 years	3,233	6.9 (5.4 – 8.9)	5,533,000
40–59 years	2,635	8.1 (6.3 – 10.5)	6,435,000
60 years and older	3,024	5.1 (3.8 – 6.8)	2,362,000
Gender			
Males	7,155	7.3 (5.9 – 9.0)	9,258,000
Females	7,424	4.8 (3.8 – 6.0)	6,476,000
Race/ethnicity			
Mexican Americans	3,628	3.1 (2.1 – 4.6)	715,000
Non-Hispanic Blacks	3,784	4.3 (3.2 – 5.7)	1,341,000
Non-Hispanic Whites	6,089	7.1 (5.8 – 8.7)	12,807,000

‡ Estimate flagged: 30% ≤ RSE < 40% for the prevalence estimate.

Table 1.8.d. Serum vitamin C: Prevalence by survey cycle

Prevalence (in percent) of low serum vitamin C concentration (< 11.4 µmol/L) for the U.S. population, National Health and Nutrition Examination Survey, 2003–2006.

	Sample size	Prevalence (95% conf. interval)	Estimated total number of persons
Total, 6 years and older			
2003–2004	7,277	7.3 (5.5 – 9.6)	19,054,000
2005–2006	7,302	4.8 (3.7 – 6.1)	12,746,000
Age group			
6–11 years			
2003–2004	823	1.5‡ (0.7 – 3.6)	372,000‡
2005–2006	880	§	§
12–19 years			
2003–2004	2,016	3.3 (1.9 – 5.7)	1,090,000
2005–2006	1,968	2.3‡ (1.2 – 4.5)	783,000‡
20–39 years			
2003–2004	1,540	9.3 (6.7 – 12.8)	7,437,000
2005–2006	1,693	4.5 (3.2 – 6.4)	3,618,000
40–59 years			
2003–2004	1,266	9.2 (6.5 – 13.0)	7,294,000
2005–2006	1,369	7.1 (4.7 – 10.5)	5,815,000
60 years and older			
2003–2004	1,632	5.5 (3.9 – 7.5)	2,543,000
2005–2006	1,392	4.7 (2.8 – 7.8)	2,272,000
Gender			
Males			
2003–2004	3,590	8.4 (6.0 – 11.8)	10,772,000
2005–2006	3,565	6.1 (4.8 – 7.7)	7,914,000
Females			
2003–2004	3,687	6.1 (4.6 – 8.0)	8,247,000
2005–2006	3,737	3.5 (2.4 – 5.1)	4,827,000
Race/ethnicity			
Mexican Americans			
2003–2004	1,766	3.7 (2.0 – 6.7)	840,000
2005–2006	1,862	2.6 (1.6 – 4.2)	627,000
Non-Hispanic Blacks			
2003–2004	1,880	4.8 (3.4 – 6.8)	1,510,000
2005–2006	1,904	3.8 (2.3 – 6.2)	1,199,000
Non-Hispanic Whites			
2003–2004	3,103	8.6 (6.4 – 11.5)	15,534,000
2005–2006	2,986	5.6 (4.2 – 7.4)	10,186,000

‡ Estimate flagged: 30% ≤ RSE < 40% for the prevalence estimate.
§ Estimate suppressed: RSE ≥ 40% for the prevalence estimate.

References

Age-Related Eye Disease Study Research Group. A randomized, placebo-controlled, clinical trial of high-dose supplementation with vitamins C and E and beta carotene for age-related cataract and vision loss: AREDS report no. 9. Arch Ophthalmol. 2001;119:1439–1452.

Gibson RS. Principles of nutritional assessment (2nd edn.). New York: Oxford University Press; 2005.

Institute of Medicine, Food and Nutrition Board. Dietary reference intakes for vitamin C, vitamin E, selenium, and carotenoids. Washington, D.C.: National Academy Press; 2000.

Jacob RA. Assessment of human vitamin C status. J Nutr. 1990;120 Suppl 11:1480–1485.

McCoy LF, Bowen MB, Xu M, Chen H, Schleicher RL. Improved HPLC assay for measuring serum vitamin C with 1-methyluric acid used as an electrochemically active internal standard. Clin Chem. 2005;51:1062–1064.

Olmedo JM, Yiannias JA, Windgassen EB, Gornet MK. Scurvy: a disease almost forgotten. Int J Dermatol. 2006;45:909–913.

Prinzo ZW. Scurvy and its prevention and control in major emergencies. Geneva, Switzerland: World Health Organization, 1999. (WHO publication WHO/NHD/99.11.)

Schleicher RL, Carroll MD, Ford ES, Lacher DA. Serum vitamin C and the prevalence of vitamin C deficiency in the United States: 2003–2004 National Health and Nutrition Examination Survey (NHANES). Am J Clin Nutr. 2009;90:1252–1263.

Shekelle P, Morton S, Hardy M. Effect of Supplemental Antioxidants Vitamin C, Vitamin E, and Coenzyme Q10 for the Prevention and Treatment of Cardiovascular Disease. Evid Report Tech Asses No. 83. AHRQ Publication No. 03-E043. Rockville, MD: Agency for Healthcare Research and Quality. July 2003.

2. Fat-Soluble Vitamins and Nutrients

Vitamins A and E and Carotenoids
- Vitamin A
- Retinyl palmitate
- Retinyl stearate
- Vitamin E
- *gamma*-Tocopherol
- *alpha*-Carotene
- *trans-beta*-Carotene
- *cis-beta*-Carotene
- *beta*-Cryptoxanthin
- Lutein and zeaxanthin
- *trans*-Lycopene
- Total lycopene *(cis-* and *trans-)*

Vitamin D
- 25-Hydroxyvitamin D

Fatty Acids
Saturated
- Myristic acid (14:0)
- Palmitic acid (16:0)
- Stearic acid (18:0)
- Arachidic acid (20:0)
- Docosanoic acid (22:0)
- Lignoceric acid (24:0)

Monounsaturated
- Myristoleic acid (14:1n-5)
- Palmitoleic acid (16:1n-7)
- *cis*-Vaccenic acid (18:1n-7)
- Oleic acid (18:1n-9)
- Eicosenoic acid (20:1n-9)
- Docosenoic acid (22:1n-9)
- Nervonic acid (24:1n-9)

Polyunsaturated
- Linoleic acid (18:2n-6)
- *alpha*-Linolenic acid (18:3n-3)
- *gamma*-Linolenic acid (18:3n-6)
- Eicosadienoic acid (20:2n-6)
- *homo-gamma*-Linolenic acid (20:3n-6)
- Arachidonic acid (20:4n-6)
- Eicosapentaenoic acid (20:5n-3)
- Docosatetraenoic acid (22:4n-6)
- Docosapentaenoic acid (22:5n-3)
- Docosapentaenoic acid (22:5n-6)
- Docosahexaenoic acid (22:6n-3)

Vitamins A, E and Carotenoids

Background Information

Sources and Physiological Functions. Vitamins A (retinol) and E (*alpha*-tocopherol) and the carotenoids are fat-soluble micronutrients found in many foods, including some vegetables, fruits, meats, and animal products. Fish-liver oils, liver, egg yolks, butter, and cream are known for their higher content of vitamin A. Nuts and seeds are particularly rich sources of vitamin E (Thomas 2006). At least 700 carotenoids—fat-soluble red and yellow pigments—are found in nature (Britton 2004). Americans consume 40–50 of these carotenoids, primarily in fruits and vegetables (Khachik 1992), and smaller amounts in poultry products, including egg yolks, as well as in seafoods (Boylston 2007). Eight different carotenoids are easily measured in human serum: *alpha*-carotene, *cis*- and *trans-beta*-carotene, *beta*-cryptoxanthin, lutein, *cis*- and *trans*-lycopene, and zeaxanthin. Main sources of carotenes are orange-colored fruits and vegetables such as carrots, pumpkins, and mangos. Lutein and zeaxanthin are also found in dark green leafy vegetables, where any orange coloring is overshadowed by chlorophyll. *Trans*-lycopene is obtained primarily from tomatoes and tomato products and some fruits. For information on the carotenoid content of U.S. foods, see the 1998 carotenoid database created by the U.S. Department of Agriculture and the Nutrition Coordinating Center at the University of Minnesota (http://www.nal.usda.gov/fnic/foodcomp/Data/car98/car98.html).

Vitamin A, found in foods that come from animal sources, is called preformed vitamin A. Some carotenoids found in colorful fruits and vegetables are called provitamin A because they are metabolized in the body to vitamin A. Among the carotenoids, *beta*-carotene, a retinol dimer consisting of two linked retinol molecules, has the most significant provitamin A activity. Approximately 12 micrograms (μg) of dietary *beta*-carotene can provide the equivalent of 1 μg of retinol. Other provitamin A carotenoids, such as *alpha*-carotene and *beta*-cryptoxanthin, are half as active as *beta*-carotene (Institute of Medicine 2000). The bioconversion of carotenoids to vitamin A is highly variable from person to person (Krinsky 2005). Retinyl esters serve as the storage form of vitamin A and are mostly concentrated in the liver.

The absorption of fat-soluble micronutrients from the gastrointestinal tract depends on processes responsible for fat absorption or metabolism. Thus, people with conditions resulting in fat malabsorption (e.g., celiac disease, Crohn's disease, pancreatic disorders) can develop vitamin A deficiency over time. Vitamin A also has interactions with other nutrients. Iron and zinc deficiency can affect vitamin A metabolism and transport of vitamin A stores from the liver to body tissues (Institute of Medicine 2001). The absorption of carotenoids from foods is highly dependent on cooking techniques that break down plant cell walls and release carotenoids; it is also dependent on the availability of dietary fat to enhance carotenoid uptake (Krinsky 2005). The liver regulates the concentration of vitamin A in the circulation by releasing stored retinyl esters as needed; only when liver reserves are nearly exhausted does serum vitamin A fall into the deficient range (Napoli 2006). The variation in serum carotenoid concentrations among people in the United States is relatively large, primarily reflecting wide-ranging differences in dietary intake (Lacher 2005).

Vitamin E activity is derived from at least eight naturally occurring tocopherols, the most potent of which is *alpha*-tocopherol. Other less active forms of vitamin E are plentiful in the U.S. diet, with *gamma*-tocopherol being the predominant form. The most commonly consumed sources of *alpha*-tocopherol in the diet of American adults are mixed foods (spaghetti sauce, pizza and chili), fried potatoes, salad dressings, and bakery goods (Ahuja 2004). Other important sources are tomatoes, eggs, nuts and seeds, and snack foods. Plasma concentrations of tocopherols vary widely among healthy individuals and are highly correlated with plasma lipid concentrations (Ford 1999; Ford 2006).

Health Effects. Inadequate or excessive intake of vitamins A or E can lead to various disorders. For example, vitamin A deficiency, considered to be the main cause of childhood blindness in low-income countries (Roodhooft 2002), is a rare condition in the United States. Prominent signs of vitamin A deficiency include night blindness, corneal thinning, and conjunctival metaplasia. Vitamin A is also essential for proper immune function, epithelial growth and repair, bone growth, reproduction, and normal embryonic and fetal development (West 2006). Acute toxicity resulting from single or short-term large doses of preformed vitamin A is characterized by nausea, vomiting, headache, vertigo, blurred vision, increased cerebrospinal fluid pressure, and lack of muscular coordination. Central nervous system effects, liver abnormalities, bone and skin changes, and other nonspecific adverse effects can be indicative of chronic hypervitaminosis A. Consuming excess amounts of vitamin A during early pregnancy may lead to serious birth defects (Institute of Medicine 2001).

Serum or plasma concentrations of carotenoids are considered among the best biological markers for fruit and vegetable intake. The strongest dietary predictors of serum carotenoid concentrations are fruits (for sources of *beta*-cryptoxanthin), carrots and root vegetables (for sources of carotenes), and tomato products (for sources of *trans*-lycopene) (Al-Delaimy 2005). Research studies have shown inconsistencies in the relation between carotenoid intake and protection from cancer. Carotenoids in foods, even when consumed over long periods and in large amounts are not known to produce adverse health effects. However, results of intervention studies of smokers who used 20–30 milligrams (mg) of *beta*-carotene per day showed that this group had more lung cancers than placebo-treated groups (Albanes 1996; Redlich 1998).

Vitamin E deficiency occurs only rarely in people, and overt deficiency symptoms in people consuming low-vitamin E diets have never been described (Institute of Medicine 2000). The main manifestation of vitamin E deficiency is peripheral neuropathy characterized by the degeneration of the large-caliber axons of sensory neurons (Institute of Medicine 2000). The upper limit (UL) for vitamin E intake (1000 mg/day) is based on hemorrhagic effects; however, a causal association between excess *alpha*-tocopherol intake in apparently healthy individuals and adverse health outcomes has not consistently been shown (Institute of Medicine 2000). Studies evaluating tocopherols to reduce the risk for cardiovascular disease demonstrated inconsistent findings (Agency for Healthcare Research and Quality 2003). The American Heart Association currently advises that antioxidant supplements (such as vitamins E and C and *beta*-carotene) should not be used for primary or secondary prevention of cardiovascular disease (Lichtenstein 2006). Nevertheless, the American Heart Association recommends consuming food sources of antioxidant nutrients, principally from a variety of plant-derived foods such as fruits, vegetables, whole grains, and vegetable oils.

Intake Recommendations. The National Academy of Sciences has established dietary-requirement intake values for vitamins A and E by determining the Adequate Intake (AI) for infants and the recommended dietary allowance (RDA) for older age groups (Institute of Medicine 2000 and 2001). The RDA for vitamin A in retinol equivalents is 900 μg/day for men and 700 μg/day for women; for children and adolescents (1–18 years), the RDA ranges from 300–900 μg/day. For infants (0–12 months), the AI is set at 400–500 μg/day of retinol equivalents. The Tolerable Upper Intake Level (UL) for adults is set at 3,000 μg/day of preformed vitamin A, whereas the UL for infants (600 μg/day), younger children 1–8 years (600-900 μg/day), older children 9–13 years (1700 μg/day), and adolescents 14–18 years (2800 µg/day) are age-dependent. For adults, the RDA for vitamin E is 15 mg/day of *alpha*-tocopherol; for children and adolescents (1–18 years), the RDA ranges from 6–15 mg/day. There is no RDA for other forms of vitamin E, such as *gamma*-tocopherol. The UL for vitamin E which applies to all eight stereoisomers of *alpha*-tocopherol is 1000 mg/day for adults; a UL for infants could not be established and thus only food and formula sources of dietary intake are recommended. The UL for children and adolescents ranges from 200-800 mg/day of vitamin E. Although no quantitative recommendations are available for the intake of carotenoids, existing recommendations support increased consumption of carotenoid-rich fruits and vegetables. Current public health guidelines advise that people consume at least 2.5 cups of fruits and vegetables a day, depending on caloric need, to ensure adequate nutrient intake (U.S. Department of Agriculture and U.S. Department of Health and Human Services 2010).

Biochemical Indicators and Methods. The best way to determine inadequate vitamin A status is through hepatic biopsy, but this invasive procedure is unsuitable for population studies. Serum or plasma retinol is measured by use of high performance liquid chromatography (HPLC) with ultraviolet (UV) detection after separation from its carrier retinol binding protein (RBP). Because retinol is closely correlated with RBP, the measurement of this transport protein through enzyme-linked immunosorbent assay (ELISA) has also been used to assess vitamin A status. In most populations, serum RBP has been shown to be a suitable surrogate for retinol. Serum or plasma concentrations of carotenoids are measured by use of HPLC and visible light (450 nm) absorbance.

Clinical laboratories typically use conventional units for serum concentrations of these fat-soluble micronutrients (µg per deciliter [dL]). Conversion factors to international system (SI) units are 1 µg/dL = 0.0349 micromole per liter (µmol/L) for vitamin A and 1 µg/dL = 0.02322 µmol/L for vitamin E. Depending on its molecular weight, each carotenoid has a specific conversion factor.

International reference materials for vitamins A and E and carotenoids are available from the U.S. National Institutes of Standards and Technology (https://www-s.nist.gov/srmors/view_detail.cfm?srm=968e). Among most laboratories participating in an external quality assurance program, standardized HPLC methods for measuring fat-soluble micronutrients show consistent agreement of values (Duewer 2000).

The diagnosis of vitamin A or E deficiency is supported by measuring these concentrations in the body. People with serum retinol concentrations of less than 20 µg/dL are considered vitamin A deficient, and those with serum concentrations of less than 10 µg/dL are considered severely deficient (West 2006). Serum retinol values do not always reflect total body status because of homeostatic

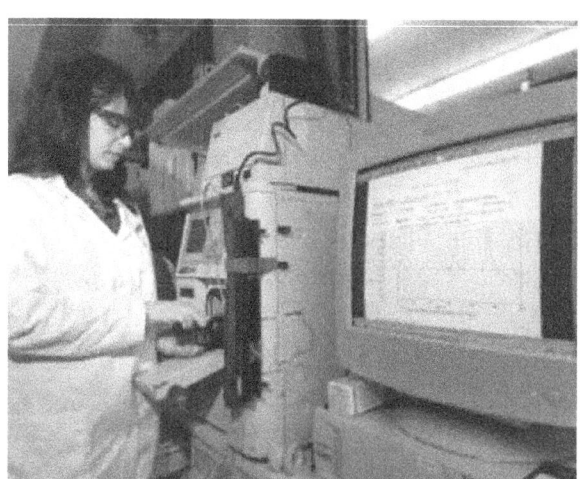

control and therefore are often not useful for assessing the vitamin A status of individuals. Additional tests may be required to confirm vitamin A deficiency when 20 µg/dL is used as a cutoff (Gibson 2005). The distribution of serum retinol values in a population together with the prevalence of individuals with serum retinol values below a given cutoff point provide important information about the vitamin A status of a population. WHO (2011) recommends using the prevalence of serum retinol concentrations of less than or equal to 20 µg/dL to define public health problems involving vitamin A deficiency as mild (2–9%), moderate (10–19%) or severe (≥20%). In chronic hypervitaminosis A, serum concentrations are generally greater than 100 µg/dL (Bendich 1989). Carotenoid deficiency has no defined serum concentrations. The laboratory diagnosis of vitamin E deficiency is based on serum concentrations of alpha-tocopherol (less than 500 µg/dL or less than 0.8 mg of alpha-tocopherol per gram of total lipids) (Beers 2006). Such concentrations are associated with in vitro hydrogen peroxide-induced red blood cell lysis, not with clinical deficiency symptoms (Institute of Medicine 2000).

Data in NHANES. The fat-soluble micronutrients vitamin A, E, and carotenoids presented in this report were measured by a single assay panel employing HPLC separation and detection by use of UV or visible light (HPLC-UV/vis). This is the same method used during the first four years of the continuous NHANES survey (1999-2002).

Since 1971, various fat-soluble micronutrients have been measured in the serum of NHANES participants. In NHANES III (1988–1994), clinically low concentrations of serum retinol were uncommon in U.S. residents aged 4 years and older, although racial/ethnic and socioeconomic differences existed (Ballew 2001). Variations in serum carotenoid concentrations by ethnicity and sex were found for adults, children, and adolescents (Ford 2000; Ford 2002). Ford *et al.* also found sociodemographic variations in serum concentrations of *alpha*-tocopherol among U.S. adults in NHANES III (1999) and *alpha-* and *gamma*-tocopherol in NHANES 1999–2000 (2006). Application of the most common cut-off value for serum *alpha*-tocopherol concentrations in NHANES 1999–2000 (500 µg/dL), demonstrated a low prevalence of vitamin E deficiency, despite the fact that the U.S. Department of Agriculture-estimated dietary intakes of vitamin E were low and that most of the U.S. population did not meet dietary intake recommendations.

For more information on these fat-soluble micronutrients, see the Institute of Medicine's Dietary Reference Intake reports (Institute of Medicine 2000 and 2001) and the vitamin fact sheets from the National Institutes of Health, Office of Dietary Supplements (http://ods.od.nih.gov/Health_Information/Vitamin_and_Mineral_Supplement_Fact_Sheets.aspx).

Highlights

Serum concentrations of fat-soluble micronutrients (vitamin A, E, and carotenoids) in the U.S. population showed the following demographic patterns and characteristics:

- With few exceptions, the highest concentrations of fat-soluble micronutrients were found in persons 60 years and older.
- No consistent pattern was observed with regard to gender or race/ethnicity.
- The likelihood of being vitamin A or E deficient was very low throughout the population.
- The likelihood of vitamin A excess was also very low, but it increased with increasing age.

For more than 20 years, the majority of the U.S. population (greater than 95%) has had adequate serum concentrations of vitamin A ($\geq$ 20 µg/dL) and vitamin E ($\geq$ 500 µg/dL).

Despite NHANES 2001–2002 dietary intake data demonstrating that 93% of the U.S. population consumed less than the Estimated Average Requirement (EAR) for vitamin E (Moshfegh 2005), for decades mean serum vitamin E concentrations have remained consistently adequate (Figure H.2.a), with less than 1% of the population vitamin E deficient. Analyses of NHANES data showed that in 1999–2000, 52% of adults (Rock 2007) and in 2003–2006, 49% of the total U.S. population (Bailey 2011) used dietary supplements; thus, the intake data (food and supplements) for vitamin E seem to be inconsistent with the biomarker data. Several explanatory possibilities have been raised, including a suggestion that the intake of fats (and fat-soluble nutrients) is under-reported in overweight and obese subjects, the database of food values is not accurate, and/or that the EAR for vitamin E needs adjustment. Low intake without widespread manifestation of deficiency suggests the need for further evaluations to determine whether improved estimates are necessary, either in the nutrient tables or in dietary intake.

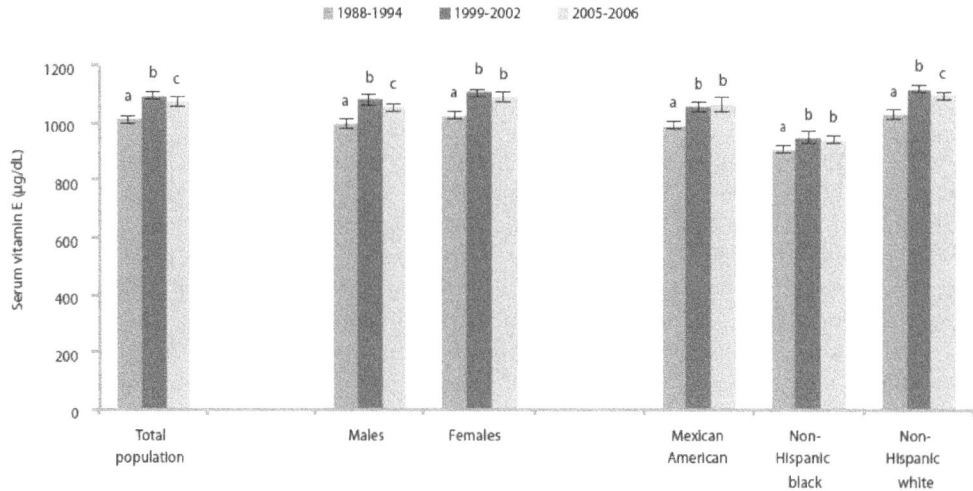

Figure H.2.a. *Age-adjusted geometric mean concentrations of serum vitamin E (alpha-tocopherol) in the U.S. population aged 6 years and older by gender or race/ethnicity, National Health and Nutrition Examination Survey, 1988–2006.*

Error bars represent 95% confidence intervals. Within a demographic group, bars not sharing a common letter differ (p < 0.05). Age adjustment was done using direct standardization.

Detailed Observations

The selected observations mentioned below are derived from the tables and figures presented next. Statements about categorical differences between demographic groups noted below are based on non-overlapping confidence limits from univariate analysis without adjusting for demographic variables (e.g., age, gender, race/ethnicity) or other blood concentration determinants (e.g., dietary intake, supplement usage, smoking, BMI). A multivariate analysis may alter the size and statistical significance of these categorical differences. Furthermore, additional significant differences of smaller magnitude may be present despite their lack of mention here (e.g., if confidence limits slightly overlap or if differences are not statistically significant before covariate adjustment has occurred). For a selection of citations of descriptive NHANES papers related to these biochemical indicators of diet and nutrition, see **Appendix G**.

Geometric mean concentrations (NHANES 2005–2006):

- Serum vitamin A concentrations increased with age (Table 2.1.a.1 and Figure 2.1.a).
- Serum retinyl palmitate concentrations were similar across age ranges, with a slight decrease in the adolescent years (Table 2.2.a.1 and Figure 2.2.a).
- Serum vitamin E concentrations decreased throughout childhood, then increased with age to concentrations higher than those seen in early childhood (Table 2.4.a.1and Figure 2.4.a), while serum *gamma*-tocopherol concentrations remained relatively constant throughout the life cycle, decreasing slightly in older persons (Table 2.5.a.1 and Figure 2.5.a).

- Serum *alpha*-carotene, *trans-beta*-carotene, and lutein/zeaxanthin concentrations decreased throughout childhood, then increased with age to concentrations higher than those seen in early childhood (Tables 2.6.a.1, 2.7.a.1, and 2.10.a.1 and Figures 2.6.a, 2.7.a, 2.10.a).

- Serum *beta*-cryptoxanthin concentrations decreased in early childhood and then remained steady (Table 2.9.a.1 and Figure 2.9.a).

- Serum *trans*-lycopene and total lycopene concentrations were highest in young adults and lowest in older persons (Tables 2.11.a.1 and 2.12.a.1 and Figures 2.11.a, 2.12.a).

- Females had higher serum vitamin E than males, while males had higher serum vitamin A concentrations than females (Tables 2.4.a.1 and 2.1.a.1).

- Females had higher serum *alpha*-carotene and *trans-beta*-carotene concentrations than males, and males had higher serum total lycopene concentrations than females (Tables 2.6.a.1, 2.7.a.1, and 2.12.a.1).

- Non-Hispanic whites had the highest concentrations of serum vitamin A and vitamin E, and the lowest concentrations of serum *gamma*-tocopherol. Non-Hispanic whites had the lowest concentrations of serum lutein/zeaxanthin. Non-Hispanic blacks had the lowest concentrations of serum *alpha*-carotene. Mexican Americans had the highest concentrations of serum *beta*-cryptoxanthin and the lowest concentrations of serum *trans*-lycopene and total lycopene. (Tables 2.1.a.1, 2.4.a.1, 2.5.a.1, 2.10.a.1, 2.6.a.1, 2.9.a.1, 2.11.a.1, and 2.12.a.1).

Changes in geometric mean concentrations across survey cycles:

- Serum vitamin A concentrations increased between 1999–2000 and 2001–2002, then held steady through the 2005–2006 survey period (Table 2.1.b).

- Serum vitamin E and *gamma*-tocopherol concentrations held steady between 1999–2000 and 2005–2006 (Tables 2.4.b and 2.5.b).

- Serum *alpha*-carotene, *trans-beta*-carotene, *beta*-cryptoxanthin, lutein/zeaxanthin, and *trans*-lycopene concentrations did not change appreciably across the survey cycles (Tables 2.6.b, 2.7.b, 2.9.b, 2.10.b, and 2.11.b).

- Prevalence estimates of low or high biochemical indicator concentrations:

- In 2005–2006, less than 1% of the population aged 6 years and older had a vitamin A or vitamin E deficiency, defined as < 20 µg/dL and < 500 µg/dL, respectively (Tables 2.1.c.1 and 2.4.c). About 2%, however, were at risk for an excess of vitamin A, or > 100 µg/dL (Table 2.1.c.2).

- Between 1999 and 2006, the prevalence of low serum vitamin A was less than 1% of all persons (Table 2.1.d.1), and the prevalence of high serum vitamin A was 1–2% of all persons (Table 2.1.d.2).

- Between 1999 and 2006, the prevalence of low serum vitamin E was 2% or less for almost all groups except for adolescents, for whom the prevalence was 2–4% (Table 2.4.d).

Table 2.1.a.1. Serum vitamin A: Concentrations

Geometric mean and selected percentiles of serum concentrations (in μg/dL) for the total U.S. population aged 6 years and older, National Health and Nutrition Examination Survey, 2005–2006.

	Geometric mean (95% conf. interval)	Selected percentiles (95% conf. interval)					Sample size
		2.5th	5th	50th	95th	97.5th	
Total, 6 years and older	54.7 (53.8 – 55.6)	29.6 (28.7 – 30.5)	32.5 (31.8 – 33.2)	55.2 (54.2 – 56.1)	87.8 (85.6 – 90.5)	96.7 (93.1 – 101)	7,254
Age group							
6–11 years	36.4 (35.6 – 37.2)	22.8 (19.9 – 24.8)	25.6 (24.3 – 26.9)	36.6 (35.9 – 37.3)	52.4 (49.1 – 54.3)	54.4 (53.3 – 57.3)	860
12–19 years	46.5 (45.4 – 47.7)	28.9 (28.6 – 29.6)	32.0 (30.6 – 33.0)	46.0 (44.6 – 47.5)	69.6 (66.9 – 73.1)	75.7 (71.4 – 82.9)	1,954
20–39 years	54.3 (53.3 – 55.3)	31.2 (29.2 – 32.1)	33.9 (32.2 – 35.1)	54.7 (53.5 – 55.6)	84.4 (81.9 – 87.9)	89.1 (87.2 – 93.3)	1,688
40–59 years	58.7 (57.7 – 59.7)	33.1 (31.4 – 34.2)	36.8 (36.0 – 38.0)	59.5 (58.1 – 60.4)	90.3 (87.2 – 94.3)	100 (94.7 – 107)	1,365
60 years and older	64.4 (62.8 – 66.1)	36.4 (31.6 – 38.8)	40.2 (38.2 – 43.0)	64.9 (63.1 – 67.0)	99.8 (96.2 – 102)	108 (105 – 115)	1,387
Gender							
Males	57.2 (56.3 – 58.2)	30.3 (29.2 – 31.2)	33.6 (32.7 – 34.8)	58.0 (57.1 – 59.0)	89.0 (86.5 – 93.0)	100 (93.3 – 104)	3,547
Females	52.4 (51.3 – 53.5)	28.9 (27.7 – 30.1)	31.9 (31.2 – 32.6)	52.4 (50.8 – 53.8)	85.9 (83.3 – 88.7)	94.8 (89.8 – 103)	3,707
Race/ethnicity							
Mexican Americans	48.4 (47.3 – 49.5)	27.8 (26.2 – 28.6)	30.3 (29.3 – 31.2)	48.8 (46.8 – 50.2)	73.7 (71.9 – 77.0)	82.1 (76.2 – 88.4)	1,844
Non-Hispanic Blacks	48.3 (47.3 – 49.3)	25.7 (23.8 – 27.5)	28.8 (27.6 – 29.8)	48.1 (47.0 – 49.5)	82.0 (78.4 – 85.5)	89.7 (86.1 – 93.6)	1,891
Non-Hispanic Whites	57.4 (56.4 – 58.4)	31.5 (30.6 – 32.4)	34.8 (33.0 – 36.2)	57.9 (56.8 – 59.0)	89.8 (87.6 – 93.3)	100 (95.6 – 104)	2,973

Figure 2.1.a. Serum vitamin A: Concentrations by age group

Geometric mean (95% confidence interval), National Health and Nutrition Examination Survey, 2005–2006

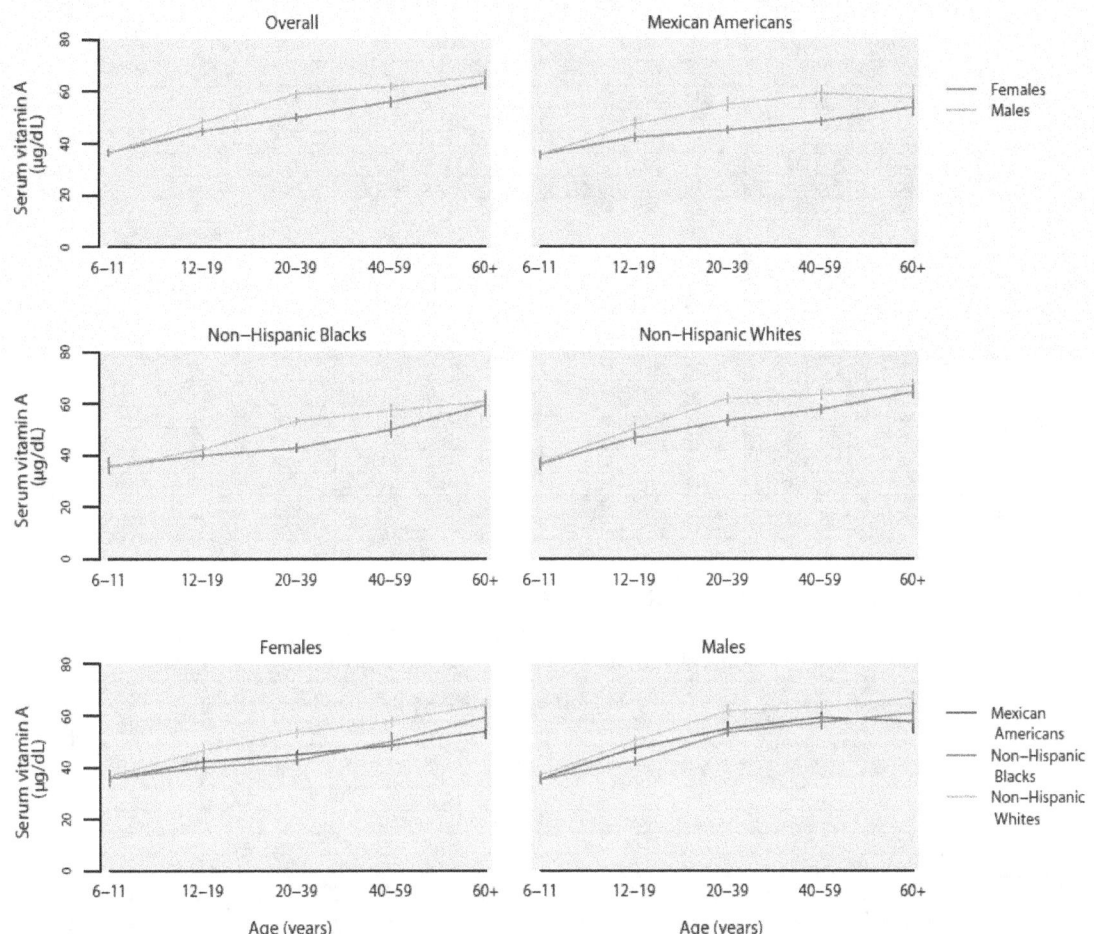

Table 2.1.a.2. Serum vitamin A: Total population

Geometric mean and selected percentiles of serum concentrations (in µg/dL) for the total U.S. population aged 6 years and older, National Health and Nutrition Examination Survey, 2005–2006.

	Geometric mean (95% conf. interval)		Selected percentiles (95% conf. interval)						Sample size
			10th		50th		90th		
Males and Females									
Total, 6 years and older	54.7	(53.8 – 55.6)	36.6	(35.8 – 37.4)	55.2	(54.2 – 56.1)	80.0	(78.1 – 82.2)	7,254
6–11 years	36.4	(35.6 – 37.2)	28.0	(27.5 – 29.1)	36.6	(35.9 – 37.3)	47.5	(45.7 – 50.1)	860
12–19 years	46.5	(45.4 – 47.7)	35.2	(33.9 – 35.9)	46.0	(44.6 – 47.5)	63.2	(60.7 – 66.9)	1,954
20–39 years	54.3	(53.3 – 55.3)	38.1	(36.5 – 39.2)	54.7	(53.5 – 55.6)	77.7	(74.1 – 81.6)	1,688
40–59 years	58.7	(57.7 – 59.7)	41.2	(39.5 – 43.0)	59.5	(58.1 – 60.4)	81.0	(79.0 – 85.2)	1,365
60 years and older	64.4	(62.8 – 66.1)	46.4	(44.7 – 47.9)	64.9	(63.1 – 67.0)	88.4	(86.0 – 91.7)	1,387
Males									
Total, 6 years and older	57.2	(56.3 – 58.2)	38.5	(37.8 – 39.2)	58.0	(57.1 – 59.0)	81.8	(79.7 – 85.0)	3,547
6–11 years	36.4	(35.4 – 37.3)	28.1	(26.4 – 29.1)	36.3	(35.0 – 37.2)	47.5	(45.7 – 51.6)	427
12–19 years	48.2	(46.9 – 49.6)	36.4	(35.3 – 37.7)	48.1	(46.3 – 49.8)	64.5	(62.9 – 67.4)	980
20–39 years	59.1	(57.7 – 60.5)	44.4	(42.3 – 46.0)	58.4	(56.8 – 60.2)	80.9	(76.8 – 84.5)	738
40–59 years	61.8	(60.7 – 63.0)	44.2	(41.6 – 47.1)	63.2	(62.4 – 64.2)	84.5	(80.1 – 92.0)	673
60 years and older	66.0	(63.9 – 68.1)	48.4	(46.0 – 50.0)	66.4	(63.7 – 68.7)	90.4	(86.3 – 97.2)	729
Females									
Total, 6 years and older	52.4	(51.3 – 53.5)	35.6	(34.3 – 36.4)	52.4	(50.8 – 53.8)	77.5	(75.0 – 79.0)	3,707
6–11 years	36.5	(35.3 – 37.8)	28.0	(27.5 – 29.4)	36.9	(35.9 – 38.0)	47.0	(45.1 – 52.3)	433
12–19 years	44.7	(43.5 – 45.9)	33.7	(33.3 – 35.0)	43.8	(42.7 – 45.1)	60.7	(57.0 – 66.6)	974
20–39 years	50.0	(48.7 – 51.3)	34.5	(32.7 – 36.1)	49.3	(48.3 – 50.9)	72.6	(69.5 – 75.9)	950
40–59 years	55.9	(54.1 – 57.7)	39.9	(36.9 – 41.2)	55.8	(53.8 – 58.5)	78.4	(74.2 – 82.8)	692
60 years and older	63.2	(61.3 – 65.2)	45.1	(43.0 – 47.2)	63.9	(62.5 – 65.7)	87.7	(84.0 – 91.2)	658

Table 2.1.a.3. Serum vitamin A: Mexican Americans

Geometric mean and selected percentiles of serum concentrations (in µg/dL) for Mexican Americans in the U.S. population aged 6 years and older, National Health and Nutrition Examination Survey, 2005–2006.

	Geometric mean (95% conf. interval)		Selected percentiles (95% conf. interval)						Sample size
			10th		50th		90th		
Males and Females									
Total, 6 years and older	48.4	(47.3 – 49.5)	33.4	(32.6 – 34.2)	48.8	(46.8 – 50.2)	68.6	(66.7 – 70.3)	1,844
6–11 years	35.6	(34.4 – 37.0)	27.6	(24.8 – 28.9)	35.8	(33.8 – 37.6)	46.2	(45.0 – 48.2)	295
12–19 years	44.9	(43.3 – 46.4)	34.1	(33.4 – 35.0)	44.4	(43.2 – 46.1)	58.8	(55.6 – 64.7)	646
20–39 years	50.1	(49.1 – 51.2)	36.0	(33.3 – 37.3)	50.3	(48.7 – 53.3)	69.1	(66.8 – 72.7)	449
40–59 years	53.6	(52.4 – 54.8)	39.0	(36.6 – 41.0)	52.6	(50.7 – 55.6)	71.7	(67.2 – 85.3)	246
60 years and older	55.5	(52.8 – 58.3)	40.8	(37.3 – 42.8)	57.0	(54.7 – 58.4)	78.1	(72.9 – 85.4)	208
Males									
Total, 6 years and older	51.9	(50.0 – 53.9)	36.5	(33.7 – 38.5)	53.3	(50.2 – 55.9)	70.7	(68.8 – 73.3)	883
6–11 years	35.6	(33.9 – 37.4)	27.2	(24.0 – 28.8)	35.4	(33.0 – 38.7)	46.8	(45.6 – 49.1)	145
12–19 years	47.4	(45.6 – 49.3)	36.1	(33.8 – 38.0)	47.0	(45.0 – 48.6)	60.9	(58.7 – 65.7)	313
20–39 years	54.8	(52.4 – 57.3)	41.3	(36.6 – 43.9)	56.0	(54.0 – 59.0)	70.6	(68.0 – 74.3)	198
40–59 years	59.1	(56.0 – 62.3)	45.8	(42.9 – 47.4)	57.9	(53.9 – 63.1)	77.7	(70.5 – 110)	122
60 years and older	57.6	(53.3 – 62.3)	42.6†	(19.8 – 47.4)	57.6	(55.1 – 62.0)	79.5†	(70.6 – 93.0)	105
Females									
Total, 6 years and older	44.7	(44.0 – 45.5)	32.1	(31.3 – 32.7)	43.7	(42.7 – 45.2)	64.2	(62.1 – 67.0)	961
6–11 years	35.7	(34.6 – 36.8)	28.0	(24.0 – 29.4)	36.0	(34.3 – 37.6)	45.7	(42.2 – 52.7)	150
12–19 years	42.3	(41.0 – 43.7)	33.3	(32.2 – 33.8)	41.6	(40.2 – 43.0)	55.9	(52.3 – 61.5)	333
20–39 years	45.0	(43.9 – 46.2)	31.9	(29.8 – 33.8)	43.2	(41.7 – 46.6)	66.6	(61.2 – 69.5)	251
40–59 years	48.4	(47.1 – 49.7)	35.6	(32.4 – 37.4)	49.1	(46.5 – 50.2)	63.9	(57.7 – 81.3)	124
60 years and older	53.8	(50.9 – 56.9)	39.4†	(32.9 – 42.3)	53.5	(51.4 – 58.9)	75.9†	(72.9 – 83.0)	103

† Estimate is subject to greater uncertainty due to small cell size.

Table 2.1.a.4. Serum vitamin A: Non-Hispanic blacks

Geometric mean and selected percentiles of serum concentrations (in µg/dL) for non-Hispanic blacks in the U.S. population aged 6 years and older, National Health and Nutrition Examination Survey, 2005–2006.

	Geometric mean (95% conf. interval)		Selected percentiles (95% conf. interval)						Sample size
			10th		50th		90th		
Males and Females									
Total, 6 years and older	48.3	(47.3 – 49.3)	32.0	(31.2 – 32.8)	48.1	(47.0 – 49.5)	72.1	(70.0 – 75.1)	1,891
6–11 years	35.6	(34.0 – 37.3)	26.6	(24.0 – 28.5)	35.7	(34.5 – 36.8)	47.3	(44.6 – 51.8)	240
12–19 years	41.1	(40.0 – 42.2)	30.5	(29.4 – 31.3)	40.9	(39.7 – 42.6)	54.2	(52.8 – 57.5)	665
20–39 years	47.3	(45.8 – 48.9)	32.3	(29.8 – 35.3)	47.9	(44.9 – 50.5)	67.7	(63.6 – 71.6)	368
40–59 years	53.2	(51.4 – 55.0)	35.4	(33.3 – 37.2)	53.7	(50.3 – 57.2)	77.1	(72.8 – 85.7)	335
60 years and older	59.9	(56.3 – 63.7)	40.1	(36.2 – 45.6)	60.7	(56.6 – 64.5)	85.1	(78.8 – 91.4)	283
Males									
Total, 6 years and older	51.2	(49.9 – 52.5)	34.0	(32.9 – 35.2)	51.9	(50.2 – 53.6)	74.8	(70.9 – 79.0)	949
6–11 years	35.4	(34.1 – 36.8)	26.2	(23.2 – 28.7)	35.3	(33.5 – 36.6)	46.2	(43.7 – 51.9)	128
12–19 years	42.2	(40.8 – 43.7)	30.6	(28.8 – 32.0)	42.0	(39.7 – 44.7)	58.1	(55.1 – 60.7)	343
20–39 years	53.3	(52.1 – 54.5)	38.9	(35.7 – 40.4)	54.1	(52.3 – 55.5)	71.2	(65.9 – 77.7)	170
40–59 years	57.3	(54.9 – 59.8)	39.0	(35.8 – 42.6)	58.4	(54.0 – 62.9)	84.8	(74.8 – 92.7)	156
60 years and older	60.8	(57.0 – 64.9)	40.0	(33.9 – 46.7)	62.5	(59.9 – 64.7)	86.0	(78.4 – 110)	152
Females									
Total, 6 years and older	45.9	(44.7 – 47.1)	31.1	(29.4 – 32.1)	44.9	(43.5 – 46.7)	70.1	(65.9 – 74.6)	942
6–11 years	35.8	(33.0 – 39.0)	26.7	(19.8 – 28.8)	36.1	(33.0 – 38.8)	47.6	(44.2 – 54.2)	112
12–19 years	39.9	(38.7 – 41.2)	30.1	(29.4 – 30.8)	40.2	(38.7 – 41.7)	51.1	(49.9 – 53.1)	322
20–39 years	42.7	(41.1 – 44.3)	29.2	(24.3 – 32.0)	42.4	(40.4 – 44.5)	60.4	(57.4 – 63.5)	198
40–59 years	49.9	(46.8 – 53.3)	33.4	(31.9 – 34.3)	48.8	(45.9 – 53.5)	73.3	(68.1 – 84.7)	179
60 years and older	59.3	(55.4 – 63.4)	39.8	(36.7 – 43.8)	60.3	(54.6 – 64.5)	84.9	(77.9 – 90.2)	131

Table 2.1.a.5. Serum vitamin A: Non-Hispanic whites

Geometric mean and selected percentiles of serum concentrations (in µg/dL) for non-Hispanic whites in the U.S. population aged 6 years and older, National Health and Nutrition Examination Survey, 2005–2006.

	Geometric mean (95% conf. interval)		Selected percentiles (95% conf. interval)						Sample size
			10th		50th		90th		
Males and Females									
Total, 6 years and older	57.4	(56.4 – 58.4)	39.0	(37.8 – 40.0)	57.9	(56.8 – 59.0)	82.0	(79.8 – 85.3)	2,973
6–11 years	36.8	(35.5 – 38.2)	28.6	(26.6 – 30.1)	37.1	(35.4 – 38.2)	47.6	(45.3 – 53.0)	231
12–19 years	48.5	(46.8 – 50.2)	37.0	(35.5 – 38.4)	48.3	(45.9 – 50.0)	66.2	(63.1 – 69.3)	499
20–39 years	57.5	(55.9 – 59.1)	41.4	(39.1 – 43.0)	57.1	(56.0 – 58.6)	81.4	(77.1 – 85.6)	714
40–59 years	60.4	(59.2 – 61.6)	43.3	(41.2 – 45.6)	60.5	(59.3 – 62.6)	81.9	(79.2 – 88.0)	683
60 years and older	65.4	(63.8 – 67.0)	47.1	(45.3 – 48.8)	66.0	(63.8 – 67.9)	89.5	(86.7 – 92.6)	846
Males									
Total, 6 years and older	59.7	(58.5 – 60.9)	40.9	(39.4 – 41.9)	60.4	(58.9 – 62.1)	84.1	(80.7 – 87.8)	1,472
6–11 years	37.0	(35.6 – 38.6)	28.6	(25.1 – 30.3)	37.0	(35.1 – 38.4)	47.4	(45.3 – 53.2)	112
12–19 years	50.2	(48.3 – 52.2)	38.5	(35.2 – 40.4)	49.8	(47.5 – 52.0)	66.8	(64.3 – 69.7)	254
20–39 years	61.8	(59.9 – 63.8)	47.1	(45.1 – 48.4)	60.8	(58.3 – 63.5)	83.8	(79.8 – 87.8)	309
40–59 years	63.3	(61.5 – 65.2)	45.3	(40.1 – 49.9)	64.0	(62.7 – 66.1)	85.0	(80.0 – 101)	351
60 years and older	66.8	(64.6 – 69.0)	49.7	(46.1 – 50.4)	67.1	(63.8 – 70.2)	90.6	(87.3 – 99.0)	446
Females									
Total, 6 years and older	55.3	(54.1 – 56.4)	37.6	(36.2 – 39.2)	55.6	(54.4 – 56.6)	79.8	(78.2 – 82.4)	1,501
6–11 years	36.6	(34.5 – 38.9)	28.2	(26.0 – 30.5)	37.1	(34.9 – 38.9)	48.1	(44.3 – 54.7)	119
12–19 years	46.6	(44.6 – 48.8)	35.9	(33.4 – 37.4)	45.5	(43.1 – 48.5)	63.7	(59.5 – 70.1)	245
20–39 years	53.5	(51.6 – 55.3)	36.7	(34.2 – 39.7)	53.1	(51.2 – 54.9)	76.1	(72.8 – 83.1)	405
40–59 years	57.7	(56.0 – 59.4)	41.6	(40.2 – 43.5)	57.7	(55.6 – 59.6)	79.1	(75.6 – 83.9)	332
60 years and older	64.3	(62.2 – 66.5)	46.4	(44.5 – 48.3)	64.8	(62.7 – 67.4)	87.9	(84.1 – 95.0)	400

Table 2.1.b. Serum vitamin A: Concentrations by survey cycle

Geometric mean and selected percentiles of serum concentrations (in µg/dL) for the U.S. population, National Health and Nutrition Examination Survey, 1999–2002 and 2005–2006.

	Geometric mean (95% conf. interval)	Selected percentiles (95% conf. interval) 5th	50th	95th	Sample size
Total, 6 years and older					
1999–2000	52.8 (51.8 – 53.8)	30.7 (29.8 – 31.6)	53.5 (52.2 – 54.9)	85.6 (83.9 – 87.2)	7,102
2001–2002	55.2 (54.1 – 56.4)	32.6 (31.8 – 33.5)	56.0 (54.7 – 57.3)	88.4 (86.6 – 91.6)	7,935
2005–2006	54.7 (53.8 – 55.6)	32.5 (31.8 – 33.2)	55.2 (54.2 – 56.1)	87.8 (85.6 – 90.5)	7,254
Age group					
3–5 years					
1999–2000	32.3 (31.6 – 33.1)	22.0 (19.0 – 23.1)	33.1 (31.5 – 34.6)	46.2 (41.1 – 66.3)	352
2001–2002	33.8 (33.1 – 34.6)	24.3 (16.5 – 25.5)	34.0 (33.1 – 35.2)	47.1 (44.3 – 50.3)	430
6–11 years					
1999–2000	35.1 (34.5 – 35.6)	25.3 (23.6 – 26.1)	35.4 (35.0 – 35.8)	48.5 (46.1 – 52.3)	866
2001–2002	37.3 (36.2 – 38.5)	26.5 (25.8 – 27.4)	37.3 (36.2 – 39.0)	51.6 (50.1 – 54.0)	1,014
2005–2006	36.4 (35.6 – 37.2)	25.6 (24.3 – 26.9)	36.6 (35.9 – 37.3)	52.4 (49.1 – 54.3)	860
12–19 years					
1999–2000	45.7 (44.7 – 46.6)	30.1 (29.1 – 30.9)	45.8 (45.0 – 46.9)	69.4 (66.9 – 71.8)	2,111
2001–2002	48.0 (47.1 – 48.9)	31.8 (30.4 – 33.3)	48.5 (47.6 – 49.3)	71.2 (69.0 – 74.2)	2,206
2005–2006	46.5 (45.4 – 47.7)	32.0 (30.6 – 33.0)	46.0 (44.6 – 47.5)	69.6 (66.9 – 73.1)	1,954
20–39 years					
1999–2000	52.1 (50.8 – 53.4)	33.0 (31.1 – 34.3)	52.8 (51.2 – 54.5)	80.3 (77.9 – 83.0)	1,461
2001–2002	54.8 (53.3 – 56.3)	34.2 (32.6 – 35.3)	55.8 (54.4 – 57.5)	83.4 (80.9 – 86.6)	1,716
2005–2006	54.3 (53.3 – 55.3)	33.9 (32.2 – 35.1)	54.7 (53.5 – 55.6)	84.4 (81.9 – 87.9)	1,688
40–59 years					
1999–2000	59.0 (57.6 – 60.6)	35.9 (34.2 – 38.1)	59.8 (57.9 – 61.5)	90.4 (86.4 – 96.8)	1,191
2001–2002	60.3 (59.2 – 61.5)	37.5 (34.8 – 39.9)	61.2 (59.8 – 62.7)	94.6 (90.3 – 97.8)	1,474
2005–2006	58.7 (57.7 – 59.7)	36.8 (36.0 – 38.0)	59.5 (58.1 – 60.4)	90.3 (87.2 – 94.3)	1,365
60 years and older					
1999–2000	62.5 (61.1 – 64.0)	39.7 (36.3 – 41.9)	63.0 (61.3 – 65.0)	94.3 (90.1 – 99.5)	1,473
2001–2002	65.0 (63.6 – 66.5)	40.3 (38.0 – 41.4)	65.4 (64.1 – 67.4)	102 (98.6 – 108)	1,525
2005–2006	64.4 (62.8 – 66.1)	40.2 (38.2 – 43.0)	64.9 (63.1 – 67.0)	99.8 (96.2 – 102)	1,387
Gender					
(6 years and older)					
Males					
1999–2000	55.8 (54.4 – 57.3)	31.9 (30.1 – 33.8)	57.5 (55.8 – 58.8)	86.3 (84.6 – 90.6)	3,450
2001–2002	58.5 (57.2 – 59.8)	34.4 (33.4 – 35.5)	59.8 (58.0 – 61.7)	91.5 (88.7 – 93.7)	3,841
2005–2006	57.2 (56.3 – 58.2)	33.6 (32.7 – 34.8)	58.0 (57.1 – 59.0)	89.0 (86.5 – 93.0)	3,547
Females					
1999–2000	50.1 (49.1 – 51.1)	30.2 (28.7 – 31.2)	50.0 (48.8 – 51.0)	84.1 (81.2 – 87.0)	3,652
2001–2002	52.3 (51.1 – 53.5)	31.7 (30.9 – 32.4)	52.5 (51.0 – 53.9)	86.6 (84.0 – 88.3)	4,094
2005–2006	52.4 (51.3 – 53.5)	31.9 (31.2 – 32.6)	52.4 (50.8 – 53.8)	85.9 (83.3 – 88.7)	3,707
Race/ethnicity					
(6 years and older)					
Mexican Americans					
1999–2000	47.0 (46.1 – 47.8)	29.0 (28.0 – 29.7)	46.9 (45.5 – 48.3)	75.6 (73.6 – 79.0)	2,410
2001–2002	48.6 (47.2 – 50.0)	29.8 (28.8 – 30.7)	48.8 (47.4 – 50.4)	76.6 (73.4 – 82.1)	1,991
2005–2006	48.4 (47.3 – 49.5)	30.3 (29.3 – 31.2)	48.8 (46.8 – 50.2)	73.7 (71.9 – 77.0)	1,844
Non-Hispanic Blacks					
1999–2000	45.8 (44.2 – 47.4)	27.8 (26.4 – 28.3)	45.4 (43.1 – 47.6)	75.7 (72.5 – 81.1)	1,590
2001–2002	47.2 (46.1 – 48.3)	28.2 (27.4 – 28.9)	47.0 (45.3 – 48.6)	80.2 (77.3 – 85.7)	1,864
2005–2006	48.3 (47.3 – 49.3)	28.8 (27.6 – 29.8)	48.1 (47.0 – 49.5)	82.0 (78.4 – 85.5)	1,891
Non-Hispanic Whites					
1999–2000	55.6 (54.2 – 57.1)	33.4 (31.2 – 34.7)	56.8 (55.0 – 58.2)	87.3 (85.4 – 90.5)	2,456
2001–2002	57.9 (56.4 – 59.5)	34.7 (33.1 – 36.2)	58.9 (56.8 – 60.7)	91.3 (88.9 – 93.5)	3,455
2005–2006	57.4 (56.4 – 58.4)	34.8 (33.0 – 36.2)	57.9 (56.8 – 59.0)	89.8 (87.6 – 93.3)	2,973

Figure 2.1.b. Serum vitamin A: Concentrations by survey cycle

Selected percentiles in µg/dL (95% confidence intervals), National Health and Nutrition Examination Survey, 1999–2002 and 2005–2006

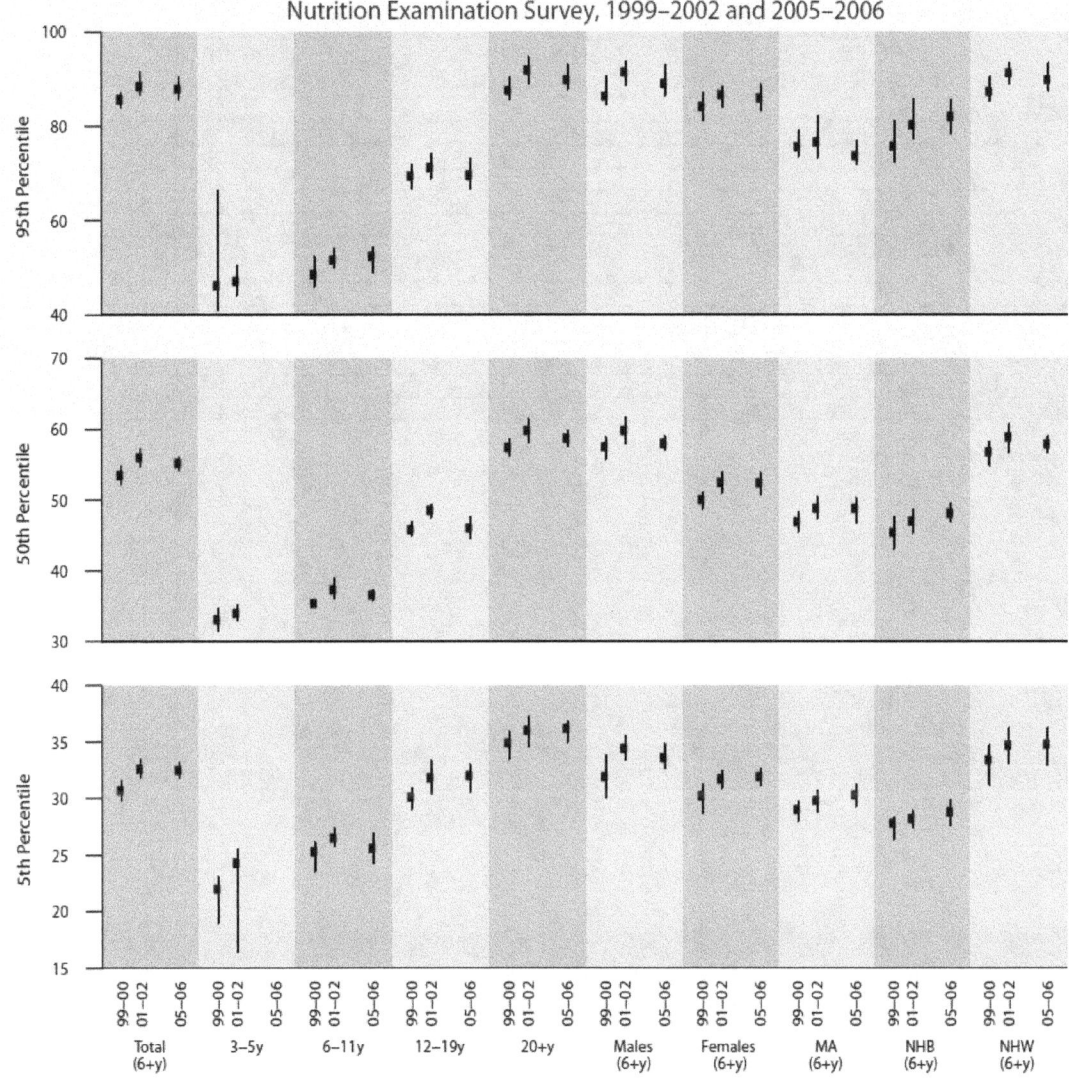

Table 2.1.c.1. Serum vitamin A: Prevalence

Prevalence (in percent) of low serum vitamin A concentration (< 20 μg/dL) for the U.S. population aged 6 years and older, National Health and Nutrition Examination Survey, 2005–2006.

	Sample size	Prevalence (95% conf. interval)	Estimated total number of persons
Total, 6 years and older	7,254	0.3 (0.1 – 0.5)	711,000
Age group			
6–11 years	860	1.0 (0.6 – 1.5)	231,000
12–19 years	1,954	§	§
20–39 years	1,688	§	§
40–59 years	1,365	§	§
60 years and older	1,387	§	§
Gender			
Males	3,547	§	§
Females	3,707	0.2‡ (0.1 – 0.4)	317,000‡
Race/ethnicity			
Mexican Americans	1,844	§	§
Non-Hispanic Blacks	1,891	0.5 (0.3 – 0.7)	145,000
Non-Hispanic Whites	2,973	0.2‡ (0.1 – 0.5)	386,000‡

‡ Estimate flagged: 30% ≤ RSE < 40% for the prevalence estimate.
§ Estimate suppressed: RSE ≥ 40% for the prevalence estimate.

Table 2.1.c.2. Serum vitamin A: Prevalence

Prevalence (in percent) of high serum vitamin A concentration (> 100 µg/dL) for the U.S. population aged 6 years and older, National Health and Nutrition Examination Survey, 2005–2006.

	Sample size	Prevalence (95% conf. interval)		Estimated total number of persons
Total, 6 years and older	7,254	2.1	(1.6 – 2.7)	5,573,000
Age group				
6–11 years	860	§		§
12–19 years	1,954	§		§
20–39 years	1,688	1.1‡	(0.5 – 2.3)	847,000‡
40–59 years	1,365	2.7	(1.8 – 3.9)	2,182,000
60 years and older	1,387	4.8	(3.8 – 6.0)	2,301,000
Gender				
Males	3,547	2.5	(1.8 – 3.4)	3,265,000
Females	3,707	1.7	(1.0 – 2.9)	2,306,000
Race/ethnicity				
Mexican Americans	1,844	0.5‡	(0.3 – 1.1)	129,000‡
Non-Hispanic Blacks	1,891	1.1	(0.6 – 2.0)	348,000
Non-Hispanic Whites	2,973	2.6	(2.0 – 3.5)	4,752,000

‡ Estimate flagged: 30% ≤ RSE < 40% for the prevalence estimate.
§ Estimate suppressed: RSE ≥ 40% for the prevalence estimate.

Table 2.1.d.1. Serum vitamin A: Prevalence by survey cycle

Prevalence (in percent) of low serum vitamin A concentration (< 20 µg/dL) for the U.S. population, National Health and Nutrition Examination Survey, 1999–2002 and 2005–2006.

	Sample size	Prevalence (95% conf. interval)	Estimated total number of persons
Total, 6 years and older			
1999–2000	7,102	0.1 (0.1 – 0.2)	360,000
2001–2002	7,935	0.3 (0.2 – 0.4)	698,000
2005–2006	7,254	0.3 (0.1 – 0.5)	711,000
Age group			
3–5 years			
1999–2000	352	§	§
2001–2002	430	§	§
6–11 years			
1999–2000	866	1.0 (0.6 – 1.6)	243,000
2001–2002	1,014	§	§
2005–2006	860	1.0 (0.6 – 1.5)	231,000
12–19 years			
1999–2000	2,111	§	§
2001–2002	2,206	§	§
2005–2006	1,954	§	§
20–39 years			
1999–2000	1,461	§	§
2001–2002	1,716	§	§
2005–2006	1,688	§	§
40–59 years			
1999–2000	1,191	§	§
2001–2002	1,474	§	§
2005–2006	1,365	§	§
60 years and older			
1999–2000	1,473	§	§
2001–2002	1,525	§	§
2005–2006	1,387	§	§
Gender			
(6 years and older)			
Males			
1999–2000	3,450	0.1‡ (0.1 – 0.3)	179,000‡
2001–2002	3,841	0.4 (0.2 – 0.7)	456,000
2005–2006	3,547	§	§
Females			
1999–2000	3,652	0.1 (0.1 – 0.2)	181,000
2001–2002	4,094	0.2‡ (0.1 – 0.4)	242,000‡
2005–2006	3,707	0.2‡ (0.1 – 0.4)	317,000‡
Race/ethnicity			
(6 years and older)			
Mexican Americans			
1999–2000	2,410	0.4‡ (0.2 – 0.8)	75,000‡
2001–2002	1,991	§	§
2005–2006	1,844	§	§
Non-Hispanic Blacks			
1999–2000	1,590	0.5 (0.3 – 0.8)	153,000
2001–2002	1,864	0.7 (0.3 – 1.2)	201,000
2005–2006	1,891	0.5 (0.3 – 0.7)	145,000
Non-Hispanic Whites			
1999–2000	2,456	§	§
2001–2002	3,455	0.2‡ (0.1 – 0.5)	398,000‡
2005–2006	2,973	0.2‡ (0.1 – 0.5)	386,000‡

‡ Estimate flagged: 30% ≤ RSE < 40% for the prevalence estimate.
§ Estimate suppressed: RSE ≥ 40% for the prevalence estimate.

Table 2.1.d.2. Serum vitamin A: Prevalence by survey cycle

Prevalence (in percent) of high serum vitamin A concentration (> 100 μg/dL) for the U.S. population, National Health and Nutrition Examination Survey, 1999–2002 and 2005–2006.

	Sample size	Prevalence (95% conf. interval)	Estimated total number of persons
Total, 6 years and older			
1999–2000	7,102	1.3 (1.0 – 1.8)	3,312,000
2001–2002	7,935	2.0 (1.6 – 2.5)	5,242,000
2005–2006	7,254	2.1 (1.6 – 2.7)	5,573,000
Age group			
3–5 years			
1999–2000	352	§	§
2001–2002	430	§	§
6–11 years			
1999–2000	866	§	§
2001–2002	1,014	§	§
2005–2006	860	§	§
12–19 years			
1999–2000	2,111	§	§
2001–2002	2,206	§	§
2005–2006	1,954	§	§
20–39 years			
1999–2000	1,461	§	§
2001–2002	1,716	0.6‡ (0.2 – 1.3)	437,000‡
2005–2006	1,688	1.1‡ (0.5 – 2.3)	847,000‡
40–59 years			
1999–2000	1,191	2.4 (1.4 – 4.0)	1,688,000
2001–2002	1,474	2.9 (2.0 – 4.4)	2,222,000
2005–2006	1,365	2.7 (1.8 – 3.9)	2,182,000
60 years and older			
1999–2000	1,473	3.2 (2.1 – 4.8)	1,381,000
2001–2002	1,525	5.9 (4.3 – 8.0)	2,628,000
2005–2006	1,387	4.8 (3.8 – 6.0)	2,301,000
Gender			
(6 years and older)			
Males			
1999–2000	3,450	1.4 (0.9 – 2.4)	1,741,000
2001–2002	3,841	2.4 (1.9 – 3.0)	3,013,000
2005–2006	3,547	2.5 (1.8 – 3.4)	3,265,000
Females			
1999–2000	3,652	1.2 (0.7 – 2.0)	1,570,000
2001–2002	4,094	1.7 (1.2 – 2.4)	2,226,000
2005–2006	3,707	1.7 (1.0 – 2.9)	2,306,000
Race/ethnicity			
(6 years and older)			
Mexican Americans			
1999–2000	2,410	§	§
2001–2002	1,991	§	§
2005–2006	1,844	0.5‡ (0.3 – 1.1)	129,000‡
Non-Hispanic Blacks			
1999–2000	1,590	1.2 (0.7 – 2.2)	376,000
2001–2002	1,864	1.7‡ (0.8 – 3.7)	519,000‡
2005–2006	1,891	1.1 (0.6 – 2.0)	348,000
Non-Hispanic Whites			
1999–2000	2,456	1.7 (1.2 – 2.4)	2,962,000
2001–2002	3,455	2.4 (1.9 – 2.9)	4,296,000
2005–2006	2,973	2.6 (2.0 – 3.5)	4,752,000

‡ Estimate flagged: 30% ≤ RSE < 40% for the prevalence estimate.
§ Estimate suppressed: RSE ≥ 40% for the prevalence estimate.

Table 2.2.a.1. Serum retinyl palmitate: Concentrations

Geometric mean and selected percentiles of serum concentrations (in µg/dL) for the total U.S. population aged 6 years and older, National Health and Nutrition Examination Survey, 2005–2006.

	Geometric mean (95% conf. interval)	Selected percentiles (95% conf. interval)						Sample size
		2.5th	5th	50th	95th	97.5th		
Total, 6 years and older	2.11 (2.05 – 2.17)	< LOD	< LOD	2.08 (1.99 – 2.17)	5.67 (5.35 – 6.03)	7.35 (6.93 – 7.96)		6,946
Age group								
6–11 years	2.15 (2.01 – 2.29)	< LOD	< LOD	2.14 (1.93 – 2.27)	5.01 (4.70 – 5.81)	6.18 (5.67 – 8.84)		827
12–19 years	1.90 (1.84 – 1.97)	< LOD	< LOD	1.83 (1.74 – 1.94)	4.78 (4.51 – 5.37)	6.19 (5.77 – 6.77)		1,865
20–39 years	2.13 (2.04 – 2.23)	< LOD	< LOD	2.18 (2.03 – 2.29)	5.00 (4.67 – 5.36)	6.31 (5.70 – 7.62)		1,620
40–59 years	2.14 (2.04 – 2.25)	< LOD	< LOD	2.12 (2.00 – 2.24)	6.15 (5.46 – 6.80)	7.58 (6.74 – 9.10)		1,315
60 years and older	2.14 (2.01 – 2.28)	< LOD	< LOD	2.04 (1.88 – 2.23)	6.87 (6.04 – 8.01)	8.80 (7.86 – 11.7)		1,319
Gender								
Males	2.15 (2.08 – 2.23)	< LOD	< LOD	2.14 (2.04 – 2.24)	5.89 (5.50 – 6.32)	7.26 (6.78 – 8.26)		3,397
Females	2.07 (2.01 – 2.12)	< LOD	< LOD	2.01 (1.94 – 2.11)	5.51 (4.96 – 6.12)	7.45 (6.53 – 8.14)		3,549
Race/ethnicity								
Mexican Americans	1.85 (1.78 – 1.91)	< LOD	< LOD	1.78 (1.69 – 1.88)	4.77 (4.40 – 5.18)	5.69 (5.19 – 7.49)		1,746
Non-Hispanic Blacks	2.04 (1.90 – 2.19)	< LOD	< LOD	2.03 (1.84 – 2.20)	5.00 (4.65 – 5.76)	6.36 (5.70 – 7.56)		1,842
Non-Hispanic Whites	2.17 (2.10 – 2.25)	< LOD	< LOD	2.17 (2.04 – 2.27)	6.02 (5.60 – 6.49)	7.82 (7.04 – 8.74)		2,838

< LOD means less than the limit of detection, which may vary for some compounds by year. See Appendix D for LOD.

Figure 2.2.a. Serum retinyl palmitate: Concentrations by age group
Geometric Mean (95% confidence interval), National Health and Nutrition Examination Survey, 2005–2006

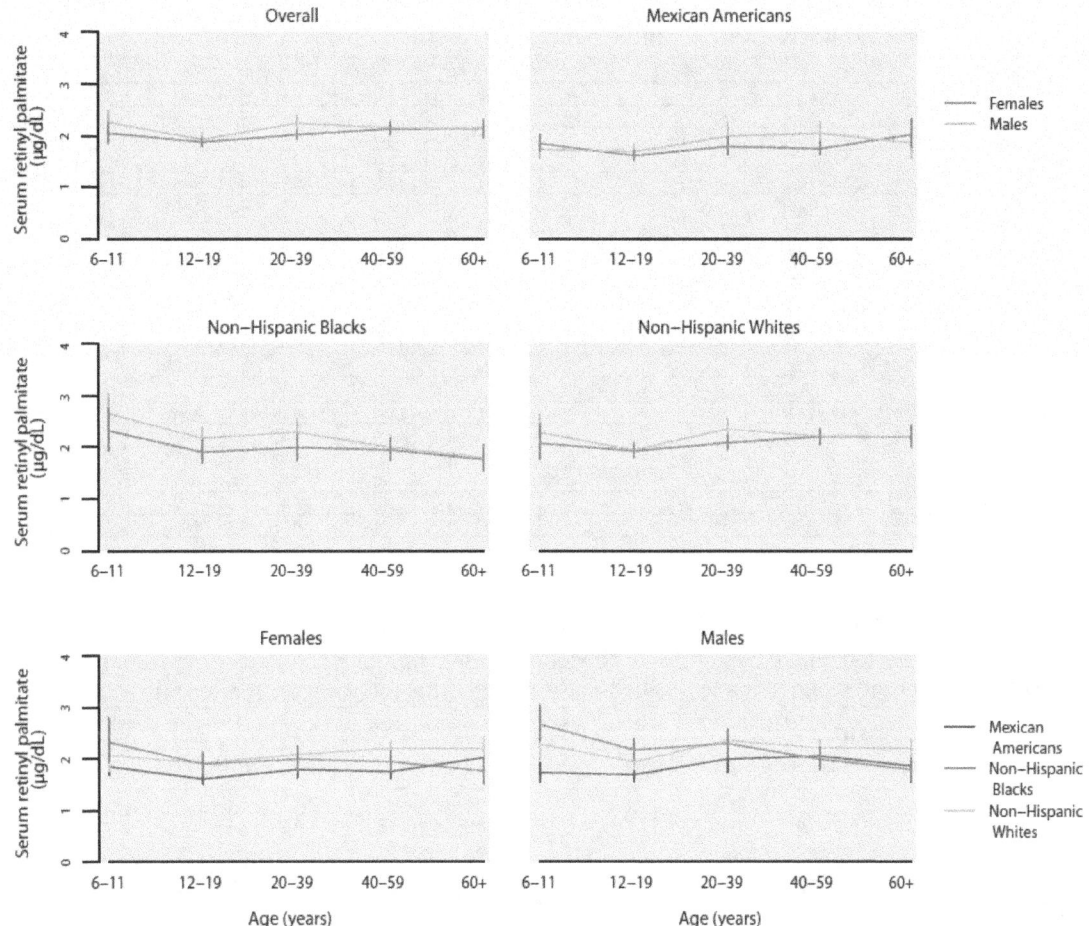

Table 2.2.a.2. Serum retinyl palmitate: Total population

Geometric mean and selected percentiles of serum concentrations (in µg/dL) for the total U.S. population aged 6 years and older, National Health and Nutrition Examination Survey, 2005–2006.

	Geometric mean (95% conf. interval)	Selected percentiles (95% conf. interval)			Sample size
		10th	50th	90th	
Males and Females					
Total, 6 years and older	2.11 (2.05 – 2.17)	< LOD	2.08 (1.99 – 2.17)	4.40 (4.28 – 4.54)	6,946
6–11 years	2.15 (2.01 – 2.29)	< LOD	2.14 (1.93 – 2.27)	4.19 (4.02 – 4.62)	827
12–19 years	1.90 (1.84 – 1.97)	< LOD	1.83 (1.74 – 1.94)	3.79 (3.60 – 4.10)	1,865
20–39 years	2.13 (2.04 – 2.23)	< LOD	2.18 (2.03 – 2.29)	4.16 (3.86 – 4.43)	1,620
40–59 years	2.14 (2.04 – 2.25)	< LOD	2.12 (2.00 – 2.24)	4.57 (4.23 – 5.15)	1,315
60 years and older	2.14 (2.01 – 2.28)	< LOD	2.04 (1.88 – 2.23)	4.99 (4.54 – 5.60)	1,319
Males					
Total, 6 years and older	2.15 (2.08 – 2.23)	< LOD	2.14 (2.04 – 2.24)	4.52 (4.39 – 4.69)	3,397
6–11 years	2.26 (2.05 – 2.48)	< LOD	2.22 (2.02 – 2.36)	4.56 (4.13 – 5.45)	411
12–19 years	1.93 (1.82 – 2.05)	< LOD	1.85 (1.72 – 2.02)	3.84 (3.55 – 4.26)	935
20–39 years	2.24 (2.09 – 2.39)	< LOD	2.30 (2.14 – 2.43)	4.42 (4.04 – 4.69)	714
40–59 years	2.15 (2.01 – 2.30)	< LOD	2.14 (2.01 – 2.27)	4.66 (4.29 – 5.53)	650
60 years and older	2.14 (2.01 – 2.28)	< LOD	2.03 (1.87 – 2.25)	5.04 (4.47 – 5.60)	687
Females					
Total, 6 years and older	2.07 (2.01 – 2.12)	< LOD	2.01 (1.94 – 2.11)	4.29 (4.13 – 4.44)	3,549
6–11 years	2.05 (1.86 – 2.25)	< LOD	2.03 (1.81 – 2.25)	4.02 (3.76 – 4.41)	416
12–19 years	1.88 (1.80 – 1.95)	< LOD	1.82 (1.69 – 1.92)	3.69 (3.44 – 4.31)	930
20–39 years	2.02 (1.94 – 2.11)	< LOD	2.03 (1.91 – 2.18)	3.87 (3.65 – 4.31)	906
40–59 years	2.13 (2.03 – 2.24)	< LOD	2.10 (1.97 – 2.24)	4.48 (4.00 – 5.50)	665
60 years and older	2.14 (1.97 – 2.33)	< LOD	2.05 (1.78 – 2.31)	4.95 (4.36 – 6.43)	632

< LOD means less than the limit of detection, which may vary for some compounds by year. See Appendix D for LOD.

Table 2.2.a.3. Serum retinyl palmitate: Mexican Americans

Geometric mean and selected percentiles of serum concentrations (in µg/dL) for Mexican Americans in the U.S. population aged 6 years and older, National Health and Nutrition Examination Survey, 2005–2006.

	Geometric mean (95% conf. interval)	Selected percentiles (95% conf. interval)			Sample size
		10th	50th	90th	
Males and Females					
Total, 6 years and older	1.85 (1.78 – 1.91)	< LOD	1.78 (1.69 – 1.88)	3.84 (3.60 – 4.09)	1,746
6–11 years	1.79 (1.67 – 1.91)	< LOD	1.68 (1.58 – 1.80)	3.66 (3.09 – 4.25)	275
12–19 years	1.65 (1.56 – 1.74)	< LOD	1.62 (1.57 – 1.67)	3.11 (2.87 – 3.51)	614
20–39 years	1.90 (1.77 – 2.04)	< LOD	1.87 (1.68 – 2.04)	3.94 (3.68 – 4.49)	432
40–59 years	1.89 (1.78 – 2.02)	< LOD	1.81 (1.67 – 2.00)	4.08 (3.50 – 4.79)	233
60 years and older	1.95 (1.78 – 2.14)	< LOD	1.79 (1.63 – 2.06)	4.57 (3.78 – 5.89)	192
Males					
Total, 6 years and older	1.91 (1.80 – 2.03)	< LOD	1.84 (1.69 – 2.00)	3.99 (3.70 – 4.70)	832
6–11 years	1.73 (1.56 – 1.91)	< LOD	1.60 (1.51 – 1.79)	3.68 (2.85 – 5.04)	136
12–19 years	1.69 (1.56 – 1.83)	< LOD	1.64 (1.56 – 1.75)	3.12 (2.70 – 3.94)	294
20–39 years	1.99 (1.74 – 2.27)	< LOD	1.95 (1.67 – 2.27)	4.21 (3.82 – 5.31)	193
40–59 years	2.05 (1.86 – 2.26)	< LOD	1.98 (1.55 – 2.44)	4.35 (3.76 – 5.44)	114
60 years and older	1.86 (1.56 – 2.22)	< LOD†	1.76 (1.35 – 2.41)	4.45† (3.55 – 5.43)	95
Females					
Total, 6 years and older	1.78 (1.70 – 1.85)	< LOD	1.72 (1.63 – 1.83)	3.56 (3.44 – 3.71)	914
6–11 years	1.85 (1.70 – 2.02)	< LOD	1.76 (1.63 – 1.94)	3.64 (3.14 – 4.87)	139
12–19 years	1.61 (1.52 – 1.70)	< LOD	1.60 (1.47 – 1.69)	3.09 (2.79 – 3.66)	320
20–39 years	1.79 (1.63 – 1.98)	< LOD	1.77 (1.53 – 2.03)	3.56 (3.32 – 3.89)	239
40–59 years	1.75 (1.63 – 1.88)	< LOD	1.72 (1.52 – 1.95)	3.52 (3.24 – 4.47)	119
60 years and older	2.02 (1.77 – 2.32)	< LOD†	1.79 (1.58 – 2.24)	4.59† (3.30 – 8.50)	97

< LOD means less than the limit of detection, which may vary for some compounds by year. See Appendix D for LOD.
† Estimate is subject to greater uncertainty due to small cell size.

Table 2.2.a.4. Serum retinyl palmitate: Non-Hispanic blacks

Geometric mean and selected percentiles of serum concentrations (in µg/dL) for non-Hispanic blacks in the U.S. population aged 6 years and older, National Health and Nutrition Examination Survey, 2005–2006.

	Geometric mean (95% conf. interval)	Selected percentiles (95% conf. interval)			Sample size
		10th	50th	90th	
Males and Females					
Total, 6 years and older	2.04 (1.90 – 2.19)	< LOD	2.03 (1.84 – 2.20)	4.13 (3.85 – 4.48)	1,842
6–11 years	2.49 (2.19 – 2.82)	< LOD	2.49 (2.13 – 3.01)	4.82 (4.58 – 5.44)	238
12–19 years	2.03 (1.88 – 2.21)	< LOD	1.99 (1.84 – 2.23)	4.05 (3.58 – 4.59)	643
20–39 years	2.12 (1.92 – 2.35)	< LOD	2.10 (1.91 – 2.27)	4.23 (3.81 – 4.67)	363
40–59 years	1.96 (1.82 – 2.12)	< LOD	1.94 (1.73 – 2.21)	3.88 (3.59 – 4.61)	326
60 years and older	1.77 (1.60 – 1.96)	< LOD	1.65 (1.44 – 1.89)	3.95 (3.26 – 4.67)	272
Males					
Total, 6 years and older	2.15 (1.99 – 2.32)	< LOD	2.16 (2.00 – 2.30)	4.45 (3.88 – 5.02)	921
6–11 years	2.66 (2.34 – 3.03)	< LOD	2.71 (2.35 – 2.96)	5.34 (4.54 – 6.33)	127
12–19 years	2.17 (1.98 – 2.38)	< LOD	2.13 (1.88 – 2.36)	4.49 (3.67 – 5.39)	330
20–39 years	2.29 (2.05 – 2.56)	< LOD	2.28 (2.05 – 2.56)	4.45 (3.73 – 5.85)	168
40–59 years	1.99 (1.80 – 2.21)	< LOD	2.12 (1.69 – 2.30)	3.84 (3.42 – 7.34)	153
60 years and older	1.79 (1.59 – 2.01)	< LOD	1.62 (1.32 – 1.99)	4.64 (3.40 – 5.35)	143
Females					
Total, 6 years and older	1.95 (1.79 – 2.12)	< LOD†	1.92 (1.74 – 2.14)	3.93 (3.80 – 4.22)	921
6–11 years	2.32 (1.94 – 2.77)	< LOD†	2.37 (1.87 – 2.87)	4.60† (4.24 – 5.12)	111
12–19 years	1.90 (1.71 – 2.12)	< LOD	1.91 (1.65 – 2.19)	3.55 (3.39 – 4.26)	313
20–39 years	1.99 (1.75 – 2.25)	< LOD	2.01 (1.73 – 2.24)	3.92 (3.70 – 4.67)	195
40–59 years	1.94 (1.76 – 2.14)	< LOD	1.88 (1.69 – 2.11)	3.92 (3.61 – 4.47)	173
60 years and older	1.76 (1.52 – 2.03)	< LOD	1.66 (1.43 – 2.02)	3.54 (3.07 – 4.22)	129

< LOD means less than the limit of detection, which may vary for some compounds by year. See Appendix D for LOD.
† Estimate is subject to greater uncertainty due to small cell size.

Table 2.2.a.5. Serum retinyl palmitate: Non-Hispanic whites

Geometric mean and selected percentiles of serum concentrations (in µg/dL) for non-Hispanic whites in the U.S. population aged 6 years and older, National Health and Nutrition Examination Survey, 2005–2006.

	Geometric mean (95% conf. interval)	Selected percentiles (95% conf. interval)			Sample size
		10th	50th	90th	
Males and Females					
Total, 6 years and older	2.17 (2.10 – 2.25)	< LOD	2.17 (2.04 – 2.27)	4.54 (4.39 – 4.71)	2,838
6–11 years	2.18 (1.97 – 2.41)	< LOD	2.16 (1.87 – 2.30)	4.19 (3.82 – 4.82)	224
12–19 years	1.93 (1.84 – 2.03)	< LOD	1.85 (1.70 – 2.01)	3.92 (3.56 – 4.47)	475
20–39 years	2.21 (2.07 – 2.36)	< LOD	2.30 (2.12 – 2.44)	4.32 (3.85 – 4.66)	676
40–59 years	2.20 (2.08 – 2.33)	< LOD	2.21 (2.02 – 2.34)	4.66 (4.33 – 5.45)	658
60 years and older	2.20 (2.05 – 2.37)	< LOD	2.12 (1.91 – 2.35)	5.16 (4.63 – 5.86)	805
Males					
Total, 6 years and older	2.22 (2.12 – 2.32)	< LOD	2.21 (2.08 – 2.30)	4.66 (4.45 – 4.99)	1,407
6–11 years	2.28 (1.97 – 2.63)	< LOD†	2.22 (1.95 – 2.61)	4.52† (3.80 – 5.92)	107
12–19 years	1.94 (1.79 – 2.10)	< LOD	1.87 (1.68 – 2.10)	3.80 (3.40 – 4.67)	245
20–39 years	2.35 (2.14 – 2.57)	< LOD	2.40 (2.22 – 2.59)	4.49 (4.09 – 5.04)	293
40–59 years	2.21 (2.06 – 2.36)	< LOD	2.20 (2.02 – 2.35)	4.77 (4.35 – 6.02)	339
60 years and older	2.20 (2.04 – 2.38)	< LOD	2.10 (1.89 – 2.36)	5.16 (4.50 – 5.79)	423
Females					
Total, 6 years and older	2.13 (2.05 – 2.21)	< LOD	2.13 (1.96 – 2.26)	4.41 (4.25 – 4.65)	1,431
6–11 years	2.07 (1.77 – 2.43)	< LOD	2.10 (1.75 – 2.39)	4.05 (3.50 – 4.51)	117
12–19 years	1.92 (1.81 – 2.04)	< LOD	1.81 (1.67 – 1.98)	3.98 (3.30 – 4.57)	230
20–39 years	2.08 (1.94 – 2.23)	< LOD	2.21 (1.91 – 2.36)	4.07 (3.57 – 4.65)	383
40–59 years	2.20 (2.06 – 2.34)	< LOD	2.21 (1.97 – 2.40)	4.54 (4.05 – 5.85)	319
60 years and older	2.20 (1.99 – 2.42)	< LOD	2.15 (1.80 – 2.41)	5.15 (4.45 – 6.71)	382

< LOD means less than the limit of detection, which may vary for some compounds by year. See Appendix D for LOD.
† Estimate is subject to greater uncertainty due to small cell size.

Table 2.2.b. Serum retinyl palmitate: Concentrations by survey cycle

Geometric mean and selected percentiles of serum concentrations (in µg/dL) for the U.S. population, National Health and Nutrition Examination Survey, 1999–2002 and 2005–2006.

	Geometric mean (95% conf. interval)	Selected percentiles (95% conf. interval) 5th	50th	95th	Sample size
Total, 6 years and older					
1999–2000	1.23 (1.04 – 1.46)	< LOD	1.47 (1.27 – 1.70)	4.95 (4.58 – 5.83)	5,589
2001–2002	1.92 (1.83 – 2.02)	.690 (.537 – .696)	1.93 (1.85 – 2.01)	5.49 (5.16 – 5.86)	7,641
2005–2006	2.11 (2.05 – 2.17)	< LOD	2.08 (1.99 – 2.17)	5.67 (5.35 – 6.03)	6,946
Age group					
3–5 years					
1999–2000	1.46 (1.16 – 1.84)	< LOD	1.67 (1.33 – 1.97)	5.39 (4.82 – 8.78)	278
2001–2002	1.88 (1.71 – 2.06)	.482 (< LOD – .710)	1.82 (1.69 – 2.02)	5.62 (4.79 – 8.77)	412
6–11 years					
1999–2000	1.33 (1.07 – 1.67)	< LOD	1.64 (1.29 – 2.02)	5.75 (4.55 – 8.88)	651
2001–2002	2.02 (1.90 – 2.15)	.700 (.462 – .801)	2.15 (2.03 – 2.25)	5.32 (4.79 – 5.85)	967
2005–2006	2.15 (2.01 – 2.29)	< LOD	2.14 (1.93 – 2.27)	5.01 (4.70 – 5.81)	827
12–19 years					
1999–2000	1.17 (.963 – 1.41)	< LOD	1.41 (1.12 – 1.68)	4.11 (3.71 – 4.77)	1,620
2001–2002	1.71 (1.61 – 1.80)	.560 (.500 – .692)	1.77 (1.66 – 1.87)	4.21 (3.98 – 4.47)	2,122
2005–2006	1.90 (1.84 – 1.97)	< LOD	1.83 (1.74 – 1.94)	4.78 (4.51 – 5.37)	1,865
20–39 years					
1999–2000	1.14 (.928 – 1.39)	< LOD	1.40 (1.21 – 1.62)	4.58 (4.14 – 5.67)	1,201
2001–2002	1.91 (1.77 – 2.06)	.643 (.543 – .720)	1.91 (1.79 – 2.03)	5.14 (4.65 – 5.79)	1,655
2005–2006	2.13 (2.04 – 2.23)	< LOD	2.18 (2.03 – 2.29)	5.00 (4.67 – 5.36)	1,620
40–59 years					
1999–2000	1.30 (1.06 – 1.59)	< LOD	1.55 (1.30 – 1.84)	5.49 (4.61 – 6.83)	959
2001–2002	1.99 (1.87 – 2.11)	.623 (.529 – .698)	1.96 (1.89 – 2.06)	5.70 (5.19 – 6.53)	1,429
2005–2006	2.14 (2.04 – 2.25)	< LOD	2.12 (2.00 – 2.24)	6.15 (5.46 – 6.80)	1,315
60 years and older					
1999–2000	1.34 (1.11 – 1.62)	< LOD	1.54 (1.29 – 1.89)	5.78 (4.87 – 6.47)	1,158
2001–2002	1.96 (1.82 – 2.11)	.522 (.453 – .580)	1.91 (1.75 – 2.13)	6.79 (6.11 – 7.83)	1,468
2005–2006	2.14 (2.01 – 2.28)	< LOD	2.04 (1.88 – 2.23)	6.87 (6.04 – 8.01)	1,319
Gender					
(6 years and older)					
Males					
1999–2000	1.38 (1.17 – 1.63)	< LOD	1.61 (1.40 – 1.82)	5.22 (4.65 – 5.94)	2,676
2001–2002	2.01 (1.90 – 2.12)	.636 (.544 – .687)	2.01 (1.91 – 2.12)	5.71 (5.31 – 6.20)	3,698
2005–2006	2.15 (2.08 – 2.23)	< LOD	2.14 (2.04 – 2.24)	5.89 (5.50 – 6.32)	3,397
Females					
1999–2000	1.11 (.922 – 1.33)	< LOD	1.36 (1.16 – 1.61)	4.79 (4.47 – 5.80)	2,913
2001–2002	1.85 (1.76 – 1.95)	.582 (.515 – .695)	1.84 (1.75 – 1.92)	5.11 (4.78 – 5.68)	3,943
2005–2006	2.07 (2.01 – 2.12)	< LOD	2.01 (1.94 – 2.11)	5.51 (4.96 – 6.12)	3,549
Race/ethnicity					
(6 years and older)					
Mexican Americans					
1999–2000	.759 (.635 – .906)	< LOD	.945 (.808 – 1.14)	3.69 (3.32 – 4.35)	1,463
2001–2002	1.62 (1.47 – 1.78)	.503 (.398 – .575)	1.65 (1.50 – 1.85)	4.28 (3.95 – 4.80)	1,980
2005–2006	1.85 (1.78 – 1.91)	< LOD	1.78 (1.69 – 1.88)	4.77 (4.40 – 5.18)	1,746
Non-Hispanic Blacks					
1999–2000	1.18 (.848 – 1.64)	< LOD	1.48 (1.07 – 1.99)	5.06 (4.41 – 5.81)	1,422
2001–2002	1.92 (1.82 – 2.02)	.628 (.390 – .709)	1.96 (1.88 – 2.06)	5.44 (4.71 – 6.44)	1,734
2005–2006	2.04 (1.90 – 2.19)	< LOD	2.03 (1.84 – 2.20)	5.00 (4.65 – 5.76)	1,842
Non-Hispanic Whites					
1999–2000	1.32 (1.08 – 1.60)	< LOD	1.57 (1.33 – 1.84)	5.12 (4.60 – 6.48)	2,121
2001–2002	1.97 (1.87 – 2.08)	.636 (.584 – .684)	1.95 (1.86 – 2.06)	5.57 (5.14 – 5.99)	3,318
2005–2006	2.17 (2.10 – 2.25)	< LOD	2.17 (2.04 – 2.27)	6.02 (5.60 – 6.49)	2,838

< LOD means less than the limit of detection, which may vary for some compounds by year. See Appendix D for LOD.

Figure 2.2.b. Serum retinyl palmitate: Concentrations by survey cycle
Selected percentiles in µg/dL (95% confidence intervals), National Health and
Nutrition Examination Survey, 1999–2002 and 2005–2006

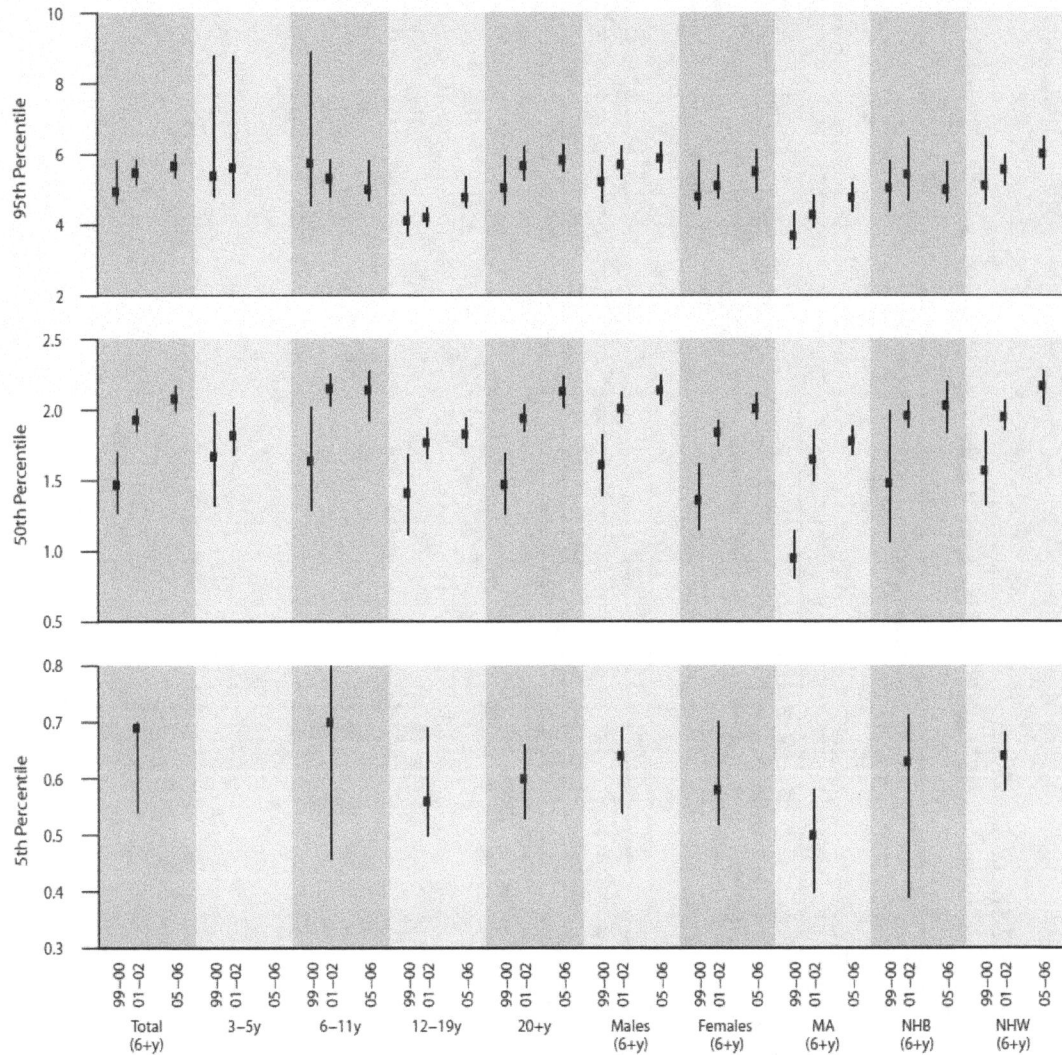

Values in the graph are suppressed if either the point estimate or the lower 95% confidence limit is noted as "< LOD" in the accompanying table.

Table 2.3.a.1. Serum retinyl stearate: Concentrations

Geometric mean and selected percentiles of serum concentrations (in µg/dL) for the total U.S. population aged 6 years and older, National Health and Nutrition Examination Survey, 2005–2006.

	Geometric mean (95% conf. interval)	Selected percentiles (95% conf. interval)					Sample size
		2.5th	5th	50th	95th	97.5th	
Total, 6 years and older	*	< LOD	< LOD	< LOD	1.31 (1.23 – 1.48)	1.95 (1.79 – 2.09)	6,698
Age group							
6–11 years	*	< LOD	< LOD	< LOD	1.33 (1.08 – 1.97)	1.97 (1.65 – 4.08)	792
12–19 years	*	< LOD	< LOD	< LOD	.911 (.743 – 1.14)	1.48 (1.18 – 2.00)	1,801
20–39 years	*	< LOD	< LOD	< LOD	.947 (.850 – 1.09)	1.32 (1.14 – 1.76)	1,555
40–59 years	*	< LOD	< LOD	< LOD	1.35 (1.23 – 1.63)	2.00 (1.68 – 2.31)	1,262
60 years and older	*	< LOD	< LOD	< LOD	1.93 (1.59 – 2.58)	2.77 (2.26 – 3.58)	1,288
Gender							
Males	*	< LOD	< LOD	< LOD	1.40 (1.29 – 1.54)	1.94 (1.86 – 2.05)	3,276
Females	*	< LOD	< LOD	< LOD	1.25 (1.09 – 1.48)	1.99 (1.62 – 2.34)	3,422
Race/ethnicity							
Mexican Americans	*	< LOD	< LOD	< LOD	.933 (.792 – 1.19)	1.35 (1.08 – 2.07)	1,739
Non-Hispanic Blacks	*	< LOD	< LOD	< LOD	.896 (.829 – 1.10)	1.38 (1.10 – 1.71)	1,699
Non-Hispanic Whites	*	< LOD	< LOD	< LOD	1.50 (1.36 – 1.64)	2.06 (1.93 – 2.36)	2,747

< LOD means less than the limit of detection, which may vary for some compounds by year. See Appendix D for LOD.
* Not calculated. Proportion of results below limit of detection was too high to provide a valid result.

No serum retinyl stearate figure for concentrations by age group is presented because the geometric means were not calculated due to the proportion of results below the limit of detection being too high for valid results (see Table 2.3.a.1).

Table 2.3.a.2. Serum retinyl stearate: Total population

Geometric mean and selected percentiles of serum concentrations (in µg/dL) for the total U.S. population aged 6 years and older, National Health and Nutrition Examination Survey, 2005–2006.

	Geometric mean (95% conf. interval)	Selected percentiles (95% conf. interval)			Sample size
		10th	50th	90th	
Males and Females					
Total, 6 years and older	*	< LOD	< LOD	.894 (.794 – 1.02)	6,698
6–11 years	*	< LOD	< LOD	.972 (.730 – 1.21)	792
12–19 years	*	< LOD	< LOD	< LOD	1,801
20–39 years	*	< LOD	< LOD	< LOD	1,555
40–59 years	*	< LOD	< LOD	.944 (.810 – 1.16)	1,262
60 years and older	*	< LOD	< LOD	1.32 (1.13 – 1.58)	1,288
Males					
Total, 6 years and older	*	< LOD	< LOD	.964 (.871 – 1.08)	3,276
6–11 years	*	< LOD	< LOD	1.03 (< LOD – 1.76)	394
12–19 years	*	< LOD	< LOD	< LOD	898
20–39 years	*	< LOD	< LOD	.813 (.709 – .968)	682
40–59 years	*	< LOD	< LOD	.993 (.842 – 1.17)	624
60 years and older	*	< LOD	< LOD	1.33 (1.16 – 1.53)	678
Females					
Total, 6 years and older	*	< LOD	< LOD	.839 (.741 – .960)	3,422
6–11 years	*	< LOD	< LOD	.896 (< LOD – 1.17)	398
12–19 years	*	< LOD	< LOD	< LOD	903
20–39 years	*	< LOD	< LOD	< LOD	873
40–59 years	*	< LOD	< LOD	.903 (.764 – 1.21)	638
60 years and older	*	< LOD	< LOD	1.32 (1.06 – 1.74)	610

< LOD means less than the limit of detection, which may vary for some compounds by year. See Appendix D for LOD.
* Not calculated. Proportion of results below limit of detection was too high to provide a valid result.

Table 2.3.a.3. Serum retinyl stearate: Mexican Americans

Geometric mean and selected percentiles of serum concentrations (in µg/dL) for Mexican Americans in the U.S. population aged 6 years and older, National Health and Nutrition Examination Survey, 2005–2006.

	Geometric mean (95% conf. interval)	Selected percentiles (95% conf. interval)			Sample size
		10th	50th	90th	
Males and Females					
Total, 6 years and older	*	< LOD	< LOD	< LOD	1,739
6–11 years	*	< LOD	< LOD	< LOD	272
12–19 years	*	< LOD	< LOD	< LOD	604
20–39 years	*	< LOD	< LOD	< LOD	428
40–59 years	*	< LOD	< LOD	.766 (< LOD – 1.23)	238
60 years and older	*	< LOD	< LOD	.902 (.707 – 1.32)	197
Males					
Total, 6 years and older	*	< LOD	< LOD	.736 (< LOD – .877)	832
6–11 years	*	< LOD	< LOD	< LOD	135
12–19 years	*	< LOD	< LOD	< LOD	290
20–39 years	*	< LOD	< LOD	.700 (< LOD – .965)	190
40–59 years	*	< LOD	< LOD	.851 (< LOD – 1.95)	118
60 years and older	*	< LOD†	< LOD	.780† (< LOD – 3.26)	99
Females					
Total, 6 years and older	*	< LOD	< LOD	< LOD	907
6–11 years	*	< LOD	< LOD	< LOD	137
12–19 years	*	< LOD	< LOD	< LOD	314
20–39 years	*	< LOD	< LOD	< LOD	238
40–59 years	*	< LOD	< LOD	< LOD	120
60 years and older	*	< LOD†	< LOD	1.02† (< LOD – 1.97)	98

< LOD means less than the limit of detection, which may vary for some compounds by year. See Appendix D for LOD.
* Not calculated. Proportion of results below limit of detection was too high to provide a valid result.
† Estimate is subject to greater uncertainty due to small cell size.

Table 2.3.a.4. Serum retinyl stearate: Non-Hispanic blacks

Geometric mean and selected percentiles of serum concentrations (in µg/dL) for non-Hispanic blacks in the U.S. population aged 6 years and older, National Health and Nutrition Examination Survey, 2005–2006.

	Geometric mean (95% conf. interval)	Selected percentiles (95% conf. interval)			Sample size
		10th	50th	90th	
Males and Females					
Total, 6 years and older	*	< LOD	< LOD	< LOD	1,699
6–11 years	*	< LOD	< LOD	< LOD	219
12–19 years	*	< LOD	< LOD	< LOD	597
20–39 years	*	< LOD	< LOD	< LOD	322
40–59 years	*	< LOD	< LOD	.781　(< LOD – .931)	301
60 years and older	*	< LOD	< LOD	.770　(< LOD – 1.39)	260
Males					
Total, 6 years and older	*	< LOD	< LOD	.746　(< LOD – .868)	849
6–11 years	*	< LOD	< LOD	< LOD	118
12–19 years	*	< LOD	< LOD	< LOD	300
20–39 years	*	< LOD	< LOD	< LOD	152
40–59 years	*	< LOD	< LOD	.813　(< LOD – 1.06)	141
60 years and older	*	< LOD	< LOD	1.06　(< LOD – 1.55)	138
Females					
Total, 6 years and older	*	< LOD	< LOD	< LOD	850
6–11 years	*	< LOD†	< LOD	< LOD†	101
12–19 years	*	< LOD	< LOD	< LOD	297
20–39 years	*	< LOD	< LOD	< LOD	170
40–59 years	*	< LOD	< LOD	.701　(< LOD – .962)	160
60 years and older	*	< LOD	< LOD	< LOD	122

< LOD means less than the limit of detection, which may vary for some compounds by year. See Appendix D for LOD.
* Not calculated. Proportion of results below limit of detection was too high to provide a valid result.
† Estimate is subject to greater uncertainty due to small cell size.

Table 2.3.a.5. Serum retinyl stearate: Non-Hispanic whites

Geometric mean and selected percentiles of serum concentrations (in µg/dL) for non-Hispanic whites in the U.S. population aged 6 years and older, National Health and Nutrition Examination Survey, 2005–2006.

	Geometric mean (95% conf. interval)	Selected percentiles (95% conf. interval)			Sample size
		10th	50th	90th	
Males and Females					
Total, 6 years and older	*	< LOD	< LOD	1.01　(.932 – 1.10)	2,747
6–11 years	*	< LOD	< LOD	1.06　(.756 – 1.99)	212
12–19 years	*	< LOD	< LOD	< LOD	465
20–39 years	*	< LOD	< LOD	.727　(< LOD – .878)	660
40–59 years	*	< LOD	< LOD	1.00　(.869 – 1.20)	627
60 years and older	*	< LOD	< LOD	1.40　(1.17 – 1.73)	783
Males					
Total, 6 years and older	*	< LOD	< LOD	1.09　(.967 – 1.18)	1,370
6–11 years	*	< LOD†	< LOD	1.09†　(< LOD – 7.58)	103
12–19 years	*	< LOD	< LOD	.740　(< LOD – 1.05)	244
20–39 years	*	< LOD	< LOD	.927　(.740 – 1.16)	283
40–59 years	*	< LOD	< LOD	1.07　(.862 – 1.24)	324
60 years and older	*	< LOD	< LOD	1.39　(1.19 – 1.65)	416
Females					
Total, 6 years and older	*	< LOD	< LOD	.948　(.855 – 1.07)	1,377
6–11 years	*	< LOD†	< LOD	1.04†　(.755 – 2.95)	109
12–19 years	*	< LOD	< LOD	< LOD	221
20–39 years	*	< LOD	< LOD	< LOD	377
40–59 years	*	< LOD	< LOD	.953　(.798 – 1.31)	303
60 years and older	*	< LOD	< LOD	1.41　(1.08 – 2.01)	367

< LOD means less than the limit of detection, which may vary for some compounds by year. See Appendix D for LOD.
* Not calculated. Proportion of results below limit of detection was too high to provide a valid result.
† Estimate is subject to greater uncertainty due to small cell size.

Table 2.3.b. Serum retinyl stearate: Concentrations by survey cycle

Geometric mean and selected percentiles of serum concentrations (in µg/dL) for the U.S. population, National Health and Nutrition Examination Survey, 1999–2002 and 2005–2006.

	Geometric mean (95% conf. interval)	Selected percentiles (95% conf. interval)			Sample size
		5th	50th	95th	
Total, 6 years and older					
1999–2000	*	< LOD	< LOD	1.12 (.983 – 1.44)	4,148
2001–2002	*	< LOD	< LOD	1.08 (.988 – 1.19)	7,690
2005–2006	*	< LOD	< LOD	1.31 (1.23 – 1.48)	6,698
Age group					
3–5 years					
1999–2000	*	< LOD†	< LOD	2.43† (1.72 – 3.65)	212
2001–2002	*	< LOD	< LOD	1.75 (1.37 – 3.49)	416
6–11 years					
1999–2000	*	< LOD	< LOD	1.74 (1.09 – 10.3)	434
2001–2002	*	< LOD	< LOD	1.14 (.964 – 1.34)	981
2005–2006	*	< LOD	< LOD	1.33 (1.08 – 1.97)	792
12–19 years					
1999–2000	*	< LOD	< LOD	.829 (< LOD – 1.30)	1,194
2001–2002	*	< LOD	< LOD	< LOD	2,145
2005–2006	*	< LOD	< LOD	.911 (.743 – 1.14)	1,801
20–39 years					
1999–2000	*	< LOD	< LOD	.928 (.651 – 1.36)	872
2001–2002	*	< LOD	< LOD	.721 (.693 – .893)	1,658
2005–2006	*	< LOD	< LOD	.947 (.850 – 1.09)	1,555
40–59 years					
1999–2000	*	< LOD	< LOD	1.32 (.944 – 2.40)	716
2001–2002	*	< LOD	< LOD	1.15 (1.04 – 1.46)	1,422
2005–2006	*	< LOD	< LOD	1.35 (1.23 – 1.63)	1,262
60 years and older					
1999–2000	*	< LOD	< LOD	1.83 (1.39 – 2.90)	932
2001–2002	*	< LOD	< LOD	1.77 (1.52 – 2.08)	1,484
2005–2006	*	< LOD	< LOD	1.93 (1.59 – 2.58)	1,288
Gender					
(6 years and older)					
Males					
1999–2000	*	< LOD	< LOD	1.13 (.987 – 1.66)	2,008
2001–2002	*	< LOD	< LOD	1.19 (1.09 – 1.42)	3,710
2005–2006	*	< LOD	< LOD	1.40 (1.29 – 1.54)	3,276
Females					
1999–2000	*	< LOD	< LOD	1.10 (.951 – 1.42)	2,140
2001–2002	*	< LOD	< LOD	.953 (.856 – 1.09)	3,980
2005–2006	*	< LOD	< LOD	1.25 (1.09 – 1.48)	3,422
Race/ethnicity					
(6 years and older)					
Mexican Americans					
1999–2000	*	< LOD	< LOD	.695 (< LOD – 2.14)	1,002
2001–2002	*	< LOD	< LOD	.587 (< LOD – .880)	1,921
2005–2006	*	< LOD	< LOD	.933 (.792 – 1.19)	1,739
Non-Hispanic Blacks					
1999–2000	*	< LOD	< LOD	.962 (.590 – 15.0)	1,060
2001–2002	*	< LOD	< LOD	.733 (.619 – .963)	1,827
2005–2006	*	< LOD	< LOD	.896 (.829 – 1.10)	1,699
Non-Hispanic Whites					
1999–2000	*	< LOD	< LOD	1.27 (1.00 – 1.81)	1,608
2001–2002	*	< LOD	< LOD	1.13 (1.02 – 1.30)	3,331
2005–2006	*	< LOD	< LOD	1.50 (1.36 – 1.64)	2,747

< LOD means less than the limit of detection, which may vary for some compounds by year. See Appendix D for LOD.
* Not calculated. Proportion of results below limit of detection was too high to provide a valid result.
† Estimate is subject to greater uncertainty due to cell size.

Figure 2.3.b. Serum retinyl stearate: Concentrations by survey cycle

Selected percentiles in μg/dL (95% confidence intervals), National Health and Nutrition Examination Survey, 1999–2002 and 2005–2006

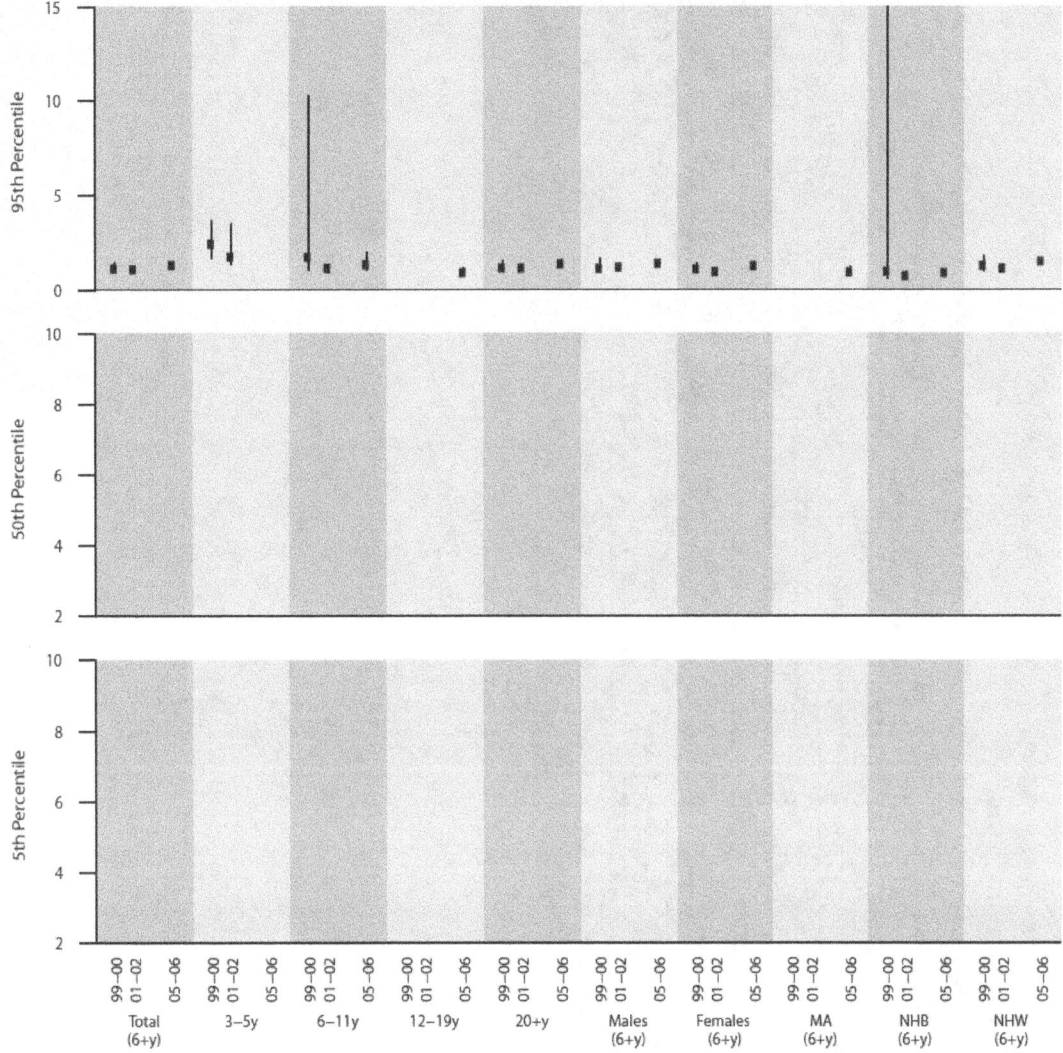

Values in the graph are suppressed if either the point estimate or the lower 95% confidence limit is noted as "< LOD" in the accompanying table.

Table 2.4.a.1. Serum vitamin E: Concentrations

Geometric mean and selected percentiles of serum concentrations (in μg/dL) for the total U.S. population aged 6 years and older, National Health and Nutrition Examination Survey, 2005–2006.

	Geometric mean (95% conf. interval)	Selected percentiles (95% conf. interval)						Sample size
		2.5th	5th	50th	95th	97.5th	
Total, 6 years and older	1,090 (1,070 – 1,120)	578 (563 – 587)	631 (620 – 642)	1,060 (1,030 – 1,080)	2,090 (2,010 – 2,180)	2,460 (2,310 – 2,600)	7,254
Age group							
6–11 years	820 (800 – 841)	546 (518 – 573)	583 (563 – 601)	806 (788 – 826)	1,200 (1,120 – 1,370)	1,360 (1,230 – 1,510)	860
12–19 years	770 (757 – 783)	497 (466 – 519)	527 (516 – 541)	759 (749 – 767)	1,160 (1,130 – 1,200)	1,320 (1,240 – 1,450)	1,954
20–39 years	1,020 (998 – 1,040)	590 (559 – 619)	645 (621 – 668)	1,000 (980 – 1,020)	1,730 (1,620 – 1,900)	1,940 (1,810 – 2,380)	1,688
40–59 years	1,230 (1,190 – 1,260)	702 (656 – 721)	749 (724 – 769)	1,200 (1,160 – 1,240)	2,210 (2,080 – 2,400)	2,510 (2,260 – 3,110)	1,365
60 years and older	1,400 (1,360 – 1,440)	704 (611 – 750)	783 (733 – 835)	1,390 (1,330 – 1,430)	2,600 (2,510 – 2,660)	2,900 (2,710 – 3,130)	1,387
Gender							
Males	1,060 (1,040 – 1,090)	559 (543 – 575)	610 (594 – 625)	1,030 (1,010 – 1,070)	2,010 (1,930 – 2,090)	2,360 (2,160 – 2,520)	3,547
Females	1,120 (1,090 – 1,140)	596 (585 – 612)	653 (639 – 664)	1,080 (1,050 – 1,100)	2,170 (2,080 – 2,260)	2,510 (2,370 – 2,660)	3,707
Race/ethnicity							
Mexican Americans	1,010 (980 – 1,040)	581 (553 – 599)	623 (602 – 637)	976 (945 – 1,000)	1,790 (1,750 – 1,870)	2,120 (1,960 – 2,330)	1,844
Non-Hispanic Blacks	933 (915 – 951)	548 (530 – 559)	588 (581 – 601)	903 (884 – 918)	1,660 (1,560 – 1,750)	1,800 (1,740 – 2,080)	1,891
Non-Hispanic Whites	1,140 (1,110 – 1,160)	584 (566 – 596)	643 (624 – 658)	1,110 (1,080 – 1,140)	2,170 (2,090 – 2,270)	2,520 (2,420 – 2,690)	2,973

Figure 2.4.a. Serum vitamin E: Concentrations by age group
Geometric mean (95% confidence interval), National Health and Nutrition Examination Survey, 2005–2006

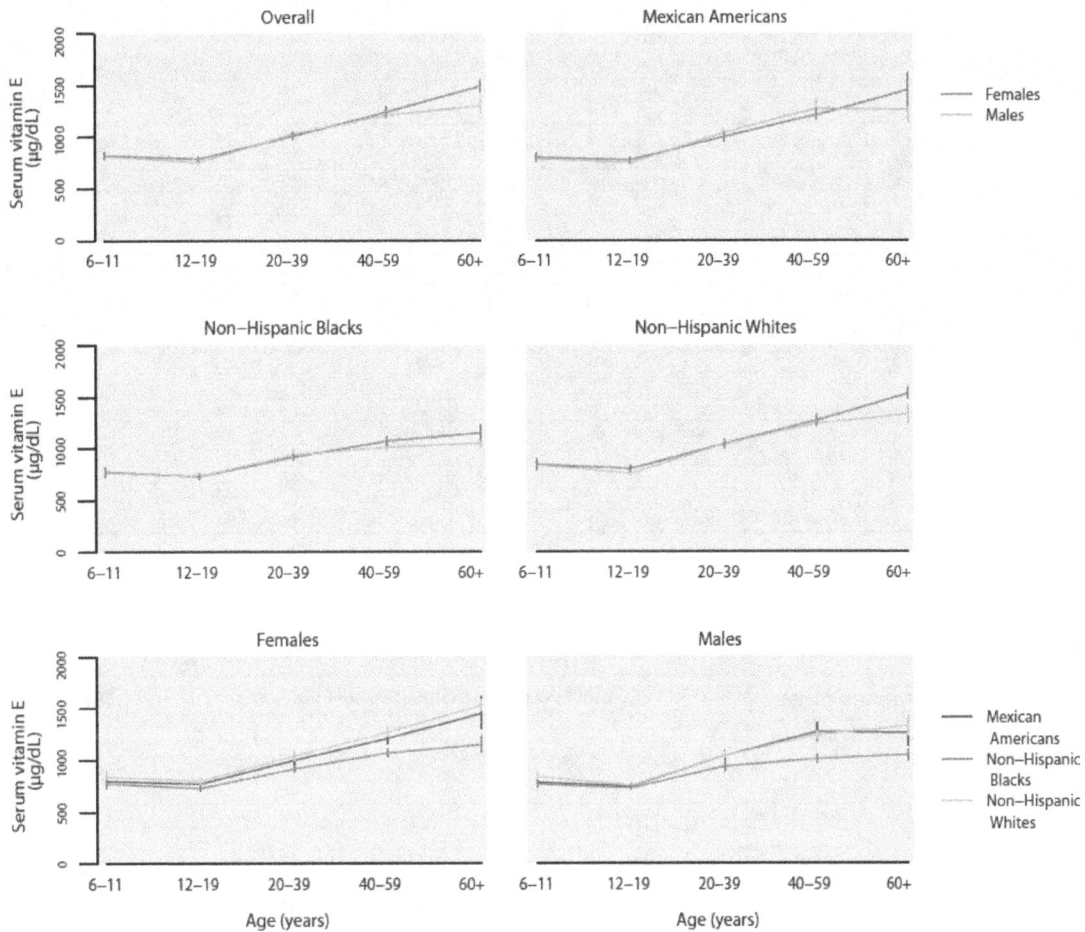

Table 2.4.a.2. Serum vitamin E: Total population

Geometric mean and selected percentiles of serum concentrations (in µg/dL) for the total U.S. population aged 6 years and older, National Health and Nutrition Examination Survey, 2005–2006.

	Geometric mean (95% conf. interval)		Selected percentiles (95% conf. interval)						Sample size
			10th		50th		90th		
Males and Females									
Total, 6 years and older	1,090	(1,070 – 1,120)	702	(686 – 716)	1,060	(1,030 – 1,080)	1,790	(1,730 – 1,840)	7,254
6–11 years	820	(800 – 841)	629	(621 – 638)	806	(788 – 826)	1,070	(1,040 – 1,180)	860
12–19 years	770	(757 – 783)	578	(557 – 587)	759	(749 – 767)	1,050	(1,000 – 1,070)	1,954
20–39 years	1,020	(998 – 1,040)	710	(683 – 727)	1,000	(980 – 1,020)	1,520	(1,410 – 1,610)	1,688
40–59 years	1,230	(1,190 – 1,260)	824	(799 – 848)	1,200	(1,160 – 1,240)	1,870	(1,790 – 2,040)	1,365
60 years and older	1,400	(1,360 – 1,440)	897	(828 – 949)	1,390	(1,330 – 1,430)	2,190	(2,130 – 2,270)	1,387
Males									
Total, 6 years and older	1,060	(1,040 – 1,090)	682	(664 – 704)	1,030	(1,010 – 1,070)	1,730	(1,640 – 1,770)	3,547
6–11 years	817	(789 – 847)	629	(593 – 642)	807	(766 – 843)	1,070	(1,030 – 1,180)	427
12–19 years	753	(739 – 768)	553	(527 – 580)	747	(733 – 759)	1,030	(986 – 1,070)	980
20–39 years	1,030	(1,010 – 1,050)	699	(671 – 728)	1,010	(984 – 1,030)	1,570	(1,440 – 1,730)	738
40–59 years	1,210	(1,180 – 1,250)	798	(767 – 848)	1,190	(1,160 – 1,240)	1,820	(1,740 – 1,950)	673
60 years and older	1,300	(1,230 – 1,370)	827	(762 – 887)	1,290	(1,220 – 1,330)	2,070	(1,950 – 2,310)	729
Females									
Total, 6 years and older	1,120	(1,090 – 1,140)	717	(705 – 723)	1,080	(1,050 – 1,100)	1,840	(1,790 – 1,910)	3,707
6–11 years	823	(792 – 856)	628	(608 – 647)	805	(784 – 837)	1,090	(1,020 – 1,230)	433
12–19 years	788	(772 – 804)	594	(570 – 611)	771	(755 – 788)	1,050	(991 – 1,120)	974
20–39 years	1,010	(981 – 1,040)	717	(679 – 738)	997	(956 – 1,030)	1,470	(1,360 – 1,580)	950
40–59 years	1,240	(1,200 – 1,290)	841	(818 – 860)	1,210	(1,160 – 1,240)	1,920	(1,820 – 2,120)	692
60 years and older	1,490	(1,440 – 1,540)	966	(926 – 987)	1,500	(1,430 – 1,540)	2,260	(2,190 – 2,470)	658

Table 2.4.a.3. Serum vitamin E: Mexican Americans

Geometric mean and selected percentiles of serum concentrations (in µg/dL) for Mexican Americans in the U.S. population aged 6 years and older, National Health and Nutrition Examination Survey, 2005–2006.

	Geometric mean (95% conf. interval)		Selected percentiles (95% conf. interval)						Sample size
			10th		50th		90th		
Males and Females									
Total, 6 years and older	1,010	(980 – 1,040)	671	(656 – 695)	976	(945 – 1,000)	1,580	(1,530 – 1,630)	1,844
6–11 years	793	(770 – 816)	623	(599 – 644)	779	(755 – 800)	1,010	(977 – 1,110)	295
12–19 years	760	(740 – 781)	587	(578 – 597)	750	(723 – 773)	991	(970 – 1,050)	646
20–39 years	1,020	(991 – 1,060)	727	(676 – 755)	997	(968 – 1,020)	1,520	(1,420 – 1,640)	449
40–59 years	1,240	(1,200 – 1,280)	836	(808 – 861)	1,220	(1,160 – 1,270)	1,790	(1,730 – 1,950)	246
60 years and older	1,360	(1,250 – 1,470)	913	(816 – 996)	1,300	(1,240 – 1,370)	2,000	(1,720 – 3,120)	208
Males									
Total, 6 years and older	1,010	(970 – 1,050)	671	(640 – 701)	972	(925 – 999)	1,570	(1,510 – 1,610)	883
6–11 years	786	(762 – 811)	622	(598 – 643)	763	(745 – 802)	989	(962 – 1,060)	145
12–19 years	748	(718 – 778)	591	(573 – 603)	733	(690 – 775)	978	(930 – 1,060)	313
20–39 years	1,040	(1,010 – 1,080)	753	(703 – 772)	990	(967 – 1,020)	1,590	(1,460 – 1,700)	198
40–59 years	1,270	(1,190 – 1,350)	863	(814 – 908)	1,260	(1,140 – 1,350)	1,670	(1,610 – 2,030)	122
60 years and older	1,260	(1,140 – 1,390)	845†	(650 – 931)	1,240	(1,100 – 1,340)	1,970†	(1,570 – 3,130)	105
Females									
Total, 6 years and older	1,010	(984 – 1,030)	670	(649 – 696)	985	(949 – 1,020)	1,610	(1,530 – 1,670)	961
6–11 years	800	(763 – 838)	625	(514 – 658)	787	(760 – 799)	1,050	(958 – 1,240)	150
12–19 years	774	(750 – 798)	583	(570 – 597)	763	(748 – 784)	1,020	(960 – 1,090)	333
20–39 years	1,000	(955 – 1,050)	700	(634 – 742)	1,000	(947 – 1,060)	1,490	(1,340 – 1,650)	251
40–59 years	1,210	(1,170 – 1,260)	808	(778 – 859)	1,200	(1,110 – 1,240)	1,840	(1,710 – 2,100)	124
60 years and older	1,450	(1,300 – 1,610)	1,000†	(872 – 1,090)	1,410	(1,240 – 1,540)	2,040†	(1,720 – 4,610)	103

† Estimate is subject to greater uncertainty due to small cell size.

Table 2.4.a.4. Serum vitamin E: Non-Hispanic blacks

Geometric mean and selected percentiles of serum concentrations (in µg/dL) for non-Hispanic blacks in the U.S. population aged 6 years and older, National Health and Nutrition Examination Survey, 2005–2006.

	Geometric mean (95% conf. interval)		Selected percentiles (95% conf. interval)						Sample size
			10th		50th		90th		
Males and Females									
Total, 6 years and older	933	(915 – 951)	644	(630 – 656)	903	(884 – 918)	1,400	(1,360 – 1,470)	1,891
6–11 years	771	(743 – 801)	587	(550 – 634)	762	(735 – 800)	1,010	(941 – 1,090)	240
12–19 years	731	(715 – 748)	575	(551 – 591)	727	(717 – 736)	945	(913 – 990)	665
20–39 years	926	(896 – 957)	665	(620 – 686)	893	(865 – 933)	1,340	(1,250 – 1,450)	368
40–59 years	1,040	(1,010 – 1,070)	736	(688 – 779)	1,010	(998 – 1,050)	1,540	(1,420 – 1,670)	335
60 years and older	1,110	(1,060 – 1,160)	752	(709 – 791)	1,080	(993 – 1,150)	1,680	(1,560 – 1,780)	283
Males									
Total, 6 years and older	915	(897 – 933)	636	(618 – 651)	882	(870 – 895)	1,390	(1,310 – 1,460)	949
6–11 years	768	(740 – 799)	588	(558 – 634)	752	(726 – 799)	1,030	(928 – 1,110)	128
12–19 years	732	(714 – 751)	582	(558 – 606)	727	(712 – 737)	940	(904 – 981)	343
20–39 years	937	(888 – 989)	650	(603 – 687)	896	(862 – 939)	1,400	(1,240 – 1,670)	170
40–59 years	1,010	(972 – 1,050)	718	(632 – 743)	988	(960 – 1,020)	1,520	(1,390 – 1,640)	156
60 years and older	1,050	(1,000 – 1,100)	726	(580 – 770)	980	(894 – 1,080)	1,680	(1,410 – 2,250)	152
Females									
Total, 6 years and older	949	(923 – 976)	651	(638 – 673)	916	(897 – 944)	1,450	(1,350 – 1,560)	942
6–11 years	775	(735 – 817)	579	(400 – 643)	776	(746 – 803)	1,000	(931 – 1,140)	112
12–19 years	731	(706 – 757)	567	(517 – 596)	726	(712 – 750)	957	(906 – 1,050)	322
20–39 years	917	(893 – 941)	677	(613 – 704)	892	(862 – 925)	1,270	(1,190 – 1,490)	198
40–59 years	1,070	(1,030 – 1,110)	761	(707 – 808)	1,040	(1,000 – 1,110)	1,540	(1,400 – 1,740)	179
60 years and older	1,150	(1,080 – 1,230)	774	(650 – 848)	1,130	(1,040 – 1,230)	1,670	(1,560 – 1,770)	131

Table 2.4.a.5. Serum vitamin E: Non-Hispanic whites

Geometric mean and selected percentiles of serum concentrations (in µg/dL) for non-Hispanic whites in the U.S. population aged 6 years and older, National Health and Nutrition Examination Survey, 2005–2006.

	Geometric mean (95% conf. interval)		Selected percentiles (95% conf. interval)						Sample size
			10th		50th		90th		
Males and Females									
Total, 6 years and older	1,140	(1,110 – 1,160)	718	(706 – 729)	1,110	(1,080 – 1,140)	1,870	(1,810 – 1,940)	2,973
6–11 years	840	(815 – 866)	627	(612 – 642)	826	(805 – 854)	1,120	(1,060 – 1,260)	231
12–19 years	779	(761 – 797)	579	(544 – 589)	765	(751 – 784)	1,060	(1,010 – 1,140)	499
20–39 years	1,040	(1,010 – 1,070)	711	(671 – 741)	1,030	(1,000 – 1,060)	1,550	(1,410 – 1,710)	714
40–59 years	1,260	(1,220 – 1,300)	846	(817 – 866)	1,230	(1,190 – 1,260)	1,910	(1,800 – 2,100)	683
60 years and older	1,430	(1,390 – 1,480)	919	(856 – 976)	1,430	(1,390 – 1,480)	2,230	(2,170 – 2,330)	846
Males									
Total, 6 years and older	1,100	(1,070 – 1,130)	703	(671 – 725)	1,080	(1,050 – 1,120)	1,770	(1,740 – 1,850)	1,472
6–11 years	839	(801 – 879)	629	(562 – 680)	830	(791 – 880)	1,080	(1,030 – 1,300)	112
12–19 years	757	(737 – 778)	542	(523 – 572)	754	(730 – 783)	1,060	(1,000 – 1,110)	254
20–39 years	1,040	(1,020 – 1,070)	687	(640 – 735)	1,030	(1,020 – 1,060)	1,590	(1,430 – 1,770)	309
40–59 years	1,240	(1,200 – 1,270)	818	(769 – 865)	1,230	(1,180 – 1,260)	1,840	(1,750 – 2,040)	351
60 years and older	1,330	(1,240 – 1,420)	862	(733 – 930)	1,300	(1,250 – 1,360)	2,100	(1,970 – 2,460)	446
Females									
Total, 6 years and older	1,170	(1,150 – 1,200)	727	(718 – 746)	1,140	(1,100 – 1,170)	1,930	(1,870 – 2,050)	1,501
6–11 years	841	(792 – 892)	624	(597 – 656)	819	(774 – 878)	1,160	(1,050 – 1,470)	119
12–19 years	803	(780 – 827)	601	(562 – 641)	779	(750 – 805)	1,060	(985 – 1,200)	245
20–39 years	1,040	(1,000 – 1,080)	720	(699 – 754)	1,020	(978 – 1,060)	1,510	(1,360 – 1,630)	405
40–59 years	1,270	(1,230 – 1,320)	862	(842 – 894)	1,240	(1,190 – 1,280)	2,000	(1,850 – 2,190)	332
60 years and older	1,530	(1,480 – 1,590)	985	(964 – 1,020)	1,530	(1,470 – 1,590)	2,320	(2,240 – 2,500)	400

Table 2.4.b. Serum vitamin E: Concentrations by survey cycle

Geometric mean and selected percentiles of serum concentrations (in µg/dL) for the U.S. population, National Health and Nutrition Examination Survey, 1999–2002 and 2005–2006.

	Geometric mean (95% conf. interval)	Selected percentiles (95% conf. interval) 5th	Selected percentiles 50th	Selected percentiles 95th	Sample size
Total, 6 years and older					
1999–2000	1,070 (1,040 – 1,110)	597 (575 – 612)	1,010 (986 – 1,040)	2,350 (2,280 – 2,500)	7,054
2001–2002	1,110 (1,090 – 1,140)	637 (623 – 649)	1,050 (1,010 – 1,090)	2,380 (2,260 – 2,520)	7,935
2005–2006	1,090 (1,070 – 1,120)	631 (620 – 642)	1,060 (1,030 – 1,080)	2,090 (2,010 – 2,180)	7,254
Age group					
3–5 years					
1999–2000	785 (752 – 820)	559 (514 – 585)	772 (734 – 829)	1,160 (1,120 – 1,400)	347
2001–2002	814 (780 – 850)	577 (553 – 601)	796 (760 – 824)	1,200 (1,090 – 1,670)	430
6–11 years					
1999–2000	783 (754 – 814)	545 (519 – 557)	781 (749 – 824)	1,130 (1,090 – 1,210)	859
2001–2002	804 (788 – 821)	576 (560 – 591)	798 (780 – 819)	1,140 (1,090 – 1,220)	1,014
2005–2006	820 (800 – 841)	583 (563 – 601)	806 (788 – 826)	1,200 (1,120 – 1,370)	860
12–19 years					
1999–2000	736 (717 – 756)	513 (491 – 530)	729 (712 – 744)	1,100 (1,020 – 1,240)	2,108
2001–2002	782 (768 – 796)	550 (540 – 559)	771 (761 – 786)	1,170 (1,110 – 1,280)	2,206
2005–2006	770 (757 – 783)	527 (516 – 541)	759 (749 – 767)	1,160 (1,130 – 1,200)	1,954
20–39 years					
1999–2000	973 (952 – 995)	615 (590 – 630)	938 (911 – 972)	1,750 (1,640 – 1,860)	1,452
2001–2002	1,010 (987 – 1,030)	646 (627 – 661)	979 (960 – 1,000)	1,720 (1,620 – 1,880)	1,716
2005–2006	1,020 (998 – 1,040)	645 (621 – 668)	1,000 (980 – 1,020)	1,730 (1,620 – 1,900)	1,688
40–59 years					
1999–2000	1,300 (1,250 – 1,360)	753 (716 – 791)	1,230 (1,200 – 1,280)	2,670 (2,470 – 2,940)	1,181
2001–2002	1,310 (1,270 – 1,340)	776 (751 – 793)	1,260 (1,220 – 1,300)	2,530 (2,380 – 3,030)	1,474
2005–2006	1,230 (1,190 – 1,260)	749 (724 – 769)	1,200 (1,160 – 1,240)	2,210 (2,080 – 2,400)	1,365
60 years and older					
1999–2000	1,510 (1,470 – 1,560)	788 (749 – 825)	1,450 (1,390 – 1,510)	3,020 (2,920 – 3,290)	1,454
2001–2002	1,540 (1,490 – 1,590)	830 (763 – 869)	1,500 (1,440 – 1,550)	3,290 (3,030 – 3,540)	1,525
2005–2006	1,400 (1,360 – 1,440)	783 (733 – 835)	1,390 (1,330 – 1,430)	2,600 (2,510 – 2,660)	1,387
Gender					
(6 years and older)					
Males					
1999–2000	1,050 (1,010 – 1,090)	580 (557 – 604)	993 (976 – 1,020)	2,280 (2,130 – 2,470)	3,426
2001–2002	1,090 (1,060 – 1,130)	623 (607 – 646)	1,030 (986 – 1,080)	2,300 (2,160 – 2,470)	3,841
2005–2006	1,060 (1,040 – 1,090)	610 (594 – 625)	1,030 (1,010 – 1,070)	2,010 (1,930 – 2,090)	3,547
Females					
1999–2000	1,100 (1,070 – 1,140)	605 (580 – 627)	1,030 (990 – 1,070)	2,450 (2,300 – 2,690)	3,628
2001–2002	1,130 (1,110 – 1,150)	646 (629 – 660)	1,060 (1,040 – 1,100)	2,480 (2,280 – 2,700)	4,094
2005–2006	1,120 (1,090 – 1,140)	653 (639 – 664)	1,080 (1,050 – 1,100)	2,170 (2,080 – 2,260)	3,707
Race/ethnicity					
(6 years and older)					
Mexican Americans					
1999–2000	962 (932 – 994)	572 (558 – 587)	918 (895 – 947)	1,810 (1,740 – 2,010)	2,410
2001–2002	994 (954 – 1,040)	606 (584 – 625)	949 (917 – 979)	1,810 (1,690 – 2,080)	1,991
2005–2006	1,010 (980 – 1,040)	623 (602 – 637)	976 (945 – 1,000)	1,790 (1,750 – 1,870)	1,844
Non-Hispanic Blacks					
1999–2000	904 (869 – 941)	566 (539 – 580)	869 (835 – 910)	1,700 (1,620 – 1,910)	1,584
2001–2002	930 (907 – 953)	601 (573 – 617)	897 (883 – 915)	1,690 (1,540 – 1,940)	1,864
2005–2006	933 (915 – 951)	588 (581 – 601)	903 (884 – 918)	1,660 (1,560 – 1,750)	1,891
Non-Hispanic Whites					
1999–2000	1,130 (1,100 – 1,170)	618 (600 – 634)	1,060 (1,040 – 1,100)	2,540 (2,380 – 2,720)	2,414
2001–2002	1,160 (1,130 – 1,200)	653 (626 – 674)	1,110 (1,060 – 1,150)	2,510 (2,380 – 2,690)	3,455
2005–2006	1,140 (1,110 – 1,160)	643 (624 – 658)	1,110 (1,080 – 1,140)	2,170 (2,090 – 2,270)	2,973

Figure 2.4.b. Serum vitamin E: Concentrations by survey cycle

Selected percentiles in µg/dL (95% confidence intervals), National Health and Nutrition Examination Survey, 1999–2002 and 2005–2006

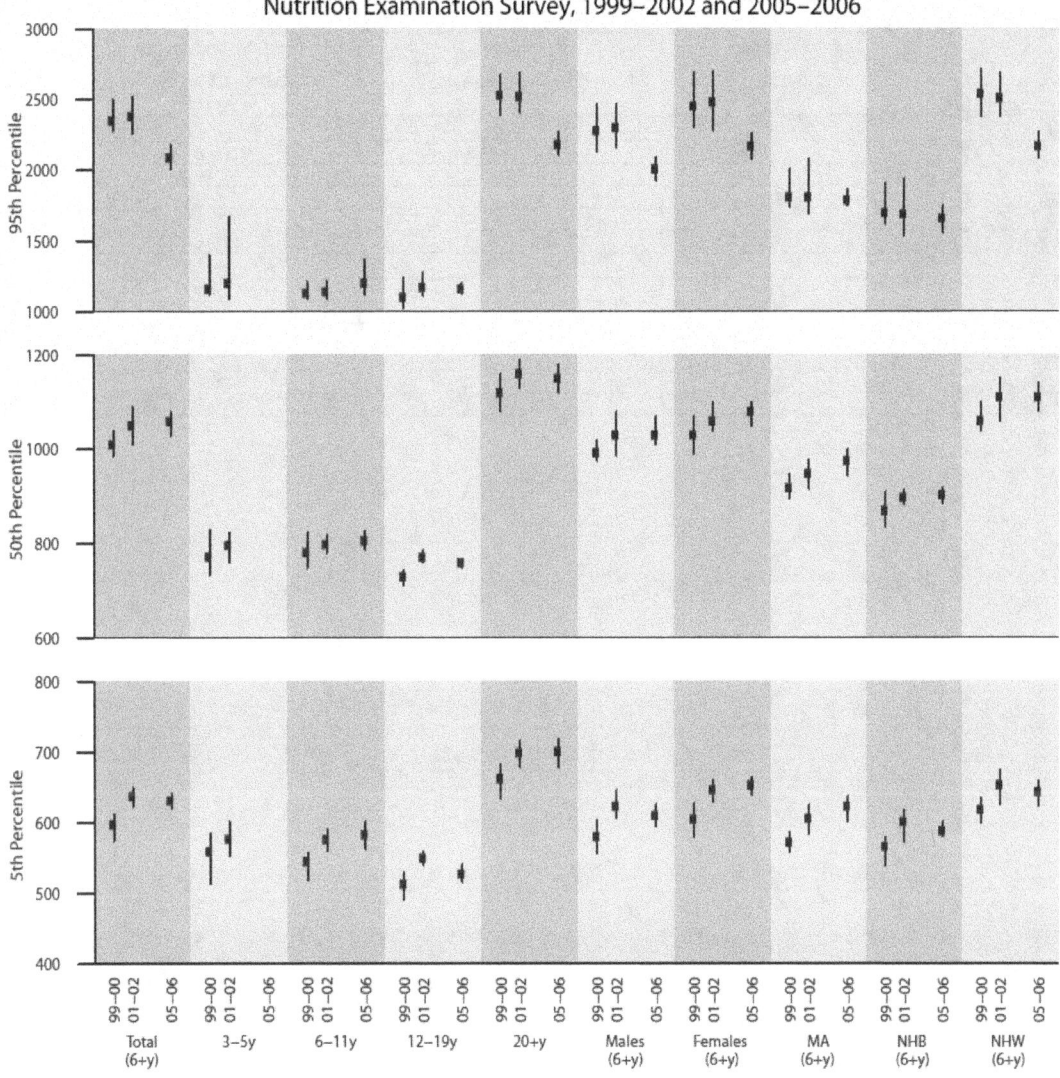

Table 2.4.c. Serum vitamin E: Prevalence

Prevalence (in percent) of low serum vitamin E concentration (< 500 µg/dL) for the U.S. population aged 6 years and older, National Health and Nutrition Examination Survey, 2005–2006.

	Sample size	Prevalence (95% conf. interval)	Estimated total number of persons
Total, 6 years and older	7,254	0.7 (0.5 – 0.9)	1,835,000
Age group			
6–11 years	860	0.9‡ (0.4 – 2.0)	221,000‡
12–19 years	1,954	2.6 (1.6 – 4.3)	885,000
20–39 years	1,688	§	§
40–59 years	1,365	0.3‡ (0.1 – 0.6)	237,000‡
60 years and older	1,387	0.4 (0.3 – 0.7)	209,000
Gender			
Males	3,547	0.9 (0.6 – 1.2)	1,110,000
Females	3,707	0.5 (0.3 – 0.8)	725,000
Race/ethnicity			
Mexican Americans	1,844	§	§
Non-Hispanic Blacks	1,891	1.2 (0.9 – 1.7)	396,000
Non-Hispanic Whites	2,973	0.6 (0.4 – 0.8)	1,059,000

‡ Estimate flagged: 30% ≤ RSE < 40% for the prevalence estimate.
§ Estimate suppressed: RSE ≥ 40% for the prevalence estimate.

Table 2.4.d. Serum vitamin E: Prevalence by survey cycle

Prevalence (in percent) of low serum vitamin E concentration (< 500 µg/dL) for the U.S. population, National Health and Nutrition Examination Survey, 1999–2002 and 2005–2006.

	Sample size	Prevalence (95% conf. interval)	Estimated total number of persons
Total, 6 years and older			
1999–2000	7,054	1.0 (0.7 – 1.6)	2,558,000
2001–2002	7,935	0.4 (0.3 – 0.6)	1,108,000
2005–2006	7,254	0.7 (0.5 – 0.9)	1,835,000
Age group			
3–5 years			
1999–2000	347	§	§
2001–2002	430	§	§
6–11 years			
1999–2000	859	2.0‡ (1.0 – 4.1)	492,000‡
2001–2002	1,014	§	
2005–2006	860	0.9‡ (0.4 – 2.0)	221,000‡
12–19 years			
1999–2000	2,108	3.8 (2.1 – 6.8)	1,202,000
2001–2002	2,206	1.6 (1.0 – 2.6)	509,000
2005–2006	1,954	2.6 (1.6 – 4.3)	885,000
20–39 years			
1999–2000	1,452	0.9‡ (0.5 – 1.8)	730,000‡
2001–2002	1,716	§	§
2005–2006	1,688	§	§
40–59 years			
1999–2000	1,181	0.1‡ (0.1 – 0.2)	80,000‡
2001–2002	1,474	§	§
2005–2006	1,365	0.3‡ (0.1 – 0.6)	237,000‡
60 years and older			
1999–2000	1,454	§	§
2001–2002	1,525	§	§
2005–2006	1,387	0.4 (0.3 – 0.7)	209,000
Gender			
(6 years and older)			
Males			
1999–2000	3,426	1.4 (0.8 – 2.3)	1,660,000
2001–2002	3,841	0.6 (0.4 – 1.0)	781,000
2005–2006	3,547	0.9 (0.6 – 1.2)	1,110,000
Females			
1999–2000	3,628	0.7 (0.4 – 1.1)	895,000
2001–2002	4,094	0.2 (0.1 – 0.5)	325,000
2005–2006	3,707	0.5 (0.3 – 0.8)	725,000
Race/ethnicity			
(6 years and older)			
Mexican Americans			
1999–2000	2,410	1.3 (0.9 – 1.8)	227,000
2001–2002	1,991	0.7‡ (0.4 – 1.5)	156,000‡
2005–2006	1,844	§	§
Non-Hispanic Blacks			
1999–2000	1,584	1.7 (0.9 – 3.2)	520,000
2001–2002	1,864	0.7 (0.4 – 1.1)	207,000
2005–2006	1,891	1.2 (0.9 – 1.7)	396,000
Non-Hispanic Whites			
1999–2000	2,414	0.8 (0.5 – 1.3)	1,491,000
2001–2002	3,455	0.3 (0.2 – 0.5)	556,000
2005–2006	2,973	0.6 (0.4 – 0.8)	1,059,000

‡ Estimate flagged: 30% ≤ RSE < 40% for the prevalence estimate.
§ Estimate suppressed: RSE ≥ 40% for the prevalence estimate.

Table 2.5.a.1. Serum gamma-tocopherol: Concentrations

Geometric mean and selected percentiles of serum concentrations (in μg/dL) for the total U.S. population aged 6 years and older, National Health and Nutrition Examination Survey, 2005–2006.

	Geometric mean (95% conf. interval)	Selected percentiles (95% conf. interval)						Sample size
		2.5th	5th	50th	95th	97.5th		
Total, 6 years and older	188 (180 – 196)	53.5 (49.6 – 59.9)	70.4 (62.9 – 75.4)	196 (187 – 204)	424 (408 – 446)	489 (464 – 519)		7,217
Age group								
6–11 years	182 (171 – 193)	68.1 (55.2 – 85.2)	91.5 (71.3 – 99.2)	179 (169 – 193)	353 (333 – 390)	392 (367 – 455)		858
12–19 years	179 (171 – 188)	75.5 (62.0 – 81.8)	89.0 (79.8 – 93.8)	184 (175 – 194)	324 (311 – 343)	376 (344 – 413)		1,942
20–39 years	194 (184 – 205)	65.4 (50.6 – 76.7)	81.9 (75.3 – 93.8)	200 (192 – 209)	423 (401 – 460)	489 (447 – 553)		1,675
40–59 years	201 (192 – 212)	53.0 (46.5 – 61.2)	69.0 (56.1 – 80.0)	213 (203 – 221)	452 (437 – 498)	545 (492 – 604)		1,358
60 years and older	165 (154 – 177)	45.1 (41.4 – 49.8)	52.4 (49.7 – 57.5)	176 (161 – 192)	422 (403 – 462)	486 (461 – 539)		1,384
Gender								
Males	192 (184 – 200)	54.9 (48.6 – 63.3)	74.5 (62.4 – 80.8)	198 (189 – 206)	434 (411 – 471)	505 (478 – 564)		3,528
Females	184 (175 – 194)	52.4 (49.4 – 58.5)	67.7 (60.1 – 73.5)	194 (183 – 203)	419 (400 – 441)	464 (444 – 497)		3,689
Race/ethnicity								
Mexican Americans	204 (192 – 217)	80.4 (64.2 – 86.3)	93.8 (84.0 – 102)	209 (195 – 222)	437 (390 – 503)	504 (463 – 585)		1,841
Non-Hispanic Blacks	214 (198 – 231)	70.6 (52.2 – 85.5)	92.0 (67.4 – 106)	219 (204 – 235)	429 (408 – 488)	509 (457 – 550)		1,865
Non-Hispanic Whites	182 (173 – 191)	51.2 (46.7 – 55.0)	65.1 (57.4 – 72.3)	190 (179 – 200)	423 (407 – 445)	485 (454 – 531)		2,965

Figure 2.5.a. Serum gamma–tocopherol: Concentrations by age group

Geometric mean (95% confidence interval), National Health and Nutrition Examination Survey, 2005–2006

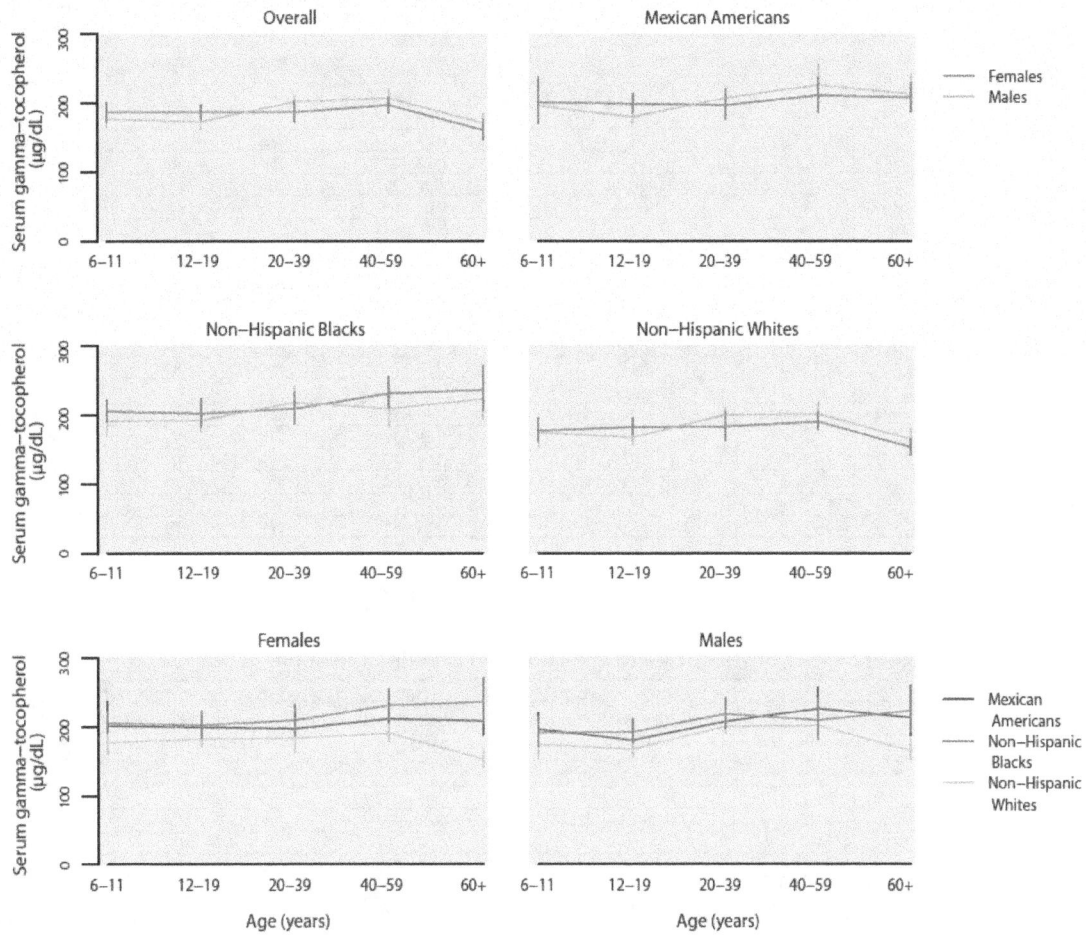

Table 2.5.a.2. Serum gamma-tocopherol: Total population

Geometric mean and selected percentiles of serum concentrations (in µg/dL) for the total U.S. population aged 6 years and older, National Health and Nutrition Examination Survey, 2005–2006.

	Geometric mean (95% conf. interval)	Selected percentiles (95% conf. interval)			Sample size
		10th	50th	90th	
Males and Females					
Total, 6 years and older	188 (180 – 196)	93.2 (86.8 – 98.0)	196 (187 – 204)	361 (347 – 385)	7,217
6–11 years	182 (171 – 193)	106 (102 – 111)	179 (169 – 193)	311 (298 – 341)	858
12–19 years	179 (171 – 188)	106 (98.1 – 114)	184 (175 – 194)	288 (276 – 304)	1,942
20–39 years	194 (184 – 205)	106 (94.7 – 114)	200 (192 – 209)	353 (330 – 393)	1,675
40–59 years	201 (192 – 212)	95.2 (84.4 – 102)	213 (203 – 221)	400 (376 – 423)	1,358
60 years and older	165 (154 – 177)	68.6 (60.9 – 73.4)	176 (161 – 192)	358 (340 – 397)	1,384
Males					
Total, 6 years and older	192 (184 – 200)	98.7 (89.3 – 107)	198 (189 – 206)	359 (349 – 389)	3,528
6–11 years	177 (166 – 189)	105 (94.0 – 109)	176 (163 – 189)	304 (276 – 349)	425
12–19 years	173 (162 – 184)	103 (89.6 – 114)	177 (168 – 188)	284 (266 – 306)	974
20–39 years	202 (193 – 211)	113 (105 – 119)	203 (194 – 215)	386 (349 – 414)	732
40–59 years	207 (194 – 221)	99.0 (86.0 – 113)	215 (202 – 230)	403 (365 – 442)	669
60 years and older	171 (157 – 185)	73.7 (66.9 – 77.2)	184 (159 – 204)	354 (336 – 396)	728
Females					
Total, 6 years and older	184 (175 – 194)	88.2 (80.0 – 93.8)	194 (183 – 203)	362 (338 – 388)	3,689
6–11 years	187 (174 – 201)	110 (93.6 – 122)	183 (169 – 199)	323 (299 – 346)	433
12–19 years	187 (177 – 197)	110 (101 – 119)	191 (184 – 201)	292 (274 – 313)	968
20–39 years	187 (173 – 202)	97.2 (79.9 – 110)	196 (180 – 207)	331 (312 – 383)	943
40–59 years	197 (186 – 208)	90.5 (75.5 – 99.0)	207 (195 – 223)	398 (377 – 423)	689
60 years and older	161 (148 – 175)	63.9 (53.9 – 72.6)	168 (155 – 188)	375 (328 – 405)	656

Table 2.5.a.3. Serum gamma-tocopherol: Mexican Americans

Geometric mean and selected percentiles of serum concentrations (in µg/dL) for Mexican Americans in the U.S. population aged 6 years and older, National Health and Nutrition Examination Survey, 2005–2006.

	Geometric mean (95% conf. interval)	Selected percentiles (95% conf. interval)			Sample size
		10th	50th	90th	
Males and Females					
Total, 6 years and older	204 (192 – 217)	113 (106 – 117)	209 (195 – 222)	363 (343 – 403)	1,841
6–11 years	199 (178 – 221)	114 (91.6 – 122)	202 (181 – 234)	323 (303 – 388)	293
12–19 years	189 (179 – 200)	115 (106 – 124)	197 (183 – 207)	292 (279 – 316)	645
20–39 years	203 (190 – 217)	111 (107 – 116)	209 (190 – 223)	366 (333 – 429)	449
40–59 years	218 (202 – 237)	114 (91.7 – 125)	226 (213 – 240)	410 (357 – 478)	246
60 years and older	210 (196 – 225)	99.7 (90.1 – 117)	211 (194 – 224)	406 (365 – 464)	208
Males					
Total, 6 years and older	206 (196 – 216)	114 (109 – 118)	210 (193 – 224)	363 (339 – 417)	881
6–11 years	196 (175 – 219)	116 (90.6 – 128)	189 (171 – 221)	329 (290 – 448)	143
12–19 years	180 (169 – 191)	109 (97.9 – 115)	187 (166 – 208)	282 (264 – 310)	313
20–39 years	207 (195 – 221)	112 (107 – 118)	216 (191 – 228)	375 (316 – 522)	198
40–59 years	226 (199 – 256)	118 (96.4 – 141)	227 (201 – 265)	376 (345 – 582)	122
60 years and older	213 (187 – 242)	100† (83.3 – 119)	205 (182 – 266)	412† (353 – 496)	105
Females					
Total, 6 years and older	202 (185 – 220)	112 (96.2 – 120)	207 (194 – 221)	363 (334 – 407)	960
6–11 years	201 (171 – 237)	113 (80.8 – 128)	219 (172 – 262)	322 (303 – 373)	150
12–19 years	199 (187 – 213)	128 (113 – 137)	202 (191 – 212)	308 (286 – 375)	332
20–39 years	197 (177 – 219)	109 (93.8 – 118)	202 (180 – 219)	362 (315 – 443)	251
40–59 years	211 (187 – 237)	103 (61.5 – 121)	223 (184 – 259)	423 (351 – 515)	124
60 years and older	208 (188 – 229)	98.8† (85.1 – 120)	213 (192 – 224)	398† (315 – 506)	103

† Estimate is subject to greater uncertainty due to small cell size.

Table 2.5.a.4. Serum gamma-tocopherol: Non-Hispanic blacks

Geometric mean and selected percentiles of serum concentrations (in µg/dL) for non-Hispanic blacks in the U.S. population aged 6 years and older, National Health and Nutrition Examination Survey, 2005–2006.

	Geometric mean (95% conf. interval)		Selected percentiles (95% conf. interval)						Sample size
			10th		50th		90th		
Males and Females									
Total, 6 years and older	214	(198 – 231)	119	(98.4 – 135)	219	(204 – 235)	383	(357 – 407)	1,865
6–11 years	198	(183 – 214)	128	(96.7 – 141)	198	(189 – 210)	317	(291 – 360)	240
12–19 years	197	(180 – 215)	126	(105 – 142)	198	(180 – 215)	308	(279 – 338)	654
20–39 years	213	(196 – 231)	114	(93.5 – 137)	216	(202 – 231)	379	(334 – 420)	359
40–59 years	221	(198 – 247)	115	(72.3 – 140)	233	(208 – 254)	404	(378 – 476)	331
60 years and older	231	(204 – 261)	109	(60.6 – 139)	255	(216 – 286)	413	(392 – 466)	281
Males									
Total, 6 years and older	209	(192 – 227)	120	(102 – 136)	210	(195 – 225)	362	(335 – 402)	935
6–11 years	191	(171 – 213)	116	(69.0 – 142)	193	(182 – 205)	297	(263 – 360)	128
12–19 years	192	(176 – 210)	127	(111 – 141)	187	(170 – 208)	302	(278 – 335)	337
20–39 years	218	(197 – 241)	119	(101 – 136)	220	(195 – 240)	386	(326 – 500)	166
40–59 years	209	(182 – 241)	109	(71.2 – 141)	213	(187 – 239)	401	(311 – 526)	153
60 years and older	223	(193 – 259)	122	(53.9 – 147)	234	(202 – 276)	393	(341 – 498)	151
Females									
Total, 6 years and older	218	(203 – 234)	116	(93.3 – 134)	228	(213 – 242)	396	(375 – 410)	930
6–11 years	205	(191 – 221)	131	(99.5 – 143)	204	(189 – 229)	327	(292 – 433)	112
12–19 years	202	(183 – 223)	123	(98.5 – 147)	205	(195 – 218)	314	(279 – 354)	317
20–39 years	209	(188 – 231)	110	(81.8 – 141)	213	(195 – 236)	377	(329 – 426)	193
40–59 years	231	(210 – 255)	116	(72.3 – 134)	249	(217 – 285)	404	(399 – 443)	178
60 years and older	236	(207 – 270)	103	(54.5 – 145)	261	(219 – 299)	448	(393 – 505)	130

Table 2.5.a.5. Serum gamma-tocopherol: Non-Hispanic whites

Geometric mean and selected percentiles of serum concentrations (in µg/dL) for non-Hispanic whites in the U.S. population aged 6 years and older, National Health and Nutrition Examination Survey, 2005–2006.

	Geometric mean (95% conf. interval)		Selected percentiles (95% conf. interval)						Sample size
			10th		50th		90th		
Males and Females									
Total, 6 years and older	182	(173 – 191)	86.4	(79.6 – 92.0)	190	(179 – 200)	356	(340 – 387)	2,965
6–11 years	175	(159 – 192)	105	(99.7 – 109)	170	(157 – 191)	304	(272 – 349)	231
12–19 years	174	(165 – 184)	102	(90.8 – 108)	179	(171 – 188)	284	(274 – 301)	499
20–39 years	191	(178 – 205)	105	(83.6 – 116)	196	(183 – 207)	349	(320 – 401)	710
40–59 years	196	(184 – 207)	91.6	(80.3 – 97.8)	207	(195 – 220)	396	(368 – 424)	680
60 years and older	158	(148 – 169)	65.9	(59.4 – 72.1)	168	(154 – 183)	353	(326 – 392)	845
Males									
Total, 6 years and older	187	(178 – 197)	94.7	(81.7 – 104)	194	(184 – 204)	355	(344 – 388)	1,469
6–11 years	174	(153 – 197)	105	(82.6 – 111)	170	(150 – 192)	307	(269 – 378)	112
12–19 years	167	(155 – 180)	95.0	(76.7 – 113)	173	(163 – 181)	280	(250 – 314)	254
20–39 years	200	(190 – 210)	117	(105 – 126)	201	(188 – 212)	370	(346 – 414)	307
40–59 years	201	(185 – 218)	95.5	(80.3 – 106)	214	(195 – 230)	398	(350 – 448)	350
60 years and older	165	(151 – 180)	71.6	(62.2 – 76.5)	177	(150 – 199)	351	(331 – 380)	446
Females									
Total, 6 years and older	177	(167 – 188)	79.9	(73.8 – 87.5)	186	(173 – 197)	359	(324 – 391)	1,496
6–11 years	177	(160 – 195)	104	(86.4 – 114)	171	(155 – 197)	300	(260 – 349)	119
12–19 years	182	(171 – 195)	103	(89.6 – 118)	187	(175 – 200)	289	(270 – 312)	245
20–39 years	183	(163 – 204)	92.8	(71.4 – 110)	191	(169 – 210)	323	(296 – 403)	403
40–59 years	190	(178 – 204)	83.6	(68.1 – 98.3)	203	(186 – 217)	392	(373 – 427)	330
60 years and older	153	(141 – 165)	61.1	(53.5 – 69.6)	161	(148 – 174)	357	(319 – 400)	399

Table 2.5.b. Serum gamma-tocopherol: Concentrations by survey cycle

Geometric mean and selected percentiles of serum concentrations (in µg/dL) for the U.S. population, National Health and Nutrition Examination Survey, 1999–2002 and 2005–2006.

	Geometric mean (95% conf. interval)	Selected percentiles (95% conf. interval)						Sample size
		5th		50th		95th		
Total, 6 years and older								
1999–2000	199 (184 – 216)	65.1	(58.2 – 71.7)	215	(197 – 230)	464	(432 – 529)	6,129
2001–2002	199 (191 – 207)	67.1	(59.4 – 73.8)	212	(204 – 220)	461	(436 – 485)	7,879
2005–2006	188 (180 – 196)	70.4	(62.9 – 75.4)	196	(187 – 204)	424	(408 – 446)	7,217
Age group								
3–5 years								
1999–2000	170 (140 – 206)	50.0	(16.2 – 90.8)	180	(158 – 200)	363	(308 – 455)	301
2001–2002	181 (170 – 193)	63.3	(52.2 – 82.2)	194	(178 – 205)	365	(342 – 430)	429
6–11 years								
1999–2000	202 (183 – 223)	93.3	(72.3 – 107)	213	(184 – 231)	407	(356 – 569)	725
2001–2002	211 (203 – 219)	102	(95.4 – 109)	218	(211 – 227)	380	(361 – 414)	1,005
2005–2006	182 (171 – 193)	91.5	(71.3 – 99.2)	179	(169 – 193)	353	(333 – 390)	858
12–19 years								
1999–2000	197 (183 – 211)	99.0	(80.4 – 112)	198	(186 – 214)	372	(363 – 389)	1,821
2001–2002	197 (190 – 205)	99.4	(90.2 – 107)	201	(191 – 209)	368	(346 – 391)	2,188
2005–2006	179 (171 – 188)	89.0	(79.8 – 93.8)	184	(175 – 194)	324	(311 – 343)	1,942
20–39 years								
1999–2000	205 (189 – 222)	75.6	(60.5 – 87.3)	220	(199 – 237)	438	(414 – 477)	1,299
2001–2002	206 (197 – 216)	85.6	(73.5 – 95.3)	217	(205 – 227)	445	(425 – 474)	1,706
2005–2006	194 (184 – 205)	81.9	(75.3 – 93.8)	200	(192 – 209)	423	(401 – 460)	1,675
40–59 years								
1999–2000	208 (185 – 232)	59.8	(51.9 – 70.0)	231	(204 – 253)	549	(507 – 631)	1,028
2001–2002	204 (192 – 217)	60.4	(52.2 – 68.3)	221	(208 – 238)	507	(463 – 576)	1,463
2005–2006	201 (192 – 212)	69.0	(56.1 – 80.0)	213	(203 – 221)	452	(437 – 498)	1,358
60 years and older								
1999–2000	178 (160 – 197)	47.6	(42.9 – 54.4)	196	(171 – 216)	496	(443 – 573)	1,256
2001–2002	172 (162 – 184)	48.2	(43.8 – 52.0)	185	(170 – 201)	497	(469 – 534)	1,517
2005–2006	165 (154 – 177)	52.4	(49.7 – 57.5)	176	(161 – 192)	422	(403 – 462)	1,384
Gender								
(6 years and older)								
Males								
1999–2000	199 (184 – 217)	65.3	(55.9 – 74.7)	213	(197 – 230)	462	(426 – 532)	2,974
2001–2002	202 (193 – 211)	66.5	(56.0 – 77.1)	213	(207 – 222)	472	(445 – 499)	3,815
2005–2006	192 (184 – 200)	74.5	(62.4 – 80.8)	198	(189 – 206)	434	(411 – 471)	3,528
Females								
1999–2000	200 (184 – 217)	64.8	(57.6 – 71.8)	217	(196 – 232)	468	(433 – 536)	3,155
2001–2002	196 (187 – 205)	67.6	(60.6 – 74.7)	210	(200 – 220)	447	(420 – 483)	4,064
2005–2006	184 (175 – 194)	67.7	(60.1 – 73.5)	194	(183 – 203)	419	(400 – 441)	3,689
Race/ethnicity								
(6 years and older)								
Mexican Americans								
1999–2000	222 (210 – 235)	104	(89.1 – 113)	225	(213 – 236)	468	(414 – 504)	1,772
2001–2002	198 (190 – 206)	89.8	(80.5 – 92.6)	203	(190 – 214)	422	(390 – 458)	1,987
2005–2006	204 (192 – 217)	93.8	(84.0 – 102)	209	(195 – 222)	437	(390 – 503)	1,841
Non-Hispanic Blacks								
1999–2000	213 (200 – 226)	94.5	(73.1 – 104)	217	(201 – 238)	437	(417 – 473)	1,515
2001–2002	235 (222 – 248)	107	(83.5 – 118)	248	(233 – 261)	450	(426 – 478)	1,843
2005–2006	214 (198 – 231)	92.0	(67.4 – 106)	219	(204 – 235)	429	(408 – 488)	1,865
Non-Hispanic Whites								
1999–2000	198 (179 – 219)	61.3	(52.8 – 70.1)	217	(192 – 234)	477	(439 – 542)	2,240
2001–2002	193 (183 – 205)	60.4	(51.4 – 68.0)	209	(198 – 220)	472	(442 – 495)	3,426
2005–2006	182 (173 – 191)	65.1	(57.4 – 72.3)	190	(179 – 200)	423	(407 – 445)	2,965

Figure 2.5.b. Serum gamma–tocopherol: Concentrations by survey cycle

Selected percentiles in μg/dL (95% confidence intervals), National Health and Nutrition Examination Survey, 1999–2002 and 2005–2006

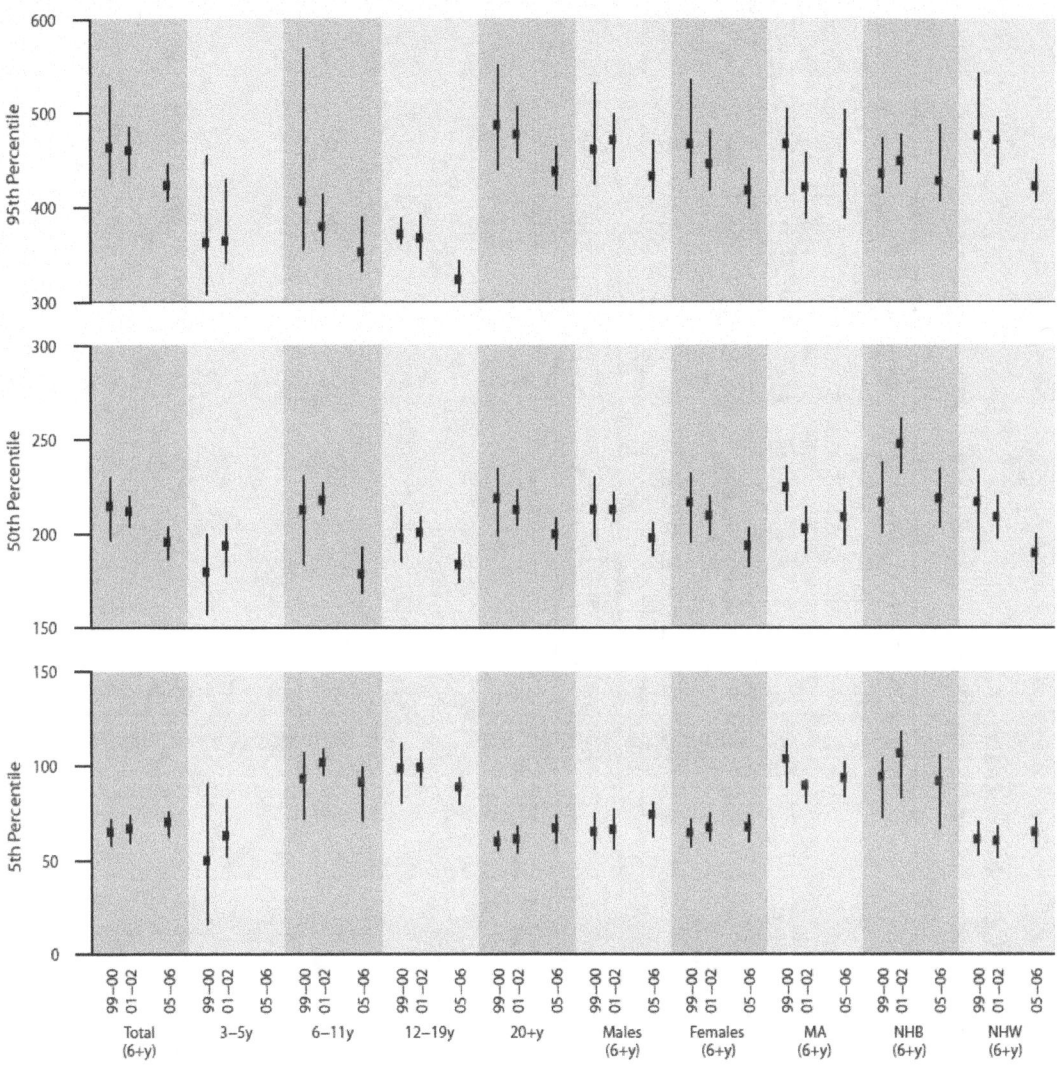

Table 2.6.a.1. Serum alpha–carotene: Concentrations

Geometric mean and selected percentiles of serum concentrations (in µg/dL) for the total U.S. population aged 6 years and older, National Health and Nutrition Examination Survey, 2005–2006.

	Geometric mean (95% conf. interval)	Selected percentiles (95% conf. interval)						Sample size
		2.5th	5th	50th	95th	97.5th		
Total, 6 years and older	2.76 (2.54 – 2.99)	< LOD	< LOD	2.63 (2.40 – 2.84)	14.1 (12.4 – 16.5)	19.5 (17.6 – 23.7)		7,246
Age group								
6–11 years	2.64 (2.32 – 3.01)	< LOD	< LOD	2.59 (2.31 – 2.90)	11.5 (9.30 – 15.1)	15.7 (11.6 – 34.7)		860
12–19 years	1.85 (1.69 – 2.03)	< LOD	< LOD	1.72 (1.53 – 1.91)	7.91 (6.65 – 10.2)	10.8 (8.96 – 15.2)		1,950
20–39 years	2.48 (2.24 – 2.74)	< LOD	< LOD	2.36 (2.06 – 2.69)	11.3 (10.1 – 14.7)	16.3 (12.7 – 23.6)		1,684
40–59 years	3.15 (2.85 – 3.47)	< LOD	< LOD	3.01 (2.72 – 3.36)	17.0 (14.5 – 21.9)	27.1 (20.3 – 35.9)		1,365
60 years and older	3.42 (3.05 – 3.83)	< LOD	.711 (< LOD – .811)	3.33 (2.86 – 3.86)	17.0 (14.0 – 19.8)	21.6 (19.3 – 25.9)		1,387
Gender								
Males	2.37 (2.20 – 2.55)	< LOD	< LOD	2.23 (2.06 – 2.39)	11.5 (9.92 – 13.9)	16.1 (13.2 – 20.9)		3,544
Females	3.18 (2.89 – 3.50)	< LOD	< LOD	3.01 (2.74 – 3.32)	16.4 (14.6 – 18.4)	23.9 (19.4 – 30.0)		3,702
Race/ethnicity								
Mexican Americans	2.99 (2.79 – 3.21)	< LOD	.824 (.749 – .889)	2.87 (2.61 – 3.21)	10.8 (10.5 – 12.5)	14.8 (13.9 – 16.6)		1,844
Non-Hispanic Blacks	1.98 (1.74 – 2.26)	< LOD	< LOD	1.71 (1.49 – 1.99)	11.0 (8.83 – 14.8)	15.2 (12.4 – 33.1)		1,890
Non-Hispanic Whites	2.80 (2.60 – 3.02)	< LOD	< LOD	2.67 (2.47 – 2.89)	14.4 (12.8 – 16.7)	20.2 (18.1 – 24.2)		2,966

< LOD means less than the limit of detection, which may vary for some compounds by year. See Appendix D for LOD.

Figure 2.6.a. Serum alpha–carotene: Concentrations by age group

Geometric mean (95% confidence interval), National Health and Nutrition Examination Survey, 2005–2006

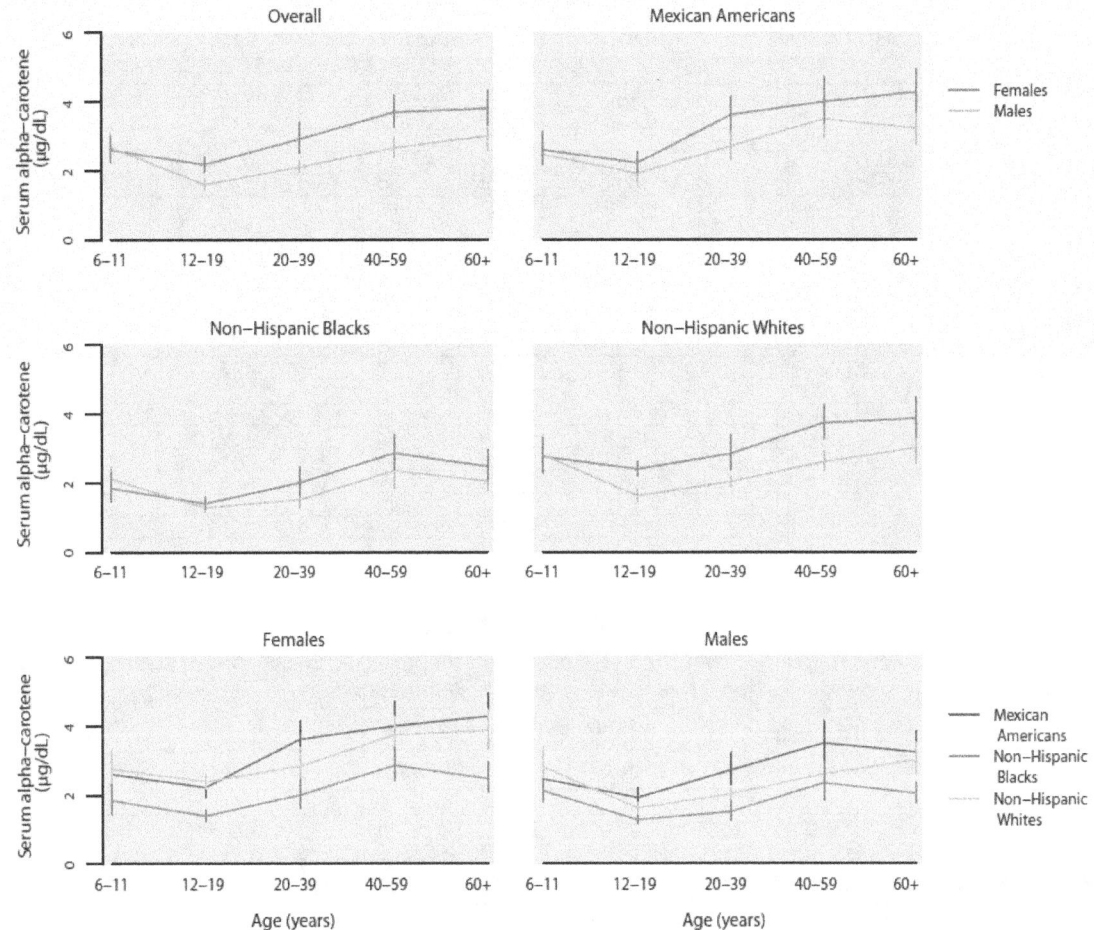

Table 2.6.a.2. Serum alpha-carotene: Total population

Geometric mean and selected percentiles of serum concentrations (in µg/dL) for the total U.S. population aged 6 years and older, National Health and Nutrition Examination Survey, 2005–2006.

	Geometric mean (95% conf. interval)		Selected percentiles (95% conf. interval)						Sample size
			10th		50th		90th		
Males and Females									
Total, 6 years and older	2.76	(2.54 – 2.99)	.772	(.718 – .823)	2.63	(2.40 – 2.84)	9.48	(8.58 – 10.6)	7,246
6–11 years	2.64	(2.32 – 3.01)	.865	(.766 – .966)	2.59	(2.31 – 2.90)	8.34	(6.74 – 10.9)	860
12–19 years	1.85	(1.69 – 2.03)	< LOD		1.72	(1.53 – 1.91)	5.55	(4.98 – 6.67)	1,950
20–39 years	2.48	(2.24 – 2.74)	.702	(< LOD – .793)	2.36	(2.06 – 2.69)	8.65	(7.55 – 9.72)	1,684
40–59 years	3.15	(2.85 – 3.47)	.836	(< LOD – .963)	3.01	(2.72 – 3.36)	11.8	(10.0 – 13.3)	1,365
60 years and older	3.42	(3.05 – 3.83)	1.02	(.832 – 1.17)	3.33	(2.86 – 3.86)	10.8	(9.64 – 13.1)	1,387
Males									
Total, 6 years and older	2.37	(2.20 – 2.55)	< LOD		2.23	(2.06 – 2.39)	7.74	(6.73 – 9.37)	3,544
6–11 years	2.68	(2.32 – 3.10)	.885	(.780 – .985)	2.59	(2.36 – 2.91)	8.27	(5.98 – 12.0)	427
12–19 years	1.60	(1.46 – 1.76)	< LOD		1.40	(1.29 – 1.61)	4.51	(3.69 – 5.54)	979
20–39 years	2.10	(1.95 – 2.27)	< LOD		2.00	(1.79 – 2.19)	6.91	(6.14 – 7.26)	736
40–59 years	2.66	(2.38 – 2.96)	.711	(< LOD – .910)	2.47	(2.24 – 2.76)	8.79	(7.13 – 11.5)	673
60 years and older	3.01	(2.61 – 3.46)	.838	(.754 – .923)	3.09	(2.55 – 3.54)	9.76	(7.73 – 12.9)	729
Females									
Total, 6 years and older	3.18	(2.89 – 3.50)	.895	(.807 – .983)	3.01	(2.74 – 3.32)	10.8	(9.83 – 12.3)	3,702
6–11 years	2.60	(2.26 – 2.99)	.854	(.712 – .972)	2.59	(2.14 – 2.97)	8.39	(6.99 – 11.1)	433
12–19 years	2.17	(1.98 – 2.39)	.709	(< LOD – .777)	2.08	(1.89 – 2.30)	6.43	(5.53 – 7.15)	971
20–39 years	2.92	(2.51 – 3.39)	.859	(< LOD – .969)	2.74	(2.41 – 3.31)	9.80	(8.53 – 11.9)	948
40–59 years	3.69	(3.25 – 4.17)	.992	(.764 – 1.23)	3.54	(3.07 – 3.97)	13.7	(11.7 – 16.7)	692
60 years and older	3.80	(3.33 – 4.32)	1.18	(1.01 – 1.32)	3.50	(2.94 – 4.36)	11.6	(10.2 – 15.0)	658

< LOD means less than the limit of detection, which may vary for some compounds by year. See Appendix D for LOD.

Table 2.6.a.3. Serum alpha-carotene: Mexican Americans

Geometric mean and selected percentiles of serum concentrations (in µg/dL) for Mexican Americans in the U.S. population aged 6 years and older, National Health and Nutrition Examination Survey, 2005–2006.

	Geometric mean (95% conf. interval)		Selected percentiles (95% conf. interval)						Sample size
			10th		50th		90th		
Males and Females									
Total, 6 years and older	2.99	(2.79 – 3.21)	1.07	(.952 – 1.21)	2.87	(2.61 – 3.21)	7.96	(7.58 – 8.67)	1,844
6–11 years	2.53	(2.21 – 2.89)	.918	(.702 – 1.14)	2.47	(2.03 – 3.00)	6.79	(5.10 – 9.28)	295
12–19 years	2.06	(1.82 – 2.33)	.847	(.723 – .952)	1.89	(1.70 – 2.22)	5.19	(4.56 – 5.91)	646
20–39 years	3.09	(2.78 – 3.42)	1.22	(1.07 – 1.33)	2.88	(2.56 – 3.37)	7.74	(7.18 – 8.74)	449
40–59 years	3.72	(3.31 – 4.19)	1.44	(.784 – 1.77)	3.57	(3.24 – 4.21)	10.5	(8.26 – 14.0)	246
60 years and older	3.76	(3.31 – 4.27)	1.28	(.767 – 1.60)	3.60	(3.22 – 4.31)	9.80	(8.51 – 16.0)	208
Males									
Total, 6 years and older	2.72	(2.50 – 2.95)	.997	(.890 – 1.09)	2.57	(2.22 – 3.00)	7.27	(6.99 – 7.73)	883
6–11 years	2.46	(2.16 – 2.81)	.904	(< LOD – 1.25)	2.49	(1.94 – 3.20)	5.58	(4.47 – 10.7)	145
12–19 years	1.92	(1.68 – 2.19)	.785	(< LOD – .874)	1.75	(1.50 – 2.05)	5.16	(3.85 – 6.20)	313
20–39 years	2.71	(2.30 – 3.20)	1.08	(.902 – 1.24)	2.47	(2.01 – 3.18)	7.32	(6.06 – 8.64)	198
40–59 years	3.49	(2.95 – 4.13)	1.43	(< LOD – 1.76)	3.35	(2.71 – 4.08)	9.79	(7.00 – 15.0)	122
60 years and older	3.23	(2.73 – 3.83)	.939†	(< LOD – 1.50)	3.18	(2.62 – 4.23)	8.07†	(6.41 – 20.8)	105
Females									
Total, 6 years and older	3.33	(3.07 – 3.61)	1.20	(1.06 – 1.30)	3.26	(2.95 – 3.50)	9.08	(8.35 – 9.84)	961
6–11 years	2.60	(2.17 – 3.12)	.923	(< LOD – 1.15)	2.43	(1.99 – 3.17)	7.44	(5.70 – 9.89)	150
12–19 years	2.22	(1.95 – 2.53)	.937	(.732 – 1.09)	2.08	(1.81 – 2.51)	5.21	(4.55 – 6.57)	333
20–39 years	3.61	(3.16 – 4.13)	1.47	(1.16 – 1.62)	3.45	(2.84 – 4.13)	9.06	(6.93 – 13.2)	251
40–59 years	3.99	(3.38 – 4.70)	1.39	(< LOD – 1.83)	3.82	(3.37 – 4.47)	10.6	(7.74 – 33.5)	124
60 years and older	4.27	(3.70 – 4.93)	1.52†	(< LOD – 2.02)	4.13	(3.36 – 5.44)	9.87†	(8.65 – 22.5)	103

< LOD means less than the limit of detection, which may vary for some compounds by year. See Appendix D for LOD.
† Estimate is subject to greater uncertainty due to small cell size.

Table 2.6.a.4. Serum alpha-carotene: Non-Hispanic blacks

Geometric mean and selected percentiles of serum concentrations (in µg/dL) for non-Hispanic blacks in the U.S. population aged 6 years and older, National Health and Nutrition Examination Survey, 2005–2006.

	Geometric mean (95% conf. interval)	Selected percentiles (95% conf. interval)						Sample size
		10th		50th		90th		
Males and Females								
Total, 6 years and older	1.98 (1.74 – 2.26)	< LOD		1.71 (1.49 – 1.99)		6.99 (5.49 – 9.49)		1,890
6–11 years	1.97 (1.68 – 2.30)	.782	(< LOD – .865)	1.73 (1.47 – 2.11)		4.97 (3.84 – 7.31)		240
12–19 years	1.33 (1.22 – 1.46)	< LOD		1.17 (1.08 – 1.27)		3.23 (2.79 – 4.25)		664
20–39 years	1.76 (1.47 – 2.10)	< LOD		1.54 (1.27 – 1.85)		5.49 (3.81 – 10.9)		368
40–59 years	2.60 (2.18 – 3.10)	< LOD		2.40 (1.86 – 3.11)		9.63 (7.77 – 12.4)		335
60 years and older	2.28 (2.05 – 2.54)	.727	(< LOD – .860)	2.09 (1.72 – 2.38)		7.35 (6.25 – 9.09)		283
Males								
Total, 6 years and older	1.79 (1.56 – 2.06)	< LOD		1.55 (1.30 – 1.84)		6.12 (4.82 – 7.67)		948
6–11 years	2.11 (1.80 – 2.46)	.934	(.761 – 1.00)	1.90 (1.51 – 2.50)		5.11 (4.03 – 6.81)		128
12–19 years	1.28 (1.17 – 1.40)	< LOD		1.18 (1.10 – 1.27)		2.65 (2.27 – 3.64)		342
20–39 years	1.51 (1.27 – 1.80)	< LOD		1.26 (1.08 – 1.43)		4.23 (3.53 – 10.1)		170
40–59 years	2.34 (1.84 – 2.96)	< LOD		2.10 (1.65 – 3.05)		8.08 (6.39 – 18.0)		156
60 years and older	2.04 (1.78 – 2.34)	< LOD		1.75 (1.48 – 2.32)		6.11 (5.37 – 7.68)		152
Females								
Total, 6 years and older	2.17 (1.91 – 2.47)	< LOD		1.91 (1.61 – 2.24)		8.09 (6.12 – 10.9)		942
6–11 years	1.84 (1.47 – 2.30)	< LOD		1.56 (1.31 – 2.06)		4.55 (3.38 – 34.6)		112
12–19 years	1.40 (1.24 – 1.57)	< LOD		1.16 (1.01 – 1.35)		3.98 (3.08 – 4.95)		322
20–39 years	2.00 (1.63 – 2.45)	< LOD		1.83 (1.46 – 2.17)		7.48 (3.92 – 14.8)		198
40–59 years	2.85 (2.40 – 3.37)	.763	(< LOD – .998)	2.59 (1.91 – 3.59)		10.2 (7.96 – 12.8)		179
60 years and older	2.47 (2.08 – 2.94)	.778	(< LOD – .932)	2.28 (1.69 – 3.06)		8.43 (5.57 – 13.9)		131

< LOD means less than the limit of detection, which may vary for some compounds by year. See Appendix D for LOD.

Table 2.6.a.5. Serum alpha-carotene: Non-Hispanic whites

Geometric mean and selected percentiles of serum concentrations (in µg/dL) for non-Hispanic whites in the U.S. population aged 6 years and older, National Health and Nutrition Examination Survey, 2005–2006.

	Geometric mean (95% conf. interval)	Selected percentiles (95% conf. interval)						Sample size
		10th		50th		90th		
Males and Females								
Total, 6 years and older	2.80 (2.60 – 3.02)	.770	(< LOD – .835)	2.67 (2.47 – 2.89)		9.64 (8.79 – 10.7)		2,966
6–11 years	2.78 (2.38 – 3.24)	.860	(.769 – .988)	2.77 (2.37 – 3.15)		8.80 (7.05 – 11.7)		231
12–19 years	1.95 (1.78 – 2.13)	< LOD		1.85 (1.65 – 2.02)		6.10 (5.30 – 7.19)		496
20–39 years	2.39 (2.16 – 2.65)	< LOD		2.31 (1.97 – 2.65)		8.10 (7.23 – 9.64)		710
40–59 years	3.12 (2.84 – 3.44)	.832	(< LOD – .971)	2.95 (2.63 – 3.36)		11.9 (10.1 – 13.5)		683
60 years and older	3.44 (3.05 – 3.88)	1.05	(.832 – 1.24)	3.34 (2.82 – 3.89)		10.7 (9.59 – 12.9)		846
Males								
Total, 6 years and older	2.38 (2.20 – 2.56)	< LOD		2.27 (2.08 – 2.42)		7.73 (6.50 – 9.42)		1,470
6–11 years	2.80 (2.34 – 3.35)	.853	(.749 – 1.02)	2.80 (2.40 – 2.99)		8.52 (5.74 – 23.7)		112
12–19 years	1.62 (1.47 – 1.78)	< LOD		1.46 (1.26 – 1.72)		4.33 (3.63 – 5.81)		254
20–39 years	2.02 (1.87 – 2.18)	< LOD		1.90 (1.65 – 2.22)		6.23 (5.68 – 7.29)		307
40–59 years	2.60 (2.33 – 2.90)	< LOD		2.42 (2.19 – 2.68)		8.71 (6.82 – 10.2)		351
60 years and older	3.00 (2.57 – 3.49)	.844	(.761 – .959)	3.09 (2.46 – 3.54)		9.36 (7.53 – 12.8)		446
Females								
Total, 6 years and older	3.28 (3.00 – 3.59)	.920	(.790 – 1.04)	3.10 (2.82 – 3.39)		11.2 (10.4 – 12.7)		1,496
6–11 years	2.75 (2.29 – 3.31)	.864	(< LOD – 1.10)	2.76 (1.93 – 3.26)		9.09 (7.10 – 12.4)		119
12–19 years	2.39 (2.19 – 2.60)	.723	(< LOD – .838)	2.22 (2.06 – 2.49)		6.93 (6.25 – 8.87)		242
20–39 years	2.83 (2.38 – 3.37)	.826	(< LOD – .962)	2.69 (2.20 – 3.36)		9.45 (7.82 – 11.8)		403
40–59 years	3.73 (3.27 – 4.26)	.964	(< LOD – 1.23)	3.57 (3.04 – 4.01)		14.4 (12.6 – 16.7)		332
60 years and older	3.86 (3.34 – 4.47)	1.24	(1.05 – 1.42)	3.54 (2.85 – 4.47)		12.0 (10.4 – 15.9)		400

Table 2.6.b. Serum alpha-carotene: Concentrations by survey cycle

Geometric mean and selected percentiles of serum concentrations (in µg/dL) for the U.S. population, National Health and Nutrition Examination Survey, 2001–2002 and 2005–2006.

	Geometric mean (95% conf. interval)	Selected percentiles (95% conf. interval)			Sample size
		5th	50th	95th	
Total, 6 years and older					
2001–2002	2.48 (2.22 – 2.77)	< LOD	2.39 (2.10 – 2.70)	12.2 (10.7 – 14.1)	7,929
2005–2006	2.76 (2.54 – 2.99)	< LOD	2.63 (2.40 – 2.84)	14.1 (12.4 – 16.5)	7,246
Age group					
3–5 years					
2001–2002	2.41 (2.13 – 2.74)	< LOD	2.14 (1.89 – 2.48)	12.2 (10.3 – 14.6)	430
6–11 years					
2001–2002	2.24 (2.00 – 2.51)	< LOD	2.04 (1.84 – 2.28)	8.54 (6.94 – 13.3)	1,014
2005–2006	2.64 (2.32 – 3.01)	< LOD	2.59 (2.31 – 2.90)	11.5 (9.30 – 15.1)	860
12–19 years					
2001–2002	1.68 (1.52 – 1.86)	< LOD	1.50 (1.37 – 1.74)	7.68 (6.61 – 9.52)	2,206
2005–2006	1.85 (1.69 – 2.03)	< LOD	1.72 (1.53 – 1.91)	7.91 (6.65 – 10.2)	1,950
20–39 years					
2001–2002	2.22 (1.93 – 2.56)	< LOD	2.11 (1.82 – 2.49)	9.80 (8.96 – 12.6)	1,716
2005–2006	2.48 (2.24 – 2.74)	< LOD	2.36 (2.06 – 2.69)	11.3 (10.1 – 14.7)	1,684
40–59 years					
2001–2002	2.98 (2.60 – 3.42)	< LOD	2.85 (2.47 – 3.28)	16.0 (12.8 – 20.7)	1,470
2005–2006	3.15 (2.85 – 3.47)	< LOD	3.01 (2.72 – 3.36)	17.0 (14.5 – 21.9)	1,365
60 years and older					
2001–2002	3.08 (2.74 – 3.46)	< LOD	3.14 (2.71 – 3.61)	12.7 (12.0 – 13.7)	1,523
2005–2006	3.42 (3.05 – 3.83)	.711 (< LOD – .811)	3.33 (2.86 – 3.86)	17.0 (14.0 – 19.8)	1,387
Gender					
(6 years and older)					
Males					
2001–2002	2.22 (1.98 – 2.49)	< LOD	2.07 (1.87 – 2.44)	10.3 (9.30 – 12.3)	3,835
2005–2006	2.37 (2.20 – 2.55)	< LOD	2.23 (2.06 – 2.39)	11.5 (9.92 – 13.9)	3,544
Females					
2001–2002	2.76 (2.47 – 3.07)	< LOD	2.67 (2.35 – 2.97)	13.3 (11.8 – 16.2)	4,094
2005–2006	3.18 (2.89 – 3.50)	< LOD	3.01 (2.74 – 3.32)	16.4 (14.6 – 18.4)	3,702
Race/ethnicity					
(6 years and older)					
Mexican Americans					
2001–2002	2.73 (2.38 – 3.14)	.726 (< LOD – .805)	2.63 (2.38 – 2.99)	10.1 (8.46 – 14.1)	1,990
2005–2006	2.99 (2.79 – 3.21)	.824 (.749 – .889)	2.87 (2.61 – 3.21)	10.8 (10.5 – 12.5)	1,844
Non-Hispanic Blacks					
2001–2002	1.77 (1.50 – 2.09)	< LOD	1.58 (1.36 – 1.91)	10.1 (7.64 – 14.5)	1,864
2005–2006	1.98 (1.74 – 2.26)	< LOD	1.71 (1.49 – 1.99)	11.0 (8.83 – 14.8)	1,890
Non-Hispanic Whites					
2001–2002	2.57 (2.25 – 2.95)	< LOD	2.48 (2.11 – 2.86)	12.8 (11.2 – 15.5)	3,450
2005–2006	2.80 (2.60 – 3.02)	< LOD	2.67 (2.47 – 2.89)	14.4 (12.8 – 16.7)	2,966

< LOD means less than the limit of detection, which may vary for some compounds by year. See Appendix D for LOD.

Figure 2.6.b. Serum alpha–carotene: Concentrations by survey cycle

Selected percentiles in µg/dL (95% confidence intervals), National Health and Nutrition Examination Survey, 2001–2002 and 2005–2006

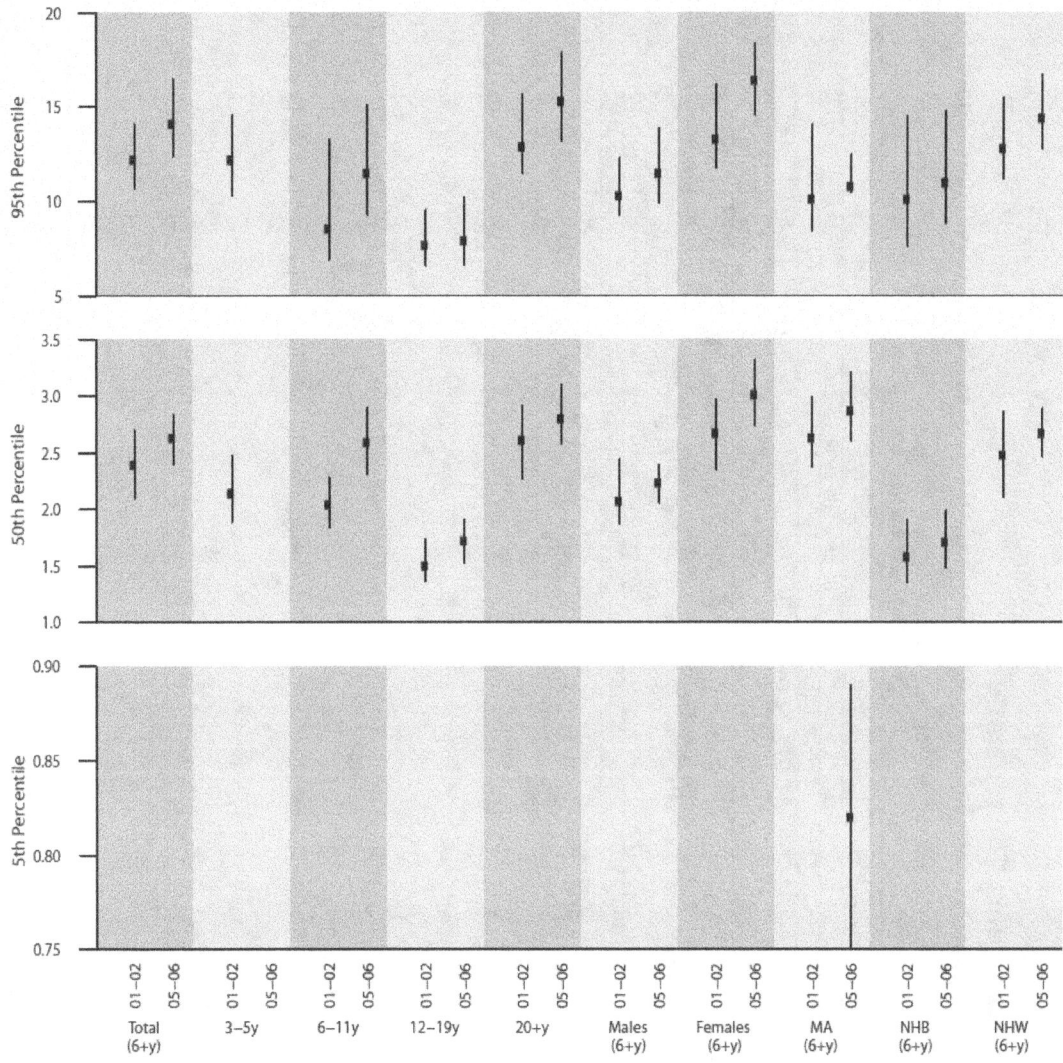

Values in the graph are suppressed if either the point estimate or the lower 95% confidence limit is noted as "< LOD" in the accompanying table.

Table 2.7.a.1. Serum trans-beta-carotene: Concentrations

Geometric mean and selected percentiles of serum concentrations (in µg/dL) for the total U.S. population aged 6 years and older, National Health and Nutrition Examination Survey, 2005–2006.

	Geometric mean (95% conf. interval)	Selected percentiles (95% conf. interval)					Sample size
		2.5th	5th	50th	95th	97.5th	
Total, 6 years and older	12.1 (11.5 – 12.8)	2.32 (1.98 – 2.67)	3.18 (2.92 – 3.42)	11.6 (11.1 – 12.3)	53.3 (49.1 – 59.3)	74.1 (68.1 – 83.3)	7,254
Age group							
6–11 years	13.0 (12.1 – 14.0)	4.14 (2.67 – 5.05)	5.15 (4.11 – 5.61)	12.7 (11.8 – 13.6)	37.7 (29.9 – 49.2)	47.6 (39.6 – 100)	860
12–19 years	9.24 (8.76 – 9.75)	2.59 (2.05 – 2.96)	3.20 (2.87 – 3.52)	8.96 (8.30 – 9.66)	28.3 (26.3 – 30.7)	35.3 (31.3 – 41.8)	1,954
20–39 years	10.4 (9.63 – 11.3)	2.41 (1.40 – 2.81)	3.01 (2.79 – 3.23)	9.97 (9.14 – 10.9)	41.6 (36.9 – 53.3)	59.5 (48.7 – 85.1)	1,688
40–59 years	12.8 (11.9 – 13.9)	1.94 (1.36 – 2.20)	2.69 (2.15 – 3.41)	12.4 (11.6 – 13.4)	63.0 (53.5 – 73.8)	79.2 (73.3 – 97.9)	1,365
60 years and older	16.4 (15.1 – 17.7)	2.80 (2.64 – 3.20)	3.90 (3.43 – 4.17)	15.9 (14.5 – 17.8)	74.6 (66.3 – 83.4)	102 (85.9 – 143)	1,387
Gender							
Males	10.3 (9.89 – 10.8)	1.96 (1.40 – 2.25)	2.77 (2.28 – 3.06)	10.3 (9.62 – 10.9)	40.8 (36.8 – 46.4)	54.3 (49.4 – 66.2)	3,547
Females	14.2 (13.3 – 15.1)	2.93 (2.45 – 3.23)	3.77 (3.51 – 4.05)	13.2 (12.0 – 14.4)	64.5 (58.3 – 73.6)	84.7 (75.9 – 102)	3,707
Race/ethnicity							
Mexican Americans	11.5 (10.5 – 12.7)	2.67 (2.19 – 3.06)	3.49 (3.15 – 3.86)	11.3 (10.4 – 12.4)	39.2 (35.1 – 46.5)	48.6 (46.2 – 59.4)	1,844
Non-Hispanic Blacks	10.8 (9.72 – 12.0)	2.29 (2.00 – 2.54)	3.02 (2.57 – 3.36)	10.5 (9.31 – 11.4)	45.0 (38.3 – 53.7)	57.4 (51.4 – 73.5)	1,891
Non-Hispanic Whites	12.3 (11.6 – 13.1)	2.20 (1.90 – 2.65)	3.06 (2.80 – 3.41)	11.8 (11.2 – 12.6)	56.9 (50.4 – 64.9)	76.2 (72.3 – 93.3)	2,973

Figure 2.7.a. Serum trans–beta–carotene: Concentrations by age group

Geometric mean (95% confidence interval), National Health and Nutrition Examination Survey, 2005–2006

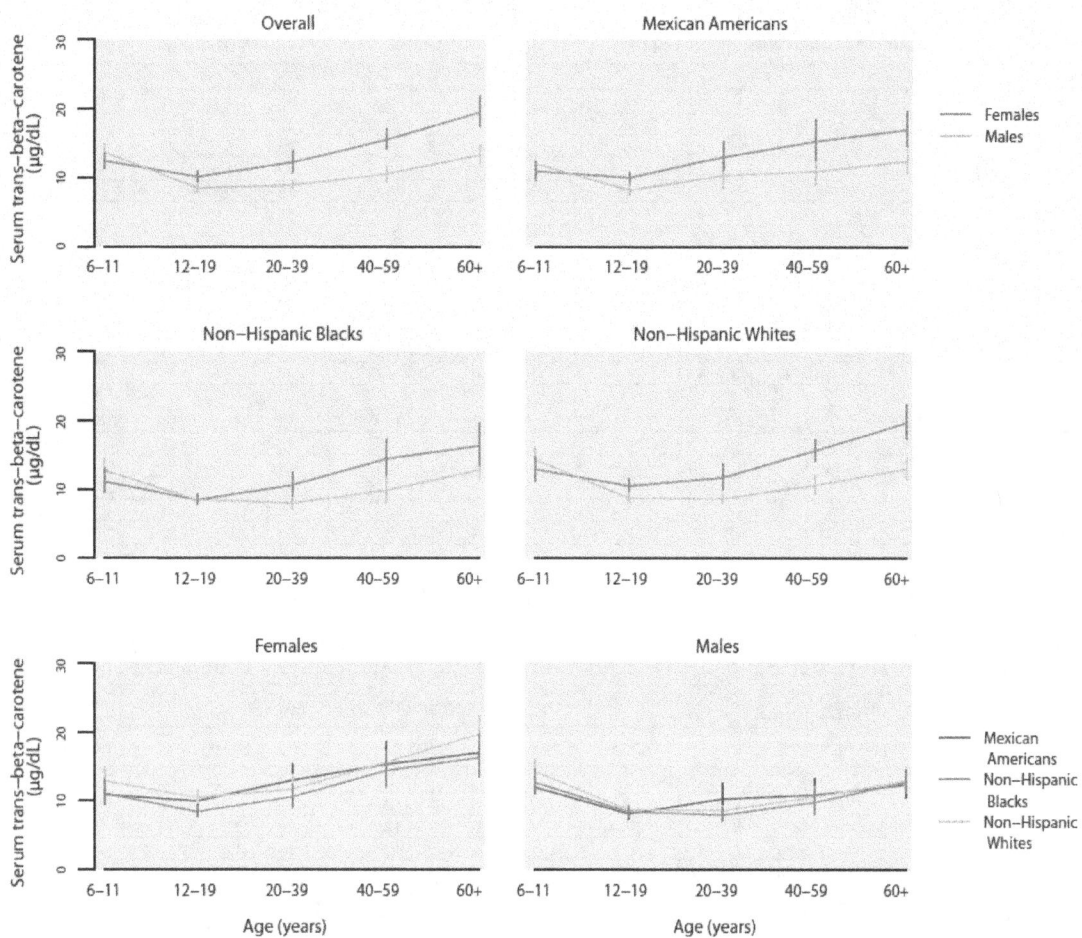

Table 2.7.a.2. Serum trans-beta-carotene: Total population

Geometric mean and selected percentiles of serum concentrations (in µg/dL) for the total U.S. population aged 6 years and older, National Health and Nutrition Examination Survey, 2005–2006.

	Geometric mean (95% conf. interval)	Selected percentiles (95% conf. interval)						Sample size
		10th		50th		90th		
Males and Females								
Total, 6 years and older	12.1 (11.5 – 12.8)	4.26	(4.02 – 4.53)	11.6	(11.1 – 12.3)	37.1	(34.2 – 40.7)	7,254
6–11 years	13.0 (12.1 – 14.0)	6.21	(5.49 – 6.89)	12.7	(11.8 – 13.6)	27.4	(25.1 – 31.7)	860
12–19 years	9.24 (8.76 – 9.75)	4.21	(3.86 – 4.52)	8.96	(8.30 – 9.66)	20.3	(18.9 – 22.7)	1,954
20–39 years	10.4 (9.63 – 11.3)	3.85	(3.50 – 4.19)	9.97	(9.14 – 10.9)	30.4	(26.5 – 35.8)	1,688
40–59 years	12.8 (11.9 – 13.9)	4.12	(3.59 – 4.55)	12.4	(11.6 – 13.4)	42.7	(39.1 – 47.5)	1,365
60 years and older	16.4 (15.1 – 17.7)	5.27	(4.47 – 6.08)	15.9	(14.5 – 17.8)	51.0	(45.9 – 59.1)	1,387
Males								
Total, 6 years and older	10.3 (9.89 – 10.8)	3.76	(3.48 – 4.02)	10.3	(9.62 – 10.9)	28.2	(26.4 – 31.4)	3,547
6–11 years	13.7 (12.6 – 15.0)	6.93	(5.62 – 7.94)	13.1	(12.1 – 14.3)	27.4	(23.5 – 34.7)	427
12–19 years	8.46 (7.93 – 9.03)	3.82	(3.27 – 4.29)	8.26	(7.75 – 8.90)	17.8	(17.2 – 18.7)	980
20–39 years	8.89 (8.36 – 9.46)	3.36	(3.02 – 3.80)	8.51	(7.91 – 9.14)	23.9	(22.2 – 26.7)	738
40–59 years	10.5 (9.38 – 11.7)	3.43	(2.20 – 4.20)	10.8	(9.45 – 12.3)	31.8	(27.9 – 36.0)	673
60 years and older	13.3 (11.9 – 14.8)	4.47	(3.75 – 5.33)	13.0	(11.5 – 14.4)	41.5	(33.8 – 51.1)	729
Females								
Total, 6 years and older	14.2 (13.3 – 15.1)	5.00	(4.60 – 5.30)	13.2	(12.0 – 14.4)	43.9	(41.2 – 48.9)	3,707
6–11 years	12.4 (11.3 – 13.5)	5.61	(4.56 – 6.75)	11.8	(10.5 – 13.6)	27.4	(24.6 – 33.5)	433
12–19 years	10.1 (9.48 – 10.9)	4.73	(4.26 – 4.95)	9.76	(8.95 – 10.7)	24.6	(20.9 – 29.1)	974
20–39 years	12.2 (10.7 – 13.9)	4.39	(3.79 – 5.08)	11.4	(10.2 – 12.9)	37.0	(28.6 – 50.2)	950
40–59 years	15.5 (14.2 – 17.0)	5.07	(4.61 – 5.33)	14.5	(12.7 – 16.2)	53.2	(44.0 – 64.4)	692
60 years and older	19.5 (17.4 – 21.8)	6.30	(5.12 – 7.04)	19.4	(16.5 – 23.1)	62.3	(50.5 – 75.2)	658

Table 2.7.a.3. Serum trans-beta-carotene: Mexican Americans

Geometric mean and selected percentiles of serum concentrations (in µg/dL) for Mexican Americans in the U.S. population aged 6 years and older, National Health and Nutrition Examination Survey, 2005–2006.

	Geometric mean (95% conf. interval)	Selected percentiles (95% conf. interval)						Sample size
		10th		50th		90th		
Males and Females								
Total, 6 years and older	11.5 (10.5 – 12.7)	4.48	(4.14 – 4.81)	11.3	(10.4 – 12.4)	29.7	(25.9 – 35.0)	1,844
6–11 years	11.4 (10.6 – 12.4)	5.74	(4.57 – 6.28)	11.0	(9.92 – 12.0)	24.2	(21.0 – 31.1)	295
12–19 years	9.02 (8.39 – 9.70)	4.07	(3.59 – 4.64)	9.05	(8.35 – 10.1)	18.6	(17.3 – 22.7)	646
20–39 years	11.5 (9.84 – 13.3)	4.45	(4.01 – 4.85)	11.3	(9.45 – 13.7)	29.9	(23.5 – 37.2)	449
40–59 years	12.8 (11.1 – 14.8)	4.15	(3.63 – 5.03)	12.7	(11.1 – 14.7)	32.5	(27.7 – 47.1)	246
60 years and older	14.8 (13.2 – 16.5)	5.31	(3.02 – 7.79)	14.7	(12.7 – 15.6)	43.1	(37.9 – 47.4)	208
Males								
Total, 6 years and older	10.4 (9.29 – 11.6)	4.15	(3.63 – 4.46)	10.3	(9.20 – 11.5)	25.3	(22.6 – 30.4)	883
6–11 years	12.0 (11.2 – 12.8)	6.15	(4.40 – 7.62)	11.5	(10.4 – 12.6)	23.1	(19.7 – 34.4)	145
12–19 years	8.18 (7.37 – 9.07)	3.71	(3.32 – 4.25)	8.34	(6.90 – 9.63)	17.7	(15.3 – 19.6)	313
20–39 years	10.3 (8.45 – 12.6)	4.20	(3.00 – 4.71)	9.64	(7.83 – 12.8)	26.6	(22.0 – 36.9)	198
40–59 years	10.9 (8.97 – 13.2)	3.82	(2.55 – 4.31)	11.3	(9.45 – 13.4)	26.3	(21.6 – 35.9)	122
60 years and older	12.4 (10.6 – 14.6)	4.47†	(2.51 – 6.70)	12.0	(9.45 – 15.9)	35.7†	(19.8 – 154)	105
Females								
Total, 6 years and older	12.9 (11.9 – 14.1)	5.08	(4.51 – 5.60)	12.5	(11.6 – 13.7)	34.4	(30.2 – 39.3)	961
6–11 years	10.9 (9.63 – 12.3)	5.10	(3.98 – 5.96)	10.2	(8.54 – 11.9)	24.3	(19.4 – 32.8)	150
12–19 years	10.0 (9.35 – 10.7)	4.83	(4.12 – 5.13)	10.2	(9.47 – 10.6)	20.9	(18.0 – 28.7)	333
20–39 years	13.0 (11.1 – 15.3)	5.15	(3.69 – 6.18)	12.6	(11.2 – 15.5)	33.8	(24.6 – 45.8)	251
40–59 years	15.3 (12.6 – 18.5)	5.06	(3.42 – 6.68)	14.4	(12.2 – 18.3)	41.2	(29.2 – 108)	124
60 years and older	17.0 (14.7 – 19.7)	5.97†	(3.10 – 8.19)	15.1	(14.3 – 19.4)	44.5†	(39.3 – 50.9)	103

† Estimate is subject to greater uncertainty due to small cell size.

Table 2.7.a.4. Serum trans-beta-carotene: Non-Hispanic blacks

Geometric mean and selected percentiles of serum concentrations (in µg/dL) for non-Hispanic blacks in the U.S. population aged 6 years and older, National Health and Nutrition Examination Survey, 2005–2006.

| | Geometric mean (95% conf. interval) | Selected percentiles (95% conf. interval) | | | Sample size |
		10th	50th	90th	
Males and Females					
Total, 6 years and older	10.8 (9.72 – 12.0)	4.00 (3.53 – 4.34)	10.5 (9.31 – 11.4)	31.2 (26.5 – 38.3)	1,891
6–11 years	11.9 (10.6 – 13.3)	6.30 (4.86 – 7.03)	11.6 (10.9 – 12.6)	23.0 (18.3 – 37.7)	240
12–19 years	8.46 (7.85 – 9.11)	4.09 (3.71 – 4.35)	8.13 (7.88 – 8.42)	17.9 (15.7 – 21.3)	665
20–39 years	9.32 (8.28 – 10.5)	3.85 (3.27 – 4.22)	8.49 (7.61 – 10.2)	23.4 (19.5 – 30.8)	368
40–59 years	12.1 (10.3 – 14.1)	3.46 (2.33 – 4.66)	12.3 (10.3 – 15.2)	40.9 (34.3 – 50.2)	335
60 years and older	14.7 (12.8 – 16.9)	4.60 (3.81 – 5.04)	15.3 (12.1 – 18.7)	44.8 (37.0 – 51.5)	283
Males					
Total, 6 years and older	9.49 (8.62 – 10.4)	3.48 (3.00 – 3.95)	8.92 (8.05 – 9.95)	26.5 (23.0 – 32.4)	949
6–11 years	12.7 (11.1 – 14.5)	6.79 (5.53 – 7.49)	12.7 (10.7 – 14.9)	22.9 (18.7 – 55.1)	128
12–19 years	8.47 (7.78 – 9.21)	4.15 (3.18 – 4.70)	8.23 (7.85 – 8.76)	17.3 (15.8 – 19.7)	343
20–39 years	8.00 (7.09 – 9.02)	3.39 (2.51 – 3.99)	7.16 (6.35 – 7.95)	22.0 (19.3 – 26.4)	170
40–59 years	9.83 (8.14 – 11.9)	2.65 (1.98 – 3.42)	9.46 (7.15 – 13.1)	36.7 (26.2 – 66.7)	156
60 years and older	12.8 (11.3 – 14.5)	3.77 (3.46 – 4.61)	12.4 (10.7 – 15.1)	35.3 (29.1 – 52.0)	152
Females					
Total, 6 years and older	12.1 (10.7 – 13.6)	4.49 (4.05 – 4.88)	11.5 (10.3 – 13.4)	35.5 (27.7 – 46.1)	942
6–11 years	11.1 (9.52 – 13.0)	5.32 (3.52 – 6.63)	11.3 (9.67 – 12.5)	22.3 (16.9 – 37.0)	112
12–19 years	8.45 (7.74 – 9.22)	4.00 (3.50 – 4.37)	8.03 (7.59 – 8.49)	18.6 (15.5 – 24.3)	322
20–39 years	10.6 (9.08 – 12.4)	4.27 (3.46 – 5.15)	10.8 (8.50 – 12.2)	25.4 (18.6 – 46.1)	198
40–59 years	14.4 (12.1 – 17.1)	4.85 (2.70 – 6.42)	14.5 (11.6 – 18.4)	44.9 (39.3 – 49.0)	179
60 years and older	16.3 (13.5 – 19.7)	4.83 (3.86 – 5.68)	17.6 (11.6 – 25.6)	46.5 (38.7 – 55.7)	131

Table 2.7.a.5. Serum trans-beta-carotene: Non-Hispanic whites

Geometric mean and selected percentiles of serum concentrations (in µg/dL) for non-Hispanic whites in the U.S. population aged 6 years and older, National Health and Nutrition Examination Survey, 2005–2006.

| | Geometric mean (95% conf. interval) | Selected percentiles (95% conf. interval) | | | Sample size |
		10th	50th	90th	
Males and Females					
Total, 6 years and older	12.3 (11.6 – 13.1)	4.21 (3.81 – 4.60)	11.8 (11.2 – 12.6)	39.0 (34.8 – 43.4)	2,973
6–11 years	13.6 (12.4 – 14.9)	6.31 (5.42 – 7.09)	13.2 (12.1 – 14.3)	27.8 (24.9 – 36.2)	231
12–19 years	9.58 (8.94 – 10.3)	4.36 (3.85 – 4.71)	9.14 (8.12 – 10.5)	20.9 (19.0 – 26.6)	499
20–39 years	10.1 (9.08 – 11.1)	3.53 (3.18 – 3.94)	9.78 (8.70 – 10.6)	30.5 (25.2 – 39.1)	714
40–59 years	12.9 (11.8 – 14.0)	4.10 (3.54 – 4.59)	12.4 (11.4 – 13.5)	43.4 (39.4 – 48.4)	683
60 years and older	16.3 (14.9 – 17.8)	5.29 (4.22 – 6.19)	15.9 (14.2 – 18.1)	50.9 (44.8 – 64.2)	846
Males					
Total, 6 years and older	10.4 (9.87 – 11.0)	3.71 (3.35 – 4.02)	10.5 (9.56 – 11.4)	28.6 (26.0 – 33.0)	1,472
6–11 years	14.3 (12.7 – 16.1)	7.16 (4.60 – 9.03)	13.4 (12.1 – 14.7)	26.3 (23.2 – 48.8)	112
12–19 years	8.77 (8.14 – 9.46)	3.91 (2.92 – 4.60)	8.49 (7.53 – 9.58)	17.9 (16.6 – 20.4)	254
20–39 years	8.65 (8.03 – 9.32)	3.13 (2.85 – 3.48)	8.30 (7.47 – 9.44)	23.8 (20.9 – 26.9)	309
40–59 years	10.6 (9.34 – 12.0)	3.45 (2.06 – 4.26)	11.0 (9.61 – 12.4)	30.6 (26.6 – 35.9)	351
60 years and older	13.0 (11.5 – 14.7)	4.39 (3.31 – 5.39)	12.6 (11.0 – 14.3)	41.0 (32.8 – 51.7)	446
Females					
Total, 6 years and older	14.5 (13.5 – 15.6)	4.95 (4.33 – 5.45)	13.4 (12.2 – 15.0)	46.4 (41.5 – 53.3)	1,501
6–11 years	12.9 (11.2 – 14.8)	5.61 (2.70 – 7.13)	12.6 (9.76 – 15.1)	27.7 (24.8 – 40.6)	119
12–19 years	10.5 (9.71 – 11.5)	4.86 (4.27 – 5.37)	9.87 (8.71 – 11.3)	26.8 (21.8 – 30.1)	245
20–39 years	11.7 (9.95 – 13.8)	4.15 (3.18 – 4.99)	10.9 (9.35 – 12.7)	36.5 (26.6 – 60.7)	405
40–59 years	15.6 (14.1 – 17.2)	5.00 (4.17 – 5.44)	14.2 (12.0 – 17.1)	57.1 (44.0 – 69.2)	332
60 years and older	19.7 (17.4 – 22.3)	6.35 (5.12 – 7.18)	19.5 (16.2 – 23.5)	64.3 (50.2 – 75.5)	400

Table 2.7.b. Serum trans-beta-carotene: Concentrations by survey cycle

Geometric mean and selected percentiles of serum concentrations (in µg/dL) for the U.S. population, National Health and Nutrition Examination Survey, 2001–2002 and 2005–2006.

	Geometric mean (95% conf. interval)		Selected percentiles (95% conf. interval)						Sample size
			5th		50th		95th		
Total, 6 years and older									
2001–2002	12.2	(11.5 – 12.9)	3.21	(2.95 – 3.46)	12.0	(11.3 – 12.6)	47.7	(44.2 – 52.1)	7,929
2005–2006	12.1	(11.5 – 12.8)	3.18	(2.92 – 3.42)	11.6	(11.1 – 12.3)	53.3	(49.1 – 59.3)	7,254
Age group									
3–5 years									
2001–2002	13.6	(12.5 – 14.6)	4.60	(3.79 – 5.00)	13.6	(12.1 – 15.2)	45.1	(35.8 – 56.3)	429
6–11 years									
2001–2002	13.3	(12.7 – 13.9)	5.44	(5.00 – 5.96)	13.2	(12.5 – 13.9)	32.9	(30.4 – 38.8)	1,012
2005–2006	13.0	(12.1 – 14.0)	5.15	(4.11 – 5.61)	12.7	(11.8 – 13.6)	37.7	(29.9 – 49.2)	860
12–19 years									
2001–2002	9.69	(9.20 – 10.2)	3.34	(2.97 – 3.59)	9.63	(8.97 – 10.4)	28.2	(25.4 – 32.5)	2,206
2005–2006	9.24	(8.76 – 9.75)	3.20	(2.87 – 3.52)	8.96	(8.30 – 9.66)	28.3	(26.3 – 30.7)	1,954
20–39 years									
2001–2002	10.3	(9.38 – 11.2)	2.90	(2.13 – 3.20)	9.81	(9.10 – 10.8)	39.8	(35.2 – 42.6)	1,716
2005–2006	10.4	(9.63 – 11.3)	3.01	(2.79 – 3.23)	9.97	(9.14 – 10.9)	41.6	(36.9 – 53.3)	1,688
40–59 years									
2001–2002	13.3	(12.1 – 14.7)	3.30	(2.74 – 3.65)	13.0	(12.0 – 14.2)	60.0	(49.9 – 79.7)	1,471
2005–2006	12.8	(11.9 – 13.9)	2.69	(2.15 – 3.41)	12.4	(11.6 – 13.4)	63.0	(53.5 – 73.8)	1,365
60 years and older									
2001–2002	16.5	(14.9 – 18.3)	3.51	(2.88 – 4.13)	17.5	(15.3 – 19.6)	61.4	(56.0 – 66.1)	1,524
2005–2006	16.4	(15.1 – 17.7)	3.90	(3.43 – 4.17)	15.9	(14.5 – 17.8)	74.6	(66.3 – 83.4)	1,387
Gender									
(6 years and older)									
Males									
2001–2002	10.9	(10.2 – 11.6)	3.01	(2.68 – 3.25)	11.0	(10.3 – 11.6)	42.1	(37.5 – 45.5)	3,837
2005–2006	10.3	(9.89 – 10.8)	2.77	(2.28 – 3.06)	10.3	(9.62 – 10.9)	40.8	(36.8 – 46.4)	3,547
Females									
2001–2002	13.6	(12.7 – 14.6)	3.57	(3.37 – 3.83)	13.1	(12.2 – 14.2)	54.1	(47.6 – 62.0)	4,092
2005–2006	14.2	(13.3 – 15.1)	3.77	(3.51 – 4.05)	13.2	(12.0 – 14.4)	64.5	(58.3 – 73.6)	3,707
Race/ethnicity									
(6 years and older)									
Mexican Americans									
2001–2002	12.5	(11.6 – 13.4)	3.56	(3.12 – 3.83)	12.9	(11.6 – 13.9)	38.5	(34.5 – 47.5)	1,990
2005–2006	11.5	(10.5 – 12.7)	3.49	(3.15 – 3.86)	11.3	(10.4 – 12.4)	39.2	(35.1 – 46.5)	1,844
Non-Hispanic Blacks									
2001–2002	10.8	(9.90 – 11.8)	2.83	(2.42 – 3.22)	10.7	(9.93 – 11.6)	40.3	(35.4 – 45.6)	1,864
2005–2006	10.8	(9.72 – 12.0)	3.02	(2.57 – 3.36)	10.5	(9.31 – 11.4)	45.0	(38.3 – 53.7)	1,891
Non-Hispanic Whites									
2001–2002	12.5	(11.5 – 13.6)	3.35	(3.06 – 3.61)	12.1	(11.3 – 13.0)	50.8	(45.8 – 56.9)	3,450
2005–2006	12.3	(11.6 – 13.1)	3.06	(2.80 – 3.41)	11.8	(11.2 – 12.6)	56.9	(50.4 – 64.9)	2,973

Figure 2.7.b. Serum trans–beta–carotene: Concentrations by survey cycle

Selected percentiles in µg/dL (95% confidence intervals), National Health and
Nutrition Examination Survey, 2001–2002 and 2005–2006

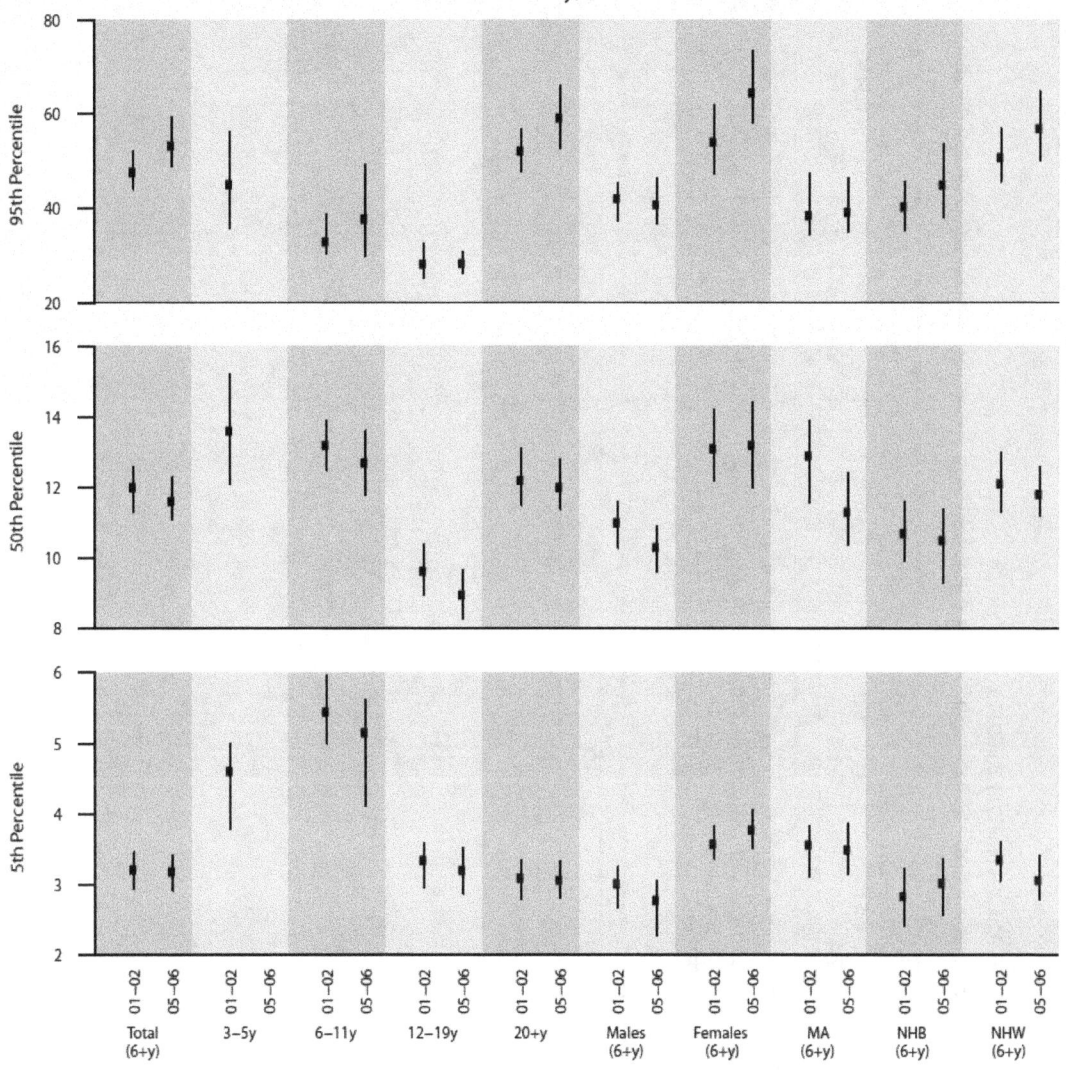

Table 2.8.a.1. Serum cis-beta-carotene: Concentrations

Geometric mean and selected percentiles of serum concentrations (in µg/dL) for the total U.S. population aged 6 years and older, National Health and Nutrition Examination Survey, 2005–2006.

	Geometric mean (95% conf. interval)	Selected percentiles (95% conf. interval)					Sample size
		2.5th	5th	50th	95th	97.5th	
Total, 6 years and older	*	< LOD	< LOD	< LOD	3.20 (2.87 – 3.64)	4.48 (3.93 – 5.11)	6,616
Age group							
6–11 years	*	< LOD	< LOD	< LOD	1.95 (1.63 – 2.68)	2.67 (2.16 – 4.22)	779
12–19 years	*	< LOD	< LOD	< LOD	1.47 (1.33 – 1.81)	1.87 (1.58 – 2.39)	1,785
20–39 years	*	< LOD	< LOD	< LOD	2.51 (2.08 – 3.19)	3.74 (2.88 – 5.09)	1,528
40–59 years	*	< LOD	< LOD	.730 (< LOD – .783)	3.73 (3.21 – 4.44)	4.84 (4.34 – 5.50)	1,254
60 years and older	1.08 (.985 – 1.17)	< LOD	< LOD	.903 (.811 – .992)	4.59 (3.93 – 5.32)	6.53 (5.17 – 8.65)	1,270
Gender							
Males	*	< LOD	< LOD	< LOD	2.26 (1.99 – 2.60)	3.09 (2.67 – 3.91)	3,204
Females	*	< LOD	< LOD	.759 (.708 – .816)	3.88 (3.60 – 4.48)	5.27 (4.71 – 6.32)	3,412
Race/ethnicity							
Mexican Americans	*	< LOD	< LOD	< LOD	2.26 (1.97 – 2.59)	2.80 (2.48 – 3.46)	1,707
Non-Hispanic Blacks	*	< LOD	< LOD	< LOD	2.81 (2.37 – 3.38)	3.51 (3.17 – 4.61)	1,673
Non-Hispanic Whites	*	< LOD	< LOD	< LOD	3.44 (3.06 – 3.82)	4.71 (4.11 – 5.20)	2,725

< LOD means less than the limit of detection, which may vary for some compounds by year. See Appendix D for LOD.
* Not calculated. Proportion of results below limit of detection was too high to provide a valid result.

No *cis-beta*-carotene figure for concentrations by age group is presented because the geometric means were not calculated due to the proportion of results below the limit of detection being too high for valid results (see Table 2.8.a.1).

Table 2.8.a.2. Serum cis-beta-carotene: Total population

Geometric mean and selected percentiles of serum concentrations (in μg/dL) for the total U.S. population aged 6 years and older, National Health and Nutrition Examination Survey, 2005–2006.

	Geometric mean (95% conf. interval)	Selected percentiles (95% conf. interval)			Sample size
		10th	50th	90th	
Males and Females					
Total, 6 years and older	*	< LOD	< LOD	2.10 (1.92 – 2.39)	6,616
6–11 years	*	< LOD	< LOD	1.47 (1.28 – 1.78)	779
12–19 years	*	< LOD	< LOD	1.12 (.995 – 1.26)	1,785
20–39 years	*	< LOD	< LOD	1.78 (1.55 – 2.03)	1,528
40–59 years	*	< LOD	.730 (< LOD – .783)	2.49 (2.18 – 2.86)	1,254
60 years and older	1.08 (.985 – 1.17)	< LOD	.903 (.811 – .992)	3.09 (2.62 – 3.64)	1,270
Males					
Total, 6 years and older	*	< LOD	< LOD	1.59 (1.43 – 1.86)	3,204
6–11 years	*	< LOD	.704 (< LOD – .757)	1.52 (1.26 – 2.33)	386
12–19 years	*	< LOD	< LOD	.935 (.878 – 1.02)	886
20–39 years	*	< LOD	< LOD	1.37 (1.23 – 1.59)	652
40–59 years	*	< LOD	< LOD	1.75 (1.50 – 2.05)	616
60 years and older	*	< LOD	.726 (< LOD – .817)	2.37 (1.91 – 2.99)	664
Females					
Total, 6 years and older	*	< LOD	.759 (.708 – .816)	2.70 (2.35 – 3.10)	3,412
6–11 years	*	< LOD	< LOD	1.44 (1.21 – 1.74)	393
12–19 years	*	< LOD	< LOD	1.35 (1.13 – 1.59)	899
20–39 years	*	< LOD	< LOD	2.15 (1.77 – 3.04)	876
40–59 years	1.04 (.954 – 1.13)	< LOD	.827 (.745 – .963)	3.30 (2.72 – 3.78)	638
60 years and older	1.26 (1.11 – 1.41)	< LOD	1.15 (.904 – 1.36)	3.69 (3.23 – 4.71)	606

< LOD means less than the limit of detection, which may vary for some compounds by year. See Appendix D for LOD.
* Not calculated. Proportion of results below limit of detection was too high to provide a valid result.

Table 2.8.a.3. Serum cis-beta-carotene: Mexican Americans

Geometric mean and selected percentiles of serum concentrations (in μg/dL) for Mexican Americans in the U.S. population aged 6 years and older, National Health and Nutrition Examination Survey, 2005–2006.

	Geometric mean (95% conf. interval)	Selected percentiles (95% conf. interval)			Sample size
		10th	50th	90th	
Males and Females					
Total, 6 years and older	*	< LOD	< LOD	1.70 (1.52 – 1.91)	1,707
6–11 years	*	< LOD	< LOD	1.34 (1.09 – 1.67)	269
12–19 years	*	< LOD	< LOD	.975 (.899 – 1.15)	609
20–39 years	*	< LOD	< LOD	1.73 (1.42 – 2.02)	402
40–59 years	.880 (.780 – .992)	< LOD	.751 (< LOD – .864)	1.97 (1.65 – 2.75)	228
60 years and older	.964 (.878 – 1.06)	< LOD	.854 (.778 – .919)	2.48 (2.05 – 3.55)	199
Males					
Total, 6 years and older	*	< LOD	< LOD	1.47 (1.21 – 1.71)	814
6–11 years	*	< LOD	< LOD	1.34 (1.06 – 1.98)	131
12–19 years	*	< LOD	< LOD	.900 (.833 – 1.09)	299
20–39 years	*	< LOD	< LOD	1.58 (1.16 – 2.07)	171
40–59 years	*	< LOD	< LOD	1.57 (1.29 – 2.19)	114
60 years and older	*	< LOD†	.718 (< LOD – .904)	1.61† (1.08 – 10.8)	99
Females					
Total, 6 years and older	*	< LOD	.720 (< LOD – .789)	1.95 (1.76 – 2.24)	893
6–11 years	*	< LOD	< LOD	1.35 (1.06 – 1.72)	138
12–19 years	*	< LOD	< LOD	1.10 (.944 – 1.46)	310
20–39 years	*	< LOD	.774 (< LOD – .960)	1.88 (1.57 – 2.36)	231
40–59 years	1.00 (.839 – 1.19)	< LOD	.870 (.703 – 1.06)	2.23 (1.71 – 6.40)	114
60 years and older	1.09 (.959 – 1.24)	< LOD†	.923 (.853 – 1.06)	2.85† (2.37 – 4.06)	100

< LOD means less than the limit of detection, which may vary for some compounds by year. See Appendix D for LOD.
* Not calculated. Proportion of results below limit of detection was too high to provide a valid result.
† Estimate is subject to greater uncertainty due to small cell size.

Table 2.8.a.4. Serum cis-beta-carotene: Non-Hispanic blacks

Geometric mean and selected percentiles of serum concentrations (in μg/dL) for non-Hispanic blacks in the U.S population aged 6 years and older, National Health and Nutrition Examination Survey, 2005–2006.

	Geometric mean (95% conf. interval)	Selected percentiles (95% conf. interval)			Sample size
		10th	50th	90th	
Males and Females					
Total, 6 years and older	*	< LOD	< LOD	1.87　(1.59 – 2.49)	1,673
6–11 years	*	< LOD	< LOD	1.33　(1.12 – 2.11)	208
12–19 years	*	< LOD	< LOD	1.05　(.916 – 1.20)	580
20–39 years	*	< LOD	< LOD	1.41　(1.24 – 1.84)	327
40–59 years	*	< LOD	.778　(< LOD – .937)	2.54　(2.16 – 3.11)	298
60 years and older	1.04　(.906 – 1.19)	< LOD	.965　(.778 – 1.09)	2.80　(2.23 – 3.45)	260
Males					
Total, 6 years and older	*	< LOD	< LOD	1.61　(1.33 – 1.94)	827
6–11 years	.807　(.695 – .937)	< LOD	.738　(< LOD – .876)	1.45　(1.13 – 6.80)	112
12–19 years	*	< LOD	< LOD	.997　(.882 – 1.17)	290
20–39 years	*	< LOD	< LOD	1.27　(.962 – 1.84)	149
40–59 years	*	< LOD	< LOD	2.28　(1.51 – 3.29)	136
60 years and older	*	< LOD	.784　(< LOD – .927)	1.95　(1.64 – 3.14)	140
Females					
Total, 6 years and older	*	< LOD	.717　(< LOD – .832)	2.20　(1.83 – 2.77)	846
6–11 years	*	< LOD†	< LOD	1.19†　(1.03 – 1.99)	96
12–19 years	*	< LOD	< LOD	1.08　(.914 – 1.42)	290
20–39 years	*	< LOD	< LOD	1.62　(1.25 – 2.76)	178
40–59 years	1.01　(.886 – 1.16)	< LOD	.877　(.765 – 1.03)	2.82　(2.25 – 3.43)	162
60 years and older	1.17　(.947 – 1.44)	< LOD	1.10　(.720 – 1.58)	3.16　(2.59 – 3.84)	120

< LOD means less than the limit of detection, which may vary for some compounds by year. See Appendix D for LOD.

* Not calculated. Proportion of results below limit of detection was too high to provide a valid result.

† Estimate is subject to greater uncertainty due to small cell size.

Table 2.8.a.5. Serum cis-beta-carotene: Non-Hispanic whites

Geometric mean and selected percentiles of serum concentrations (in μg/dL) for non-Hispanic whites in the U.S. population aged 6 years and older, National Health and Nutrition Examination Survey, 2005–2006.

	Geometric mean (95% conf. interval)	Selected percentiles (95% conf. interval)			Sample size
		10th	50th	90th	
Males and Females					
Total, 6 years and older	*	< LOD	< LOD	2.17　(1.92 – 2.55)	2,725
6–11 years	*	< LOD	< LOD	1.46　(1.21 – 2.42)	212
12–19 years	*	< LOD	< LOD	1.16　(.979 – 1.39)	462
20–39 years	*	< LOD	< LOD	1.74　(1.44 – 2.15)	653
40–59 years	*	< LOD	.720　(< LOD – .779)	2.50　(2.11 – 3.14)	634
60 years and older	1.07　(.967 – 1.18)	< LOD	.892　(.783 – 1.00)	3.09　(2.57 – 3.70)	764
Males					
Total, 6 years and older	*	< LOD	< LOD	1.59　(1.42 – 1.92)	1,336
6–11 years	*	< LOD†	< LOD	1.49†　(1.16 – 5.17)	102
12–19 years	*	< LOD	< LOD	.926　(.842 – 1.19)	231
20–39 years	*	< LOD	< LOD	1.35　(1.18 – 1.59)	278
40–59 years	*	< LOD	< LOD	1.69　(1.46 – 1.99)	324
60 years and older	*	< LOD	< LOD	2.39　(1.82 – 3.14)	401
Females					
Total, 6 years and older	*	< LOD	.761　(.704 – .828)	2.79　(2.34 – 3.48)	1,389
6–11 years	*	< LOD†	< LOD	1.43†　(1.19 – 1.98)	110
12–19 years	*	< LOD	< LOD	1.39　(1.12 – 1.85)	231
20–39 years	*	< LOD	< LOD	2.14　(1.62 – 3.70)	375
40–59 years	1.03　(.941 – 1.13)	< LOD	.795　(.718 – .966)	3.55　(2.73 – 3.96)	310
60 years and older	1.26　(1.10 – 1.45)	< LOD	1.16　(.875 – 1.38)	3.70　(3.16 – 4.80)	363

< LOD means less than the limit of detection, which may vary for some compounds by year. See Appendix D for LOD.

* Not calculated. Proportion of results below limit of detection was too high to provide a valid result.

† Estimate is subject to greater uncertainty due to small cell size.

Table 2.8.b. Serum cis-beta-carotene: Concentrations by survey cycle

Geometric mean and selected percentiles of serum concentrations (in µg/dL) for the U.S. population, National Health and Nutrition Examination Survey, 2001–2002 and 2005–2006.

| | Geometric mean (95% conf. interval) | Selected percentiles (95% conf. interval) | | | Sample size |
		5th	50th	95th	
Total, 6 years and older					
2001–2002	*	< LOD	< LOD	2.64 (2.41 – 2.87)	7,929
2005–2006	*	< LOD	< LOD	3.20 (2.87 – 3.64)	6,616
Age group					
3–5 years					
2001–2002	*	< LOD	< LOD	2.07 (1.88 – 2.62)	430
6–11 years					
2001–2002	*	< LOD	< LOD	1.64 (1.50 – 1.84)	1,014
2005–2006	*	< LOD	< LOD	1.95 (1.63 – 2.68)	779
12–19 years					
2001–2002	*	< LOD	< LOD	1.39 (1.30 – 1.55)	2,206
2005–2006	*	< LOD	< LOD	1.47 (1.33 – 1.81)	1,785
20–39 years					
2001–2002	*	< LOD	< LOD	2.05 (1.82 – 2.46)	1,716
2005–2006	*	< LOD	< LOD	2.51 (2.08 – 3.19)	1,528
40–59 years					
2001–2002	*	< LOD	< LOD	3.30 (2.77 – 4.39)	1,470
2005–2006	*	< LOD	.730 (< LOD – .783)	3.73 (3.21 – 4.44)	1,254
60 years and older					
2001–2002	1.02 (.943 – 1.11)	< LOD	.899 (.803 – 1.02)	3.50 (3.11 – 3.94)	1,523
2005–2006	1.08 (.985 – 1.17)	< LOD	.903 (.811 – .992)	4.59 (3.93 – 5.32)	1,270
Gender					
(6 years and older)					
Males					
2001–2002	*	< LOD	< LOD	2.13 (1.94 – 2.41)	3,835
2005–2006	*	< LOD	< LOD	2.26 (1.99 – 2.60)	3,204
Females					
2001–2002	*	< LOD	< LOD	3.08 (2.73 – 3.70)	4,094
2005–2006	*	< LOD	.759 (.708 – .816)	3.88 (3.60 – 4.48)	3,412
Race/ethnicity					
(6 years and older)					
Mexican Americans					
2001–2002	*	< LOD	< LOD	2.06 (1.85 – 2.42)	1,990
2005–2006	*	< LOD	< LOD	2.26 (1.97 – 2.59)	1,707
Non-Hispanic Blacks					
2001–2002	*	< LOD	< LOD	2.29 (1.96 – 2.69)	1,864
2005–2006	*	< LOD	< LOD	2.81 (2.37 – 3.38)	1,673
Non-Hispanic Whites					
2001–2002	*	< LOD	< LOD	2.79 (2.48 – 3.28)	3,450
2005–2006	*	< LOD	< LOD	3.44 (3.06 – 3.82)	2,725

< LOD means less than the limit of detection, which may vary for some compounds by year. See Appendix D for LOD.
* Not calculated. Proportion of results below limit of detection was too high to provide a valid result.

Figure 2.8.b. Serum cis–beta–carotene: Concentrations by survey cycle

Selected percentiles in µg/dL (95% confidence intervals), National Health and Nutrition Examination Survey, 2001–2002 and 2005–2006

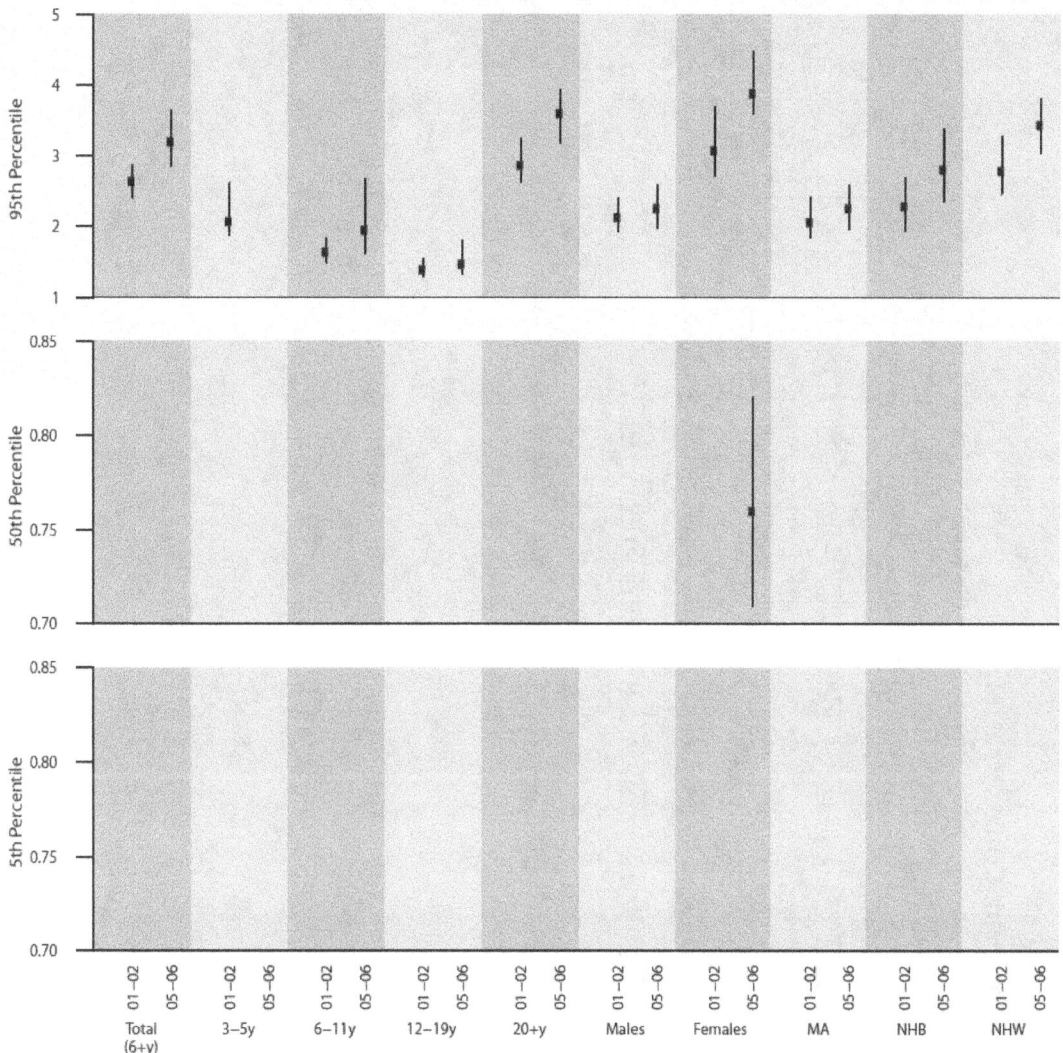

Values in the graph are suppressed if either the point estimate or the lower 95% confidence limit is noted as "< LOD" in the accompanying table.

Table 2.9.a.1. Serum beta-cryptoxanthin: Concentrations

Geometric mean and selected percentiles of serum concentrations (in µg/dL) for the total U.S. population aged 6 years and older, National Health and Nutrition Examination Survey, 2005–2006.

	Geometric mean (95% conf. interval)	Selected percentiles (95% conf. interval)					Sample size
		2.5th	5th	50th	95th	97.5th	
Total, 6 years and older	7.70 (7.34 – 8.08)	1.90 (1.63 – 2.06)	2.46 (2.26 – 2.63)	7.62 (7.24 – 7.99)	24.1 (22.5 – 26.4)	30.5 (28.7 – 33.2)	7,195
Age group							
6–11 years	9.47 (8.88 – 10.1)	3.41 (2.68 – 3.69)	3.90 (3.32 – 4.23)	9.14 (8.52 – 9.66)	24.9 (23.0 – 28.7)	30.4 (27.1 – 42.3)	855
12–19 years	7.82 (7.42 – 8.23)	2.56 (2.13 – 2.97)	3.20 (2.91 – 3.50)	7.49 (7.01 – 7.99)	20.3 (18.8 – 23.4)	25.5 (23.6 – 27.2)	1,924
20–39 years	7.95 (7.52 – 8.40)	2.33 (1.84 – 2.53)	2.78 (2.50 – 2.97)	7.81 (7.31 – 8.18)	24.5 (21.7 – 28.8)	31.7 (28.8 – 38.0)	1,679
40–59 years	7.24 (6.60 – 7.94)	1.48 (1.14 – 1.92)	2.16 (1.80 – 2.40)	7.03 (6.50 – 7.82)	24.8 (21.5 – 29.2)	30.3 (27.7 – 41.1)	1,357
60 years and older	7.39 (6.86 – 7.97)	1.52 (1.38 – 1.62)	1.98 (1.62 – 2.25)	7.48 (7.03 – 8.13)	24.2 (22.7 – 27.6)	31.9 (27.8 – 35.2)	1,380
Gender							
Males	7.51 (7.10 – 7.94)	1.86 (1.42 – 2.14)	2.41 (2.10 – 2.70)	7.49 (7.12 – 7.88)	22.8 (21.5 – 25.0)	28.4 (26.4 – 30.9)	3,514
Females	7.89 (7.53 – 8.27)	1.93 (1.68 – 2.10)	2.54 (2.24 – 2.69)	7.74 (7.28 – 8.14)	25.5 (23.4 – 28.1)	32.5 (30.0 – 37.1)	3,681
Race/ethnicity							
Mexican Americans	13.0 (11.8 – 14.3)	3.45 (3.15 – 3.89)	4.42 (3.87 – 4.86)	12.9 (11.9 – 14.2)	36.2 (32.4 – 45.4)	46.2 (40.7 – 63.0)	1,842
Non-Hispanic Blacks	8.34 (7.88 – 8.84)	2.32 (2.02 – 2.51)	2.89 (2.59 – 3.11)	8.23 (7.80 – 8.81)	23.6 (20.8 – 27.8)	29.8 (26.9 – 35.6)	1,848
Non-Hispanic Whites	6.94 (6.59 – 7.32)	1.66 (1.47 – 1.92)	2.26 (2.07 – 2.44)	6.96 (6.62 – 7.38)	20.5 (19.7 – 21.9)	25.5 (23.3 – 28.2)	2,960

Figure 2.9.a. Serum beta–cryptoxanthin: Concentrations by age group

Geometric mean (95% confidence interval), National Health and Nutrition Examination Survey, 2005–2006

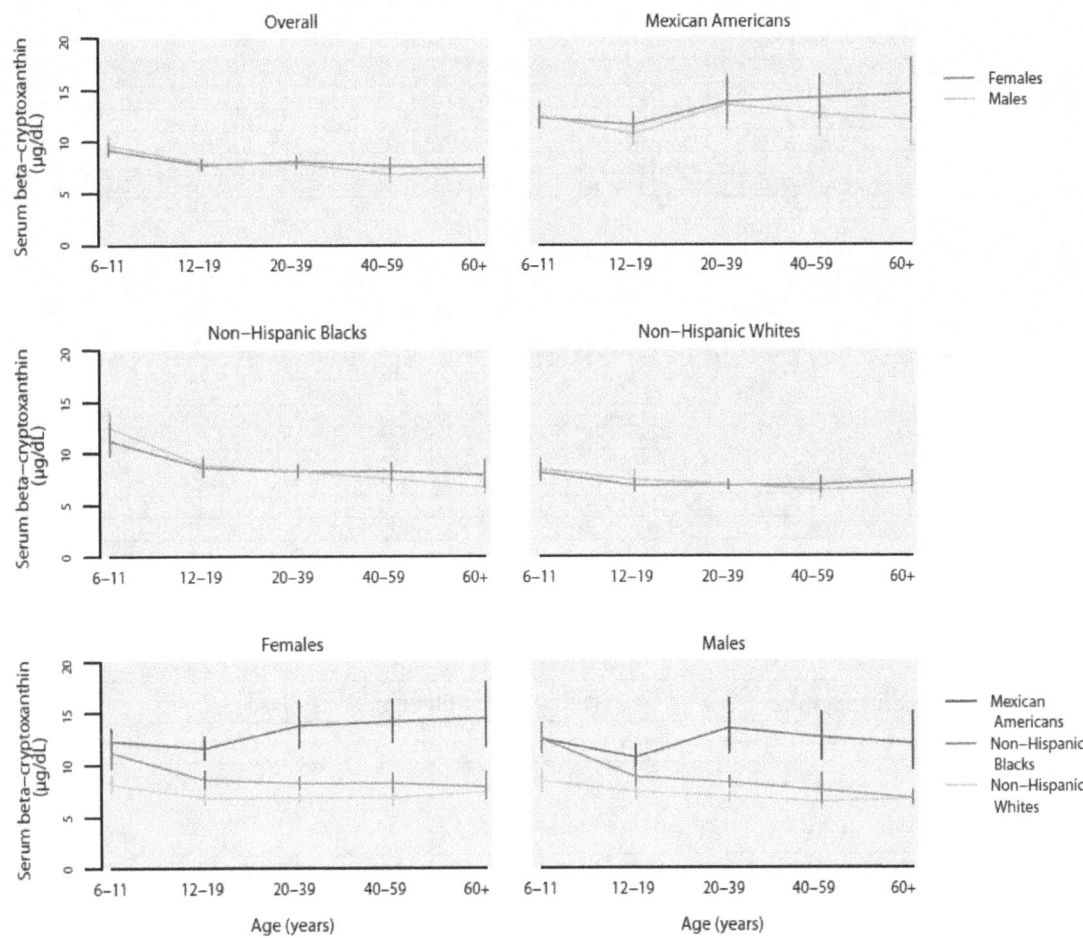

Table 2.9.a.2. Serum beta-cryptoxanthin: Total population

Geometric mean and selected percentiles of serum concentrations (in µg/dL) for the total U.S. population aged 6 years and older, National Health and Nutrition Examination Survey, 2005–2006.

	Geometric mean (95% conf. interval)		Selected percentiles (95% conf. interval)						Sample size
			10th		50th		90th		
Males and Females									
Total, 6 years and older	7.70	(7.34 – 8.08)	3.17	(2.95 – 3.36)	7.62	(7.24 – 7.99)	18.5	(17.5 – 19.7)	7,195
6–11 years	9.47	(8.88 – 10.1)	4.47	(3.95 – 5.23)	9.14	(8.52 – 9.66)	19.5	(17.8 – 21.7)	855
12–19 years	7.82	(7.42 – 8.23)	3.86	(3.64 – 4.01)	7.49	(7.01 – 7.99)	16.5	(15.2 – 17.8)	1,924
20–39 years	7.95	(7.52 – 8.40)	3.42	(3.06 – 3.76)	7.81	(7.31 – 8.18)	18.2	(16.7 – 20.0)	1,679
40–59 years	7.24	(6.60 – 7.94)	2.76	(2.48 – 3.06)	7.03	(6.50 – 7.82)	19.3	(17.2 – 21.2)	1,357
60 years and older	7.39	(6.86 – 7.97)	2.82	(2.40 – 3.01)	7.48	(7.03 – 8.13)	19.0	(17.4 – 20.7)	1,380
Males									
Total, 6 years and older	7.51	(7.10 – 7.94)	3.13	(2.87 – 3.38)	7.49	(7.12 – 7.88)	18.0	(17.1 – 19.3)	3,514
6–11 years	9.70	(8.87 – 10.6)	4.86	(3.91 – 5.70)	9.33	(8.48 – 10.2)	19.2	(17.3 – 21.7)	426
12–19 years	7.89	(7.36 – 8.46)	3.95	(3.55 – 4.37)	7.65	(7.02 – 8.42)	16.9	(15.0 – 18.6)	961
20–39 years	7.86	(7.38 – 8.38)	3.49	(3.11 – 3.88)	7.74	(7.16 – 8.22)	17.9	(16.0 – 19.5)	735
40–59 years	6.84	(6.09 – 7.69)	2.58	(2.16 – 2.91)	6.74	(6.12 – 7.68)	18.8	(16.7 – 21.9)	668
60 years and older	7.01	(6.37 – 7.70)	2.87	(2.36 – 3.05)	7.16	(6.44 – 7.89)	17.6	(16.7 – 20.5)	724
Females									
Total, 6 years and older	7.89	(7.53 – 8.27)	3.21	(2.99 – 3.40)	7.74	(7.28 – 8.14)	19.1	(17.9 – 20.2)	3,681
6–11 years	9.23	(8.67 – 9.83)	4.21	(3.49 – 4.98)	8.82	(8.30 – 9.60)	19.7	(17.8 – 23.4)	429
12–19 years	7.73	(7.26 – 8.23)	3.77	(3.48 – 3.96)	7.32	(6.78 – 8.01)	16.3	(14.9 – 17.8)	963
20–39 years	8.04	(7.52 – 8.59)	3.32	(2.93 – 3.81)	7.87	(7.27 – 8.51)	19.3	(17.3 – 23.4)	944
40–59 years	7.63	(6.94 – 8.39)	3.08	(2.66 – 3.33)	7.35	(6.62 – 8.25)	19.7	(17.2 – 20.9)	689
60 years and older	7.73	(7.04 – 8.48)	2.79	(2.34 – 3.03)	7.73	(7.23 – 8.79)	20.0	(18.1 – 22.9)	656

Table 2.9.a.3. Serum beta-cryptoxanthin: Mexican Americans

Geometric mean and selected percentiles of serum concentrations (in µg/dL) for Mexican Americans in the U.S. population aged 6 years and older, National Health and Nutrition Examination Survey, 2005–2006.

	Geometric mean (95% conf. interval)		Selected percentiles (95% conf. interval)						Sample size
			10th		50th		90th		
Males and Females									
Total, 6 years and older	13.0	(11.8 – 14.3)	5.53	(5.21 – 5.91)	12.9	(11.9 – 14.2)	29.7	(25.9 – 34.0)	1,842
6–11 years	12.4	(11.4 – 13.5)	6.01	(4.82 – 6.78)	12.3	(11.0 – 14.0)	24.8	(23.0 – 27.8)	295
12–19 years	11.1	(10.3 – 12.1)	5.77	(5.11 – 6.34)	11.0	(10.2 – 12.1)	22.8	(19.2 – 26.1)	646
20–39 years	13.6	(11.7 – 16.0)	5.47	(4.92 – 6.41)	13.5	(11.7 – 15.7)	31.9	(26.5 – 45.3)	448
40–59 years	13.3	(11.7 – 15.2)	5.34	(4.80 – 5.81)	13.6	(11.9 – 15.8)	29.8	(25.8 – 35.3)	245
60 years and older	13.3	(11.4 – 15.6)	5.60	(2.79 – 7.53)	13.4	(11.3 – 15.8)	29.7	(24.7 – 42.9)	208
Males									
Total, 6 years and older	12.6	(11.2 – 14.1)	5.38	(4.94 – 5.92)	12.7	(11.4 – 14.4)	27.9	(24.5 – 32.7)	881
6–11 years	12.5	(11.3 – 13.8)	6.02	(3.82 – 6.86)	12.5	(11.2 – 14.4)	24.3	(22.2 – 32.0)	145
12–19 years	10.7	(9.74 – 11.9)	6.00	(5.02 – 6.51)	10.5	(9.42 – 11.6)	21.7	(18.5 – 26.0)	313
20–39 years	13.5	(11.1 – 16.4)	5.38	(4.43 – 6.71)	13.8	(11.6 – 16.0)	29.6	(22.6 – 45.6)	197
40–59 years	12.6	(10.5 – 15.0)	5.06	(3.45 – 5.65)	13.0	(10.4 – 15.5)	30.6	(25.0 – 45.0)	121
60 years and older	12.0	(9.50 – 15.1)	4.24†	(1.40 – 7.66)	11.4	(9.88 – 15.0)	26.9†	(21.1 – 37.5)	105
Females									
Total, 6 years and older	13.4	(12.2 – 14.6)	5.64	(5.31 – 6.10)	13.1	(12.2 – 14.2)	30.8	(26.8 – 39.3)	961
6–11 years	12.3	(11.3 – 13.5)	5.87	(4.89 – 6.83)	11.8	(10.9 – 13.3)	26.0	(21.9 – 28.8)	150
12–19 years	11.6	(10.6 – 12.7)	5.49	(4.35 – 6.31)	12.1	(10.9 – 13.0)	23.4	(19.9 – 30.4)	333
20–39 years	13.8	(11.7 – 16.2)	5.49	(4.69 – 6.54)	13.0	(11.0 – 16.0)	34.7	(29.7 – 47.2)	251
40–59 years	14.2	(12.2 – 16.4)	5.67	(3.59 – 7.24)	13.7	(12.5 – 16.3)	29.5	(24.9 – 36.5)	124
60 years and older	14.5	(11.8 – 18.0)	5.79†	(3.11 – 7.70)	15.4	(12.2 – 17.4)	30.1†	(25.5 – 59.9)	103

† Estimate is subject to greater uncertainty due to small cell size.

Table 2.9.a.4. Serum beta-cryptoxanthin: Non-Hispanic blacks

Geometric mean and selected percentiles of serum concentrations (in µg/dL) for non-Hispanic blacks in the U.S. population aged 6 years and older, National Health and Nutrition Examination Survey, 2005–2006.

	Geometric mean (95% conf. interval)		Selected percentiles (95% conf. interval)						Sample size
			10th		50th		90th		
Males and Females									
Total, 6 years and older	8.34	(7.88 – 8.84)	3.72	(3.51 – 4.02)	8.23	(7.80 – 8.81)	18.1	(17.2 – 19.3)	1,848
6–11 years	11.9	(11.1 – 12.8)	6.05	(5.13 – 6.76)	11.7	(10.6 – 13.2)	22.8	(19.7 – 25.0)	237
12–19 years	8.69	(7.99 – 9.46)	4.54	(4.16 – 4.92)	8.47	(7.65 – 9.40)	17.4	(15.7 – 19.0)	637
20–39 years	8.26	(7.76 – 8.78)	3.97	(3.62 – 4.26)	7.95	(7.47 – 8.71)	16.3	(15.0 – 18.9)	363
40–59 years	7.89	(6.95 – 8.97)	2.90	(2.54 – 3.55)	7.98	(6.88 – 9.10)	18.8	(17.2 – 22.3)	332
60 years and older	7.38	(6.55 – 8.31)	3.16	(2.61 – 3.71)	7.31	(6.35 – 8.23)	16.8	(15.5 – 21.8)	279
Males									
Total, 6 years and older	8.23	(7.64 – 8.87)	3.58	(3.20 – 3.89)	8.03	(7.38 – 8.90)	19.0	(17.7 – 20.9)	922
6–11 years	12.5	(11.2 – 14.0)	6.69	(4.92 – 7.69)	12.6	(10.6 – 14.7)	23.9	(21.5 – 25.6)	127
12–19 years	8.80	(8.01 – 9.67)	4.43	(3.92 – 4.96)	8.50	(7.75 – 9.40)	18.2	(15.8 – 20.7)	325
20–39 years	8.26	(7.73 – 8.83)	4.00	(3.65 – 4.31)	7.41	(7.04 – 7.98)	18.2	(15.3 – 21.6)	168
40–59 years	7.49	(6.22 – 9.03)	2.63	(2.42 – 2.81)	7.64	(6.42 – 9.09)	19.0	(17.1 – 24.6)	153
60 years and older	6.73	(6.08 – 7.45)	2.92	(2.43 – 3.29)	6.06	(5.09 – 7.20)	17.0	(15.6 – 17.8)	149
Females									
Total, 6 years and older	8.44	(8.04 – 8.86)	3.87	(3.56 – 4.40)	8.39	(8.01 – 8.86)	17.3	(16.4 – 18.5)	926
6–11 years	11.2	(9.74 – 13.0)	5.33†	(4.18 – 6.55)	10.8	(9.90 – 12.2)	19.6†	(17.8 – 30.0)	110
12–19 years	8.59	(7.79 – 9.46)	4.66	(4.22 – 5.04)	8.46	(7.40 – 9.63)	16.6	(14.9 – 18.0)	312
20–39 years	8.25	(7.69 – 8.86)	3.73	(3.50 – 4.18)	8.14	(7.80 – 8.94)	15.6	(13.7 – 20.1)	195
40–59 years	8.24	(7.42 – 9.14)	3.64	(2.54 – 4.52)	8.22	(6.90 – 9.23)	18.5	(16.3 – 21.5)	179
60 years and older	7.89	(6.67 – 9.33)	3.67	(2.29 – 4.00)	7.96	(6.64 – 9.20)	16.5	(14.7 – 26.2)	130

† Estimate is subject to greater uncertainty due to small cell size.

Table 2.9.a.5. Serum beta-cryptoxanthin: Non-Hispanic whites

Geometric mean and selected percentiles of serum concentrations (in µg/dL) for non-Hispanic whites in the U.S. population aged 6 years and older, National Health and Nutrition Examination Survey, 2005–2006.

	Geometric mean (95% conf. interval)		Selected percentiles (95% conf. interval)						Sample size
			10th		50th		90th		
Males and Females									
Total, 6 years and older	6.94	(6.59 – 7.32)	2.93	(2.72 – 3.14)	6.96	(6.62 – 7.38)	16.3	(15.3 – 17.4)	2,960
6–11 years	8.29	(7.73 – 8.89)	4.21	(3.43 – 4.88)	8.12	(7.60 – 8.69)	15.7	(14.5 – 17.9)	230
12–19 years	7.12	(6.60 – 7.68)	3.72	(3.31 – 3.93)	6.82	(6.07 – 7.64)	14.2	(13.1 – 16.1)	497
20–39 years	6.90	(6.60 – 7.21)	3.01	(2.73 – 3.40)	6.93	(6.69 – 7.24)	15.1	(13.3 – 16.5)	711
40–59 years	6.63	(5.99 – 7.33)	2.63	(2.35 – 2.88)	6.61	(6.11 – 7.28)	17.2	(14.6 – 20.0)	679
60 years and older	7.05	(6.51 – 7.64)	2.75	(2.28 – 2.96)	7.26	(6.66 – 7.79)	17.7	(16.8 – 19.6)	843
Males									
Total, 6 years and older	6.83	(6.42 – 7.28)	2.92	(2.50 – 3.23)	6.90	(6.58 – 7.29)	15.9	(14.6 – 17.5)	1,468
6–11 years	8.45	(7.44 – 9.60)	4.43	(3.50 – 5.65)	7.99	(7.29 – 9.15)	15.9	(14.0 – 21.0)	112
12–19 years	7.38	(6.60 – 8.26)	3.87	(3.20 – 4.40)	7.10	(6.14 – 8.39)	14.5	(12.6 – 17.5)	253
20–39 years	6.94	(6.51 – 7.40)	3.15	(2.80 – 3.53)	7.06	(6.75 – 7.53)	14.0	(12.1 – 16.7)	309
40–59 years	6.39	(5.62 – 7.26)	2.42	(1.99 – 2.82)	6.31	(5.75 – 6.96)	17.6	(14.6 – 21.6)	350
60 years and older	6.66	(6.02 – 7.37)	2.78	(2.23 – 3.04)	6.94	(5.82 – 7.73)	17.0	(15.2 – 18.8)	444
Females									
Total, 6 years and older	7.05	(6.69 – 7.43)	2.94	(2.70 – 3.20)	7.04	(6.59 – 7.55)	16.6	(15.4 – 18.1)	1,492
6–11 years	8.11	(7.34 – 8.95)	3.85	(3.04 – 4.45)	8.14	(7.69 – 8.60)	15.0	(13.3 – 22.0)	118
12–19 years	6.84	(6.25 – 7.48)	3.57	(2.93 – 3.86)	6.57	(5.73 – 7.38)	14.0	(12.8 – 16.4)	244
20–39 years	6.86	(6.45 – 7.28)	2.92	(2.53 – 3.38)	6.73	(6.29 – 7.41)	15.7	(13.5 – 18.2)	402
40–59 years	6.87	(6.18 – 7.64)	2.84	(2.52 – 3.24)	6.84	(6.09 – 7.85)	16.5	(14.4 – 19.9)	329
60 years and older	7.39	(6.69 – 8.17)	2.73	(2.26 – 2.94)	7.50	(6.74 – 8.69)	19.5	(17.0 – 21.2)	399

Table 2.9.b. Serum beta-cryptoxanthin: Concentrations by survey cycle

Geometric mean and selected percentiles of serum concentrations (in µg/dL) for the U.S. population, National Health and Nutrition Examination Survey, 2001–2002 and 2005–2006.

	Geometric mean (95% conf. interval)	Selected percentiles (95% conf. interval)						Sample size
		5th		50th		95th		
Total, 6 years and older								
2001–2002	7.46	(7.06 – 7.87)	2.45	(2.20 – 2.68)	7.40	(7.00 – 7.82)	23.0	(20.9 – 25.5)	7,890
2005–2006	7.70	(7.34 – 8.08)	2.46	(2.26 – 2.63)	7.62	(7.24 – 7.99)	24.1	(22.5 – 26.4)	7,195
Age group								
3–5 years								
2001–2002	9.43	(8.40 – 10.6)	3.30	(1.88 – 3.96)	9.09	(7.81 – 10.4)	30.7	(25.3 – 43.1)	427
6–11 years								
2001–2002	9.40	(8.71 – 10.2)	3.92	(3.28 – 4.22)	9.05	(8.29 – 10.2)	26.1	(21.9 – 31.6)	1,006
2005–2006	9.47	(8.88 – 10.1)	3.90	(3.32 – 4.23)	9.14	(8.52 – 9.66)	24.9	(23.0 – 28.7)	855
12–19 years								
2001–2002	7.63	(7.20 – 8.08)	3.05	(2.58 – 3.31)	7.45	(7.00 – 7.99)	19.8	(18.5 – 22.3)	2,199
2005–2006	7.82	(7.42 – 8.23)	3.20	(2.91 – 3.50)	7.49	(7.01 – 7.99)	20.3	(18.8 – 23.4)	1,924
20–39 years								
2001–2002	7.11	(6.57 – 7.69)	2.40	(2.04 – 2.73)	6.83	(6.25 – 7.50)	22.9	(20.0 – 26.6)	1,707
2005–2006	7.95	(7.52 – 8.40)	2.78	(2.50 – 2.97)	7.81	(7.31 – 8.18)	24.5	(21.7 – 28.8)	1,679
40–59 years								
2001–2002	7.28	(6.75 – 7.86)	2.39	(2.02 – 2.71)	7.16	(6.66 – 7.77)	23.2	(20.4 – 26.1)	1,459
2005–2006	7.24	(6.60 – 7.94)	2.16	(1.80 – 2.40)	7.03	(6.50 – 7.82)	24.8	(21.5 – 29.2)	1,357
60 years and older								
2001–2002	7.44	(6.84 – 8.09)	1.94	(1.71 – 2.22)	7.64	(7.06 – 8.28)	23.5	(20.9 – 27.8)	1,519
2005–2006	7.39	(6.86 – 7.97)	1.98	(1.62 – 2.25)	7.48	(7.03 – 8.13)	24.2	(22.7 – 27.6)	1,380
Gender								
(6 years and older)								
Males								
2001–2002	7.28	(6.89 – 7.69)	2.41	(2.10 – 2.66)	7.32	(6.82 – 7.81)	22.3	(20.4 – 25.0)	3,815
2005–2006	7.51	(7.10 – 7.94)	2.41	(2.10 – 2.70)	7.49	(7.12 – 7.88)	22.8	(21.5 – 25.0)	3,514
Females								
2001–2002	7.63	(7.20 – 8.08)	2.48	(2.29 – 2.75)	7.45	(7.05 – 7.84)	23.8	(21.1 – 26.2)	4,075
2005–2006	7.89	(7.53 – 8.27)	2.54	(2.24 – 2.69)	7.74	(7.28 – 8.14)	25.5	(23.4 – 28.1)	3,681
Race/ethnicity								
(6 years and older)								
Mexican Americans								
2001–2002	12.1	(11.2 – 13.2)	4.14	(3.71 – 4.53)	12.1	(10.9 – 13.5)	34.5	(32.1 – 38.5)	1,988
2005–2006	13.0	(11.8 – 14.3)	4.42	(3.87 – 4.86)	12.9	(11.9 – 14.2)	36.2	(32.4 – 45.4)	1,842
Non-Hispanic Blacks								
2001–2002	8.03	(7.38 – 8.74)	2.99	(2.66 – 3.27)	7.92	(7.32 – 8.55)	23.0	(19.9 – 27.7)	1,859
2005–2006	8.34	(7.88 – 8.84)	2.89	(2.59 – 3.11)	8.23	(7.80 – 8.81)	23.6	(20.8 – 27.8)	1,848
Non-Hispanic Whites								
2001–2002	6.80	(6.43 – 7.19)	2.36	(2.05 – 2.53)	6.71	(6.29 – 7.16)	19.6	(18.2 – 22.2)	3,422
2005–2006	6.94	(6.59 – 7.32)	2.26	(2.07 – 2.44)	6.96	(6.62 – 7.38)	20.5	(19.7 – 21.9)	2,960

Figure 2.9.b. Serum beta–cryptoxanthin: Concentrations by survey cycle

Selected percentiles in µg/dL (95% confidence intervals), National Health and Nutrition Examination Survey, 2001–2002 and 2005–2006

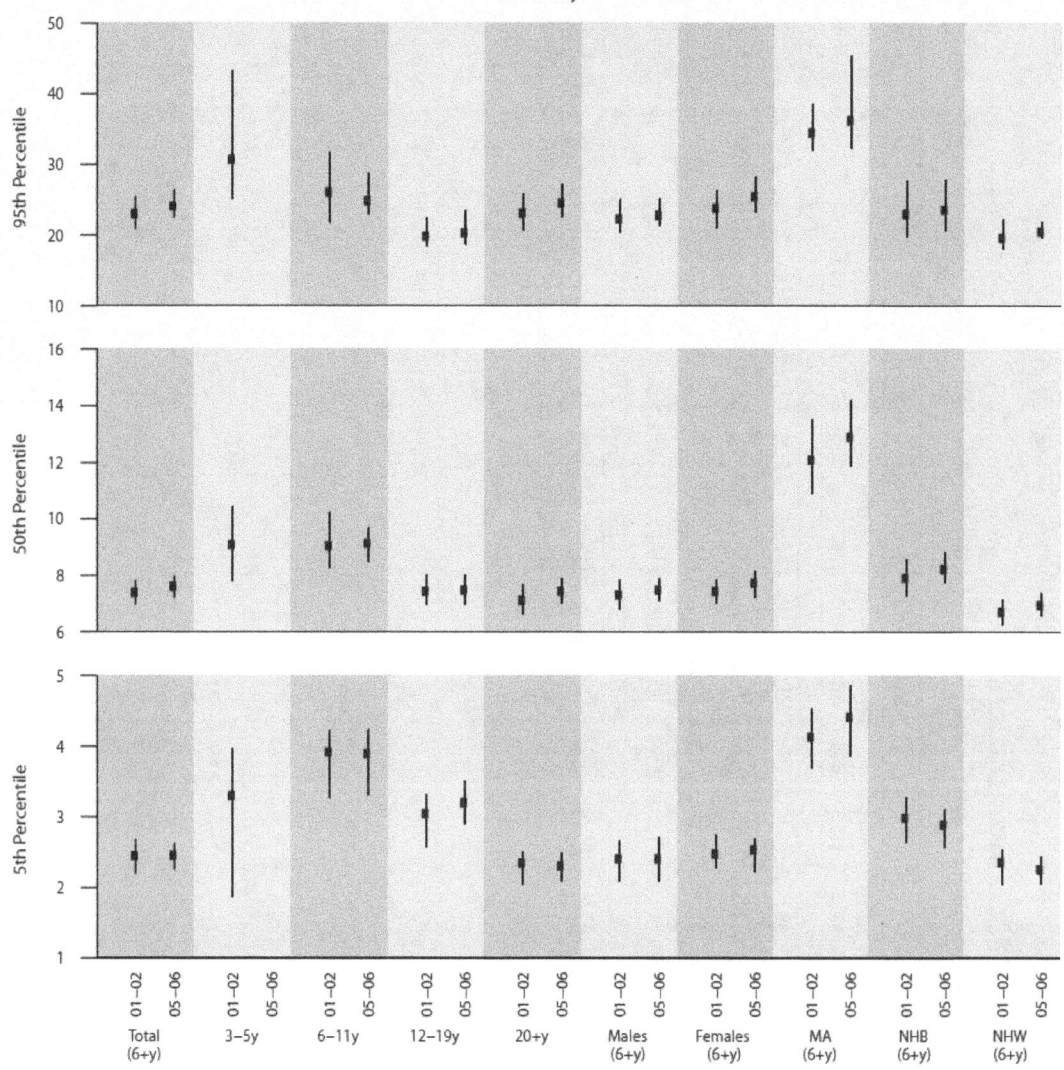

Table 2.10.a.1. Serum lutein/zeaxanthin: Concentrations

Geometric mean and selected percentiles of serum concentrations (in µg/dL) for the total U.S. population aged 6 years and older, National Health and Nutrition Examination Survey, 2005–2006.

	Geometric mean (95% conf. interval)	Selected percentiles (95% conf. interval)					Sample size
		2.5th	5th	50th	95th	97.5th	
Total, 6 years and older	13.8 (13.4 – 14.2)	4.95 (4.69 – 5.19)	5.90 (5.68 – 6.18)	13.7 (13.2 – 14.1)	31.3 (30.3 – 33.2)	38.5 (37.0 – 40.0)	7,254
Age group							
6–11 years	13.1 (12.6 – 13.7)	5.74 (4.13 – 6.47)	6.70 (5.50 – 7.67)	13.3 (12.8 – 13.9)	24.5 (23.5 – 27.4)	29.0 (27.3 – 30.2)	860
12–19 years	10.7 (10.3 – 11.1)	4.91 (4.39 – 5.18)	5.67 (5.21 – 5.91)	10.6 (10.0 – 11.1)	20.0 (19.1 – 21.1)	22.7 (21.4 – 25.1)	1,954
20–39 years	13.6 (13.1 – 14.1)	4.94 (4.24 – 5.46)	5.91 (5.19 – 6.41)	13.6 (12.9 – 14.4)	29.3 (27.7 – 32.1)	35.2 (31.7 – 40.0)	1,688
40–59 years	14.5 (13.8 – 15.2)	4.62 (4.02 – 5.31)	5.82 (5.28 – 6.13)	14.5 (13.7 – 15.2)	35.7 (33.3 – 37.8)	40.8 (38.5 – 46.1)	1,365
60 years and older	15.5 (14.9 – 16.2)	5.27 (4.72 – 5.83)	6.44 (6.02 – 6.69)	15.7 (15.0 – 16.5)	35.9 (32.8 – 40.3)	42.5 (39.7 – 51.2)	1,387
Gender							
Males	13.6 (13.1 – 14.0)	4.92 (4.48 – 5.30)	5.93 (5.42 – 6.35)	13.5 (13.0 – 14.1)	30.7 (28.7 – 31.4)	35.7 (33.3 – 39.0)	3,547
Females	14.0 (13.5 – 14.4)	4.98 (4.62 – 5.26)	5.89 (5.69 – 6.13)	13.8 (13.3 – 14.4)	32.8 (31.0 – 35.7)	39.9 (38.4 – 41.5)	3,707
Race/ethnicity							
Mexican Americans	15.1 (14.5 – 15.8)	6.36 (5.62 – 6.79)	7.41 (6.79 – 7.83)	15.0 (14.4 – 15.6)	31.3 (29.2 – 34.1)	35.5 (33.2 – 40.8)	1,844
Non-Hispanic Blacks	15.3 (14.8 – 15.8)	5.88 (5.20 – 6.37)	7.03 (6.33 – 7.71)	15.4 (15.0 – 15.8)	31.5 (29.4 – 35.1)	38.0 (34.8 – 41.7)	1,891
Non-Hispanic Whites	13.2 (12.8 – 13.6)	4.74 (4.46 – 4.96)	5.70 (5.33 – 5.88)	12.9 (12.5 – 13.4)	30.9 (29.1 – 32.8)	37.5 (34.4 – 39.9)	2,973

Figure 2.10.a. Serum lutein/zeaxanthin: Concentrations by age group

Geometric Mean (95% confidence interval), National Health and Nutrition Examination Survey, 2005–2006

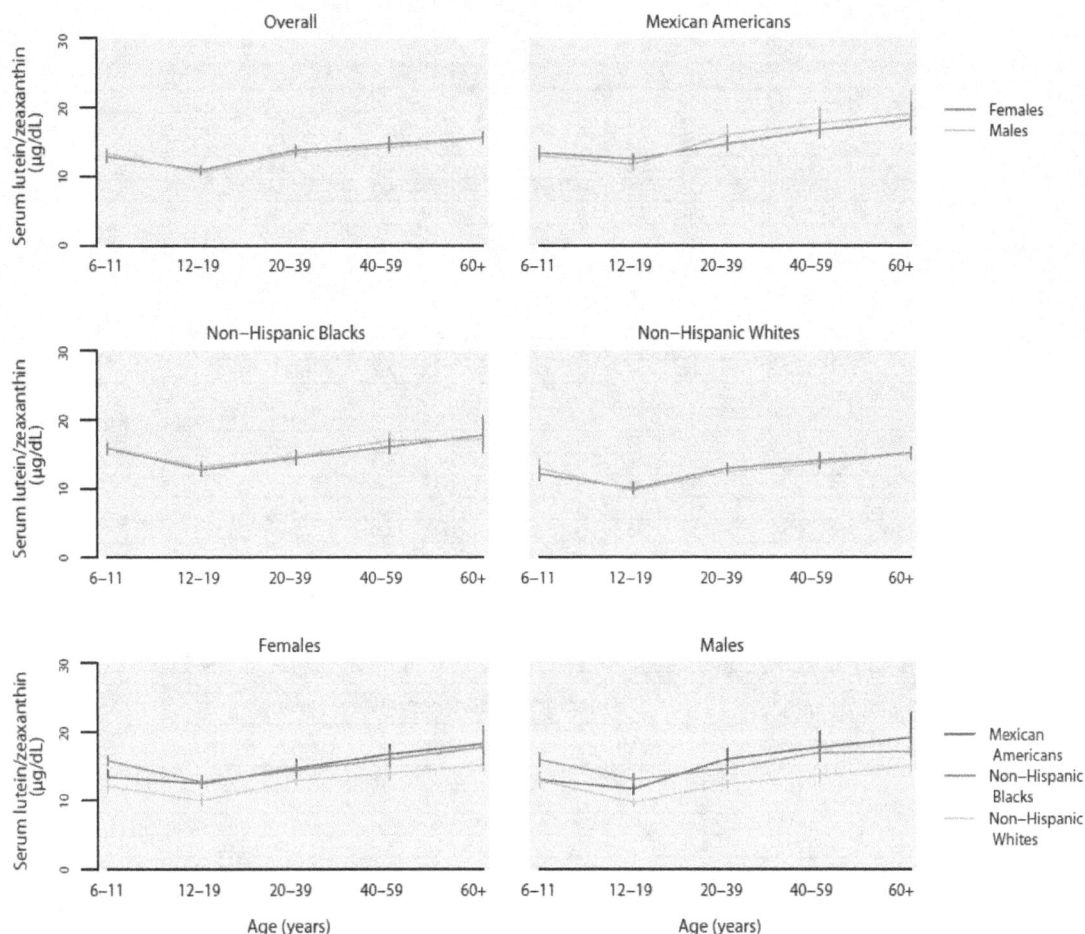

Table 2.10.a.2. Serum lutein/zeaxanthin: Total population

Geometric mean and selected percentiles of serum concentrations (in µg/dL) for the total U.S. population aged 6 years and older, National Health and Nutrition Examination Survey, 2005–2006.

| | Geometric mean (95% conf. interval) | Selected percentiles (95% conf. interval) | | | Sample size |
		10th	50th	90th	
Males and Females					
Total, 6 years and older	13.8 (13.4 – 14.2)	7.24 (6.91 – 7.49)	13.7 (13.2 – 14.1)	26.5 (25.7 – 27.3)	7,254
6–11 years	13.1 (12.6 – 13.7)	7.93 (6.84 – 8.54)	13.3 (12.8 – 13.9)	20.7 (20.1 – 22.0)	860
12–19 years	10.7 (10.3 – 11.1)	6.50 (6.19 – 6.74)	10.6 (10.0 – 11.1)	17.6 (16.9 – 18.4)	1,954
20–39 years	13.6 (13.1 – 14.1)	7.40 (6.64 – 7.83)	13.6 (12.9 – 14.4)	25.1 (23.4 – 27.1)	1,688
40–59 years	14.5 (13.8 – 15.2)	7.23 (6.70 – 7.58)	14.5 (13.7 – 15.2)	29.4 (27.5 – 31.0)	1,365
60 years and older	15.5 (14.9 – 16.2)	7.89 (7.52 – 8.13)	15.7 (15.0 – 16.5)	29.0 (27.3 – 31.9)	1,387
Males					
Total, 6 years and older	13.6 (13.1 – 14.0)	7.22 (6.78 – 7.61)	13.5 (13.0 – 14.1)	25.6 (24.5 – 26.2)	3,547
6–11 years	13.4 (12.7 – 14.1)	8.08 (7.62 – 8.69)	13.6 (12.5 – 14.2)	20.5 (19.0 – 22.5)	427
12–19 years	10.5 (10.1 – 10.9)	6.49 (6.06 – 6.86)	10.3 (9.91 – 10.9)	17.3 (16.7 – 18.3)	980
20–39 years	13.4 (12.8 – 14.0)	7.26 (6.51 – 7.96)	13.4 (12.8 – 14.2)	23.8 (22.4 – 26.0)	738
40–59 years	14.2 (13.4 – 15.0)	7.22 (5.99 – 7.90)	14.1 (13.1 – 15.1)	27.6 (26.6 – 31.0)	673
60 years and older	15.5 (14.7 – 16.4)	7.94 (7.26 – 8.26)	15.9 (15.2 – 17.0)	27.8 (26.2 – 31.2)	729
Females					
Total, 6 years and older	14.0 (13.5 – 14.4)	7.27 (6.77 – 7.56)	13.8 (13.3 – 14.4)	27.5 (26.7 – 28.5)	3,707
6–11 years	12.9 (12.1 – 13.7)	7.63 (5.98 – 8.50)	13.1 (12.6 – 13.7)	21.4 (19.9 – 23.6)	433
12–19 years	10.9 (10.3 – 11.4)	6.52 (5.98 – 6.93)	10.8 (10.1 – 11.5)	18.0 (16.9 – 19.1)	974
20–39 years	13.8 (13.2 – 14.5)	7.42 (6.59 – 7.80)	13.8 (12.9 – 14.8)	25.7 (23.9 – 28.0)	950
40–59 years	14.7 (13.9 – 15.6)	7.17 (6.76 – 7.56)	15.0 (13.8 – 16.2)	29.6 (28.9 – 32.2)	692
60 years and older	15.6 (14.8 – 16.4)	7.80 (7.40 – 8.17)	15.6 (14.1 – 16.7)	29.8 (28.0 – 32.8)	658

Table 2.10.a.3. Serum lutein/zeaxanthin: Mexican Americans

Geometric mean and selected percentiles of serum concentrations (in µg/dL) for Mexican Americans in the U.S. population aged 6 years and older, National Health and Nutrition Examination Survey, 2005–2006.

| | Geometric mean (95% conf. interval) | Selected percentiles (95% conf. interval) | | | Sample size |
		10th	50th	90th	
Males and Females					
Total, 6 years and older	15.1 (14.5 – 15.8)	8.60 (8.07 – 9.17)	15.0 (14.4 – 15.6)	26.8 (25.2 – 28.6)	1,844
6–11 years	13.2 (12.4 – 14.0)	8.43 (6.89 – 9.35)	13.3 (12.2 – 14.1)	21.1 (19.3 – 23.5)	295
12–19 years	12.1 (11.5 – 12.7)	7.64 (7.22 – 8.01)	12.3 (11.7 – 12.9)	18.9 (18.0 – 20.0)	646
20–39 years	15.4 (14.3 – 16.6)	8.96 (8.09 – 9.65)	15.4 (14.2 – 17.3)	26.2 (23.4 – 30.5)	449
40–59 years	17.2 (16.0 – 18.5)	9.78 (7.36 – 11.0)	17.2 (16.2 – 18.5)	30.4 (27.3 – 36.3)	246
60 years and older	18.6 (16.7 – 20.7)	9.96 (7.59 – 12.0)	18.7 (16.9 – 20.3)	32.2 (30.1 – 34.4)	208
Males					
Total, 6 years and older	15.4 (14.5 – 16.3)	8.81 (8.00 – 9.51)	15.1 (14.4 – 16.0)	28.1 (25.6 – 31.1)	883
6–11 years	13.0 (12.1 – 13.9)	8.75 (6.33 – 9.71)	13.1 (12.1 – 13.9)	19.6 (17.5 – 22.0)	145
12–19 years	11.7 (11.0 – 12.5)	7.62 (6.85 – 8.20)	12.0 (10.9 – 12.9)	18.2 (17.4 – 19.2)	313
20–39 years	16.0 (14.6 – 17.5)	9.47 (8.02 – 10.1)	15.8 (14.9 – 17.4)	28.5 (24.2 – 33.1)	198
40–59 years	17.7 (15.7 – 19.9)	8.69 (5.55 – 11.6)	17.6 (16.1 – 19.9)	31.1 (27.0 – 52.1)	122
60 years and older	19.1 (16.0 – 22.7)	10.7† (6.38 – 12.2)	18.5 (14.5 – 25.4)	34.1† (29.9 – 45.4)	105
Females					
Total, 6 years and older	14.9 (14.2 – 15.6)	8.46 (7.68 – 9.34)	14.7 (14.1 – 15.5)	24.4 (23.3 – 27.0)	961
6–11 years	13.4 (12.5 – 14.4)	7.94 (6.66 – 8.97)	13.6 (11.9 – 14.4)	23.4 (19.8 – 27.1)	150
12–19 years	12.5 (11.9 – 13.1)	7.61 (7.08 – 8.14)	12.8 (12.3 – 13.1)	19.7 (18.3 – 20.8)	333
20–39 years	14.7 (13.7 – 15.9)	8.18 (7.42 – 9.74)	14.7 (13.1 – 16.9)	23.1 (22.2 – 27.0)	251
40–59 years	16.7 (15.6 – 18.0)	10.1 (7.40 – 10.9)	16.6 (14.5 – 18.4)	28.6 (23.7 – 44.2)	124
60 years and older	18.2 (16.1 – 20.7)	9.82† (7.45 – 11.7)	18.8 (16.2 – 21.7)	30.6† (28.3 – 33.6)	103

† Estimate is subject to greater uncertainty due to small cell size.

Table 2.10.a.4. Serum lutein/zeaxanthin: Non-Hispanic blacks

Geometric mean and selected percentiles of serum concentrations (in μg/dL) for non-Hispanic blacks in the U.S. population aged 6 years and older, National Health and Nutrition Examination Survey, 2005–2006.

	Geometric mean (95% conf. interval)	Selected percentiles (95% conf. interval)						Sample size
		10th		50th		90th		
Males and Females								
Total, 6 years and older	15.3	(14.8 – 15.8)	8.61	(8.21 – 9.04)	15.4	(15.0 – 15.8)	26.6 (25.2 – 28.4)	1,891
6–11 years	15.8	(15.3 – 16.4)	10.5	(9.30 – 11.0)	16.2	(15.6 – 16.8)	23.9 (22.5 – 27.4)	240
12–19 years	12.9	(12.3 – 13.5)	7.94	(7.37 – 8.38)	13.0	(12.1 – 13.7)	20.9 (19.5 – 22.1)	665
20–39 years	14.5	(13.7 – 15.3)	8.29	(6.74 – 9.45)	14.4	(13.5 – 15.4)	25.3 (24.0 – 28.3)	368
40–59 years	16.4	(15.5 – 17.4)	8.77	(7.81 – 9.51)	17.0	(15.8 – 18.2)	28.6 (26.6 – 30.2)	335
60 years and older	17.4	(16.0 – 19.1)	8.99	(8.24 – 10.1)	17.7	(16.0 – 19.1)	31.5 (27.1 – 36.5)	283
Males								
Total, 6 years and older	15.4	(14.9 – 15.9)	8.69	(8.26 – 9.42)	15.6	(14.9 – 16.3)	26.6 (25.6 – 28.4)	949
6–11 years	15.9	(14.9 – 16.9)	11.1	(10.3 – 11.9)	15.9	(15.0 – 17.2)	23.1 (21.9 – 26.9)	128
12–19 years	13.1	(12.4 – 13.8)	8.08	(7.27 – 8.68)	13.3	(12.2 – 14.6)	20.8 (19.6 – 21.9)	343
20–39 years	14.6	(13.8 – 15.5)	8.48	(6.56 – 9.65)	14.2	(13.1 – 15.7)	26.3 (23.2 – 29.1)	170
40–59 years	16.9	(15.8 – 18.1)	9.21	(7.66 – 9.97)	18.2	(15.6 – 19.3)	30.6 (27.5 – 36.0)	156
60 years and older	17.1	(16.2 – 18.1)	8.83	(7.79 – 9.64)	17.9	(17.2 – 18.8)	29.0 (25.9 – 34.0)	152
Females								
Total, 6 years and older	15.2	(14.5 – 15.8)	8.51	(7.69 – 9.12)	15.3	(14.8 – 15.9)	26.4 (24.6 – 29.1)	942
6–11 years	15.8	(15.1 – 16.5)	9.57	(7.86 – 10.7)	16.5	(14.8 – 17.1)	24.0 (22.3 – 28.9)	112
12–19 years	12.7	(11.9 – 13.6)	7.70	(6.62 – 8.68)	12.7	(11.4 – 13.6)	21.1 (19.1 – 23.5)	322
20–39 years	14.4	(13.4 – 15.5)	8.03	(5.21 – 9.63)	14.7	(13.6 – 15.4)	24.6 (23.2 – 28.5)	198
40–59 years	16.0	(15.0 – 17.1)	8.72	(7.23 – 9.34)	16.6	(15.6 – 17.6)	26.9 (24.6 – 29.9)	179
60 years and older	17.7	(15.2 – 20.5)	9.08	(7.95 – 10.6)	17.3	(15.1 – 20.2)	33.2 (26.3 – 57.9)	131

Table 2.10.a.5. Serum lutein/zeaxanthin: Non-Hispanic whites

Geometric mean and selected percentiles of serum concentrations (in μg/dL) for non-Hispanic whites in the U.S. population aged 6 years and older, National Health and Nutrition Examination Survey, 2005–2006.

	Geometric mean (95% conf. interval)	Selected percentiles (95% conf. interval)						Sample size
		10th		50th		90th		
Males and Females								
Total, 6 years and older	13.2	(12.8 – 13.6)	6.80	(6.48 – 7.16)	12.9	(12.5 – 13.4)	25.8 (25.1 – 26.9)	2,973
6–11 years	12.5	(11.8 – 13.3)	7.68	(6.04 – 8.34)	12.7	(12.2 – 13.6)	19.8 (18.3 – 23.1)	231
12–19 years	9.88	(9.46 – 10.3)	6.16	(5.75 – 6.48)	9.80	(9.34 – 10.3)	16.2 (15.0 – 17.1)	499
20–39 years	12.7	(12.2 – 13.1)	6.56	(5.93 – 7.39)	12.4	(11.7 – 13.2)	23.6 (22.1 – 26.9)	714
40–59 years	13.8	(13.0 – 14.6)	6.87	(6.26 – 7.25)	13.7	(12.6 – 15.1)	27.9 (26.7 – 30.2)	683
60 years and older	15.0	(14.4 – 15.7)	7.59	(7.25 – 7.97)	15.2	(14.2 – 15.8)	28.5 (26.4 – 31.4)	846
Males								
Total, 6 years and older	13.0	(12.5 – 13.4)	6.87	(6.45 – 7.22)	12.8	(12.2 – 13.5)	24.4 (23.5 – 25.7)	1,472
6–11 years	12.9	(11.8 – 14.2)	7.95	(5.77 – 8.67)	13.0	(12.2 – 14.1)	18.9 (17.1 – 31.9)	112
12–19 years	9.75	(9.24 – 10.3)	6.23	(5.55 – 6.75)	9.71	(9.33 – 10.0)	15.6 (14.3 – 16.9)	254
20–39 years	12.4	(11.9 – 12.9)	6.55	(5.75 – 7.69)	12.3	(11.7 – 13.0)	22.7 (21.8 – 24.8)	309
40–59 years	13.6	(12.8 – 14.4)	6.96	(5.83 – 7.71)	13.4	(12.3 – 14.9)	26.6 (24.5 – 29.9)	351
60 years and older	15.0	(14.2 – 15.9)	7.59	(7.11 – 8.05)	15.4	(14.4 – 16.5)	26.6 (25.5 – 30.6)	446
Females								
Total, 6 years and older	13.4	(12.9 – 13.8)	6.75	(6.20 – 7.26)	13.0	(12.4 – 13.7)	27.4 (26.0 – 28.1)	1,501
6–11 years	12.1	(11.1 – 13.2)	6.73	(5.07 – 8.32)	12.4	(11.1 – 13.2)	19.9 (18.2 – 28.1)	119
12–19 years	10.0	(9.21 – 10.9)	6.08	(5.23 – 6.57)	9.90	(9.18 – 11.1)	16.5 (15.3 – 18.1)	245
20–39 years	12.9	(12.2 – 13.6)	6.60	(5.82 – 7.42)	12.6	(11.2 – 14.4)	25.0 (22.3 – 28.5)	405
40–59 years	14.0	(13.0 – 15.0)	6.78	(5.98 – 7.28)	14.0	(12.5 – 15.7)	29.2 (27.5 – 30.7)	332
60 years and older	15.1	(14.3 – 15.9)	7.58	(6.96 – 8.05)	14.7	(13.6 – 16.2)	29.2 (27.6 – 32.6)	400

Table 2.10.b. Serum lutein/zeaxanthin: Concentrations by survey cycle

Geometric mean and selected percentiles of serum concentrations (in µg/dL) for the U.S. population, National Health and Nutrition Examination Survey, 2001–2002 and 2005–2006.

	Geometric mean (95% conf. interval)	Selected percentiles (95% conf. interval)						Sample size
		5th		50th		95th		
Total, 6 years and older								
2001–2002	13.1 (12.5 – 13.6)	5.77	(5.53 – 6.00)	12.9	(12.2 – 13.5)	30.4	(28.6 – 32.2)	7,923
2005–2006	13.8 (13.4 – 14.2)	5.90	(5.68 – 6.18)	13.7	(13.2 – 14.1)	31.3	(30.3 – 33.2)	7,254
Age group								
3–5 years								
2001–2002	12.5 (11.8 – 13.2)	6.38	(5.82 – 7.04)	12.5	(12.0 – 13.1)	24.6	(22.2 – 31.5)	430
6–11 years								
2001–2002	12.5 (11.9 – 13.2)	6.61	(5.88 – 7.06)	12.3	(11.6 – 13.1)	24.8	(22.4 – 26.0)	1,014
2005–2006	13.1 (12.6 – 13.7)	6.70	(5.50 – 7.67)	13.3	(12.8 – 13.9)	24.5	(23.5 – 27.4)	860
12–19 years								
2001–2002	10.4 (9.91 – 11.0)	4.99	(4.64 – 5.54)	10.4	(9.80 – 11.0)	20.9	(19.4 – 23.2)	2,205
2005–2006	10.7 (10.3 – 11.1)	5.67	(5.21 – 5.91)	10.6	(10.0 – 11.1)	20.0	(19.1 – 21.1)	1,954
20–39 years								
2001–2002	12.1 (11.5 – 12.9)	5.47	(5.16 – 5.73)	12.0	(11.2 – 12.7)	27.1	(25.7 – 30.7)	1,714
2005–2006	13.6 (13.1 – 14.1)	5.91	(5.19 – 6.41)	13.6	(12.9 – 14.4)	29.3	(27.7 – 32.1)	1,688
40–59 years								
2001–2002	14.4 (13.6 – 15.2)	6.47	(5.69 – 7.04)	14.1	(13.5 – 14.9)	32.6	(31.0 – 35.5)	1,468
2005–2006	14.5 (13.8 – 15.2)	5.82	(5.28 – 6.13)	14.5	(13.7 – 15.2)	35.7	(33.3 – 37.8)	1,365
60 years and older								
2001–2002	15.2 (14.3 – 16.2)	6.14	(5.54 – 6.68)	15.3	(14.3 – 16.6)	35.1	(33.3 – 41.0)	1,522
2005–2006	15.5 (14.9 – 16.2)	6.44	(6.02 – 6.69)	15.7	(15.0 – 16.5)	35.9	(32.8 – 40.3)	1,387
Gender								
(6 years and older)								
Males								
2001–2002	13.0 (12.5 – 13.6)	5.67	(5.35 – 6.01)	13.0	(12.4 – 13.6)	29.8	(28.3 – 31.7)	3,832
2005–2006	13.6 (13.1 – 14.0)	5.93	(5.42 – 6.35)	13.5	(13.0 – 14.1)	30.7	(28.7 – 31.4)	3,547
Females								
2001–2002	13.1 (12.5 – 13.7)	5.87	(5.59 – 6.03)	12.7	(12.1 – 13.5)	31.4	(28.8 – 33.0)	4,091
2005–2006	14.0 (13.5 – 14.4)	5.89	(5.69 – 6.13)	13.8	(13.3 – 14.4)	32.8	(31.0 – 35.7)	3,707
Race/ethnicity								
(6 years and older)								
Mexican Americans								
2001–2002	13.7 (13.3 – 14.2)	6.58	(6.15 – 6.84)	13.6	(13.2 – 14.1)	28.5	(26.8 – 30.7)	1,988
2005–2006	15.1 (14.5 – 15.8)	7.41	(6.79 – 7.83)	15.0	(14.4 – 15.6)	31.3	(29.2 – 34.1)	1,844
Non-Hispanic Blacks								
2001–2002	14.2 (13.1 – 15.5)	6.80	(6.20 – 7.20)	14.1	(12.8 – 15.5)	30.7	(28.5 – 34.6)	1,864
2005–2006	15.3 (14.8 – 15.8)	7.03	(6.33 – 7.71)	15.4	(15.0 – 15.8)	31.5	(29.4 – 35.1)	1,891
Non-Hispanic Whites								
2001–2002	12.6 (12.0 – 13.2)	5.60	(5.14 – 5.90)	12.4	(11.7 – 13.1)	28.8	(27.2 – 31.8)	3,447
2005–2006	13.2 (12.8 – 13.6)	5.70	(5.33 – 5.88)	12.9	(12.5 – 13.4)	30.9	(29.1 – 32.8)	2,973

Figure 2.10.b. Serum lutein/zeaxanthin: Concentrations by survey cycle

Selected percentiles in μg/dL (95% confidence intervals), National Health and Nutrition Examination Survey, 2001–2002 and 2005–2006

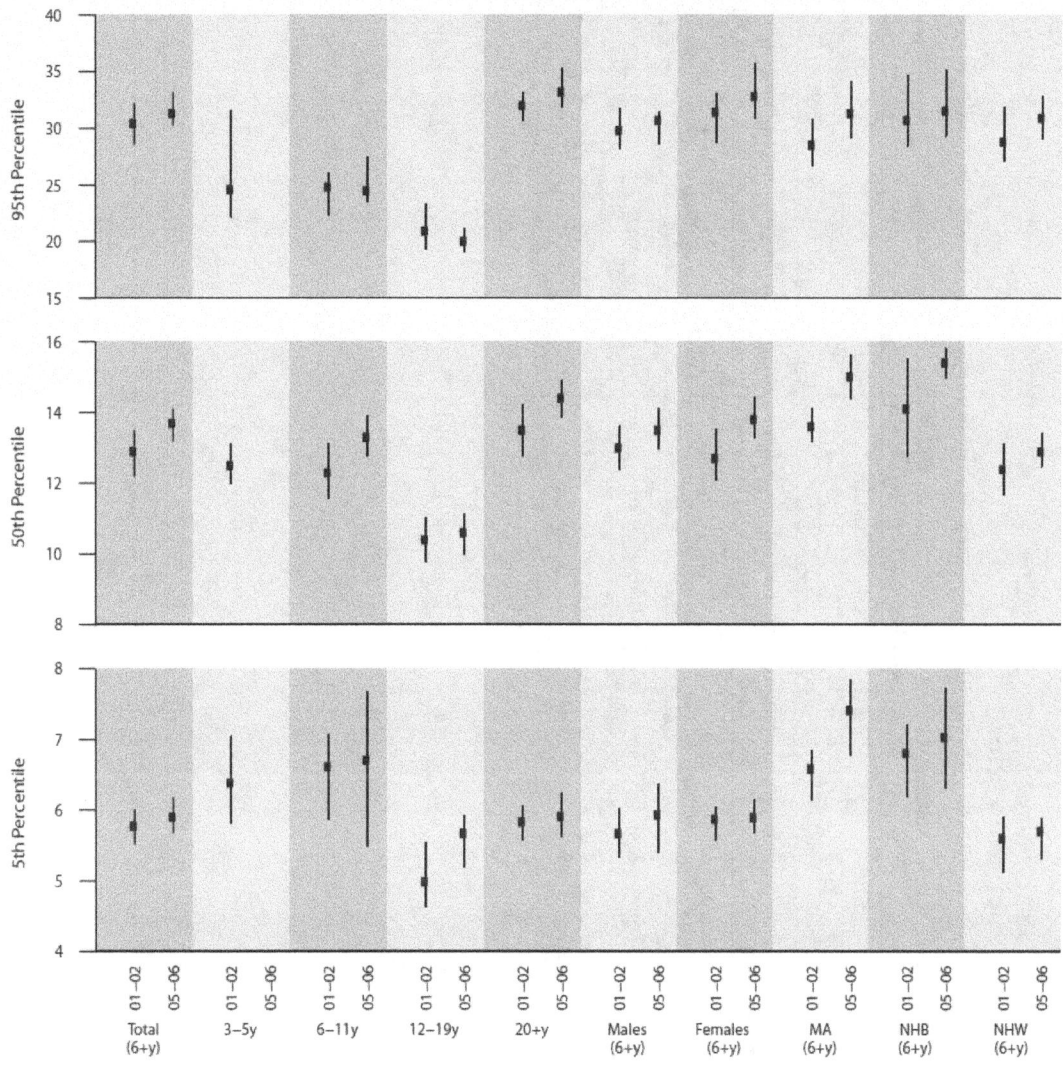

Table 2.11.a.1. Serum trans-lycopene: Concentrations

Geometric mean and selected percentiles of serum concentrations (in µg/dL) for the total U.S. population aged 6 years and older, National Health and Nutrition Examination Survey, 2005–2006.

	Geometric mean (95% conf. interval)	Selected percentiles (95% conf. interval)						Sample size
		2.5th	5th	50th	95th	97.5th		
Total, 6 years and older	21.2 (20.7 – 21.7)	5.64 (4.99 – 6.25)	7.81 (7.33 – 8.40)	22.7 (22.2 – 23.2)	43.6 (42.4 – 44.9)	48.4 (47.5 – 49.8)		7,254
Age group								
6–11 years	21.7 (20.5 – 22.9)	7.67 (5.27 – 9.29)	9.48 (7.38 – 10.9)	22.5 (21.1 – 23.7)	42.8 (40.0 – 46.0)	46.1 (44.0 – 54.8)		860
12–19 years	21.9 (21.1 – 22.6)	8.42 (7.31 – 8.78)	9.91 (8.98 – 11.0)	22.3 (21.8 – 22.9)	42.6 (40.2 – 45.1)	46.8 (44.4 – 52.7)		1,954
20–39 years	23.9 (23.3 – 24.4)	8.24 (7.38 – 8.96)	10.7 (8.97 – 11.4)	25.1 (24.3 – 25.6)	46.1 (44.1 – 47.2)	51.6 (48.9 – 53.5)		1,688
40–59 years	21.6 (20.4 – 22.8)	5.13 (3.76 – 6.34)	7.69 (6.02 – 8.98)	23.2 (22.1 – 24.4)	44.6 (42.5 – 47.1)	50.0 (47.2 – 55.9)		1,365
60 years and older	16.4 (15.4 – 17.4)	3.75 (2.69 – 4.36)	5.19 (4.32 – 5.97)	17.8 (16.8 – 19.0)	38.8 (37.3 – 40.7)	44.4 (40.7 – 46.5)		1,387
Gender								
Males	21.8 (21.0 – 22.6)	5.79 (4.54 – 6.70)	7.85 (6.99 – 8.89)	23.4 (22.6 – 24.3)	44.7 (43.7 – 47.0)	52.1 (49.0 – 55.7)		3,547
Females	20.6 (20.0 – 21.2)	5.47 (4.93 – 6.39)	7.76 (7.09 – 8.40)	22.2 (21.5 – 22.6)	42.3 (41.2 – 43.9)	46.3 (45.1 – 48.8)		3,707
Race/ethnicity								
Mexican Americans	19.5 (19.1 – 20.0)	7.04 (6.09 – 7.33)	8.80 (7.83 – 9.29)	20.2 (19.6 – 20.9)	38.0 (36.4 – 40.2)	42.5 (39.8 – 49.9)		1,844
Non-Hispanic Blacks	22.0 (20.9 – 23.2)	6.29 (5.46 – 6.99)	8.11 (7.39 – 8.77)	23.5 (22.6 – 24.7)	47.0 (44.7 – 49.5)	53.5 (51.0 – 57.3)		1,891
Non-Hispanic Whites	21.3 (20.8 – 21.9)	5.46 (4.83 – 6.26)	7.69 (7.04 – 8.47)	23.0 (22.4 – 23.5)	43.8 (42.4 – 45.2)	48.5 (47.3 – 50.6)		2,973

Figure 2.11.a. Serum trans–lycopene: Concentrations by age group

Geometric mean (95% confidence interval), National Health and Nutrition Examination Survey, 2005–2006

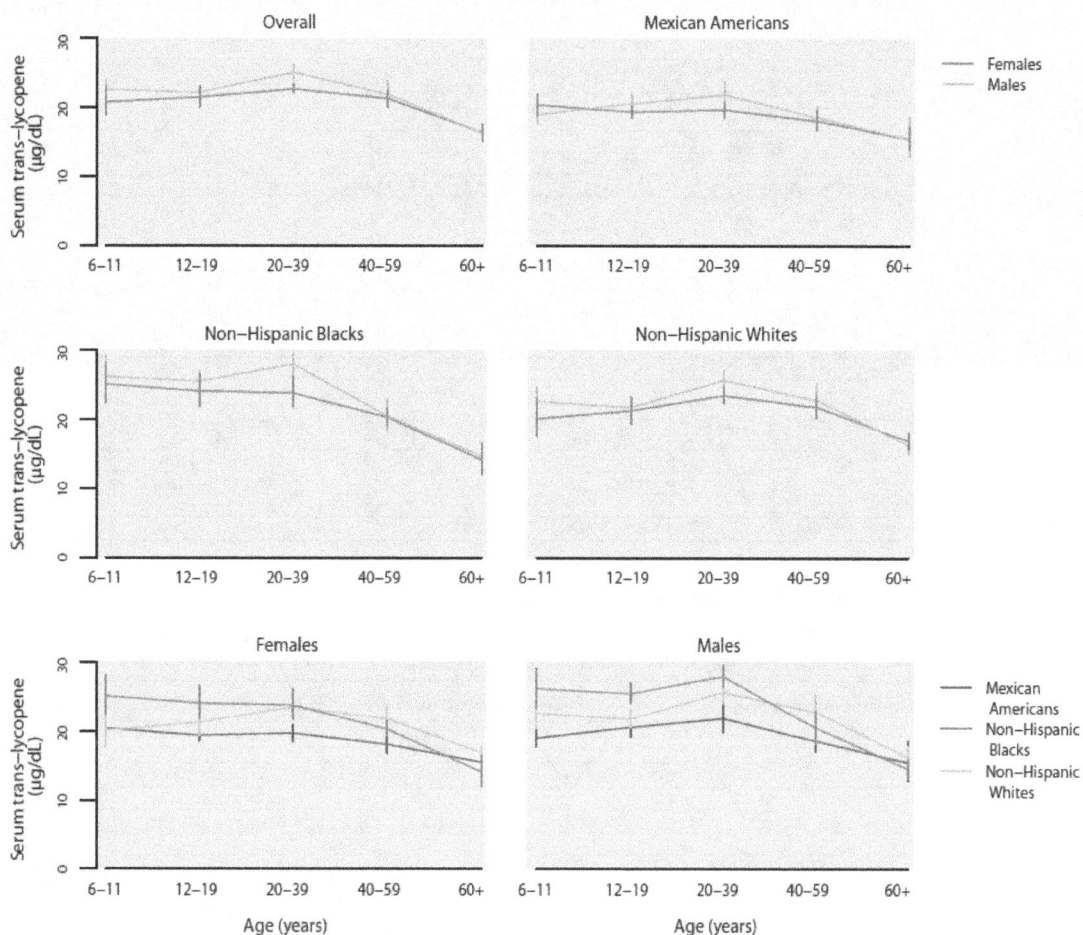

Table 2.11.a.2. Serum trans-lycopene: Total population

Geometric mean and selected percentiles of serum concentrations (in µg/dL) for the total U.S. population aged 6 years and older, National Health and Nutrition Examination Survey, 2005–2006.

	Geometric mean (95% conf. interval)	Selected percentiles (95% conf. interval)			Sample size
		10th	50th	90th	
Males and Females					
Total, 6 years and older	21.2 (20.7 – 21.7)	10.7 (10.1 – 11.3)	22.7 (22.2 – 23.2)	38.9 (37.7 – 39.8)	7,254
6–11 years	21.7 (20.5 – 22.9)	11.6 (10.5 – 12.9)	22.5 (21.1 – 23.7)	38.3 (36.3 – 40.3)	860
12–19 years	21.9 (21.1 – 22.6)	12.9 (12.2 – 13.6)	22.3 (21.8 – 22.9)	37.2 (35.8 – 39.1)	1,954
20–39 years	23.9 (23.3 – 24.4)	13.4 (11.8 – 14.8)	25.1 (24.3 – 25.6)	40.2 (39.5 – 41.2)	1,688
40–59 years	21.6 (20.4 – 22.8)	11.0 (9.50 – 11.9)	23.2 (22.1 – 24.4)	39.9 (38.4 – 41.8)	1,365
60 years and older	16.4 (15.4 – 17.4)	7.14 (6.48 – 7.69)	17.8 (16.8 – 19.0)	33.7 (32.3 – 36.1)	1,387
Males					
Total, 6 years and older	21.8 (21.0 – 22.6)	11.2 (10.3 – 11.8)	23.4 (22.6 – 24.3)	39.6 (38.1 – 41.0)	3,547
6–11 years	22.6 (21.4 – 23.9)	12.8 (11.0 – 14.4)	23.1 (21.8 – 24.3)	38.6 (36.9 – 40.8)	427
12–19 years	22.2 (21.4 – 23.0)	13.4 (11.5 – 14.2)	22.7 (22.0 – 23.6)	37.2 (36.3 – 38.7)	980
20–39 years	25.1 (24.0 – 26.2)	14.6 (11.9 – 15.8)	26.2 (24.9 – 27.4)	41.4 (40.0 – 43.7)	738
40–59 years	21.9 (20.1 – 23.9)	10.9 (8.58 – 12.4)	23.9 (22.3 – 25.6)	40.6 (37.3 – 43.9)	673
60 years and older	16.3 (15.1 – 17.6)	7.44 (6.33 – 7.78)	17.8 (16.4 – 19.1)	33.5 (31.3 – 36.8)	729
Females					
Total, 6 years and older	20.6 (20.0 – 21.2)	10.3 (9.56 – 11.1)	22.2 (21.5 – 22.6)	38.2 (36.7 – 39.5)	3,707
6–11 years	20.8 (18.9 – 22.8)	10.4 (8.68 – 12.8)	21.7 (20.3 – 23.5)	37.3 (35.2 – 41.9)	433
12–19 years	21.5 (20.1 – 23.0)	12.8 (10.7 – 13.7)	21.9 (21.0 – 23.2)	37.1 (34.6 – 40.6)	974
20–39 years	22.7 (22.1 – 23.3)	12.9 (11.1 – 14.2)	23.7 (23.0 – 24.6)	39.0 (35.9 – 41.3)	950
40–59 years	21.3 (20.1 – 22.5)	11.0 (9.50 – 11.9)	22.4 (21.0 – 24.3)	39.3 (38.6 – 40.8)	692
60 years and older	16.4 (15.3 – 17.6)	6.89 (6.29 – 7.73)	17.9 (16.6 – 19.3)	34.2 (31.5 – 38.3)	658

Table 2.11.a.3. Serum trans-lycopene: Mexican Americans

Geometric mean and selected percentiles of serum concentrations (in µg/dL) for Mexican Americans in the U.S. population aged 6 years and older, National Health and Nutrition Examination Survey, 2005–2006.

	Geometric mean (95% conf. interval)	Selected percentiles (95% conf. interval)			Sample size
		10th	50th	90th	
Males and Females					
Total, 6 years and older	19.5 (19.1 – 20.0)	10.7 (10.1 – 11.2)	20.2 (19.6 – 20.9)	33.7 (32.8 – 34.4)	1,844
6–11 years	19.6 (18.5 – 20.8)	11.0 (9.47 – 13.0)	20.1 (19.1 – 21.2)	32.4 (31.2 – 34.0)	295
12–19 years	20.0 (19.2 – 20.9)	12.0 (10.1 – 12.8)	20.9 (19.8 – 22.1)	33.5 (32.3 – 35.2)	646
20–39 years	20.9 (19.7 – 22.1)	11.6 (9.65 – 13.5)	22.0 (21.0 – 23.3)	34.7 (33.4 – 38.1)	449
40–59 years	18.4 (17.3 – 19.5)	10.0 (9.04 – 11.0)	18.8 (18.2 – 19.4)	32.8 (30.6 – 37.0)	246
60 years and older	15.5 (14.0 – 17.1)	7.71 (5.24 – 8.87)	16.1 (14.7 – 17.7)	28.6 (26.1 – 33.2)	208
Males					
Total, 6 years and older	20.1 (19.4 – 20.8)	11.0 (9.96 – 12.0)	21.1 (20.1 – 22.2)	34.4 (32.2 – 37.6)	883
6–11 years	19.0 (17.8 – 20.2)	10.9 (9.33 – 12.7)	19.5 (18.2 – 20.5)	32.1 (28.9 – 36.1)	145
12–19 years	20.6 (19.2 – 22.1)	12.3 (8.72 – 13.6)	22.1 (19.9 – 23.4)	34.0 (32.7 – 35.5)	313
20–39 years	21.9 (20.0 – 23.9)	13.2 (8.92 – 15.1)	23.1 (21.5 – 24.9)	35.1 (32.1 – 44.4)	198
40–59 years	18.6 (17.1 – 20.2)	10.1 (7.36 – 11.3)	19.3 (17.8 – 20.7)	32.7 (28.9 – 39.9)	122
60 years and older	15.5 (12.9 – 18.6)	7.41† (2.71 – 8.77)	16.2 (13.9 – 19.3)	31.3† (25.2 – 56.0)	105
Females					
Total, 6 years and older	19.0 (18.4 – 19.5)	10.5 (10.0 – 11.0)	19.4 (18.5 – 20.2)	33.3 (32.1 – 34.1)	961
6–11 years	20.4 (18.9 – 22.0)	11.4 (9.53 – 13.4)	21.2 (19.3 – 23.0)	32.5 (31.2 – 35.0)	150
12–19 years	19.4 (18.6 – 20.3)	11.8 (10.1 – 12.2)	20.0 (19.4 – 20.9)	32.9 (31.5 – 35.7)	333
20–39 years	19.7 (18.6 – 20.8)	10.8 (9.95 – 12.7)	20.0 (18.5 – 23.4)	34.1 (32.5 – 36.7)	251
40–59 years	18.1 (16.8 – 19.6)	10.0 (9.01 – 11.0)	18.0 (16.9 – 19.1)	32.8 (30.5 – 34.5)	124
60 years and older	15.5 (14.0 – 17.2)	7.98† (5.24 – 10.5)	16.0 (13.3 – 18.1)	26.7† (25.0 – 31.2)	103

† Estimate is subject to greater uncertainty due to small cell size.

Table 2.11.a.4. Serum trans-lycopene: Non-Hispanic blacks

Geometric mean and selected percentiles of serum concentrations (in µg/dL) for non-Hispanic blacks in the U.S. population aged 6 years and older, National Health and Nutrition Examination Survey, 2005–2006.

	Geometric mean (95% conf. interval)	Selected percentiles (95% conf. interval)						Sample size
		10th		50th		90th		
Males and Females								
Total, 6 years and older	22.0 (20.9 – 23.2)	10.8	(9.77 – 11.8)	23.5	(22.6 – 24.7)	40.0	(39.1 – 41.7)	1,891
6–11 years	25.6 (23.3 – 28.2)	13.7	(11.1 – 17.0)	27.0	(24.6 – 28.9)	41.8	(38.7 – 45.9)	240
12–19 years	24.8 (23.5 – 26.2)	14.3	(12.9 – 15.4)	25.8	(23.6 – 27.4)	41.6	(39.1 – 44.9)	665
20–39 years	25.7 (24.2 – 27.2)	14.5	(12.4 – 15.6)	26.3	(25.0 – 27.8)	42.4	(39.6 – 47.1)	368
40–59 years	20.4 (19.1 – 21.8)	9.89	(8.68 – 10.8)	21.3	(19.9 – 23.3)	38.6	(36.2 – 43.4)	335
60 years and older	14.3 (13.1 – 15.7)	6.20	(4.94 – 6.93)	15.3	(14.5 – 16.5)	31.2	(27.5 – 35.7)	283
Males								
Total, 6 years and older	23.1 (21.9 – 24.3)	11.2	(9.87 – 12.4)	24.9	(23.3 – 26.4)	41.8	(39.8 – 44.9)	949
6–11 years	26.2 (23.4 – 29.2)	16.4	(10.4 – 18.0)	27.0	(23.4 – 29.8)	40.1	(38.4 – 46.3)	128
12–19 years	25.5 (24.1 – 27.0)	14.9	(13.5 – 16.1)	26.2	(23.9 – 27.8)	43.2	(39.5 – 51.7)	343
20–39 years	28.0 (26.5 – 29.6)	15.3	(13.6 – 16.8)	27.9	(26.2 – 30.2)	47.8	(42.5 – 52.7)	170
40–59 years	20.5 (18.3 – 22.9)	9.19	(6.70 – 10.9)	22.1	(18.9 – 26.4)	38.6	(35.6 – 51.3)	156
60 years and older	14.6 (13.3 – 15.9)	5.56	(4.94 – 6.14)	15.5	(15.0 – 17.1)	32.1	(30.0 – 38.1)	152
Females								
Total, 6 years and older	21.2 (19.8 – 22.7)	10.6	(9.30 – 11.6)	22.5	(21.1 – 23.7)	39.0	(37.2 – 41.0)	942
6–11 years	25.1 (22.4 – 28.1)	12.4	(9.15 – 15.1)	26.7	(24.9 – 28.9)	42.1	(38.4 – 49.7)	112
12–19 years	24.1 (21.9 – 26.6)	13.9	(10.5 – 15.5)	24.8	(22.1 – 27.6)	39.8	(36.6 – 43.9)	322
20–39 years	23.8 (21.8 – 26.1)	13.6	(10.9 – 15.7)	25.0	(22.1 – 27.2)	39.1	(37.4 – 41.6)	198
40–59 years	20.3 (19.2 – 21.6)	9.99	(9.03 – 11.3)	20.9	(18.1 – 23.3)	39.0	(34.8 – 44.3)	179
60 years and older	14.1 (12.1 – 16.5)	6.71	(3.54 – 7.89)	15.0	(13.0 – 17.4)	28.1	(24.6 – 39.1)	131

Table 2.11.a.5. Serum trans-lycopene: Non-Hispanic whites

Geometric mean and selected percentiles of serum concentrations (in µg/dL) for non-Hispanic whites in the U.S. population aged 6 years and older, National Health and Nutrition Examination Survey, 2005–2006.

	Geometric mean (95% conf. interval)	Selected percentiles (95% conf. interval)						Sample size
		10th		50th		90th		
Males and Females								
Total, 6 years and older	21.3 (20.8 – 21.9)	10.8	(10.1 – 11.3)	23.0	(22.4 – 23.5)	39.1	(37.5 – 40.6)	2,973
6–11 years	21.4 (19.6 – 23.4)	11.1	(9.63 – 12.9)	22.1	(20.4 – 24.0)	37.5	(33.7 – 42.4)	231
12–19 years	21.6 (20.6 – 22.6)	13.0	(11.1 – 13.7)	22.1	(21.4 – 22.7)	37.0	(35.0 – 39.9)	499
20–39 years	24.6 (23.6 – 25.6)	13.7	(11.4 – 16.4)	25.6	(24.8 – 26.4)	40.7	(39.6 – 42.3)	714
40–59 years	22.3 (20.9 – 23.9)	11.7	(9.54 – 13.0)	24.2	(22.9 – 25.3)	40.5	(38.3 – 42.2)	683
60 years and older	16.6 (15.6 – 17.6)	7.32	(6.45 – 8.11)	18.0	(16.9 – 19.2)	34.2	(32.3 – 37.0)	846
Males								
Total, 6 years and older	21.9 (21.0 – 22.9)	11.3	(10.3 – 11.9)	23.6	(22.7 – 24.8)	39.6	(37.9 – 41.6)	1,472
6–11 years	22.6 (20.7 – 24.6)	12.8	(8.41 – 14.9)	23.0	(21.1 – 24.8)	38.3	(33.4 – 43.2)	112
12–19 years	21.8 (20.6 – 23.2)	13.2	(10.0 – 14.3)	22.5	(21.1 – 24.3)	36.6	(35.8 – 38.4)	254
20–39 years	25.7 (24.2 – 27.2)	14.8	(11.8 – 17.1)	26.5	(25.1 – 28.4)	41.5	(39.6 – 46.1)	309
40–59 years	22.8 (20.6 – 25.2)	11.8	(8.02 – 14.0)	25.0	(23.2 – 27.0)	41.2	(38.1 – 44.0)	351
60 years and older	16.3 (15.0 – 17.8)	7.49	(6.36 – 8.08)	17.7	(16.0 – 19.2)	33.7	(31.3 – 37.0)	446
Females								
Total, 6 years and older	20.8 (20.0 – 21.7)	10.2	(9.48 – 11.1)	22.4	(21.5 – 23.1)	38.5	(36.5 – 40.3)	1,501
6–11 years	20.1 (17.6 – 23.1)	9.66	(4.60 – 12.9)	20.7	(19.2 – 23.2)	36.7	(30.8 – 50.0)	119
12–19 years	21.3 (19.4 – 23.3)	12.7	(9.21 – 14.2)	21.6	(20.3 – 23.5)	37.2	(33.9 – 41.5)	245
20–39 years	23.5 (22.5 – 24.5)	13.0	(10.2 – 16.2)	24.6	(23.3 – 25.3)	40.2	(35.9 – 42.7)	405
40–59 years	21.8 (20.3 – 23.6)	11.7	(9.46 – 12.9)	23.4	(21.4 – 25.3)	39.7	(37.9 – 41.1)	332
60 years and older	16.9 (15.8 – 18.0)	7.00	(6.17 – 8.28)	18.3	(17.1 – 20.1)	34.4	(32.1 – 38.5)	400

Table 2.11.b. Serum trans-lycopene: Concentrations by survey cycle

Geometric mean and selected percentiles of serum concentrations (in µg/dL) for the U.S. population, National Health and Nutrition Examination Survey, 2001–2002 and 2005–2006.

	Geometric mean (95% conf. interval)	Selected percentiles (95% conf. interval)						Sample size
		5th		50th		95th		
Total, 6 years and older								
2001–2002	20.6 (19.9 – 21.3)	7.87	(7.49 – 8.27)	22.2	(21.3 – 23.1)	42.5	(41.0 – 43.9)	7,921
2005–2006	21.2 (20.7 – 21.7)	7.81	(7.33 – 8.40)	22.7	(22.2 – 23.2)	43.6	(42.4 – 44.9)	7,254
Age group								
3–5 years								
2001–2002	16.1 (15.2 – 17.1)	6.16	(3.73 – 7.47)	17.3	(16.2 – 18.1)	33.9	(32.8 – 37.9)	427
6–11 years								
2001–2002	21.6 (20.7 – 22.5)	9.31	(8.20 – 9.83)	22.7	(21.4 – 23.6)	40.5	(37.7 – 47.0)	1,012
2005–2006	21.7 (20.5 – 22.9)	9.48	(7.38 – 10.9)	22.5	(21.1 – 23.7)	42.8	(40.0 – 46.0)	860
12–19 years								
2001–2002	21.6 (21.1 – 22.1)	10.5	(9.69 – 11.1)	22.2	(21.8 – 22.7)	40.5	(38.1 – 43.2)	2,205
2005–2006	21.9 (21.1 – 22.6)	9.91	(8.98 – 11.0)	22.3	(21.8 – 22.9)	42.6	(40.2 – 45.1)	1,954
20–39 years								
2001–2002	22.7 (21.5 – 23.9)	10.3	(9.02 – 11.5)	23.7	(22.5 – 24.9)	44.9	(42.4 – 47.1)	1,714
2005–2006	23.9 (23.3 – 24.4)	10.7	(8.97 – 11.4)	25.1	(24.3 – 25.6)	46.1	(44.1 – 47.2)	1,688
40–59 years								
2001–2002	21.1 (20.1 – 22.1)	7.82	(7.02 – 8.61)	22.7	(21.4 – 24.1)	42.6	(41.2 – 43.8)	1,468
2005–2006	21.6 (20.4 – 22.8)	7.69	(6.02 – 8.98)	23.2	(22.1 – 24.4)	44.6	(42.5 – 47.1)	1,365
60 years and older								
2001–2002	15.4 (14.6 – 16.3)	4.15	(2.92 – 5.13)	17.1	(16.1 – 17.9)	39.0	(36.4 – 41.3)	1,522
2005–2006	16.4 (15.4 – 17.4)	5.19	(4.32 – 5.97)	17.8	(16.8 – 19.0)	38.8	(37.3 – 40.7)	1,387
Gender								
(6 years and older)								
Males								
2001–2002	21.4 (20.6 – 22.3)	8.02	(7.31 – 8.80)	23.3	(22.3 – 24.2)	44.2	(42.8 – 46.3)	3,832
2005–2006	21.8 (21.0 – 22.6)	7.85	(6.99 – 8.89)	23.4	(22.6 – 24.3)	44.7	(43.7 – 47.0)	3,547
Females								
2001–2002	19.8 (19.2 – 20.5)	7.82	(7.13 – 8.34)	21.2	(20.4 – 22.0)	40.3	(38.9 – 42.1)	4,089
2005–2006	20.6 (20.0 – 21.2)	7.76	(7.09 – 8.40)	22.2	(21.5 – 22.6)	42.3	(41.2 – 43.9)	3,707
Race/ethnicity								
(6 years and older)								
Mexican Americans								
2001–2002	20.0 (19.2 – 20.8)	8.89	(7.84 – 9.62)	20.7	(20.1 – 21.7)	39.8	(38.1 – 42.0)	1,987
2005–2006	19.5 (19.1 – 20.0)	8.80	(7.83 – 9.29)	20.2	(19.6 – 20.9)	38.0	(36.4 – 40.2)	1,844
Non-Hispanic Blacks								
2001–2002	21.7 (21.0 – 22.3)	8.03	(6.83 – 9.11)	23.4	(22.2 – 24.3)	46.6	(44.9 – 49.0)	1,864
2005–2006	22.0 (20.9 – 23.2)	8.11	(7.39 – 8.77)	23.5	(22.6 – 24.7)	47.0	(44.7 – 49.5)	1,891
Non-Hispanic Whites								
2001–2002	20.8 (20.1 – 21.6)	8.17	(7.55 – 8.72)	22.4	(21.3 – 23.5)	42.5	(40.9 – 44.0)	3,446
2005–2006	21.3 (20.8 – 21.9)	7.69	(7.04 – 8.47)	23.0	(22.4 – 23.5)	43.8	(42.4 – 45.2)	2,973

Figure 2.11.b. Serum trans–lycopene: Concentrations by survey cycle

Selected percentiles in µg/dL (95% confidence intervals), National Health and
Nutrition Examination Survey, 2001–2002 and 2005–2006

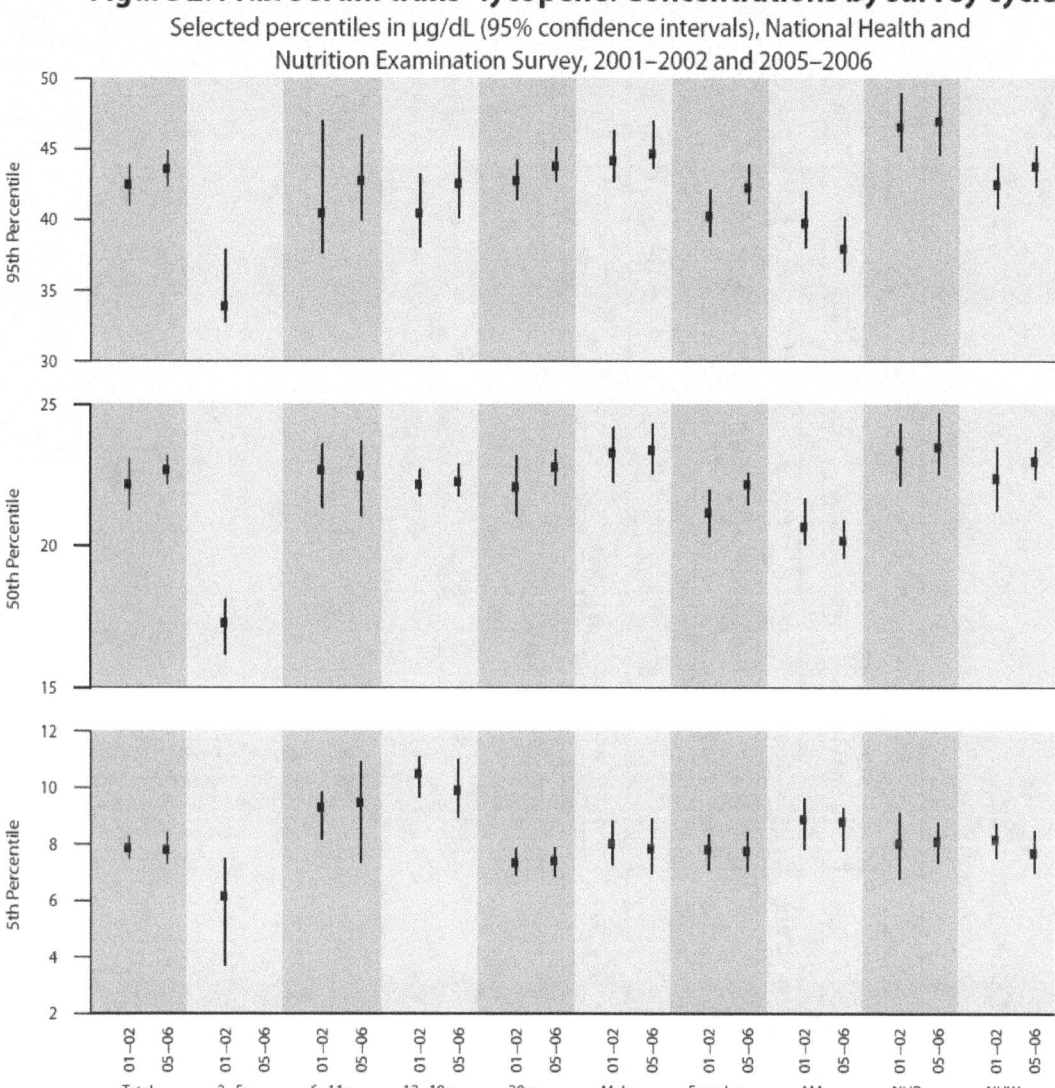

Table 2.12.a.1. Serum total lycopene: Concentrations

Geometric mean and selected percentiles of serum concentrations (in µg/dL) for the total U.S. population aged 6 years and older, National Health and Nutrition Examination Survey, 2005–2006.

	Geometric mean (95% conf. interval)	Selected percentiles (95% conf. interval)						Sample size
		2.5th	5th	50th	95th	97.5th		
Total, 6 years and older	39.4 (38.5 – 40.2)	11.3 (10.4 – 12.6)	15.4 (14.6 – 16.1)	41.8 (41.0 – 42.6)	80.8 (78.8 – 82.5)	90.7 (87.9 – 94.7)		7,149
Age group								
6–11 years	39.7 (37.5 – 42.0)	14.9 (10.7 – 17.8)	18.8 (15.1 – 19.9)	40.9 (38.5 – 44.1)	78.4 (74.8 – 82.5)	83.0 (80.6 – 105)		851
12–19 years	39.5 (38.2 – 40.8)	15.4 (12.9 – 17.4)	19.1 (17.2 – 20.9)	40.6 (39.6 – 42.0)	73.9 (71.5 – 79.0)	82.8 (78.1 – 93.4)		1,907
20–39 years	43.8 (42.7 – 44.9)	15.9 (14.0 – 17.8)	20.0 (17.0 – 21.8)	45.2 (43.8 – 46.6)	83.3 (81.4 – 86.1)	92.7 (87.4 – 99.3)		1,667
40–59 years	40.5 (38.2 – 42.9)	10.6 (7.35 – 13.2)	15.0 (12.4 – 17.1)	43.1 (41.1 – 45.3)	84.1 (79.9 – 89.2)	97.2 (90.7 – 103)		1,346
60 years and older	31.5 (29.8 – 33.2)	8.08 (6.96 – 9.57)	10.7 (9.50 – 12.4)	33.5 (31.4 – 35.9)	72.8 (69.5 – 76.4)	81.7 (76.3 – 89.4)		1,378
Gender								
Males	40.6 (39.3 – 42.0)	11.4 (9.28 – 13.2)	15.6 (13.9 – 17.3)	43.5 (42.2 – 44.7)	84.5 (81.6 – 86.9)	95.2 (89.9 – 103)		3,493
Females	38.2 (37.1 – 39.3)	11.1 (10.3 – 12.9)	15.3 (14.2 – 16.4)	40.1 (38.9 – 41.6)	77.6 (75.1 – 80.5)	86.0 (81.9 – 92.1)		3,656
Race/ethnicity								
Mexican Americans	36.2 (35.3 – 37.1)	13.7 (11.8 – 14.3)	16.6 (15.3 – 17.9)	37.4 (36.1 – 38.9)	70.5 (67.0 – 74.0)	79.3 (74.1 – 91.3)		1,818
Non-Hispanic Blacks	41.3 (39.2 – 43.5)	12.9 (10.9 – 14.2)	16.7 (14.3 – 18.0)	43.1 (41.1 – 45.5)	86.4 (83.0 – 89.5)	97.2 (91.5 – 107)		1,846
Non-Hispanic Whites	39.6 (38.6 – 40.6)	10.9 (9.72 – 12.5)	15.1 (14.2 – 16.0)	42.4 (41.3 – 43.3)	81.1 (78.9 – 82.9)	89.7 (87.2 – 94.8)		2,943

Figure 2.12.a. Serum total lycopene: Concentrations by age group

Geometric mean (95% confidence interval), National Health and Nutrition Examination Survey, 2005–2006

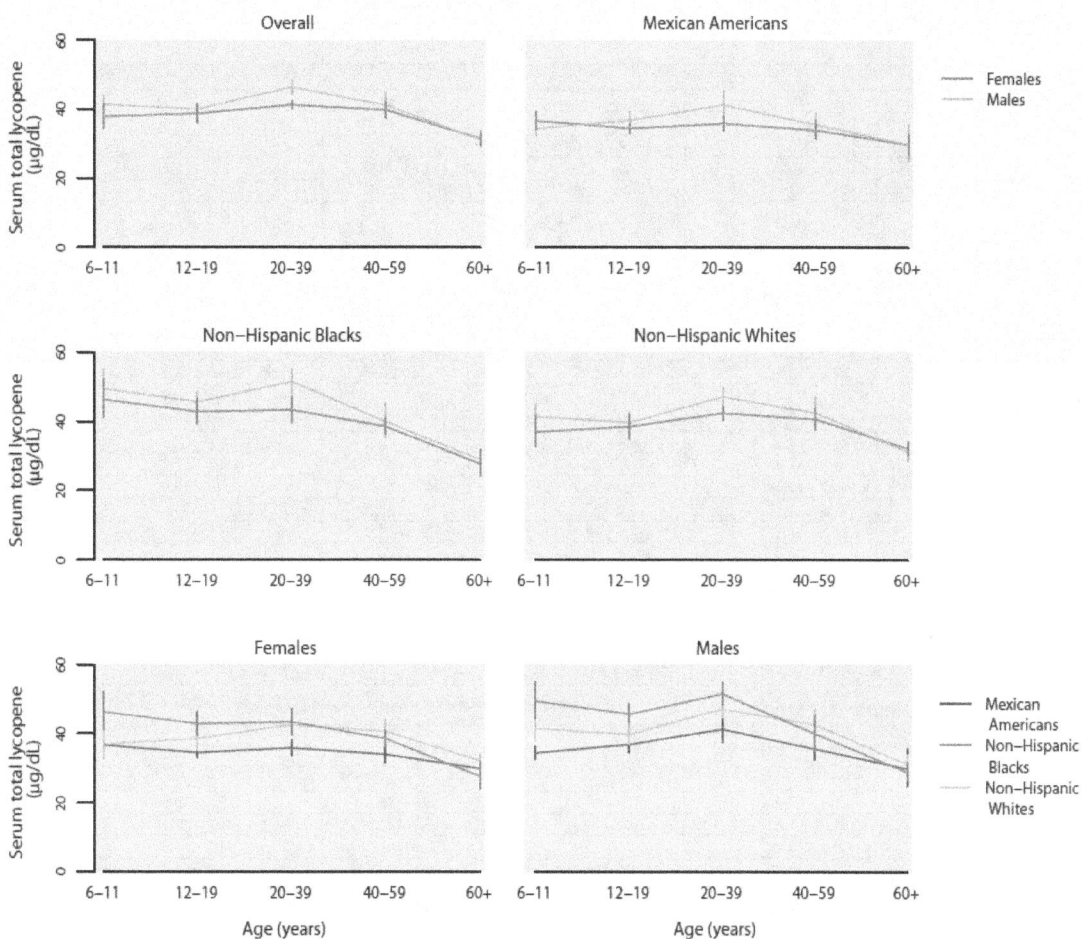

Table 2.12.a.2. Serum total lycopene: Total population

Geometric mean and selected percentiles of serum concentrations (in μg/dL) for the total U.S. population aged 6 years and older, National Health and Nutrition Examination Survey, 2005–2006.

	Geometric mean (95% conf. interval)	Selected percentiles (95% conf. interval)			Sample size
		10th	50th	90th	
Males and Females					
Total, 6 years and older	39.4 (38.5 – 40.2)	20.5 (19.5 – 21.3)	41.8 (41.0 – 42.6)	71.2 (69.5 – 72.7)	7,149
6–11 years	39.7 (37.5 – 42.0)	21.5 (19.3 – 25.4)	40.9 (38.5 – 44.1)	67.6 (63.5 – 74.9)	851
12–19 years	39.5 (38.2 – 40.8)	23.5 (21.8 – 24.6)	40.6 (39.6 – 42.0)	66.3 (63.1 – 69.6)	1,907
20–39 years	43.8 (42.7 – 44.9)	24.6 (21.9 – 27.2)	45.2 (43.8 – 46.6)	74.0 (72.5 – 75.8)	1,667
40–59 years	40.5 (38.2 – 42.9)	21.0 (18.6 – 22.9)	43.1 (41.1 – 45.3)	72.8 (70.3 – 77.1)	1,346
60 years and older	31.5 (29.8 – 33.2)	14.3 (13.3 – 15.9)	33.5 (31.4 – 35.9)	62.8 (60.2 – 67.5)	1,378
Males					
Total, 6 years and older	40.6 (39.3 – 42.0)	21.2 (20.1 – 22.2)	43.5 (42.2 – 44.7)	72.9 (70.9 – 75.6)	3,493
6–11 years	41.4 (39.2 – 43.8)	23.7 (20.3 – 26.4)	42.1 (39.7 – 44.9)	69.5 (63.4 – 78.2)	421
12–19 years	40.1 (38.5 – 41.8)	23.8 (21.3 – 26.0)	41.1 (40.0 – 42.5)	66.3 (64.6 – 69.4)	955
20–39 years	46.4 (44.5 – 48.5)	26.8 (22.9 – 30.6)	48.3 (45.5 – 51.0)	78.5 (74.6 – 81.9)	730
40–59 years	41.2 (37.7 – 45.0)	20.9 (15.2 – 23.9)	44.9 (42.6 – 47.1)	75.0 (71.0 – 81.4)	663
60 years and older	31.3 (29.1 – 33.7)	14.3 (12.6 – 15.9)	34.4 (31.6 – 36.4)	62.0 (59.0 – 69.3)	724
Females					
Total, 6 years and older	38.2 (37.1 – 39.3)	19.9 (18.8 – 21.1)	40.1 (38.9 – 41.6)	69.3 (67.0 – 71.7)	3,656
6–11 years	37.9 (34.8 – 41.3)	19.4 (16.3 – 24.7)	39.8 (35.7 – 43.9)	66.2 (59.8 – 74.0)	430
12–19 years	38.8 (36.2 – 41.5)	23.4 (20.0 – 24.6)	40.1 (37.8 – 42.4)	65.3 (60.1 – 72.6)	952
20–39 years	41.3 (40.2 – 42.4)	22.6 (20.7 – 26.2)	42.7 (41.5 – 43.7)	71.6 (66.4 – 74.0)	937
40–59 years	39.8 (37.6 – 42.1)	20.9 (18.9 – 22.8)	41.1 (37.8 – 45.0)	71.3 (68.8 – 75.6)	683
60 years and older	31.6 (29.7 – 33.5)	14.2 (12.9 – 16.4)	33.0 (30.8 – 35.8)	64.6 (58.0 – 69.7)	654

Table 2.12.a.3. Serum total lycopene: Mexican Americans

Geometric mean and selected percentiles of serum concentrations (in μg/dL) for Mexican Americans in the U.S. population aged 6 years and older, National Health and Nutrition Examination Survey, 2005–2006.

	Geometric mean (95% conf. interval)	Selected percentiles (95% conf. interval)			Sample size
		10th	50th	90th	
Males and Females					
Total, 6 years and older	36.2 (35.3 – 37.1)	20.5 (19.5 – 21.7)	37.4 (36.1 – 38.9)	61.5 (58.8 – 63.5)	1,818
6–11 years	35.5 (33.8 – 37.3)	21.0 (18.7 – 22.5)	35.5 (33.8 – 37.3)	58.4 (55.7 – 63.1)	292
12–19 years	35.7 (34.5 – 37.0)	21.8 (19.6 – 23.4)	37.4 (36.0 – 38.7)	58.5 (55.6 – 61.8)	639
20–39 years	38.8 (36.5 – 41.1)	22.7 (18.7 – 24.7)	41.0 (39.1 – 42.5)	63.8 (58.8 – 71.2)	441
40–59 years	34.8 (32.7 – 37.1)	19.6 (17.4 – 21.1)	35.1 (32.6 – 38.5)	60.7 (57.3 – 65.5)	240
60 years and older	29.9 (27.3 – 32.8)	14.7 (11.9 – 17.9)	30.1 (27.9 – 33.8)	54.7 (48.8 – 65.8)	206
Males					
Total, 6 years and older	37.6 (36.3 – 39.0)	21.4 (19.9 – 23.0)	39.2 (36.9 – 40.8)	63.1 (59.5 – 68.0)	867
6–11 years	34.4 (32.6 – 36.4)	20.2 (17.8 – 22.4)	34.3 (31.7 – 36.1)	57.4 (50.5 – 73.4)	142
12–19 years	36.9 (34.6 – 39.4)	22.5 (19.2 – 24.6)	39.1 (36.8 – 40.7)	59.7 (55.9 – 63.9)	310
20–39 years	41.3 (37.8 – 45.1)	24.6 (16.6 – 27.7)	42.6 (40.6 – 45.4)	66.1 (58.3 – 94.4)	192
40–59 years	35.6 (32.6 – 38.8)	19.0 (14.4 – 22.6)	36.4 (33.4 – 40.5)	58.7 (56.0 – 74.3)	120
60 years and older	29.9 (25.1 – 35.7)	14.5† (5.80 – 18.2)	30.2 (26.0 – 36.1)	61.9† (48.0 – 86.3)	103
Females					
Total, 6 years and older	34.8 (33.8 – 35.8)	20.0 (18.7 – 21.4)	35.3 (33.5 – 37.3)	59.5 (56.8 – 62.0)	951
6–11 years	36.7 (34.4 – 39.1)	21.1 (17.7 – 24.4)	36.7 (34.3 – 40.4)	58.8 (56.3 – 62.2)	150
12–19 years	34.5 (33.2 – 35.8)	20.6 (19.0 – 22.6)	34.8 (33.8 – 36.8)	57.8 (51.9 – 62.0)	329
20–39 years	35.9 (33.9 – 38.1)	20.2 (17.5 – 22.7)	37.4 (33.3 – 41.9)	61.4 (56.1 – 68.6)	249
40–59 years	34.0 (31.6 – 36.7)	19.6 (16.1 – 21.4)	33.0 (30.2 – 38.3)	61.0 (55.9 – 67.8)	120
60 years and older	29.9 (27.3 – 32.8)	16.1† (12.1 – 20.5)	29.2 (26.6 – 35.7)	52.7† (48.0 – 59.9)	103

† Estimate is subject to greater uncertainty due to small cell size.

Table 2.12.a.4. Serum total lycopene: Non-Hispanic blacks

Geometric mean and selected percentiles of serum concentrations (in µg/dL) for non-Hispanic blacks in the U.S. population aged 6 years and older, National Health and Nutrition Examination Survey, 2005–2006.

	Geometric mean (95% conf. interval)	Selected percentiles (95% conf. interval)						Sample size
		10th		50th		90th		
Males and Females								
Total, 6 years and older	41.3 (39.2 – 43.5)	21.4	(19.5 – 23.1)	43.1	(41.1 – 45.5)	75.5	(72.1 – 79.6)	1,846
6–11 years	47.9 (43.3 – 52.9)	27.4	(20.5 – 31.8)	49.6	(44.6 – 56.3)	78.5	(73.9 – 84.4)	236
12–19 years	44.3 (42.3 – 46.4)	26.9	(23.9 – 29.0)	45.8	(42.8 – 47.8)	73.1	(69.2 – 78.2)	636
20–39 years	47.0 (44.2 – 50.1)	26.4	(23.2 – 29.6)	49.0	(45.5 – 52.3)	79.6	(76.1 – 82.9)	363
40–59 years	39.2 (36.4 – 42.2)	20.0	(17.1 – 21.4)	40.8	(37.7 – 43.4)	73.7	(66.9 – 84.2)	331
60 years and older	28.2 (26.0 – 30.6)	12.7	(10.4 – 15.4)	29.1	(26.6 – 32.7)	59.0	(53.0 – 68.4)	280
Males								
Total, 6 years and older	43.6 (41.0 – 46.3)	22.9	(19.5 – 24.5)	45.8	(42.8 – 48.4)	81.2	(76.4 – 87.8)	922
6–11 years	49.5 (44.4 – 55.1)	30.6	(15.3 – 35.9)	50.4	(42.4 – 58.7)	76.8	(70.9 – 91.8)	126
12–19 years	45.7 (43.1 – 48.6)	28.9	(25.6 – 30.2)	46.7	(43.6 – 50.4)	76.3	(69.3 – 90.2)	324
20–39 years	51.6 (48.4 – 55.1)	29.7	(25.9 – 31.9)	51.4	(48.1 – 54.9)	86.3	(81.2 – 90.5)	169
40–59 years	40.0 (35.3 – 45.3)	18.4	(13.2 – 22.9)	41.1	(36.8 – 47.4)	82.9	(67.2 – 97.5)	153
60 years and older	28.9 (26.5 – 31.6)	12.5	(11.1 – 13.0)	31.1	(28.3 – 34.7)	59.5	(52.9 – 66.0)	150
Females								
Total, 6 years and older	39.3 (37.0 – 41.8)	20.8	(18.5 – 22.2)	41.0	(39.4 – 43.0)	71.4	(68.7 – 74.1)	924
6–11 years	46.3 (41.2 – 52.1)	24.6†	(17.9 – 27.5)	48.5	(44.6 – 54.8)	78.5†	(72.8 – 84.6)	110
12–19 years	42.9 (39.5 – 46.4)	25.6	(20.1 – 28.1)	44.1	(39.8 – 48.0)	70.4	(67.3 – 75.3)	312
20–39 years	43.4 (39.8 – 47.3)	23.6	(21.0 – 28.0)	44.5	(40.4 – 50.6)	72.6	(68.4 – 76.7)	194
40–59 years	38.6 (36.3 – 41.0)	20.1	(17.1 – 21.5)	40.2	(36.7 – 43.0)	68.6	(63.6 – 75.8)	178
60 years and older	27.7 (24.1 – 31.9)	12.8	(8.09 – 17.2)	28.6	(24.8 – 32.4)	57.6	(45.4 – 82.2)	130

† Estimate is subject to greater uncertainty due to small cell size.

Table 2.12.a.5. Serum total lycopene: Non-Hispanic whites

Geometric mean and selected percentiles of serum concentrations (in µg/dL) for non-Hispanic whites in the U.S. population aged 6 years and older, National Health and Nutrition Examination Survey, 2005–2006.

	Geometric mean (95% conf. interval)	Selected percentiles (95% conf. interval)						Sample size
		10th		50th		90th		
Males and Females								
Total, 6 years and older	39.6 (38.6 – 40.6)	20.4	(19.4 – 21.3)	42.4	(41.3 – 43.3)	71.5	(69.4 – 73.8)	2,943
6–11 years	39.3 (35.9 – 43.1)	20.7	(18.9 – 24.9)	40.6	(37.7 – 44.9)	64.8	(58.7 – 78.0)	230
12–19 years	39.2 (37.5 – 40.9)	23.3	(20.8 – 24.8)	40.7	(39.3 – 42.1)	66.2	(62.8 – 70.2)	489
20–39 years	44.8 (43.2 – 46.5)	25.3	(21.5 – 29.3)	45.9	(44.0 – 48.4)	75.4	(72.5 – 77.8)	706
40–59 years	41.6 (38.8 – 44.6)	22.2	(17.8 – 24.4)	44.7	(42.6 – 47.0)	73.9	(70.4 – 78.5)	674
60 years and older	31.7 (30.0 – 33.5)	14.4	(13.3 – 16.2)	33.9	(31.7 – 36.7)	62.9	(60.2 – 67.4)	844
Males								
Total, 6 years and older	40.7 (39.2 – 42.3)	21.0	(19.7 – 22.0)	43.9	(42.5 – 45.2)	73.2	(70.9 – 76.0)	1,461
6–11 years	41.5 (38.1 – 45.3)	23.6†	(19.7 – 26.4)	42.3	(39.5 – 45.7)	66.0†	(58.8 – 81.5)	111
12–19 years	39.8 (37.1 – 42.6)	23.2	(19.9 – 27.0)	41.0	(38.4 – 43.0)	66.3	(63.5 – 69.8)	251
20–39 years	47.2 (44.7 – 49.8)	26.8	(21.7 – 31.6)	49.4	(45.9 – 52.3)	78.7	(73.9 – 85.0)	308
40–59 years	42.6 (38.4 – 47.1)	22.4	(15.0 – 27.3)	46.3	(44.0 – 49.0)	75.3	(70.9 – 82.7)	346
60 years and older	31.2 (28.6 – 34.0)	14.4	(12.3 – 16.1)	33.9	(30.8 – 36.5)	62.0	(58.8 – 69.7)	445
Females								
Total, 6 years and older	38.5 (36.9 – 40.1)	19.7	(18.2 – 21.3)	40.7	(38.9 – 42.5)	69.6	(66.8 – 72.6)	1,482
6–11 years	37.0 (32.7 – 41.8)	19.1	(13.7 – 25.3)	39.1	(33.8 – 43.3)	61.9	(54.6 – 78.0)	119
12–19 years	38.6 (35.1 – 42.3)	23.6	(18.0 – 25.6)	40.4	(37.0 – 43.4)	64.4	(57.9 – 75.6)	238
20–39 years	42.5 (40.6 – 44.4)	22.9	(19.9 – 28.7)	43.2	(41.9 – 44.2)	72.1	(66.5 – 77.0)	398
40–59 years	40.7 (37.6 – 44.0)	21.6	(17.5 – 24.5)	42.4	(39.0 – 47.4)	72.1	(68.7 – 78.7)	328
60 years and older	32.2 (30.3 – 34.2)	14.3	(12.9 – 16.6)	33.8	(31.6 – 37.1)	64.5	(59.0 – 68.7)	399

† Estimate is subject to greater uncertainty due to small cell size.

References

Agency for Healthcare Research and Quality. Effect of supplemental antioxidants vitamin C, vitamin E, and coenzyme Q10 for the prevention and treatment of cardiovascular disease. Evidence Report/Technology Assessment Number 83, 2003.

Ahuja JK, Goldman JD, Moshfegh AJ. Current status of vitamin E nurture. Ann N Y Acad Sci. 2004;1031:387–390.

Albanes D, Heinonen OP, Taylor PR, Virtamo J, Edwards BK, Rautalahti M, et al. Alpha-tocopherol and beta-carotene supplement and lung cancer incidence in the alpha-tocopherol, beta-carotene cancer prevention study: effects of base-line characteristics and study compliance. J Natl Cancer Inst.1996;88:1560–1570.

Al-Delaimy WK, Ferrari P, Slimani N, Pala V, Johansson I, Nilsson S, et al. Plasma carotenoids as biomarkers of intake of fruits and vegetables: individual-level correlations in the European Prospective Investigation into Cancer and Nutrition (EPIC). Eur J Clin Nutr. 2005;59:1387–1396.

Bailey RL, Gahche JJ, Lentino CV, Dwyer JT, Engel JS, Thomas PT, et al. Dietary Supplement Use in the United States, 2003-2006. Journal of Nutrition 2011;141:261-6.

Ballew C, Bowman BA, Sowell AL, Gillespie C. Serum retinol distributions in residents of the United States: Third National Health and Nutrition Examination Survey, 1988–1994. Am J Clin Nutr. 2001;73:586–593.

Beers MH, editor. Vitamin deficiency, dependency, and toxicity. In: Merck Manual of Diagnosis and Therapy. 18th ed. Whitehouse Station, (NJ): Merck & Co., Inc.; 2006 [cited 2011]. Available at: http://www.merck.com/mmpe/sec01/ch004/ch004l.html.

Bendich A, Langseth L. Safety of vitamin A. Am J Clin Nutr. 1989 Feb;49(2):358-71.

Boylston T, Nollet LML. Chemical and biochemical aspects of color in muscle foods. In: Perez-Alvarez JA and Fernandez-Lopez J, editors. Handbook of meat, poultry and seafood quality. Ames (IA): Blackwell Publishing; 2007. pp. 25–44.

Britton G, Liaaen-Jensen S, Pfander H., editors. Carotenoids handbook. Basel (Switzerland): Birkhäuser; 2004.

Duewer DL, Kline MC, Sharpless KE, Thomas JB. NIST micronutrients measurement quality assurance program: characterizing the measurement community's performance over time. Anal Chem. 2000;72:4163–4170.

Ford ES, Sowell A. Serum α-tocopherol status in the United States population: findings from the Third National Health and Nutrition Examination Survey. Am J Epidemiol. 1999;150:290–300.

Ford ES. Variations in serum carotenoid concentrations among United States adults by ethnicity and sex. Ethn Dis. 2000;10:208–217.

Ford ES, Gillespie C, Ballew C, Sowell A, Mannino DM. Serum carotenoid concentrations in U.S. children and adolescents. Am J Clin Nutr. 2002;76:818–827.

Ford ES, Schleicher RL, Mokdad AH, Ajani UA, Liu S. Distribution of serum concentrations of alpha-tocopherol and gamma-tocopherol in the US population. Am J Clin Nutr. 2006;84:375–383.

Gibson RS. Principles of nutritional assessment (2nd edn.). New York: Oxford University Press; 2005.

Institute of Medicine, Food and Nutrition Board. Dietary reference intakes: vitamin C, vitamin E, selenium, and carotenoids. Washington, D.C.: National Academy Press; 2000.

Institute of Medicine, Food and Nutrition Board. Dietary reference intakes: vitamin A, vitamin K, arsenic, boron, chromium, copper, iodine, iron, manganese, molybdenum, nickel, silicon, vanadium, and zinc. Washington, D.C.: National Academy Press; 2001.

Khachik F, Beecher GR, Goli MB, Lusby WR. Separation and quantitation of carotenoids in foods. Methods Enzymol. 1992;213:347–359.

Krinsky NI, Johnson EJ. Carotenoid actions and their relation to health and disease. Mol Aspects Med. 2005;26:459–516.

Lacher DA, Hughes JP, Carroll MD. Estimate of biological variation of laboratory analytes based on the Third National Health and Nutrition Examination Survey. Clin Chem. 2005;51:450–452.

Lichtenstein AH, Appel LJ, Brands M, Carnethon M, Daniels S, Franch HA, *et al.* Summary of American Heart Association diet and lifestyle recommendations revision. Arterioscler Thromb Vasc Biol. 2006;26:2186–2191.

Moshfegh A, Goldman J, Cleveland L. What we eat in America, NHANES 2001–02: Usual nutrient intakes from food compared to dietary reference intakes. Beltsville (MD): U.S. Department of Agriculture, Agricultural Research Service; 2005 [cited 2011]. Available at: http://www.ars.usda.gov/SP2UserFiles/Place/12355000/pdf/0102/usualintaketables2001-02.pdf.

Napoli JL. Vitamin A: biochemistry and physiological role. In: Caballero B, Allen L, Prentice A, editors. Encyclopedia of human nutrition. 2nd ed. Amsterdam: Elsevier Ltd.; 2006. pp. 339–347.

Redlich CA, Blaner WS, Van Bennekum AM, Chung JS, Clever SL, Holm CT, *et al.* Effect of supplementation with beta-carotene and vitamin A on lung nutrient levels. Cancer Epidemiol Biomarkers Prev. 1998;7:211–214.

Rock CL. Multivitamin-multimineral supplements: who uses them? Am J Clin Nutr 2007;85(suppl):277S-9S.

Roodhooft JM. Leading causes of blindness worldwide. Bull Soc Belge Ophthalmol. 2002;283:19–25.

Thomas, RG, Gebhardt, SE. Nuts and seeds as sources of alpha and gamma tocopherols. ICR/WCRF International Research Conference, 2006 Jul 13-14; Washington, D.C. [cited 2011]. Available at: http://www.ars.usda.gov/SP2UserFiles/Place/12354500/Articles/AICR06_NutSeed.pdf.

U.S. Department of Agriculture and U.S. Department of Health and Human Services. *Dietary Guidelines for Americans, 2010.* 7th Edition, Washington, DC: U.S. Government Printing Office, December 2010 [cited 2011]. Available at: http://www.cnpp.usda.gov/DGAs2010-PolicyDocument.htm.

West Jr, KP. Vitamin A: deficiency and interventions. In: Caballero B, Allen L, Prentice A, editors. Encyclopedia of human nutrition. 2nd ed. Amsterdam: Elsevier Ltd.; 2006. pp. 348–359.

WHO. Serum retinol concentrations for determining the prevalence of vitamin A deficiency in populations. Vitamin and Mineral Nutrition Information System. Geneva, World Health Organization, 2011 (WHO/NMH/NHD/MNM/11.3). Available at: http://www.who.int/vmnis/indicators/retinol.pdf.

Vitamin D

Background Information

Sources and Physiological Functions. Vitamin D (calciferol) comprises a group of fat soluble seco-sterols found naturally in only a few foods, such as fish-liver oils, fatty fishes, mushrooms, egg yolks, and liver. The two major physiologically relevant forms of vitamin D are D_2 (ergocalciferol) and D_3 (cholecalciferol). Vitamin D_3 is photosynthesized in the skin of vertebrates by the action of solar ultraviolet (UV) B radiation on 7-dehydrocholesterol present in the skin (Fieser 1959). Vitamin D_2 is produced by UV irradiation of ergosterol, which occurs in molds, yeast, and higher-order plants. Under conditions of regular sun exposure, dietary vitamin D intake is of minor importance. However, latitude, season, aging, sunscreen use, and skin pigmentation influence the production of vitamin D_3 by the skin (Institute of Medicine 2011). In the United States, most of the dietary intake of vitamin D comes from fortified milk products and other fortified foods such as breakfast cereals and orange juice (Institute of Medicine 2011). Both vitamin D_2 and D_3 are used in nonprescription vitamin D supplements, but vitamin D_2 is the only form available by prescription in the United States (Holick 2007).

Vitamin D without a subscript represents either D_2 or D_3 or both. Vitamin D, *per se*, is biologically inert. Whether derived from the skin or diet, vitamin D is only short-lived in circulation (with a half-life of 1–2 days), as it is either stored in fat cells or metabolized in the liver (Mawer 1972). In circulation, vitamin D is bound to vitamin D-binding protein and transported to the liver, where it is converted to 25-hydroxyvitamin D [25(OH)D] (DeLuca 1984). This major circulating form of vitamin D is a good reflection of cumulative effects of exposure to sunlight and dietary intake of vitamin D (Haddad 1973; Holick 1995) and is therefore used by clinicians to determine vitamin D status. To be biologically activated at physiologic concentrations, 25(OH)D must be converted in the kidneys to 1,25-dihydroxyvitamin D [1,25(OH)$_2$D], which is thought to be responsible for most, if not all, of the biologic functions of vitamin D (DeLuca 1988; Reichel 1989). The production of 25(OH)D in the liver is a function of vitamin D availability from dietary intake and sun exposure whereas production of 1,25(OH)$_2$D in the kidney is tightly regulated by mineral requirements. In the liver, vitamin D-25-hydroxylase is down-regulated by vitamin D and its metabolites, thereby limiting any increase in the circulating concentration of 25(OH)D following intakes or following production of vitamin D after exposure to sunlight. In the kidney, in response to serum calcium and phosphorus concentrations, the production of 1,25(OH)$_2$D is regulated through the action of parathyroid hormone (PTH) (DeLuca 1988; Reichel 1989).

Health Effects. Active vitamin D (1,25-dihydroxyvitamin D) functions as a hormone, and its main biologic function in people is to maintain serum calcium and phosphorus concentrations within the normal range by enhancing the efficiency of the small intestine to absorb these minerals from the diet (DeLuca 1988; Reichel 1989). When dietary calcium intake is inadequate to satisfy the body's calcium requirement, 1,25(OH)$_2$D, along with PTH, mobilizes calcium stores from the bone. In the kidney, 1,25(OH)$_2$D increases calcium reabsorption by the distal renal tubules. Apart from these traditional calcium-related actions, 1,25(OH)$_2$D and its synthetic analogs are increasingly recognized for their potent anti-proliferative, pro-differentiative, and immunomodulatory activities (Nagpal 2005).

Vitamin D deficiency is characterized by inadequate mineralization or by demineralization of the skeleton. Among children, vitamin D deficiency is a common cause of bone deformities known as rickets. Vitamin D deficiency in adults leads to a mineralization defect in the skeleton, causing osteomalacia, and it induces secondary hyperparathyroidism with consequent bone loss and osteoporosis. Potential roles for vitamin D beyond bone health, such as effects on muscle strength, the risk for cancer, and the risk for type 2 diabetes, are under intense investigation. The Agency for Healthcare Research and Quality (AHRQ) reviewed the effectiveness and safety of vitamin D on outcomes related to bone health (Cranney 2007). The report suggests that vitamin D supplementation has positive effects on bone health in postmenopausal women and older men. Another AHRQ systematic review of vitamin D status and health outcomes found no significant associations between vitamin D status and total cancer mortality, nor did it find any conclusive evidence for the association of vitamin D status with cancer risk or cancer outcome (Chung 2009). It also found no clear association between vitamin D status and cardiometabolic outcomes including fasting glucose, blood pressure, myocardial infarction or stroke. Randomized trials showed no clinically significant consistent effects of vitamin D supplementation at the dosages given (Pittas 2010).

Intake Recommendations. What constitutes the optimal intake of vitamin D remains a matter of some disagreement. Current recommendations from the Institute of Medicine (2011) call for 400 international units (IU) [10 micrograms (μg)] of vitamin D daily from birth through age 1 year for adequate intake (AI)]. The Recommended Dietary Allowance (RDA) for those aged 1–70 years is 600 IU (15 μg) and 800 IU (20 μg) for those older than 70 years. According to the Dietary Guidelines for Americans (U.S. Department of Agriculture and U.S. Department of Health Human Services 2010), moderate evidence shows that intake of milk and milk products is linked to improved bone health, especially in children and adolescents. In the United States, most dietary vitamin D is obtained from fortified foods, especially milk. The Tolerable Upper Intake Level for vitamin D is 4000 IU (100 μg) per day in North America for individuals 9 years of age and older and ranges from 1000 IU to 3000 IU for infants and children less than 9 years of age; as intake increases above this amount, the potential risk for adverse consequences increases.

Biochemical Indicators and Methods. To assess vitamin D status, one measures the concentration of 25(OH)D in serum, using either antibody-based methods such as radioisotope-, enzyme-linked- or chemiluminescence- immunoassays, or using chemistry-based methods such as HPLC separation with UV or tandem mass spectrometry detection. Studies have shown that standardized chemistry-based methods are equivalent but that antibody-based methods may show significant bias. Some clinical laboratories use conventional units for 25(OH)D (nanogram per

milliliter [ng/mL]), whereas other laboratories use international system (SI) units (nanomole per liter [nmol/L]). The conversion factor to SI units is: 1 ng/mL = 2.5 nmol/L.

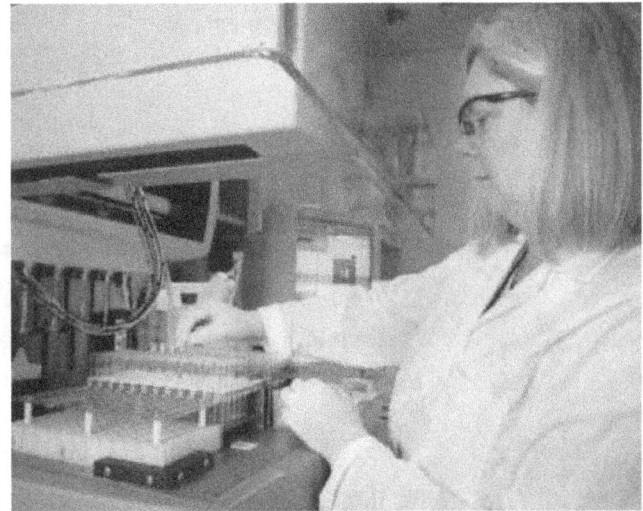

The Institute of Medicine (2011) committee to review dietary reference intakes for vitamin D and calcium suggested that persons with serum 25(OH) D concentrations of less than 30 nmol/L (12 ng/mL) are at risk for deficiency; those with concentrations of at least 30 but less than 50 nmol/L (12 to less than 20 ng/mL) are at risk for inadequacy; and those with concentrations between 50–75 nmol/L (20–30 ng/mL) are considered sufficient. The Committee indicated that concentrations greater than 125 nmol/L (50 ng/mL) may be reason for concern. Of interest to public health scientists, the report indicated that a serum 25(OH)D level consistent with the Estimated Average Requirement for dietary intake (EAR) lies between 30 and 50 nmol/L and that 40 nmol/L was selected from the middle of the range to serve as the targeted level for median dietary requirements (Institute of Medicine 2011).

A number of external quality assurance programs exist for serum or plasma 25(OH)D concentration measurements, including those sponsored by DEQAS (Vitamin D External Quality Assessment Scheme), College of American Pathologists (Bone and Growth Survey and Accuracy-Based Vitamin D Survey), and NIST/NIH (Vitamin D Metabolites Quality Assurance Program). Standard reference materials (SRM 972) with certified values for $25(OH)D_2$, $25(OH)D_3$ and C3-epimer of $25(OH)D_3$ are available from the U.S. National Institute of Standards and Technology (NIST). An additional solvent-based reference material set (SRM 2972) with certified values for $25(OH)D_2$ and $25(OH)D_3$ is also available (https://www-s.nist.gov/srmors/view_detail.cfm?srm=972). Further improvement in the agreement between laboratories and methods is expected as more laboratories use these SRMs.

Data in NHANES. The data in this report were obtained by use of an antibody-based method, specifically a radioimmunoassay (DiaSorin, Stillwater, MN). The manufacturer reformulated the kit in the late 1990s, resulting in data that were on average 12% lower than those generated with the original kit. To make NHANES III data (original kit) comparable to data from 2001–2006 (reformulated kit), we followed the recommendations of a panel of experts (Yetley 2010) to use a published adjustment equation for the NHANES III data (see Analytic Note at http://www.cdc.gov/nchs/nhanes/nhanes2005-2006/VID_D.htm). The Analytic Note also reported that the reformulated kit showed some assay drifts between 2001 and 2006. To generate 2003–2004 and 2005–2006 tables and figures, we used the public release data files from November 2010. Using data that were already adjusted for these assay drifts was the most appropriate way to make comparisons across survey cycles.

Since 1988, NHANES has monitored the vitamin D status of the U.S. population. By design, this survey collects information and biological samples in the summer from people living at higher latitudes and in the winter from people living at lower latitudes. Because the different racial and ethnic groups are not evenly distributed across all geographic regions in the United States, the season-latitude structure of the survey can affect comparisons by race or ethnicity. In two seasonal subpopulations from NHANES III (1988–1994), Looker *et al.* (2002) showed that in the winter and lower latitude subpopulation, 1–5% and 25–57% had 25(OH)D concentrations less than 25 nmol/L (10 ng/mL) and less than 62.5 nmol/L (25 ng/mL), respectively. In the summer and higher latitude subpopulation, 1–3% and 21–49% had 25(OH)D concentrations below these cutoffs. Mean 25(OH)D concentrations were highest in non-Hispanic whites, intermediate in Mexican Americans, and lowest in non-Hispanic blacks. A more recent analysis of NHANES III and NHANES 2000–2004 (Looker 2008) demonstrated that overall, mean serum 25(OH)D were 5–9 nmol/L lower in 2000–2004 than in 1988–1994 in most males, but not in most females. Factors related to changes in vitamin D status were increased body mass index, decreased milk intake, and increased usage of sun protection in the more recent surveys.

For more information about vitamin D, see the Institute of Medicine's Dietary Reference Intake reports (Institute of Medicine 2011), fact sheets from the National Institutes of Health, Office of Dietary Supplements

(http://ods.od.nih.gov/Health_Information/Information_About_Individual_Dietary_Supplements.aspx).

Highlights

Serum 25-hydroxyvitamin D [25(OH)D] concentrations in the U.S. population showed the following demographic patterns and characteristics:

- Concentrations generally decreased with increasing age.
- No consistent pattern was observed with regard to gender.
- Among the three race/ethnic groups, non-Hispanic blacks had the lowest 25(OH)D concentrations and non-Hispanic whites had the highest concentrations.
- The likelihood of being vitamin D deficient was significantly influenced by race/ethnicity.

During the past several years, the vitamin D status of the U.S. population was under intensive investigation to determine whether a downward trend was apparent. In the analysis below, we used data that were adjusted for radioimmunoassay reformulation and assay drifts according to recommendations made by a panel of experts (Yetley 2010). The age-adjusted mean 25(OH)D concentrations in the U.S. population decreased by approximately 10% between NHANES III and the periods 2001–2002 and 2003–2006 (Figure H.2.b). Decreases were seen in all groups shown (total or stratified by gender or race/ethnicity). Similarly, a recent report found that the age- and season-adjusted prevalence at risk of deficiency (serum 25(OH)D concentrations less than 30 nmol/L) increased between 1988–1994 and 2001–2002 from 4% to 7% for males aged 12 years and older and from 7% to 11% for females aged 12 years and older (Looker 2011).

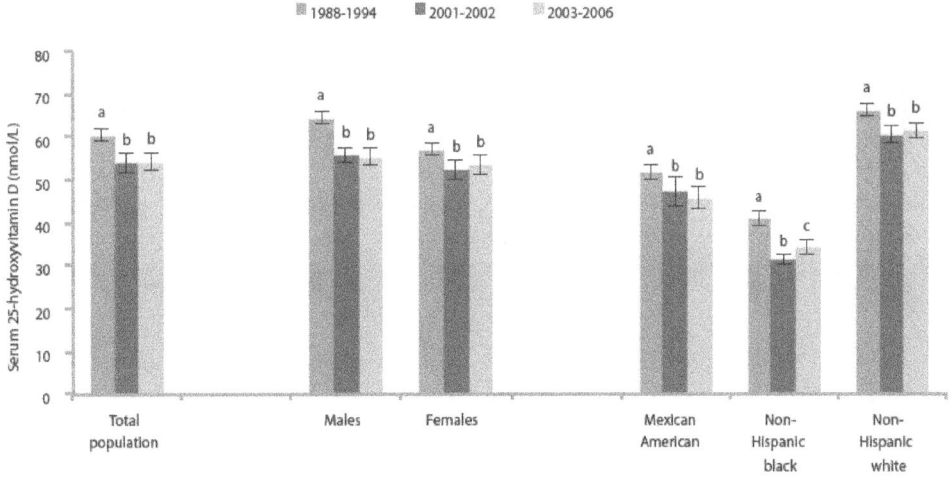

Figure H.2.b. Age-adjusted geometric mean concentrations of serum 25-hydroxyvitamin D in the U.S. population aged 12 years and older by gender or race/ethnicity, National Health and Nutrition Examination Survey, 1988–2006.

Error bars represent 95% confidence intervals. Within a demographic group, bars not sharing a common letter differ (p < 0.05). Age adjustment was done using direct standardization.

It is interesting to note that non-Hispanic blacks one year and older had the highest prevalence of vitamin D deficiency (serum 25(OH)D concentrations less than 30 nmol/L) (Figure H.2.c), despite clinical data showing superior bone health with greater density and fewer fractures than other race/ethnic groups; further research is needed to explain this unusual finding (Aloia 2008). Higher peak bone mass, higher obesity rates, greater muscle mass and lower bone turnover are some of the factors that have been suggested to protect African Americans against fracture

(Aloia 2008). Non-Hispanic blacks and Mexican Americans had the highest prevalence of low serum 25(OH)D concentrations categorized at risk for inadequacy (30 to less than 50 nmol/L) compared to non-Hispanic whites (Figure H.2.c).

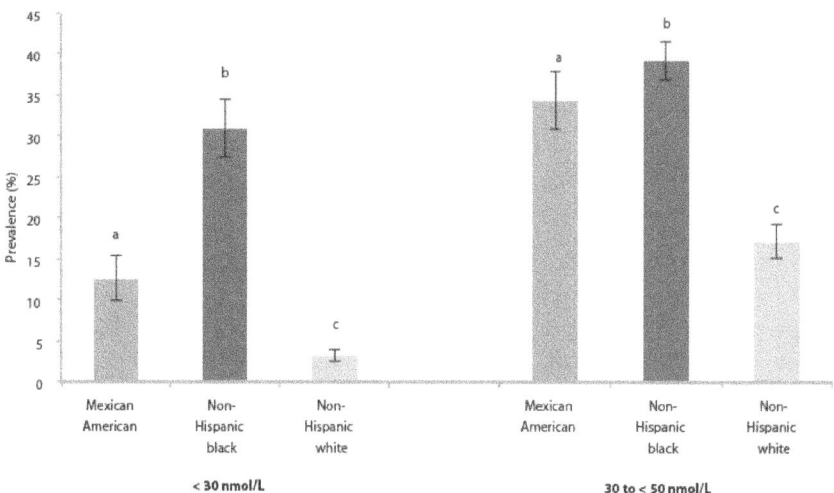

Figure H.2.c. *Age-adjusted prevalence estimates of serum 25-hydroxyvitamin D concentrations less than 30 and 30 to less than 50 nmol/L in the U.S. population aged 1 year and older by race/ethnicity, National Health and Nutrition Examination Survey, 2003–2006.*

Error bars represent 95% confidence intervals. Within each vitamin D status category, bars not sharing a common letter differ (p < 0.05). Age adjustment was done using direct standardization.

The Institute of Medicine (2011) report concluded that serum 25(OH)D levels of 40 nmol/L are at a level consistent with a desirable median intake of vitamin D. Non-Hispanic blacks had significantly higher prevalence of serum concentrations less than 40 nmol/L (Figure H.2.d) which corresponds to the targeted level for the median dietary requirement. The median meets the requirement of approximately half the population thus individuals with concentrations less than 40 nmol/L are at increased risk of adverse health outcomes.

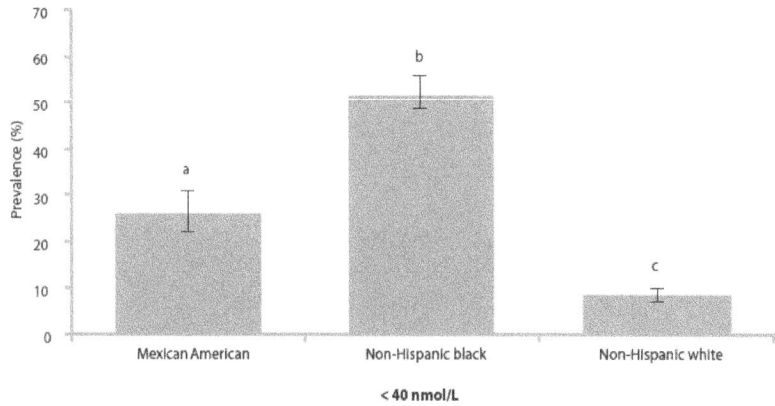

Figure H.2.d. *Age-adjusted prevalence estimates of serum 25-hydroxyvitamin D concentrations less than 40 nmol/L in the U.S. population aged 1 years and older by race/ethnicity, National Health and Nutrition Examination Survey, 2003–2006.*

Error bars represent 95% confidence intervals. Bars not sharing a common letter differ (p < 0.05). Age adjustment was done using direct standardization.

Detailed Observations

The selected observations mentioned below are derived from the tables and figures presented next. Statements about categorical differences between demographic groups noted below are based on non-overlapping confidence limits from univariate analysis without adjusting for demographic variables (e.g., age, gender, race/ethnicity) or other blood concentration determinants (e.g., dietary intake, supplement usage, smoking, BMI). A multivariate analysis may alter the size and statistical significance of these categorical differences. Furthermore, additional significant differences of smaller magnitude may be present despite their lack of mention here (e.g., if confidence limits slightly overlap or if differences are not statistically significant before covariate adjustment has occurred). For a selection of citations of descriptive NHANES papers related to these biochemical indicators of diet and nutrition, see **Appendix G**.

Geometric mean concentrations (NHANES 2003–2006):

- Serum 25(OH)D concentrations decreased through adolescence and then stabilized (Table 2.13.a.1).

- Non-Hispanic blacks had the lowest concentrations of serum 25(OH)D (Table 2.13.a.1).

Changes in geometric mean concentrations across surveys:

- Geometric mean 25(OH)D concentrations remained steady across the survey cycles from 2001–2006 (Table 2.13.b).

Prevalence estimates of low or high biochemical indicator concentrations:

- Between 2003 and 2006, 8% of the population aged 1 year and older were at risk for vitamin D deficiency, as defined by a serum concentration < 30 nmol/L, whereas 24% had serum concentrations between 30 and less than 50 nmol/L, levels that placed them at risk for inadequacy (Tables 2.13.c.1 and 2.13.c.2). Approximately 17% of the population had concentrations < 40 nmol/L which is considered the level associated with desirable intake (Tables 2.13.c.3). Less than 1% had serum concentrations > 125 nmol/L, a level that may be reason for concern about excess (Tables 2.13.c.4).

- Less than 2% of children (1–11 years) were at risk for vitamin D deficiency (Table 2.13.c.1).

- More females (10%) than males (6%) were at risk for vitamin D deficiency (Table 2.13.c.1).

- More non-Hispanic blacks (31%) were at risk for vitamin D deficiency than non-Hispanic whites (4%) or Mexican Americans (11%) (Table 2.13.c.1).

- The prevalence of risk for vitamin D deficiency remained steady across the 2001–2006 survey cycles (Table 2.13.d.1).

Table 2.13.a.1. Serum 25-hydroxyvitamin D: Concentrations

Geometric mean and selected percentiles of serum concentrations (in nmol/L) for the total U.S. population aged 1 year and older, National Health and Nutrition Examination Survey, 2003–2006.

	Geometric mean (95% conf. interval)	Selected percentiles (95% conf. interval)					Sample size
		2.5th	5th	50th	95th	97.5th	
Total, 1 year and older	55.6 (53.6 – 57.6)	18.5 (17.4 – 19.7)	23.2 (21.4 – 25.0)	58.0 (56.3 – 59.9)	96.6 (93.9 – 101)	108 (105 – 112)	16,604
Age group							
1–5 years	68.6 (66.7 – 70.5)	36.9 (32.9 – 38.8)	41.6 (39.5 – 43.4)	68.8 (66.9 – 70.6)	99.6 (95.7 – 107)	107 (102 – 121)	1,799
6–11 years	63.8 (61.6 – 66.1)	30.5 (27.3 – 31.6)	35.3 (32.0 – 38.7)	64.5 (63.0 – 66.1)	97.2 (92.5 – 108)	105 (98.4 – 122)	1,768
12–19 years	55.1 (52.4 – 58.0)	18.0 (15.6 – 20.1)	22.7 (19.8 – 25.1)	57.6 (55.3 – 60.1)	98.4 (94.3 – 108)	111 (106 – 123)	4,044
20–39 years	54.5 (52.1 – 57.0)	17.6 (15.9 – 19.0)	21.8 (20.3 – 23.3)	56.6 (54.4 – 58.9)	102 (97.2 – 108)	115 (110 – 122)	3,262
40–59 years	53.6 (51.3 – 56.0)	17.8 (16.3 – 18.9)	21.7 (19.8 – 23.6)	56.0 (54.1 – 58.1)	94.3 (90.5 – 98.3)	103 (98.0 – 110)	2,660
60 years and older	54.1 (52.4 – 55.8)	19.1 (18.1 – 20.1)	23.1 (21.6 – 24.6)	56.9 (55.4 – 58.5)	91.9 (89.5 – 95.0)	100 (96.6 – 106)	3,071
Gender							
Males	56.7 (54.7 – 58.7)	20.7 (18.6 – 22.3)	25.8 (23.8 – 27.3)	58.9 (57.1 – 60.7)	94.0 (90.7 – 97.7)	103 (98.6 – 109)	8,145
Females	54.5 (52.5 – 56.6)	17.6 (16.2 – 18.5)	21.2 (19.8 – 22.5)	57.2 (55.2 – 59.2)	99.4 (96.1 – 106)	112 (108 – 117)	8,459
Race/ethnicity							
Mexican Americans	48.7 (46.3 – 51.2)	18.2 (16.8 – 19.4)	21.5 (19.6 – 23.3)	49.9 (47.7 – 53.4)	81.8 (79.2 – 84.7)	88.2 (85.4 – 92.0)	4,275
Non-Hispanic Blacks	36.1 (34.3 – 38.0)	12.0 (11.0 – 12.8)	14.3 (13.5 – 15.1)	36.6 (34.2 – 39.1)	70.9 (68.5 – 73.7)	79.0 (74.9 – 82.2)	4,349
Non-Hispanic Whites	61.9 (60.3 – 63.4)	24.9 (23.3 – 25.9)	31.0 (29.1 – 32.6)	63.2 (61.8 – 64.6)	102 (97.8 – 106)	113 (110 – 117)	6,698

Figure 2.13.a. Serum 25–hydroxyvitamin D: Concentrations by age group
Geometric mean (95% confidence interval), National Health and Nutrition Examination Survey, 2003–2006

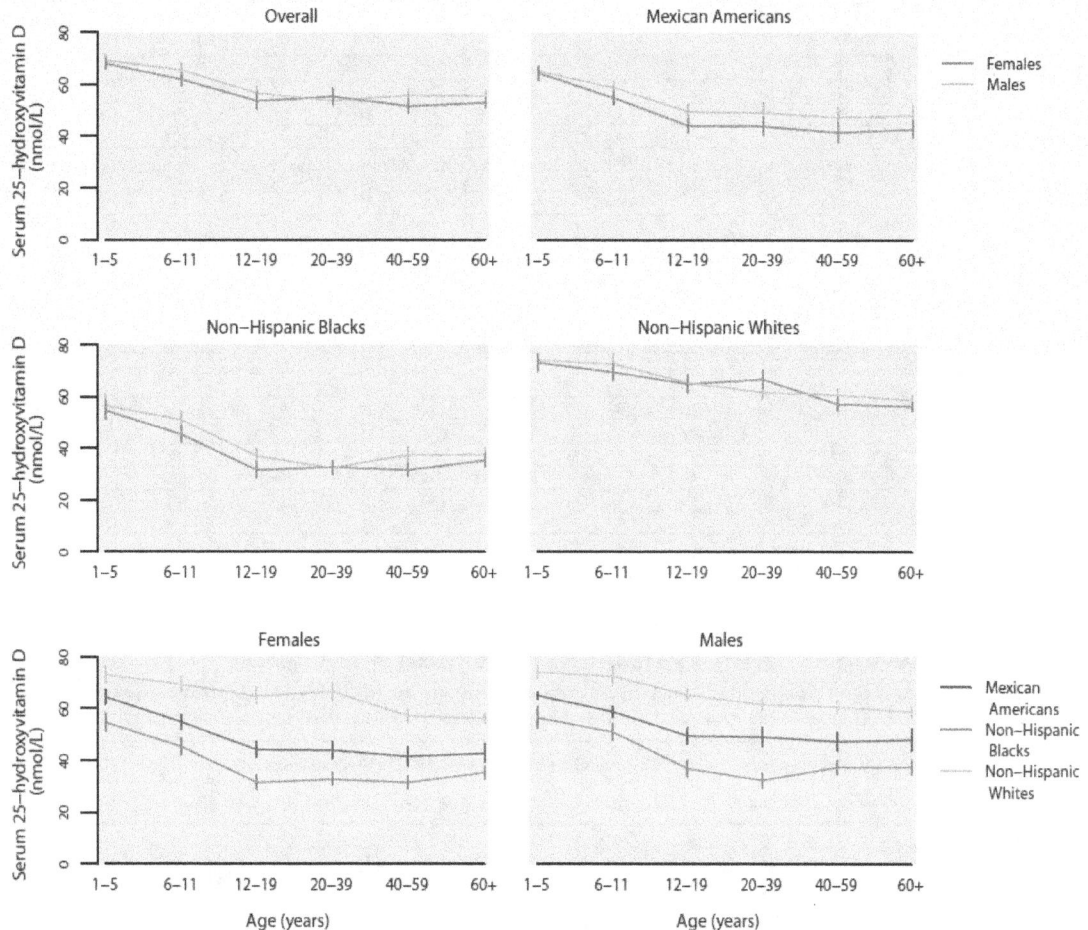

Table 2.13.a.2. Serum 25-hydroxyvitamin D: Total population

Geometric mean and selected percentiles of serum concentrations (in nmol/L) for the total U.S. population aged 1 year and older, National Health and Nutrition Examination Survey, 2003–2006.

	Geometric mean (95% conf. interval)	Selected percentiles (95% conf. interval)						Sample size
		5th		50th		95th		
Males and Females								
Total, 1 year and older	55.6	(53.6 – 57.6)	23.2	(21.4 – 25.0)	58.0	(56.3 – 59.9)	96.6	(93.9 – 101)	16,604
1–5 years	68.6	(66.7 – 70.5)	41.6	(39.5 – 43.4)	68.8	(66.9 – 70.6)	99.6	(95.7 – 107)	1,799
6–11 years	63.8	(61.6 – 66.1)	35.3	(32.0 – 38.7)	64.5	(63.0 – 66.1)	97.2	(92.5 – 108)	1,768
12–19 years	55.1	(52.4 – 58.0)	22.7	(19.8 – 25.1)	57.6	(55.3 – 60.1)	98.4	(94.3 – 108)	4,044
20–39 years	54.5	(52.1 – 57.0)	21.8	(20.3 – 23.3)	56.6	(54.4 – 58.9)	102	(97.2 – 108)	3,262
40–59 years	53.6	(51.3 – 56.0)	21.7	(19.8 – 23.6)	56.0	(54.1 – 58.1)	94.3	(90.5 – 98.3)	2,660
60 years and older	54.1	(52.4 – 55.8)	23.1	(21.6 – 24.6)	56.9	(55.4 – 58.5)	91.9	(89.5 – 95.0)	3,071
Males								
Total, 1 year and older	56.7	(54.7 – 58.7)	25.8	(23.8 – 27.3)	58.9	(57.1 – 60.7)	94.0	(90.7 – 97.7)	8,145
1–5 years	69.2	(67.0 – 71.5)	41.7	(40.1 – 43.5)	69.3	(66.7 – 71.6)	101	(96.7 – 106)	904
6–11 years	65.5	(63.2 – 67.9)	36.9	(32.5 – 40.3)	65.8	(64.3 – 67.6)	98.0	(92.4 – 116)	862
12–19 years	56.6	(54.0 – 59.3)	25.3	(22.5 – 28.0)	58.7	(56.4 – 61.2)	95.2	(88.8 – 105)	2,049
20–39 years	53.7	(51.4 – 56.1)	23.6	(20.9 – 25.7)	55.9	(53.7 – 57.8)	90.6	(87.7 – 96.7)	1,472
40–59 years	55.8	(53.3 – 58.4)	25.3	(22.4 – 27.0)	58.0	(55.8 – 60.8)	92.4	(88.1 – 98.7)	1,311
60 years and older	55.6	(53.7 – 57.7)	26.0	(23.8 – 27.9)	57.5	(55.6 – 59.7)	91.9	(89.1 – 97.2)	1,547
Females								
Total, 1 year and older	54.5	(52.5 – 56.6)	21.2	(19.8 – 22.5)	57.2	(55.2 – 59.2)	99.4	(96.1 – 106)	8,459
1–5 years	67.9	(65.8 – 70.0)	41.3	(37.4 – 44.3)	68.4	(66.3 – 70.3)	98.1	(93.3 – 113)	895
6–11 years	61.9	(59.6 – 64.4)	34.0	(31.4 – 37.6)	62.8	(60.1 – 65.3)	96.4	(92.5 – 103)	906
12–19 years	53.6	(50.6 – 56.9)	20.6	(18.0 – 22.9)	56.4	(53.1 – 59.5)	106	(96.5 – 114)	1,995
20–39 years	55.3	(52.4 – 58.3)	20.5	(19.1 – 21.8)	57.6	(54.4 – 60.7)	110	(106 – 116)	1,790
40–59 years	51.6	(49.2 – 54.2)	19.4	(18.3 – 20.6)	54.1	(50.8 – 57.0)	95.1	(91.5 – 99.2)	1,349
60 years and older	52.9	(51.1 – 54.7)	21.7	(20.2 – 23.2)	56.4	(54.5 – 58.2)	92.0	(89.1 – 95.8)	1,524

Table 2.13.a.3. Serum 25-hydroxyvitamin D: Mexican Americans

Geometric mean and selected percentiles of serum concentrations (in nmol/L) for Mexican Americans in the U.S. population aged 1 year and older, National Health and Nutrition Examination Survey, 2003–2006.

	Geometric mean (95% conf. interval)	Selected percentiles (95% conf. interval)						Sample size
		5th		50th		95th		
Males and Females								
Total, 1 year and older	48.7	(46.3 – 51.2)	21.5	(19.6 – 23.3)	49.9	(47.7 – 53.4)	81.8	(79.2 – 84.7)	4,275
1–5 years	64.8	(63.1 – 66.6)	42.5	(39.4 – 44.7)	64.3	(62.3 – 66.1)	93.8	(89.5 – 99.7)	584
6–11 years	56.9	(55.0 – 58.8)	32.7	(30.9 – 34.9)	58.2	(56.3 – 59.8)	82.9	(80.7 – 86.9)	589
12–19 years	46.8	(44.2 – 49.6)	22.0	(20.2 – 23.4)	47.8	(45.6 – 50.7)	74.8	(71.2 – 83.6)	1,288
20–39 years	46.6	(43.6 – 49.7)	20.6	(17.6 – 23.5)	48.0	(45.4 – 51.5)	78.0	(75.6 – 83.1)	789
40–59 years	44.4	(41.4 – 47.7)	19.4	(17.4 – 21.2)	45.8	(41.9 – 49.0)	79.8	(72.4 – 87.7)	472
60 years and older	45.0	(42.4 – 47.8)	20.1	(17.6 – 21.4)	45.9	(43.6 – 48.1)	79.5	(73.4 – 89.5)	553
Males								
Total, 1 year and older	51.1	(48.7 – 53.7)	24.5	(21.7 – 26.6)	52.7	(49.4 – 55.5)	81.7	(79.0 – 85.2)	2,073
1–5 years	65.2	(63.9 – 66.5)	44.6	(40.5 – 45.8)	64.4	(63.1 – 65.6)	94.9	(88.6 – 109)	282
6–11 years	58.8	(56.8 – 60.8)	36.0	(32.3 – 38.8)	59.7	(57.8 – 62.3)	83.3	(80.5 – 92.2)	286
12–19 years	49.5	(46.6 – 52.6)	23.8	(21.5 – 26.2)	50.0	(47.4 – 54.0)	78.0	(72.7 – 85.8)	641
20–39 years	49.1	(45.5 – 52.8)	24.3	(19.7 – 26.2)	49.8	(47.1 – 54.1)	77.0	(73.1 – 86.5)	353
40–59 years	47.4	(44.0 – 51.0)	20.9	(15.3 – 25.9)	47.4	(44.6 – 54.3)	79.8	(72.2 – 92.8)	239
60 years and older	48.0	(44.0 – 52.2)	21.4	(18.3 – 25.0)	48.3	(43.6 – 54.3)	81.2	(74.4 – 96.7)	272
Females								
Total, 1 year and older	46.2	(43.7 – 48.8)	19.8	(18.9 – 20.6)	47.7	(45.4 – 50.3)	82.1	(78.6 – 85.4)	2,202
1–5 years	64.5	(61.8 – 67.2)	40.5	(36.0 – 44.3)	64.2	(59.9 – 67.5)	92.9	(89.1 – 98.6)	302
6–11 years	54.8	(52.3 – 57.5)	31.1	(25.0 – 33.7)	56.6	(54.0 – 58.8)	82.3	(74.5 – 93.8)	303
12–19 years	44.1	(41.4 – 47.1)	20.4	(17.3 – 22.5)	45.6	(42.4 – 48.0)	73.2	(67.7 – 80.3)	647
20–39 years	43.9	(40.7 – 47.3)	18.5	(16.4 – 20.4)	44.9	(41.6 – 48.2)	80.2	(74.8 – 87.1)	436
40–59 years	41.5	(37.9 – 45.3)	18.7	(17.5 – 20.0)	42.8	(37.3 – 46.8)	79.6	(70.9 – 85.0)	233
60 years and older	42.7	(39.6 – 46.1)	19.1	(15.4 – 21.1)	44.3	(40.5 – 47.0)	78.0	(71.5 – 88.9)	281

Table 2.13.a.4. Serum 25-hydroxyvitamin D: Non-Hispanic blacks

Geometric mean and selected percentiles of serum concentrations (in nmol/L) for non-Hispanic blacks in the U.S. population aged 1 year and older, National Health and Nutrition Examination Survey, 2003–2006.

	Geometric mean (95% conf. interval)	Selected percentiles (95% conf. interval)			Sample size
		5th	50th	95th	
Males and Females					
Total, 1 year and older	36.1 (34.3 – 38.0)	14.3 (13.5 – 15.1)	36.6 (34.2 – 39.1)	70.9 (68.5 – 73.7)	4,349
1–5 years	55.5 (52.7 – 58.5)	29.4 (21.0 – 33.4)	57.5 (54.5 – 59.6)	86.6 (82.1 – 91.3)	503
6–11 years	48.1 (45.7 – 50.6)	24.8 (23.4 – 25.7)	49.4 (47.3 – 52.2)	73.8 (71.5 – 80.2)	561
12–19 years	34.2 (31.4 – 37.2)	13.8 (13.0 – 14.6)	34.6 (31.3 – 38.2)	68.3 (64.2 – 72.2)	1,421
20–39 years	32.5 (30.4 – 34.8)	13.7 (12.7 – 14.8)	31.5 (29.2 – 34.2)	64.0 (61.1 – 70.4)	716
40–59 years	34.1 (32.0 – 36.3)	13.3 (11.6 – 14.8)	34.7 (32.4 – 37.7)	66.2 (62.0 – 71.6)	626
60 years and older	36.2 (34.1 – 38.3)	15.0 (13.2 – 15.9)	36.3 (33.8 – 39.7)	72.9 (67.6 – 80.3)	522
Males					
Total, 1 year and older	38.0 (35.9 – 40.3)	15.5 (14.0 – 16.6)	38.6 (35.9 – 41.4)	71.8 (69.0 – 78.6)	2,166
1–5 years	56.5 (52.5 – 60.7)	30.0 (21.7 – 34.0)	58.4 (54.3 – 61.6)	89.1 (81.9 – 98.4)	248
6–11 years	51.0 (48.1 – 54.1)	26.0 (23.0 – 28.4)	53.0 (49.3 – 56.5)	75.0 (70.5 – 88.7)	277
12–19 years	36.9 (34.0 – 40.0)	14.6 (13.2 – 15.9)	38.1 (34.9 – 41.0)	70.8 (66.6 – 75.9)	745
20–39 years	32.4 (29.8 – 35.1)	13.8 (11.6 – 15.2)	30.5 (28.4 – 33.3)	64.9 (59.0 – 82.3)	339
40–59 years	37.4 (34.8 – 40.2)	15.9 (14.0 – 17.1)	38.2 (34.2 – 42.2)	69.6 (62.4 – 77.2)	293
60 years and older	37.5 (34.9 – 40.3)	15.0 (12.8 – 16.6)	38.5 (34.7 – 42.7)	72.3 (66.1 – 79.2)	264
Females					
Total, 1 year and older	34.5 (32.7 – 36.3)	13.6 (12.9 – 14.3)	34.9 (32.4 – 37.7)	69.6 (65.9 – 73.0)	2,183
1–5 years	54.6 (51.2 – 58.2)	28.4 (13.2 – 35.2)	56.0 (53.3 – 58.8)	83.1 (79.7 – 94.4)	255
6–11 years	45.3 (42.3 – 48.4)	23.6 (19.4 – 25.3)	46.0 (42.4 – 49.7)	73.0 (71.0 – 76.9)	284
12–19 years	31.5 (28.8 – 34.5)	13.3 (12.5 – 14.2)	31.3 (27.7 – 34.3)	64.7 (59.3 – 71.5)	676
20–39 years	32.7 (30.4 – 35.1)	13.7 (11.8 – 15.1)	32.4 (29.3 – 36.2)	63.0 (60.6 – 70.6)	377
40–59 years	31.5 (29.2 – 34.0)	12.2 (10.5 – 13.2)	32.5 (28.6 – 35.2)	63.2 (58.7 – 75.3)	333
60 years and older	35.3 (32.8 – 37.9)	15.0 (13.0 – 15.8)	34.7 (31.6 – 39.3)	73.5 (64.4 – 96.3)	258

Table 2.13.a.5. Serum 25-hydroxyvitamin D: Non-Hispanic whites

Geometric mean and selected percentiles of serum concentrations (in nmol/L) for non-Hispanic whites in the U.S. population aged 1 year and older, National Health and Nutrition Examination Survey, 2003–2006.

	Geometric mean (95% conf. interval)	Selected percentiles (95% conf. interval)			Sample size
		5th	50th	95th	
Males and Females					
Total, 1 year and older	61.9 (60.3 – 63.4)	31.0 (29.1 – 32.6)	63.2 (61.8 – 64.6)	102 (97.8 – 106)	6,698
1–5 years	73.6 (71.3 – 76.0)	49.0 (44.1 – 51.7)	72.3 (70.7 – 74.2)	105 (97.8 – 118)	516
6–11 years	71.1 (68.2 – 74.1)	46.1 (43.5 – 48.1)	69.6 (67.5 – 71.8)	103 (96.1 – 119)	457
12–19 years	65.2 (63.0 – 67.4)	37.4 (35.6 – 40.1)	64.7 (62.9 – 66.6)	107 (100 – 113)	1,050
20–39 years	64.1 (61.8 – 66.5)	33.3 (29.8 – 36.3)	64.3 (61.8 – 66.6)	110 (107 – 115)	1,458
40–59 years	58.9 (56.8 – 61.0)	27.4 (25.9 – 30.2)	60.4 (58.0 – 63.2)	96.7 (92.5 – 103)	1,360
60 years and older	57.4 (55.9 – 58.9)	26.0 (24.2 – 27.7)	59.7 (58.3 – 61.1)	92.9 (90.8 – 97.2)	1,857
Males					
Total, 1 year and older	62.4 (60.8 – 64.1)	33.7 (31.8 – 35.4)	63.6 (62.1 – 65.0)	97.4 (93.9 – 103)	3,303
1–5 years	74.1 (71.7 – 76.6)	47.1 (41.5 – 52.3)	72.7 (70.4 – 74.8)	105 (99.2 – 116)	279
6–11 years	72.6 (69.1 – 76.3)	47.1† (41.6 – 52.5)	70.9 (68.0 – 74.8)	105† (96.4 – 136)	219
12–19 years	65.4 (63.2 – 67.7)	40.6 (37.3 – 42.7)	65.3 (63.5 – 67.1)	99.6 (93.5 – 112)	528
20–39 years	61.6 (59.5 – 63.8)	33.5 (30.7 – 36.5)	62.3 (59.6 – 64.7)	96.8 (90.9 – 104)	641
40–59 years	60.7 (58.5 – 63.0)	31.8 (28.4 – 34.0)	62.6 (59.9 – 64.8)	96.1 (90.0 – 104)	691
60 years and older	58.7 (56.9 – 60.5)	30.5 (26.7 – 33.3)	60.0 (58.1 – 61.5)	92.7 (90.1 – 98.7)	945
Females					
Total, 1 year and older	61.3 (59.6 – 63.1)	27.9 (25.6 – 30.3)	62.9 (61.0 – 64.5)	107 (102 – 111)	3,395
1–5 years	73.1 (69.8 – 76.5)	49.8 (45.5 – 52.8)	71.9 (69.3 – 75.8)	105 (94.9 – 122)	237
6–11 years	69.4 (66.6 – 72.4)	45.6 (42.7 – 47.6)	68.3 (65.6 – 70.8)	99.9 (94.8 – 109)	238
12–19 years	64.9 (61.7 – 68.3)	34.9 (31.1 – 37.5)	63.9 (61.4 – 67.0)	112 (106 – 127)	522
20–39 years	66.7 (63.5 – 70.0)	33.0 (26.4 – 37.1)	66.6 (63.5 – 69.6)	117 (112 – 128)	817
40–59 years	57.1 (54.6 – 59.7)	24.8 (19.9 – 27.0)	58.4 (55.6 – 61.9)	97.2 (93.4 – 105)	669
60 years and older	56.3 (54.6 – 58.0)	23.9 (22.0 – 25.7)	59.5 (57.8 – 61.2)	93.1 (90.0 – 99.8)	912

† Estimate is subject to greater uncertainty due to small cell size.

Table 2.13.b. Serum 25-hydroxyvitamin D: Concentrations by survey cycle

Geometric mean and selected percentiles of serum concentrations (in nmol/L) for the U.S. population, National Health and Nutrition Examination Survey, 2001–2006.

	Geometric mean (95% conf. interval)	Selected percentiles (95% conf. interval) 5th	Selected percentiles 50th	Selected percentiles 95th	Sample size
Total, 6 years and older					
2001–2002	54.7 (52.6 – 56.8)	22.6 (20.4 – 24.9)	57.1 (55.1 – 59.3)	96.8 (92.4 – 105)	7,807
2003–2004	55.5 (52.5 – 58.7)	24.2 (20.9 – 26.3)	57.5 (54.7 – 60.6)	97.2 (92.8 – 104)	7,403
2005–2006	54.3 (51.5 – 57.3)	21.8 (20.1 – 23.5)	57.2 (54.8 – 59.7)	95.9 (91.9 – 103)	7,402
Age group					
1–5 years					
2003–2004	68.2 (65.9 – 70.5)	41.3 (37.6 – 44.4)	68.7 (66.8 – 70.6)	97.8 (96.3 – 101)	895
2005–2006	69.0 (65.7 – 72.5)	41.8 (39.3 – 44.0)	69.1 (64.7 – 72.1)	103 (94.2 – 121)	904
6–11 years					
2001–2002	63.8 (60.5 – 67.3)	36.9 (31.9 – 39.7)	63.7 (60.4 – 66.8)	101 (90.1 – 138)	991
2003–2004	63.4 (60.2 – 66.7)	34.8 (31.2 – 40.5)	64.5 (61.8 – 66.9)	94.3 (87.5 – 109)	846
2005–2006	64.2 (60.8 – 67.7)	35.8 (31.9 – 38.6)	64.4 (62.6 – 66.8)	98.8 (92.5 – 129)	922
12–19 years					
2001–2002	55.1 (52.5 – 57.8)	24.5 (20.8 – 27.2)	56.7 (54.2 – 59.1)	96.1 (91.8 – 102)	2,167
2003–2004	56.2 (52.2 – 60.6)	24.8 (21.0 – 27.3)	57.9 (53.9 – 61.8)	101 (94.1 – 112)	2,059
2005–2006	54.0 (50.1 – 58.3)	21.2 (17.6 – 23.9)	57.3 (54.0 – 60.7)	96.3 (88.6 – 111)	1,985
20–39 years					
2001–2002	54.1 (51.8 – 56.5)	21.2 (19.4 – 23.1)	56.4 (54.0 – 59.0)	102 (94.8 – 110)	1,691
2003–2004	54.4 (50.9 – 58.1)	22.5 (19.0 – 25.4)	56.1 (51.9 – 59.9)	104 (95.9 – 110)	1,559
2005–2006	54.6 (51.1 – 58.4)	21.1 (19.0 – 23.3)	57.0 (54.2 – 60.1)	99.2 (95.5 – 113)	1,703
40–59 years					
2001–2002	54.0 (51.4 – 56.6)	21.4 (18.7 – 24.4)	56.8 (54.6 – 59.8)	94.9 (90.5 – 104)	1,449
2003–2004	54.7 (51.1 – 58.5)	23.6 (18.7 – 26.9)	56.5 (53.6 – 60.2)	94.5 (89.0 – 102)	1,278
2005–2006	52.6 (49.6 – 55.9)	20.8 (18.8 – 22.8)	55.5 (52.9 – 58.4)	94.1 (88.9 – 100)	1,382
60 years and older					
2001–2002	52.5 (49.9 – 55.3)	23.1 (21.1 – 24.4)	55.1 (52.4 – 57.7)	91.8 (88.4 – 95.0)	1,509
2003–2004	55.2 (52.9 – 57.5)	24.2 (21.8 – 25.8)	57.6 (55.2 – 59.7)	94.1 (90.1 – 102)	1,661
2005–2006	53.1 (50.4 – 55.9)	22.3 (20.4 – 24.3)	56.4 (54.1 – 58.9)	90.4 (87.5 – 93.9)	1,410
Gender					
(6 years and older)					
Males					
2001–2002	56.5 (54.5 – 58.6)	25.8 (23.8 – 27.2)	58.3 (56.3 – 60.7)	96.0 (91.2 – 105)	3,782
2003–2004	56.8 (53.6 – 60.2)	27.0 (23.7 – 29.4)	58.6 (55.8 – 61.7)	92.1 (88.8 – 98.2)	3,638
2005–2006	55.1 (52.4 – 58.0)	23.8 (21.5 – 25.6)	57.7 (55.7 – 60.1)	94.1 (88.1 – 102)	3,603
Females					
2001–2002	53.0 (50.6 – 55.5)	20.5 (18.0 – 22.7)	55.8 (53.5 – 58.1)	98.4 (92.6 – 108)	4,025
2003–2004	54.3 (51.4 – 57.3)	21.3 (19.2 – 23.5)	56.3 (53.3 – 59.5)	103 (97.3 – 109)	3,765
2005–2006	53.6 (50.5 – 56.9)	20.5 (18.6 – 22.3)	56.6 (53.8 – 59.5)	97.1 (93.1 – 107)	3,799
Race/ethnicity					
(6 years and older)					
Mexican Americans					
2001–2002	48.9 (46.2 – 51.8)	23.0 (21.3 – 24.5)	50.1 (47.1 – 52.7)	81.6 (77.3 – 91.2)	1,961
2003–2004	48.7 (46.0 – 51.6)	22.8 (19.4 – 25.5)	50.2 (47.1 – 53.4)	80.5 (77.2 – 84.1)	1,802
2005–2006	45.9 (41.9 – 50.2)	20.0 (16.3 – 22.6)	47.3 (43.3 – 52.8)	78.5 (73.0 – 84.5)	1,889
Non-Hispanic Blacks					
2001–2002	32.6 (31.3 – 34.0)	13.3 (10.9 – 14.4)	32.5 (31.1 – 34.2)	66.2 (63.9 – 68.5)	1,821
2003–2004	36.3 (33.5 – 39.4)	14.3 (12.8 – 15.6)	37.0 (34.0 – 40.7)	69.1 (65.8 – 73.9)	1,914
2005–2006	33.8 (31.6 – 36.2)	13.9 (13.0 – 14.8)	33.4 (30.7 – 37.1)	68.4 (64.5 – 71.1)	1,932
Non-Hispanic Whites					
2001–2002	60.9 (58.7 – 63.1)	29.9 (28.2 – 31.2)	62.2 (60.2 – 64.2)	102 (95.9 – 110)	3,416
2003–2004	61.7 (59.3 – 64.2)	30.2 (27.0 – 33.6)	63.2 (60.8 – 65.2)	103 (97.3 – 109)	3,155
2005–2006	61.0 (59.0 – 63.1)	31.0 (27.5 – 32.4)	62.3 (60.3 – 64.1)	99.0 (95.9 – 108)	3,027

Figure 2.13.b. Serum 25–hydroxyvitamin D: Concentrations by survey cycle

Selected percentiles in nmol/L (95% confidence intervals), National Health and Nutrition Examination Survey, 2001–2006

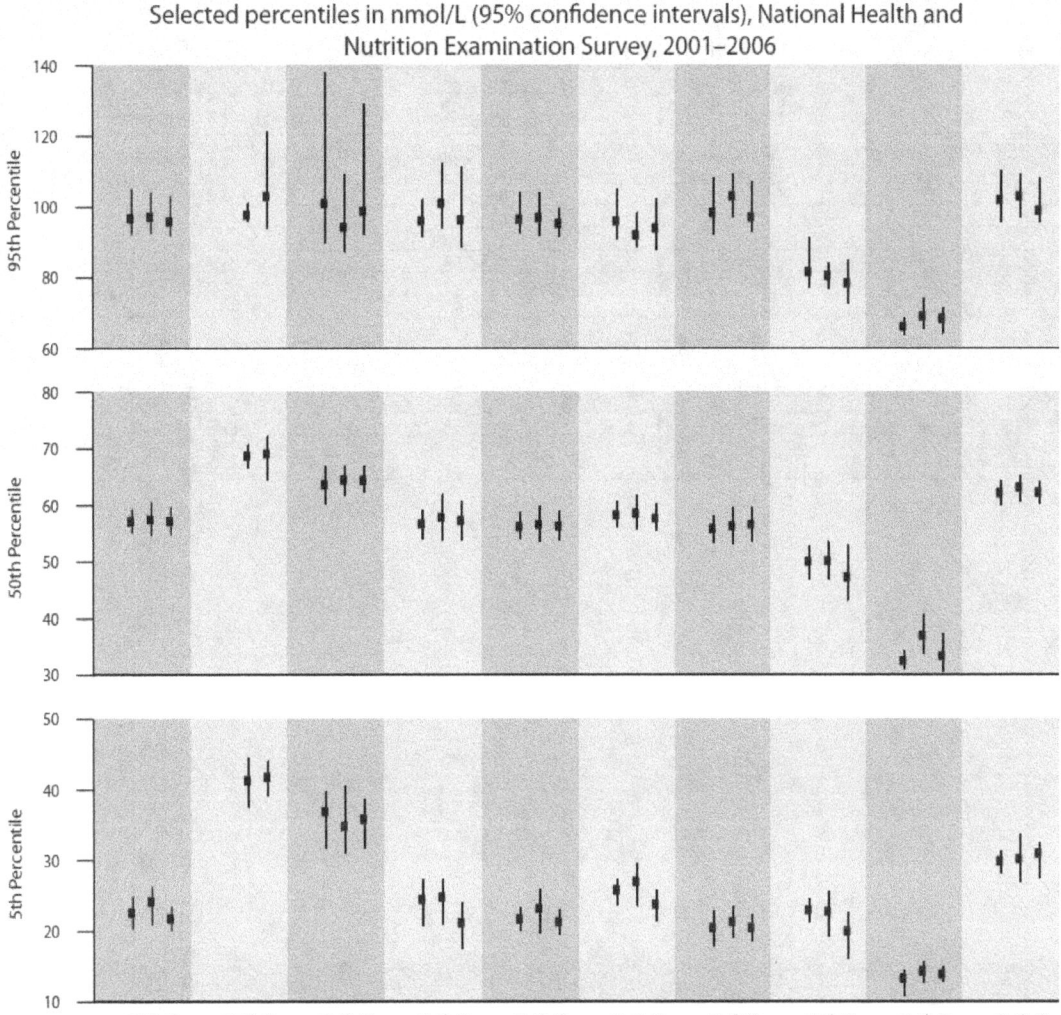

Table 2.13.c.1. Serum 25-hydroxyvitamin D: Prevalence

Prevalence (in percent) of low serum 25-hydroxyvitamin D concentration (< 30 nmol/L) for the U.S. population aged 1 year and older, National Health and Nutrition Examination Survey, 2003–2006.

	Sample size	Prevalence (95% conf. interval)	Estimated total number of persons
Total, 1 year and older	16,604	8.1 (6.7 – 9.8)	23,004,000
Age group			
1–5 years	1,799	0.7 (0.4 – 1.3)	146,000
6–11 years	1,768	1.8 (1.3 – 2.6)	442,000
12–19 years	4,044	8.5 (6.5 – 11.2)	2,823,000
20–39 years	3,262	9.5 (7.6 – 11.8)	7,538,000
40–59 years	2,660	9.3 (7.4 – 11.7)	7,343,000
60 years and older	3,071	8.8 (7.3 – 10.5)	4,084,000
Gender			
Males	8,145	6.3 (5.0 – 7.9)	8,735,000
Females	8,459	9.9 (8.1 – 11.9)	14,288,000
Race/ethnicity			
Mexican Americans	4,275	11.3 (8.7 – 14.6)	2,919,000
Non-Hispanic Blacks	4,349	31.1 (27.4 – 35.1)	10,623,000
Non-Hispanic Whites	6,698	3.6 (3.0 – 4.4)	6,929,000

Table 2.13.c.2. Serum 25-hydroxyvitamin D: Prevalence

Prevalence (in percent) of low serum 25-hydroxyvitamin D concentration (between 30–50 nmol/L) for the U.S. population aged 1 year and older, National Health and Nutrition Examination Survey, 2003–2006.

	Sample size	Prevalence (95% conf. interval)	Estimated total number of persons
Total, 1 year and older	16,604	23.6 (21.6 – 25.8)	66,859,000
Age group			
1–5 years	1,799	8.9 (7.1 – 11.0)	1,799,000
6–11 years	1,768	14.1 (11.5 – 17.2)	3,407,000
12–19 years	4,044	24.2 (21.3 – 27.3)	8,005,000
20–39 years	3,262	26.2 (23.6 – 29.0)	20,908,000
40–59 years	2,660	25.0 (22.2 – 28.0)	19,729,000
60 years and older	3,071	25.5 (23.7 – 27.4)	11,879,000
Gender			
Males	8,145	23.1 (20.8 – 25.6)	31,909,000
Females	8,459	24.1 (22.1 – 26.3)	34,955,000
Race/ethnicity			
Mexican Americans	4,275	32.9 (29.6 – 36.4)	8,514,000
Non-Hispanic Blacks	4,349	39.5 (37.3 – 41.7)	13,483,000
Non-Hispanic Whites	6,698	18.1 (16.2 – 20.2)	34,769,000

Table 2.13.c.3. Serum 25-hydroxyvitamin D: Prevalence

Prevalence (in percent) of low serum 25-hydroxyvitamin D concentration (< 40 nmol/L) for the U.S. population aged 1 year and older, National Health and Nutrition Examination Survey, 2003–2006.

	Sample size	Prevalence (95% conf. interval)	Estimated total number of persons
Total, 1 year and older	16,604	17.2 (14.7 – 20.0)	49,431,000
Age group			
1–5 years	1,799	2.7 (1.8 – 4.0)	541,000
6–11 years	1,768	5.7 (4.2 – 7.7)	1,358,000
12–19 years	4,044	17.1 (13.8 – 21.0)	5,729,000
20–39 years	3,262	19.7 (16.4 – 23.4)	15,722,000
40–59 years	2,660	20.0 (16.6 – 23.9)	16,400,000
60 years and older	3,071	17.8 (15.5 – 20.4)	8,602,000
Gender			
Males	8,145	14.6 (12.3 – 17.4)	20,576,000
Females	8,459	19.6 (16.9 – 22.7)	28,869,000
Race/ethnicity			
Mexican Americans	4,275	24.4 (20.1 – 29.3)	6,635,000
Non-Hispanic Blacks	4,349	51.6 (46.7 – 56.5)	17,968,000
Non-Hispanic Whites	6,698	9.4 (7.9 – 11.2)	18,114,000

Table 2.13.c.4. Serum 25-hydroxyvitamin D: Prevalence

Prevalence (in percent) of high serum 25-hydroxyvitamin D concentration (> 125 nmol/L) for the U.S. population aged 1 year and older, National Health and Nutrition Examination Survey, 2003–2006.

	Sample size	Prevalence (95% conf. interval)	Estimated total number of persons
Total, 1 year and older	16,604	0.9 (0.6 – 1.2)	2,449,000
Age group			
1–5 years	1,799	§	§
6–11 years	1,768	§	§
12–19 years	4,044	1.4 (0.9 – 2.1)	450,000
20–39 years	3,262	1.5 (0.9 – 2.4)	1,193,000
40–59 years	2,660	0.6‡ (0.3 – 1.2)	498,000‡
60 years and older	3,071	0.3‡ (0.1 – 0.6)	134,000‡
Gender			
Males	8,145	0.4 (0.3 – 0.7)	587,000
Females	8,459	1.3 (0.9 – 1.9)	1,867,000
Race/ethnicity			
Mexican Americans	4,275	§	§
Non-Hispanic Blacks	4,349	§	§
Non-Hispanic Whites	6,698	1.2 (0.8 – 1.7)	2,283,000

‡ Estimate flagged: 30% ≤ RSE < 40% for the prevalence estimate.
§ Estimate suppressed: RSE ≥ 40% for the prevalence estimate.

Table 2.13.d.1. Serum 25-hydroxyvitamin D: Prevalence by survey cycle

Prevalence (in percent) of low serum 25-hydroxyvitamin D concentration (< 30 nmol/L) for the U.S. population, National Health and Nutrition Examination Survey, 2001–2006.

	Sample size	Prevalence (95% conf. interval)	Estimated total number of persons
Total, 6 years and older			
2001–2002	7,807	8.4 (6.8 – 10.3)	21,467,000
2003–2004	7,403	7.6 (5.5 – 10.5)	20,049,000
2005–2006	7,402	9.5 (7.3 – 12.2)	25,318,000
Age group			
1–5 years			
2003–2004	895	§	§
2005–2006	904	0.7‡ (0.3 – 1.5)	137,000‡
6–11 years			
2001–2002	991	§	§
2003–2004	846	1.5 (0.8 – 2.6)	350,000
2005–2006	922	2.2 (1.4 – 3.5)	524,000
12–19 years			
2001–2002	2,167	7.0 (4.4 – 11.1)	2,266,000
2003–2004	2,059	7.0 (4.6 – 10.7)	2,327,000
2005–2006	1,985	10.0 (6.8 – 14.5)	3,353,000
20–39 years			
2001–2002	1,691	9.5 (7.7 – 11.5)	7,498,000
2003–2004	1,559	9.3 (6.6 – 12.8)	7,391,000
2005–2006	1,703	9.6 (6.9 – 13.3)	7,700,000
40–59 years			
2001–2002	1,449	9.4 (7.2 – 12.2)	7,125,000
2003–2004	1,278	7.5 (4.8 – 11.4)	5,910,000
2005–2006	1,382	11.0 (8.3 – 14.5)	9,054,000
60 years and older			
2001–2002	1,509	8.8 (6.7 – 11.3)	3,921,000
2003–2004	1,661	8.3 (6.1 – 11.1)	3,841,000
2005–2006	1,410	9.3 (7.2 – 11.8)	4,488,000
Gender			
(6 years and older)			
Males			
2001–2002	3,782	6.2 (4.9 – 7.9)	7,774,000
2003–2004	3,638	5.3 (3.5 – 8.1)	6,830,000
2005–2006	3,603	8.0 (6.0 – 10.6)	10,419,000
Females			
2001–2002	4,025	10.4 (8.2 – 13.0)	13,726,000
2003–2004	3,765	9.8 (7.3 – 13.1)	13,254,000
2005–2006	3,799	10.9 (8.2 – 14.2)	14,894,000
Race/ethnicity			
(6 years and older)			
Mexican Americans			
2001–2002	1,961	8.9 (6.7 – 11.6)	1,863,000
2003–2004	1,802	9.7 (7.1 – 13.3)	2,218,000
2005–2006	1,889	15.0 (10.2 – 21.5)	3,604,000
Non-Hispanic Blacks			
2001–2002	1,821	37.8 (34.5 – 41.2)	11,654,000
2003–2004	1,914	28.5 (22.6 – 35.2)	8,872,000
2005–2006	1,932	37.4 (32.2 – 42.9)	11,915,000
Non-Hispanic Whites			
2001–2002	3,416	3.7 (2.9 – 4.7)	6,654,000
2003–2004	3,155	3.6 (2.6 – 4.9)	6,423,000
2005–2006	3,027	4.0 (3.1 – 5.1)	7,240,000

‡ Estimate flagged: 30% ≤ RSE < 40% for the prevalence estimate.
§ Estimate suppressed: RSE ≥ 40% for the prevalence estimate.

Table 2.13.d.2. Serum 25-hydroxyvitamin D: Prevalence by survey cycle

Prevalence (in percent) of low serum 25-hydroxyvitamin D concentration (between 30–50 nmol/L) for the U.S. population, National Health and Nutrition Examination Survey, 2001–2006.

	Sample size	Prevalence (95% conf. interval)		Estimated total number of persons
Total, 6 years and older				
2001–2002	7,807	24.0	(21.7 – 26.4)	61,533,000
2003–2004	7,403	24.5	(21.2 – 28.1)	64,338,000
2005–2006	7,402	24.5	(21.7 – 27.5)	65,423,000
Age group				
1–5 years				
2003–2004	895	8.6	(6.4 – 11.5)	1,741,000
2005–2006	904	9.2	(6.5 – 12.8)	1,857,000
6–11 years				
2001–2002	991	14.7	(10.9 – 19.6)	3,639,000
2003–2004	846	13.3	(9.4 – 18.4)	3,199,000
2005–2006	922	15.0	(11.5 – 19.3)	3,558,000
12–19 years				
2001–2002	2,167	23.6	(20.4 – 27.1)	7,638,000
2003–2004	2,059	23.8	(19.4 – 28.9)	7,881,000
2005–2006	1,985	24.6	(20.8 – 28.8)	8,214,000
20–39 years				
2001–2002	1,691	24.8	(21.8 – 28.1)	19,655,000
2003–2004	1,559	27.5	(23.1 – 32.4)	21,959,000
2005–2006	1,703	24.9	(21.9 – 28.1)	19,866,000
40–59 years				
2001–2002	1,449	24.3	(21.3 – 27.5)	18,368,000
2003–2004	1,278	25.1	(21.0 – 29.6)	19,828,000
2005–2006	1,382	24.8	(20.8 – 29.4)	20,365,000
60 years and older				
2001–2002	1,509	26.9	(23.0 – 31.2)	12,040,000
2003–2004	1,661	23.8	(21.6 – 26.0)	11,054,000
2005–2006	1,410	27.3	(24.1 – 30.6)	13,167,000
Gender				
(6 years and older)				
Males				
2001–2002	3,782	22.8	(20.4 – 25.4)	28,420,000
2003–2004	3,638	23.6	(19.8 – 27.9)	30,162,000
2005–2006	3,603	24.3	(21.2 – 27.8)	31,683,000
Females				
2001–2002	4,025	25.1	(22.5 – 27.9)	33,130,000
2003–2004	3,765	25.4	(22.1 – 28.9)	34,190,000
2005–2006	3,799	24.6	(21.6 – 27.8)	33,739,000
Race/ethnicity				
(6 years and older)				
Mexican Americans				
2001–2002	1,961	35.6	(31.0 – 40.5)	7,496,000
2003–2004	1,802	34.9	(30.6 – 39.5)	7,963,000
2005–2006	1,889	35.5	(30.0 – 41.3)	8,515,000
Non-Hispanic Blacks				
2001–2002	1,821	40.0	(37.5 – 42.6)	12,350,000
2003–2004	1,914	42.2	(38.1 – 46.3)	13,140,000
2005–2006	1,932	39.0	(36.1 – 42.0)	12,422,000
Non-Hispanic Whites				
2001–2002	3,416	18.7	(16.6 – 21.0)	33,627,000
2003–2004	3,155	18.6	(15.6 – 22.1)	33,594,000
2005–2006	3,027	18.9	(16.0 – 22.2)	34,271,000

Table 2.13.d.3. Serum 25-hydroxyvitamin D: Prevalence by survey cycle

Prevalence (in percent) of low serum 25-hydroxyvitamin D concentration (< 40 nmol/L) for the U.S. population, National Health and Nutrition Examination Survey, 2001–2006.

	Sample size	Prevalence (95% conf. interval)	Estimated total number of persons
Total, 6 years and older			
2001–2002	7,807	18.2 (15.5 – 21.3)	46,723,000
2003–2004	7,403	17.2 (13.3 – 21.9)	45,025,000
2005–2006	7,402	18.9 (15.3 – 23.1)	50,461,000
Age group			
1–5 years			
2003–2004	895	3.0 (1.6 – 5.5)	612,000
2005–2006	904	2.3 (1.4 – 3.7)	467,000
6–11 years			
2001–2002	991	5.3 (3.2 – 8.7)	1,313,000
2003–2004	846	5.8 (3.4 – 9.7)	1,399,000
2005–2006	922	5.6 (4.0 – 7.9)	1,338,000
12–19 years			
2001–2002	2,167	17.5 (13.2 – 22.8)	5,660,000
2003–2004	2,059	15.3 (11.2 – 20.6)	5,078,000
2005–2006	1,985	18.9 (13.8 – 25.4)	6,325,000
20–39 years			
2001–2002	1,691	19.7 (16.2 – 23.6)	15,557,000
2003–2004	1,559	19.9 (15.1 – 25.6)	15,829,000
2005–2006	1,703	19.5 (14.9 – 25.2)	15,587,000
40–59 years			
2001–2002	1,449	19.1 (16.0 – 22.7)	14,488,000
2003–2004	1,278	18.5 (13.6 – 24.6)	14,620,000
2005–2006	1,382	21.5 (16.8 – 27.0)	17,595,000
60 years and older			
2001–2002	1,509	20.9 (16.9 – 25.7)	9,371,000
2003–2004	1,661	16.4 (13.4 – 20.0)	7,646,000
2005–2006	1,410	19.1 (15.5 – 23.4)	9,241,000
Gender			
(6 years and older)			
Males			
2001–2002	3,782	14.8 (12.6 – 17.3)	18,450,000
2003–2004	3,638	14.2 (10.4 – 19.1)	18,138,000
2005–2006	3,603	16.6 (13.4 – 20.4)	21,606,000
Females			
2001–2002	4,025	21.4 (18.1 – 25.3)	28,325,000
2003–2004	3,765	20.0 (15.9 – 24.8)	26,932,000
2005–2006	3,799	21.0 (16.8 – 26.0)	28,849,000
Race/ethnicity			
(6 years and older)			
Mexican Americans			
2001–2002	1,961	23.3 (19.0 – 28.2)	4,904,000
2003–2004	1,802	24.5 (19.1 – 30.8)	5,582,000
2005–2006	1,889	28.9 (21.3 – 37.9)	6,943,000
Non-Hispanic Blacks			
2001–2002	1,821	60.6 (57.1 – 64.1)	18,708,000
2003–2004	1,914	51.0 (43.9 – 58.1)	15,900,000
2005–2006	1,932	57.7 (50.3 – 64.7)	18,374,000
Non-Hispanic Whites			
2001–2002	3,416	10.4 (8.6 – 12.4)	18,638,000
2003–2004	3,155	9.5 (7.0 – 12.8)	17,121,000
2005–2006	3,027	10.1 (8.1 – 12.6)	18,342,000

Table 2.13.d.4. Serum 25-hydroxyvitamin D: Prevalence by survey cycle

Prevalence (in percent) of high serum 25-hydroxyvitamin D concentration (> 125 nmol/L) for the U.S. population, National Health and Nutrition Examination Survey, 2001–2006.

	Sample size	Prevalence (95% conf. interval)	Estimated total number of persons
Total, 6 years and older			
2001–2002	7,807	0.8 (0.5 – 1.2)	1,998,000
2003–2004	7,403	1.0 (0.5 – 1.7)	2,547,000
2005–2006	7,402	0.8 (0.6 – 1.2)	2,224,000
Age group			
1–5 years			
2003–2004	895	§	§
2005–2006	904	§	§
6–11 years			
2001–2002	991	§	§
2003–2004	846	§	§
2005–2006	922	§	§
12–19 years			
2001–2002	2,167	§	§
2003–2004	2,059	1.3 (0.7 – 2.3)	427,000
2005–2006	1,985	1.4‡ (0.7 – 2.9)	478,000‡
20–39 years			
2001–2002	1,691	1.0 (0.6 – 1.8)	821,000
2003–2004	1,559	1.7‡ (0.8 – 3.4)	1,334,000‡
2005–2006	1,703	1.3 (0.7 – 2.4)	1,050,000
40–59 years			
2001–2002	1,449	0.8‡ (0.4 – 1.6)	616,000‡
2003–2004	1,278	§	§
2005–2006	1,382	§	§
60 years and older			
2001–2002	1,509	§	§
2003–2004	1,661	§	§
2005–2006	1,410	§	§
Gender			
(6 years and older)			
Males			
2001–2002	3,782	§	§
2003–2004	3,638	§	§
2005–2006	3,603	0.5‡ (0.2 – 1.0)	649,000‡
Females			
2001–2002	4,025	1.1 (0.7 – 1.7)	1,395,000
2003–2004	3,765	1.5 (0.8 – 2.9)	2,071,000
2005–2006	3,799	1.1 (0.7 – 1.9)	1,574,000
Race/ethnicity			
(6 years and older)			
Mexican Americans			
2001–2002	1,961	§	§
2003–2004	1,802	§	§
2005–2006	1,889	§	§
Non-Hispanic Blacks			
2001–2002	1,821	§	§
2003–2004	1,914	§	§
2005–2006	1,932	§	§
Non-Hispanic Whites			
2001–2002	3,416	1.0 (0.7 – 1.5)	1,859,000
2003–2004	3,155	1.3 (0.7 – 2.5)	2,391,000
2005–2006	3,027	1.1 (0.7 – 1.7)	2,047,000

‡ Estimate flagged: 30% ≤ RSE < 40% for the prevalence estimate.
§ Estimate suppressed: RSE ≥ 40% for the prevalence estimate.

References

Aloia JF. African Americans, 25-hydroxyvitamin D, and osteoporosis: a paradox. Am J Clin Nutr. 2008;88(2):545S–550S.

Chung M, Balk EM, Brendel M, Ip S, Lau J, Lee J, et al. Vitamin D and calcium: Systematic review of health outcomes. Evid Rep Technol Assess No. 183. AHRQ Publication No. 09-E015, Rockville, MD: Agency for Healthcare Research and Quality. August 2009.

Cranney A, Horsley T, O'Donnell S, Weiler HA, Puil L, Ooi DS, et al. Effectiveness and safety of vitamin D in relation to bone health. Evid Rep Technol Assess No. 158 AHRQ Publication No. 07-E013, Rockville, MD: Agency for Healthcare Research and Quality. August 2007.

DeLuca HF. The metabolism, physiology, and function of vitamin D. In: Kumar R, editor. Vitamin D: basic and clinical aspects. Boston (MA): M. Nijhoff Publishers; 1984. pp. 1–68.

DeLuca HF. The vitamin D story: a collaborative effort of basic science and clinical medicine. FASEB J. 1988;2:224–236.

Fieser LF, Fieser M. Vitamin D. In: Steroids. 1st ed. New York: Reinhold Publishing Corporation;1959. pp. 90–168.

Haddad JG, Hahn TJ. Natural and synthetic sources of circulating 25-hydroxy-vitamin D in man. Nature. 1973;244:515–517.

Holick MF. Vitamin D: photobiology, metabolism, and clinical applications. In: DeGroot LJ, editor. Endocrinology, Vol 2, 3rd ed. Philadelphia (PA): WB Saunders; 1995. pp. 990–1013.

Holick MF. Vitamin D deficiency. N Engl J Med. 2007;357:266–281.

Institute of Medicine. Food and Nutrition Board. Dietary reference intakes for calcium and vitamin D. Washington, D.C.: National Academies Press; 2011.

Looker AC, Dawson-Hughs B, Calvo MS, Gunter EW, Sayhoun NR. Serum 25-hydroxyvitamin D status of adolescents and adults in two seasonal subpopulations from NHANES III. Bone. 2002;30:771–777.

Looker AC, Pfeiffer CM, Lacher DA, Schleicher RL, Picciano MF, Yetley EA. Serum 25-hydroxyvitamin D status of the US population: 1988–1994 compared with 2000–2004. Am J Clin Nutr. 2008;88:1519–1527.

Looker AC, Johnson CL, Lacher DA, Pfeiffer CM, Schleicher RL, Sempos CT. Vitamin D status: United States, 2001–2006. NCHS Data Brief, No 59. Hyattsville, MD: National Center for Health Statistics. 2011.

Mawer EB, Blackhouse J, Holman CA, Lumb GA, Stanbury DW. The distribution and storage of vitamin D and its metabolites in human tissues. Clin Sci. 1972;43:413–431.

Nagpal S, Na S, Rathnachalam R. Noncalcemic actions of vitamin D receptor ligands. Endocr Rev. 2005;26:662–687.

Pittas AG, Chung M, Trikalinos T, Mitri J, Brendel M, Patel K, et al. Systematic review: Vitamin D and cardiometabolic outcomes. Ann Intern Med. 2010;152:307–314.

Reichel H, Koeffler HP, Norman AW. The role of vitamin D endocrine system in health and disease. N Engl J Med. 1989;320:980–991.

U.S. Department of Agriculture and U.S. Department of Health and Human Services. *Dietary Guidelines for Americans, 2010.* 7th Edition, Washington, DC: U.S. Government Printing Office, December 2010 [cited 2011]. Available at: http://www.cnpp.usda.gov/DGAs2010-PolicyDocument.htm.

Yetley EA, Pfeiffer CM, Schleicher RL, Phinney KW, Lacher DA, Christakos S, et al. NHANES monitoring of serum 25-hydroxyvitamin D: a roundtable summary. J Nutr. 2010;140:2030S–2045S.

Fatty Acids

Background Information

Nomenclature. Fatty acids are organic acids characterized by long unbranched aliphatic tails (4-28 carbons) attached to a carboxyl group. Fatty acids usually possess an even number of carbon atoms; and the carbon chain may contain several unsaturated or exclusively saturated bonds. Thus, fatty acids differ in chain length, degree of saturation, location of the double bond(s) along the chain, and whether the orientation of hydrogen atoms adjacent to the double bond is *cis* or *trans*. Fatty acids with no double bonds are referred to as saturated fatty acids (SFA) while those with one double bond are monounsaturated fatty acids (MUFA). Fatty acids with two or more double bonds are termed polyunsaturated fatty acids (PUFA). PUFA are most often categorized into two groups distinguished by a difference in location of the first double bond from the methyl end of the acyl chain, namely, n-6 and n-3. Linoleic acid (18:2n-6) and alpha-linolenic acid (18:3n-3) are representatives of these two groups. Each contains 18 carbon atoms but differs in the number of double bonds (18:**2**n-6 vs 18:**3**n-3) and the location of the first double bond (18:2**n-6** vs 18:3**n-3**). In this report, unless marked, all unsaturated fatty acids are assumed to be in the *cis* configuration.

Sources and Physiological Functions. Good sources of PUFA include soybean, corn and cottonseed oils (U.S. Department of Agriculture and U.S. Department of Health and Human Services 2010). Oils that are rich in MUFA include olive, canola and safflower oils (U.S. Department of Agriculture and U.S. Department of Health and Human Services 2010). Recent NHANES data provide information on the major food sources of various fatty acids consumed in the United States (U.S. National Institutes of Health 2010a and 2010b). Chicken dishes, desserts, salad dressings, chips, nuts, seeds and pizza are the main sources of n-6 PUFA. The main sources of n-3 PUFA (C18:3n-3) in the American diet are salad dressings, chicken dishes, desserts, pizza, bread, mayonnaise and pasta dishes; whereas, the main sources of long-chain n-3 PUFA (C20:5n-3 and C22:6n-3) are fish and fish mixed dishes. The chief dietary sources of MUFA (C18:1) are desserts, meats, nuts, seeds, pizza, French fries and Mexican foods. The main sources of SFA in the American diet are full-fat cheese, pizza and desserts; other sources include chicken dishes, cured meats, ribs and burgers.

Triacylglycerols (triglycerides), the basic building blocks of fats and oils, are made up of three fatty acids esterified to a glycerol molecule (Lichtenstein 2005). They are usually composed of 2–3 different kinds of fatty acids per molecule. During digestion, dietary triglycerides from animal and vegetable fats are hydrolyzed in the small intestine to release free fatty acids. These acids enter the intestinal cells and are used to resynthesize triglycerides, which become incorporated into large lipoprotein particles called chylomicrons; these in turn are released into the lymph prior to entering the plasma. Fatty acids with 10 or fewer carbon atoms can be absorbed from the gut directly into the bloodstream where they are bound to albumin in the plasma. At distal sites, triglycerides are again hydrolyzed by lipases before fatty acids can enter cells for further metabolism. Once inside peripheral cells, free fatty acids provide an immediate source of energy (fatty acids are the body's major fuel source) or act as substrate for the biosynthesis of signaling molecules such as eicosanoids. Free fatty acids are also incorporated into other lipid classes, such as phospholipids, sphingolipids, and cholesteryl esters, or they may be resynthesized into triglycerides and stored for later use. Phospholipids, which are critical structural components of cellular membranes, tend to incorporate unsaturated fatty acids and so serve as a reservoir for MUFA and PUFA.

Humans are incapable of *de novo* synthesis of n-6 and n-3 PUFA because they lack the ability to insert a double bond any closer than 9 carbons from the methyl end. Thus, linoleic (18:2n-6) and alpha-linolenic (18:3n-3) acid are called "essential" PUFA in that they are required for good health but must be derived from food sources rather than through endogenous biosynthesis or metabolism. Both of these fatty acids are metabolized to longer-chain, more highly unsaturated forms. Note that SFA and MUFA in plasma are not expected to closely reflect dietary intake because these two classes of fatty acids can be endogenously synthesized from carbohydrates. The strongest correlations with dietary intake are provided by plasma concentrations of n-3 PUFA and *trans*-fatty acids (Sun 2007).

Health Effects. The most common MUFA is oleic acid (C18:1n-9); although humans can synthesize this fatty acid, it is obtained largely through the diet. Evidence suggests that replacing dietary carbohydrates with MUFA decreases LDL-cholesterol concentration, but there is little evidence that MUFA are associated with coronary heart disease (Astrup 2011). Currently, intense debate surrounds the question whether reduction in dietary SFA reduces risk of cardiovascular disease (Zelman 2011). At present, the Dietary Guidelines for Americans recommend reduced intake of SFA (U.S. Department of Agriculture and U.S. Department of Health and Human Services 2010). Restricting fat intake and replacing SFA with other nutrients has revealed added complexity in the diet-heart issue. According to evidence from human studies, replacing SFA with PUFA lowers coronary heart disease risk, whereas replacing SFA with carbohydrate either has no benefit (Micha 2010) or may be harmful or beneficial depending upon the quality of the carbohydrate (Jakobsen 2009; Jakobsen 2010). Carbohydrates either rapidly or slowly increase blood glucose; highly refined carbohydrates are amongst the former, and higher intake of these is associated with greater risk for development of diabetes. Replacing SFA with highly refined carbohydrates and added sugars may be increasing heart disease risk through promotion of obesity and diabetes (Hu 2010).

The heart healthy effects of PUFA are most often assessed based on their effects on the concentrations of total cholesterol, HDL- and LDL-cholesterol, cholesterol ratios and/or triglycerides. Intake of n-6 PUFA helps to lower total cholesterol and LDL-cholesterol, however, high intake of n-6 fatty acids may suppress HDL-cholesterol levels. In contrast, n-3 fatty acid consumption has been shown to maintain and even increase HDL status (International Life Sciences Institute 2001). In the United States, the FDA permits qualified health claims to be made about a diet-disease relationship for cardiovascular disease; currently, 6 of the 7 permitted claims for cardiovascular disease are related to the MUFA or PUFA content of nuts, oils and spreads, or fish oil supplements.

Deficiency in the essential fatty acids is determined by use of a plasma triene-to-tetraene ratio (eicosatrienoic [C20:3n-9]:arachidonic [C20:4n-6] acid); a ratio greater than 0.2 indicates deficiency (Institute of Medicine 2005). (Note: eicosatrienoic was not part of the plasma fatty acid profile measured for NHANES 2003-2004.) PUFA deficiency may manifest with neuropathy and skin problems, such as rough or scaly skin and dermatitis (International Life Sciences Institute 2001).

Intake Recommendations. Because the body makes more than enough SFA to meet metabolic needs, people have no requirement for these fatty acids. Evidence suggests that SFA are positively associated with total cholesterol and LDL-cholesterol concentrations and thus with cardiovascular disease risk. Lowering dietary intake of SFA to no more than 10% of caloric intake and replacing them with MUFA and PUFA is recommended to reduce the risk of cardiovascular disease; moreover, lowering the percentage of calories derived from SFA to 7% of calories, can further reduce risk of cardiovascular disease (U.S. Department of Agriculture and U.S. Department of Health and Human Services 2010; Cleeman 2001). The National Cholesterol Education Program Expert Panel on Detection, Evaluation, and Treatment of High Blood Cholesterol in Adults (ATP III) recommends that MUFA not exceed 20% of calories (Cleeman 2001). Guidance about adequate intake (AI) is available for the essential fatty acids. The AI of linoleic acid is 17 g/d for men and 12 g/d for women. For alpha-linolenic acid, the AI is 1.6 g/d for men and 1.1 g/d for women. Moderate evidence shows that consumption of about 8 oz of seafood per week, which provides an average of 250 mg per day of eicosapentaenoic acid (C20:5n-3) and docosahexaenoic acid (C22:6n-3), reduces cardiac deaths among persons with and without cardiovascular disease (U.S. Department of Agriculture and U.S. Department of Health and Human Services 2010). This amount of seafood is also associated with improved infant health outcomes such as visual and cognitive development, when consumed by pregnant or lactating women (U.S. Department of Agriculture and U.S. Department of Health and Human Services 2010). Currently, there is not enough evidence to establish upper tolerable limits for n-3 or n-6 PUFA (Institute of Medicine 2005).

According to the American Heart Association, patients with coronary heart disease should be encouraged to increase their consumption of eicosapentaenoic acid (C20:5n-3) and docosahexaenoic acid (C22:6n-3) to about 1 gram per day preferably from oily fish. The American Heart Association Dietary Guidelines recommend at least two servings of fish per week (particularly fatty fish) for patients without documented coronary heart disease. In addition, inclusion of vegetable oils (e.g., soybean, canola, walnut, flaxseed) and food sources (e.g., walnuts, flaxseeds) high in alpha-linolenic acid (C18:3n-3) is recommended in a healthy diet for the general population (*Kris-Etherton 2002*). The American Heart Association recommends 5-10% of energy from n-6 fatty acids (Harris 2009) while Adult Treatment Panel III recommends up to 10% of total calories may be consumed from polyunsaturated fats (Cleeman 2001).

Biochemical Indicators and Methods. The long term fatty acid content of the diet is best represented by the adipose tissue triglyceride content owing to the two-year half-life of adipose tissue fatty acids. Erythrocytes, due to their 120 day half-life, reflect intermediate term (weeks-to-months) dietary intake, although this idea has been challenged by data demonstrating large changes in the fatty acid composition of erthyrocytes within days of altering dietary fat intake (Hodson 2008). Serum or plasma concentrations represent more recent intake (days-to-weeks). Few studies have compared the fatty acid composition of plasma with red blood cells to assess which substrate best reflects dietary intake. In one study, fatty acid correlations with food frequency questionnaire data were only slightly stronger for erythrocytes than for plasma (Sun 2007). The triglyceride fraction of plasma appears to demonstrate the greatest day-to-day variation of any circulating lipid fraction. Thus, whenever serum or plasma is collected for fatty acid analysis, fasting is preferred to minimize the within- and between-person variability at the time of specimen collection.

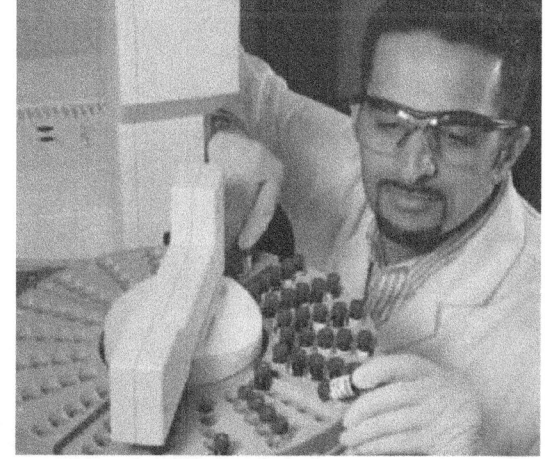

Capillary gas chromatography (GC) is the technique most frequently used to separate fatty acids for quantitative analysis. Detection methods include flame ionization or electron capture negative chemical ionization mass spectrometry. Internal standards are used to correct for losses during sample preparation and improve the accuracy and precision of measurements.

Data in NHANES. The data in this report were generated for fasted (≥ 8 hours) adults (≥ 20 years) by use of gas chromatography-mass spectrometry (GC-MS) based on a modification of the method of Lagerstedt *et al.* (2001). Plasma fatty acid concentrations are reported in μmol/L units.

Generally, fatty acid data are expressed as percentage by weight of total fatty acids (wt%) although percentage by mole (mol%) would be more meaningful. The possible advantages of using absolute concentrations of individual fatty acids have not been well investigated (Hodson 2008). No data exist on plasma concentrations of fatty acids in NHANES prior to 2003. This report shows first-time NHANES data for 24 plasma fatty acids including 6 SFA, 7 MUFA, and 11 PUFA; these data were acquired using surplus plasma from NHANES 2003-2004. The serum specimens were stored at -70°C until fatty acids were measured during the period 2010–2011. Based on limited information in the literature about absolute concentrations, these 24 fatty acids are estimated to comprise at least 90% of the total fatty acids circulating in the plasma in all lipid classes (fatty acyls, glycerolipids, glycerophospholipids, sphingolipids and sterols). All unsaturated fatty acids are assumed to be in the *cis* configuration; *trans*-fatty acids were not measured.

For more information about polyunsaturated fatty acids, see the Institute of Medicine's Dietary Reference Intake reports (Institute of Medicine 2005) and fact sheets from the National Institutes of Health, Office of Dietary Supplements (http://ods.od.nih.gov/FactSheets/Omega3FattyAcidsandHealth.asp).

Highlights

These first-time plasma concentrations of saturated (SFA), monounsaturated (MUFA), and polyunsaturated (PUFA) fatty acids in the U.S. population showed the following demographic patterns and characteristics:

- In general, fatty acids circulated at lower concentrations in younger adults.
- Plasma concentrations of individual fatty acids were generally similar in men and women.
- No consistent race/ethnic pattern was observed for plasma fatty acid concentrations, however heart-healthy polyunsaturated fatty acids showed race/ethnic differences.

All three classes of fatty acids contained representatives at low (< 100 µmol/L) and high concentrations (> 1,000 µmol/L) (Figure H.2.e).

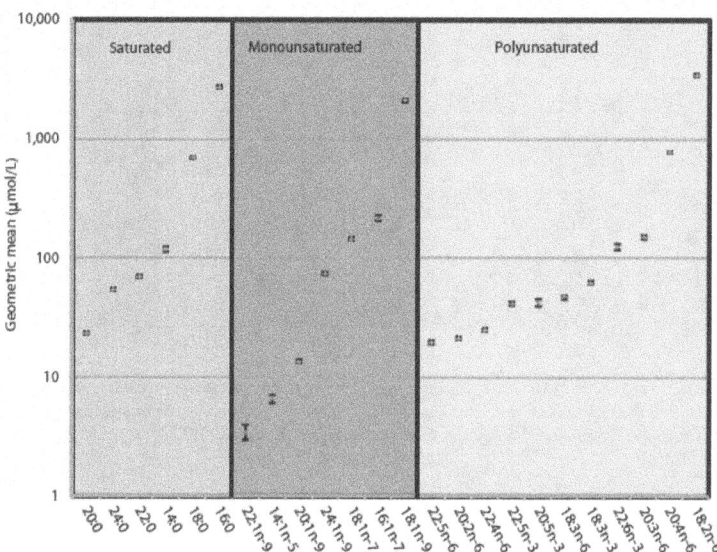

Figure H.2.e. Geometric mean plasma concentrations of individual fatty acids in the U.S. population from fasted adults aged 20 years and older by race/ethnicity, National Health and Nutrition Examination Survey, 2003-2004.

Error bars represent 95% confidence intervals. The y-axis is displayed on the logarithmic scale.

Saturated (SFA)	Monounsaturated (MUFA)	Polyunsaturated (PUFA)
20:0 Arachidic acid	22:1n-9 Docosenoic acid	22:5n-6 Docosapentaenoic acid
24:0 Lignoceric acid	14:1n-5 Myristoleic acid	20:2n-6 Eicosadienoic acid
22:0 Doconsanoic acid	20:1n-9 Eicosenoic acid	22:4n-6 Docosatetraenoic acid
14:0 Myristic acid	24:1n-9 Nervonic acid	22:5n-3 Docosapentaenoic acid
18:0 Stearic acid	18:1n-9 *cis*-Vaccenic acid	20:5n-3 Eicosapentaenoic acid
16:0 Palmitic acid	16:1n-9 Palmitoleic acid	18:3n-6 *gamma*-Linolenic acid
	18:1n-9 Oleic acid	18:3n-3 *alpha*-Linolenic acid
		22:6n-3 Docosahexaenoic acid
		20:3n-6 *homo-gamma*-Linolenic acid
		20:4n-6 Arachidonic acid
		18:2n-6 Linoleic acid

Plasma concentrations of heart-healthy PUFA showed race/ethnic differences. Geometric mean concentrations of eicosapentaenoic acid (EPA), which is typically derived from seafood and supplements, were higher in fasted non-Hispanic blacks and whites compared with Mexican-American adults (Figure H.2.f).

In addition, plasma concentrations of the related long-chain polyunsaturated docosahexaenoic acid (DHA) were higher in non-Hispanic black compared with Mexican-American and non-Hispanic white adults (Figure H.2.g).

Tracking plasma fatty acid concentrations over time will show progress toward more heart-healthy diets.

A.

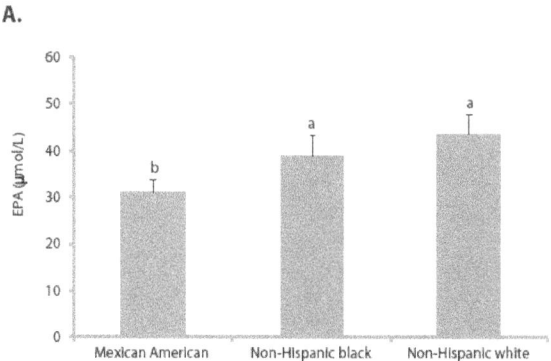

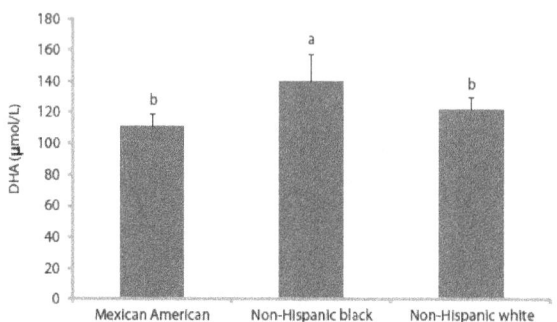

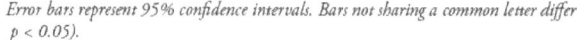

Figure H.2.f. *Geometric mean plasma concentrations of eicosapentaenoic acid (EPA) in the U.S. population from fasted adults aged 20 years and older by race/ethnicity, National Health and Nutrition Examination Survey, 2003-2004.*

Error bars represent 95% confidence intervals. Bars not sharing a common letter differ p < 0.05).

Figure H.2.g. *Geometric mean plasma concentrations of docosahexaenoic acid (DHA) in the U.S. population from fasted adults aged 20 years and older by race/ethnicity, National Health and Nutrition Examination Survey, 2003-2004.*

Error bars represent 95% confidence intervals. Bars not sharing a common letter differ (p < 0.05).

Detailed Observations

The selected observations mentioned below are taken from the tables and figures presented next. Statements about categorical differences between demographic groups noted below are based on non-overlapping confidence limits from univariate analysis without adjusting for demographic variables e.g., age, gender, race/ethnicity) or other blood concentration determinants e.g., dietary intake, supplement usage, smoking, BMI). A multivariate analysis may alter the size and statistical significance of these categorical differences. Furthermore, additional significant differences of smaller magnitude may be present despite their lack of mention here e.g., if confidence limits slightly overlap or if differences are not statistically significant before covariate adjustment has occurred). For a selection of citations of descriptive NHANES papers related to these biochemical indicators of diet and nutrition, see **Appendix G**.

Geometric mean concentrations (NHANES 2003–2004):

- The majority of fatty acids circulated in plasma at lower concentrations in younger adults 20-29 y) compared with those in the older age groups 40-59 and/or 60+ y) Tables 2.14.a.1-2.37.a.1).

- (While in general, plasma concentrations of fatty acids were similar in men and women, there were a few long chain C20-C24) exceptions in which concentrations were higher in women than in men Tables 2.14.a.1-2.37.a.1).

- (Plasma concentrations of approximately one-third of SFA and three-quarters of MUFA were found at lower concentrations in non-Hispanic blacks compared with non-Hispanic whites and/or Mexican Americans. Notably, non-Hispanic blacks had substantially lower plasma concentrations of myristic SFA) and myristoleic MUFA) acid than non-Hispanic whites or Mexican Americans Tables 2.14.a.1 and 2.20.a.1). For PUFA, the picture was mixed with each race/ethnic group having higher or lower concentrations of at least one PUFA compared with one or both race/ethnic groups.

Table 2.14.a.1. Plasma myristic acid (14:0): Concentrations

Geometric mean and selected percentiles of plasma concentrations (in μmol/L) for the fasted U.S. population aged 20 years and older, National Health and Nutrition Examination Survey, 2003–2004.

	Geometric mean (95% conf. interval)	Selected percentiles (95% conf. interval)					Sample size
		2.5th	5th	50th	95th	97.5th	
Total, 20 years and older	119 (113 – 125)	42.5 (39.9 – 45.1)	48.1 (46.2 – 50.5)	116 (108 – 123)	308 (282 – 353)	392 (360 – 438)	1,796
Age group							
20–39 years	110 (104 – 117)	39.0 (31.1 – 42.5)	45.0 (42.5 – 46.8)	106 (99.0 – 118)	301 (252 – 370)	370 (330 – 533)	603
40–59 years	126 (117 – 136)	46.2 (41.4 – 47.9)	51.8 (47.2 – 56.4)	120 (109 – 132)	329 (287 – 401)	410 (383 – 481)	514
60 years and older	121 (112 – 131)	44.5 (37.9 – 47.5)	50.2 (46.3 – 54.5)	120 (112 – 127)	300 (243 – 366)	329 (307 – 426)	679
Gender							
Males	120 (112 – 129)	40.6 (34.0 – 45.1)	47.6 (44.8 – 52.6)	118 (105 – 129)	320 (285 – 384)	414 (366 – 508)	856
Females	117 (111 – 124)	44.6 (39.5 – 45.9)	48.3 (45.9 – 50.8)	115 (107 – 121)	303 (258 – 359)	365 (325 – 434)	940
Race/ethnicity							
Mexican Americans	126 (110 – 144)	41.6† (39.1 – 47.5)	48.5 (40.6 – 52.3)	124 (108 – 144)	342 (304 – 470)	408† (349 – 1,810)	375
Non-Hispanic Blacks	85.8 (78.9 – 93.3)	32.8† (27.9 – 38.3)	39.8 (30.2 – 43.5)	84.3 (72.0 – 95.0)	223 (178 – 283)	261† (229 – 410)	309
Non-Hispanic Whites	123 (116 – 131)	45.6 (38.4 – 47.8)	50.9 (46.5 – 55.8)	119 (110 – 127)	310 (286 – 364)	396 (358 – 464)	982

† Estimate is subject to greater uncertainty due to small cell size.

Figure 2.14.a. Plasma myristic acid (14:0): Concentrations by age group

Geometric mean (95% confidence interval), National Health and Nutrition Examination Survey, 2003–2004

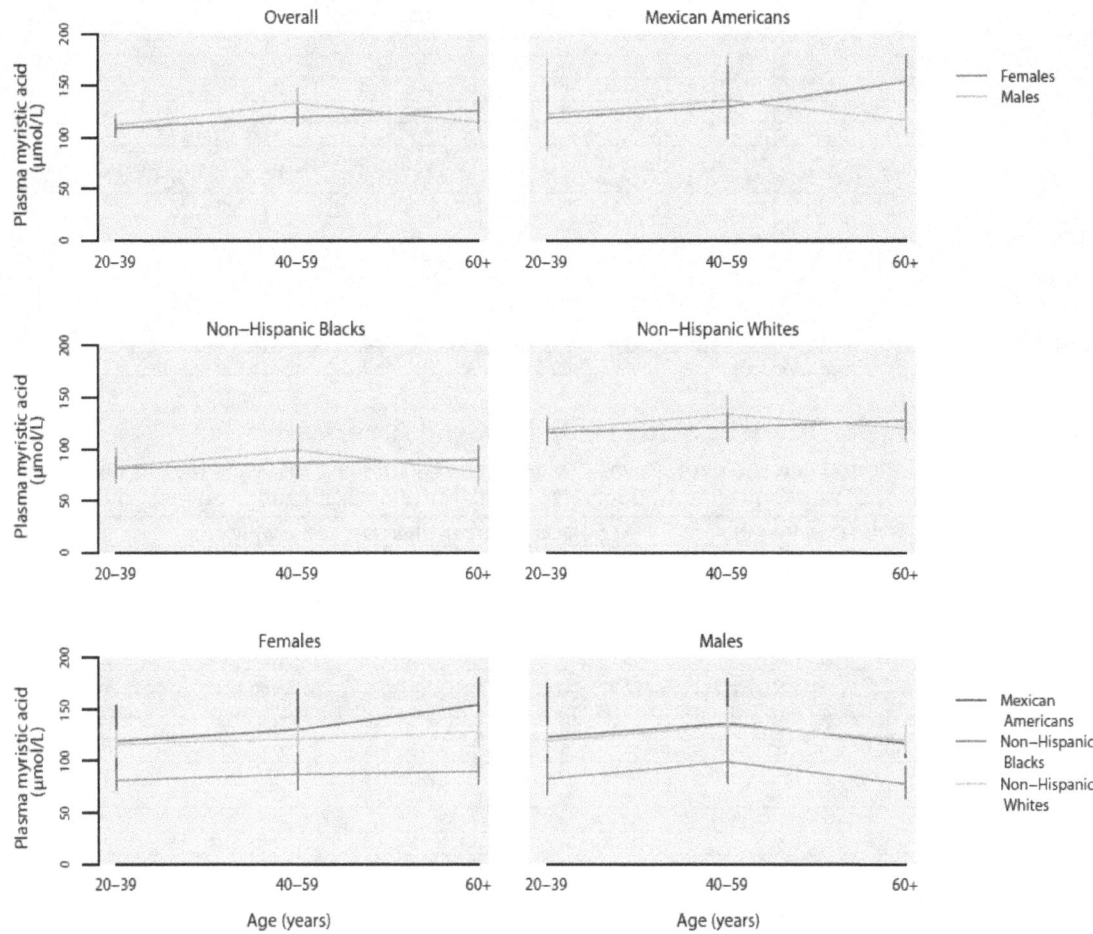

Table 2.14.a.2. Plasma myristic acid (14:0): Total population

Geometric mean and selected percentiles of plasma concentrations (in µmol/L) for the fasted U.S. population aged 20 years and older, National Health and Nutrition Examination Survey, 2003–2004.

| | Geometric mean (95% conf. interval) | Selected percentiles (95% conf. interval) | | | Sample size |
		10th	50th	90th	
Males and Females					
Total, 20 years and older	119 (113 – 125)	57.9 (55.2 – 61.1)	116 (108 – 123)	248 (237 – 266)	1,796
20–39 years	110 (104 – 117)	52.8 (49.4 – 55.9)	106 (99.0 – 118)	240 (209 – 260)	603
40–59 years	126 (117 – 136)	61.8 (56.1 – 66.0)	120 (109 – 132)	266 (248 – 294)	514
60 years and older	121 (112 – 131)	61.4 (54.6 – 67.0)	120 (112 – 127)	238 (224 – 256)	679
Males					
Total, 20 years and older	120 (112 – 129)	58.8 (54.7 – 61.5)	118 (105 – 129)	260 (243 – 272)	856
20–39 years	112 (102 – 122)	53.4 (47.6 – 57.8)	106 (93.5 – 122)	245 (209 – 284)	277
40–59 years	133 (120 – 147)	61.8 (57.5 – 70.6)	124 (109 – 154)	279 (265 – 336)	247
60 years and older	115 (106 – 126)	58.2 (47.3 – 67.9)	119 (112 – 123)	226 (201 – 244)	332
Females					
Total, 20 years and older	117 (111 – 124)	56.6 (53.6 – 61.5)	115 (107 – 121)	242 (225 – 270)	940
20–39 years	109 (101 – 117)	51.3 (49.2 – 55.4)	106 (95.9 – 119)	226 (193 – 308)	326
40–59 years	120 (111 – 131)	61.5 (51.6 – 64.9)	115 (107 – 123)	249 (226 – 301)	267
60 years and older	126 (114 – 139)	64.1 (51.0 – 73.7)	121 (109 – 143)	244 (227 – 302)	347

Table 2.14.a.3. Plasma myristic acid (14:0): Mexican Americans

Geometric mean and selected percentiles of plasma concentrations (in µmol/L) for fasted Mexican Americans in the U.S. population aged 20 years and older, National Health and Nutrition Examination Survey, 2003–2004.

| | Geometric mean (95% conf. interval) | Selected percentiles (95% conf. interval) | | | Sample size |
		10th	50th	90th	
Males and Females					
Total, 20 years and older	126 (110 – 144)	54.6 (49.2 – 62.0)	124 (108 – 144)	277 (244 – 352)	375
20–39 years	122 (95.1 – 155)	51.0 (45.4 – 56.1)	123 (83.9 – 158)	259 (212 – 1,990)	132
40–59 years	133 (112 – 159)	61.2† (46.5 – 76.0)	130 (95.3 – 155)	313† (248 – 387)	93
60 years and older	135 (124 – 146)	68.0 (64.2 – 75.1)	133 (112 – 160)	252 (224 – 315)	150
Males					
Total, 20 years and older	126 (102 – 156)	56.3 (49.6 – 62.4)	123 (95.9 – 153)	282 (228 – 410)	188
20–39 years	123 (86.4 – 175)	51.8† (46.6 – 57.2)	123 (67.8 – 214)	274† (202 – 556)	67
40–59 years	136 (104 – 179)	68.5† (54.1 – 82.7)	125 (90.5 – 177)	305† (201 – 721)	48
60 years and older	117 (104 – 131)	65.6† (48.2 – 71.4)	117 (104 – 135)	199† (164 – 390)	73
Females					
Total, 20 years and older	126 (110 – 145)	51.4 (40.7 – 65.3)	127 (108 – 152)	268 (240 – 339)	187
20–39 years	119 (92.9 – 153)	50.5† (39.7 – 66.1)	121 (93.6 – 150)	245† (173 – 2,410)	65
40–59 years	130 (99.5 – 169)	50.0† (36.9 – 74.6)	134 (83.1 – 193)	313† (248 – 460)	45
60 years and older	154 (131 – 180)	81.6† (54.5 – 95.1)	153 (120 – 195)	274† (228 – 391)	77

† Estimate is subject to greater uncertainty due to small cell size.

Table 2.14.a.4. Plasma myristic acid (14:0): Non-Hispanic blacks

Geometric mean and selected percentiles of plasma concentrations (in μmol/L) for fasted non-Hispanic blacks in the U.S. population aged 20 years and older, National Health and Nutrition Examination Survey, 2003–2004.

	Geometric mean (95% conf. interval)		Selected percentiles (95% conf. interval)						Sample size
			10th		50th		90th		
Males and Females									
Total, 20 years and older	85.8	(78.9 – 93.3)	44.8	(38.0 – 50.1)	84.3	(72.0 – 95.0)	161	(146 – 201)	309
20–39 years	81.9	(72.7 – 92.2)	43.6	(33.7 – 48.1)	76.7	(66.9 – 92.1)	149	(128 – 249)	125
40–59 years	91.9	(82.8 – 102)	44.5†	(28.4 – 51.6)	93.4	(82.5 – 106)	184†	(150 – 249)	98
60 years and older	84.9	(76.3 – 94.5)	46.9†	(36.2 – 58.7)	79.7	(71.8 – 95.2)	154†	(129 – 188)	86
Males									
Total, 20 years and older	87.3	(76.6 – 99.4)	40.9	(31.8 – 46.6)	85.3	(67.2 – 98.7)	170	(148 – 270)	142
20–39 years	82.7	(67.7 – 101)	39.7†	(28.5 – 47.0)	71.6	(61.5 – 101)	167†	(128 – 466)	57
40–59 years	98.8	(78.8 – 124)	41.2†	(29.2 – 55.7)	97.8	(84.0 – 115)	229†	(148 – 479)	42
60 years and older	78.0	(64.2 – 94.6)	43.7†	(36.0 – 52.8)	67.4	(58.9 – 104)	143†	(121 – 187)	43
Females									
Total, 20 years and older	84.7	(76.2 – 94.2)	46.5	(39.2 – 51.8)	83.0	(69.2 – 99.1)	153	(135 – 189)	167
20–39 years	81.2	(72.4 – 91.2)	44.2†	(33.9 – 51.5)	78.8	(64.6 – 98.7)	144†	(110 – 259)	68
40–59 years	87.0	(72.2 – 105)	46.6†	(27.8 – 51.5)	86.5	(64.8 – 106)	160†	(123 – 690)	56
60 years and older	89.6	(78.3 – 103)	53.5†	(39.8 – 63.8)	82.6	(73.5 – 103)	158†	(120 – 194)	43

† Estimate is subject to greater uncertainty due to small cell size.

Table 2.14.a.5. Plasma myristic acid (14:0): Non-Hispanic whites

Geometric mean and selected percentiles of plasma concentrations (in μmol/L) for fasted non-Hispanic whites in the U.S. population aged 20 years and older, National Health and Nutrition Examination Survey, 2003–2004.

	Geometric mean (95% conf. interval)		Selected percentiles (95% conf. interval)						Sample size
			10th		50th		90th		
Males and Females									
Total, 20 years and older	123	(116 – 131)	61.6	(56.2 – 65.5)	119	(110 – 127)	250	(236 – 280)	982
20–39 years	118	(110 – 126)	56.9	(50.1 – 64.0)	115	(103 – 123)	244	(216 – 303)	294
40–59 years	127	(115 – 140)	63.8	(56.4 – 69.1)	120	(108 – 136)	266	(238 – 299)	279
60 years and older	124	(114 – 136)	61.8	(53.5 – 70.8)	121	(116 – 134)	241	(225 – 301)	409
Males									
Total, 20 years and older	126	(115 – 137)	61.5	(56.0 – 67.2)	121	(107 – 141)	263	(243 – 273)	465
20–39 years	119	(107 – 133)	58.3	(35.4 – 67.0)	115	(98.2 – 140)	245	(206 – 337)	124
40–59 years	134	(120 – 151)	65.6	(57.8 – 72.3)	124	(108 – 163)	272	(264 – 317)	139
60 years and older	120	(108 – 134)	58.8	(46.7 – 72.3)	121	(115 – 127)	229	(203 – 262)	202
Females									
Total, 20 years and older	121	(114 – 128)	61.5	(55.6 – 64.2)	118	(110 – 123)	247	(223 – 303)	517
20–39 years	116	(104 – 129)	55.5	(48.9 – 63.3)	114	(97.3 – 128)	240	(197 – 361)	170
40–59 years	121	(108 – 135)	62.2	(48.3 – 69.0)	115	(104 – 123)	237	(195 – 399)	140
60 years and older	128	(114 – 145)	64.1	(47.6 – 74.7)	124	(110 – 146)	248	(229 – 314)	207

Table 2.15.a.1. Plasma palmitic acid (16:0): Concentrations

Geometric mean and selected percentiles of plasma concentrations (in µmol/L) for the fasted U.S. population aged 20 years and older, National Health and Nutrition Examination Survey, 2003–2004.

| | Geometric mean (95% conf. interval) | | Selected percentiles (95% conf. interval) | | | | | | | | | | Sample size |
			2.5th		5th		50th		95th		97.5th		
Total, 20 years and older	2,710	(2,640 – 2,780)	1,570	(1,420 – 1,610)	1,690	(1,610 – 1,770)	2,630	(2,540 – 2,730)	4,710	(4,500 – 5,030)	5,370	(5,180 – 5,630)	1,805
Age group													
20–39 years	2,540	(2,470 – 2,610)	1,440	(1,330 – 1,550)	1,590	(1,480 – 1,670)	2,450	(2,380 – 2,540)	4,550	(4,000 – 5,330)	5,340	(4,740 – 6,860)	609
40–59 years	2,780	(2,680 – 2,880)	1,600	(1,330 – 1,750)	1,830	(1,650 – 1,910)	2,650	(2,530 – 2,800)	4,750	(4,560 – 5,320)	5,410	(5,260 – 5,760)	514
60 years and older	2,890	(2,790 – 2,990)	1,750	(1,610 – 1,860)	1,910	(1,760 – 1,970)	2,820	(2,740 – 2,940)	4,630	(4,390 – 5,160)	5,220	(4,830 – 5,790)	682
Gender													
Males	2,700	(2,590 – 2,810)	1,560	(1,380 – 1,650)	1,670	(1,570 – 1,790)	2,610	(2,500 – 2,710)	4,730	(4,400 – 5,320)	5,630	(5,090 – 6,090)	863
Females	2,720	(2,640 – 2,800)	1,570	(1,400 – 1,610)	1,710	(1,660 – 1,780)	2,640	(2,540 – 2,760)	4,660	(4,450 – 5,270)	5,350	(4,970 – 5,500)	942
Race/ethnicity													
Mexican Americans	2,880	(2,710 – 3,050)	1,500†	(1,310 – 1,710)	1,750	(1,500 – 1,830)	2,750	(2,620 – 2,970)	5,430	(4,580 – 6,310)	5,980†	(5,640 – 6,380)	374
Non-Hispanic Blacks	2,450	(2,340 – 2,570)	1,540†	(1,250 – 1,580)	1,590	(1,320 – 1,730)	2,330	(2,240 – 2,480)	4,020	(3,610 – 4,510)	4,570†	(4,050 – 8,480)	310
Non-Hispanic Whites	2,720	(2,630 – 2,810)	1,570	(1,380 – 1,610)	1,690	(1,600 – 1,780)	2,650	(2,550 – 2,730)	4,720	(4,430 – 5,270)	5,350	(4,930 – 5,640)	991

† Estimate is subject to greater uncertainty due to small cell size.

Figure 2.15.a. Plasma palmitic acid (16:0): Concentrations by age group

Geometric mean (95% confidence interval), National Health and Nutrition Examination Survey, 2003–2004

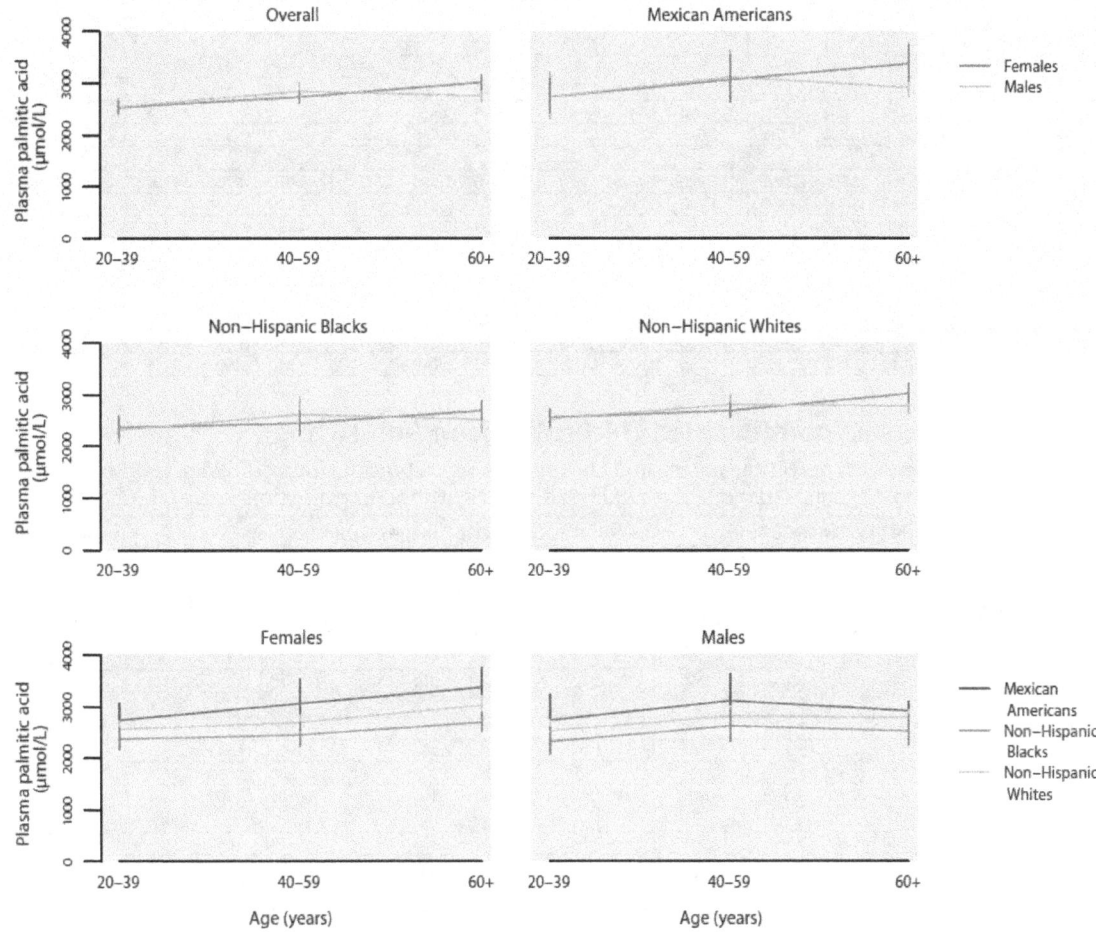

Table 2.15.a.2. Plasma palmitic acid (16:0): Total population

Geometric mean and selected percentiles of plasma concentrations (in µmol/L) for the fasted U.S. population aged 20 years and older, National Health and Nutrition Examination Survey, 2003–2004.

	Geometric mean (95% conf. interval)		Selected percentiles (95% conf. interval)						Sample size
			10th		50th		90th		
Males and Females									
Total, 20 years and older	2,710	(2,640 – 2,780)	1,890	(1,820 – 1,930)	2,630	(2,540 – 2,730)	3,990	(3,820 – 4,360)	1,805
20–39 years	2,540	(2,470 – 2,610)	1,750	(1,660 – 1,810)	2,450	(2,380 – 2,540)	3,790	(3,540 – 4,260)	609
40–59 years	2,780	(2,680 – 2,880)	1,950	(1,910 – 1,990)	2,650	(2,530 – 2,800)	4,160	(3,840 – 4,570)	514
60 years and older	2,890	(2,790 – 2,990)	2,050	(1,960 – 2,140)	2,820	(2,740 – 2,940)	4,050	(3,840 – 4,430)	682
Males									
Total, 20 years and older	2,700	(2,590 – 2,810)	1,880	(1,760 – 1,920)	2,610	(2,500 – 2,710)	4,010	(3,790 – 4,430)	863
20–39 years	2,540	(2,400 – 2,690)	1,740	(1,580 – 1,820)	2,470	(2,340 – 2,600)	3,690	(3,420 – 4,540)	282
40–59 years	2,840	(2,690 – 3,000)	1,950	(1,890 – 2,010)	2,700	(2,480 – 2,870)	4,420	(4,030 – 4,760)	247
60 years and older	2,750	(2,640 – 2,860)	1,960	(1,820 – 2,070)	2,730	(2,620 – 2,830)	3,790	(3,530 – 4,380)	334
Females									
Total, 20 years and older	2,720	(2,640 – 2,800)	1,920	(1,820 – 1,970)	2,640	(2,540 – 2,760)	3,960	(3,810 – 4,370)	942
20–39 years	2,530	(2,440 – 2,640)	1,760	(1,670 – 1,840)	2,440	(2,350 – 2,580)	3,870	(3,510 – 4,530)	327
40–59 years	2,730	(2,620 – 2,840)	1,960	(1,820 – 2,090)	2,590	(2,530 – 2,760)	3,850	(3,620 – 4,630)	267
60 years and older	3,010	(2,870 – 3,150)	2,180	(2,050 – 2,230)	2,950	(2,760 – 3,150)	4,340	(4,000 – 4,570)	348

Table 2.15.a.3. Plasma palmitic acid (16:0): Mexican Americans

Geometric mean and selected percentiles of plasma concentrations (in µmol/L) for fasted Mexican Americans in the U.S. population aged 20 years and older, National Health and Nutrition Examination Survey, 2003–2004.

	Geometric mean (95% conf. interval)		Selected percentiles (95% conf. interval)						Sample size
			10th		50th		90th		
Males and Females									
Total, 20 years and older	2,880	(2,710 – 3,050)	1,900	(1,720 – 2,050)	2,750	(2,620 – 2,970)	4,540	(4,130 – 5,550)	374
20–39 years	2,730	(2,510 – 2,970)	1,820	(1,390 – 1,970)	2,700	(2,350 – 2,890)	4,410	(3,700 – 5,680)	131
40–59 years	3,090	(2,820 – 3,380)	2,000†	(1,480 – 2,330)	2,840	(2,610 – 3,290)	4,940†	(4,130 – 6,470)	93
60 years and older	3,140	(3,010 – 3,280)	2,250	(1,970 – 2,420)	3,150	(3,010 – 3,300)	4,530	(3,910 – 5,350)	150
Males									
Total, 20 years and older	2,850	(2,580 – 3,160)	1,890	(1,570 – 2,010)	2,690	(2,510 – 3,180)	4,500	(4,020 – 5,950)	188
20–39 years	2,730	(2,320 – 3,220)	1,770†	(1,460 – 1,940)	2,540	(2,090 – 3,270)	4,400†	(3,600 – 6,350)	67
40–59 years	3,110	(2,670 – 3,630)	1,950†	(1,790 – 2,530)	2,830	(2,580 – 3,400)	4,580†	(3,880 – 7,970)	48
60 years and older	2,910	(2,740 – 3,080)	2,090†	(1,500 – 2,420)	2,900	(2,580 – 3,230)	3,810†	(3,500 – 5,010)	73
Females									
Total, 20 years and older	2,900	(2,660 – 3,170)	1,930	(1,330 – 2,180)	2,790	(2,450 – 3,280)	4,570	(4,060 – 5,360)	186
20–39 years	2,730	(2,430 – 3,070)	1,840†	(1,300 – 2,150)	2,740	(2,230 – 3,080)	4,330†	(3,560 – 6,760)	64
40–59 years	3,060	(2,650 – 3,530)	2,050†	(1,480 – 2,330)	2,890	(2,460 – 3,500)	4,950†	(3,540 – 6,010)	45
60 years and older	3,370	(3,050 – 3,740)	2,370†	(2,060 – 2,540)	3,370	(2,780 – 3,790)	5,020†	(4,210 – 6,170)	77

† Estimate is subject to greater uncertainty due to small cell size.

Table 2.15.a.4. Plasma palmitic acid (16:0): Non-Hispanic blacks

Geometric mean and selected percentiles of plasma concentrations (in µmol/L) for fasted non-Hispanic blacks in the U.S. population aged 20 years and older, National Health and Nutrition Examination Survey, 2003–2004.

	Geometric mean (95% conf. interval)		Selected percentiles (95% conf. interval)						Sample size
			10th		50th		90th		
Males and Females									
Total, 20 years and older	2,450	(2,340 – 2,570)	1,750	(1,600 – 1,830)	2,330	(2,240 – 2,480)	3,430	(3,330 – 3,630)	310
20–39 years	2,350	(2,170 – 2,530)	1,680	(1,410 – 1,810)	2,190	(2,070 – 2,480)	3,390	(3,140 – 3,730)	126
40–59 years	2,520	(2,370 – 2,680)	1,790†	(1,620 – 1,890)	2,350	(2,270 – 2,590)	3,430†	(3,370 – 4,090)	98
60 years and older	2,620	(2,490 – 2,760)	2,030†	(1,870 – 2,180)	2,510	(2,430 – 2,760)	3,450†	(3,280 – 3,770)	86
Males									
Total, 20 years and older	2,450	(2,280 – 2,640)	1,690	(1,550 – 1,810)	2,340	(2,180 – 2,500)	3,550	(3,170 – 4,270)	143
20–39 years	2,320	(2,080 – 2,600)	1,570†	(1,310 – 1,770)	2,140	(1,930 – 2,710)	3,410†	(2,940 – 9,940)	58
40–59 years	2,620	(2,330 – 2,940)	1,770†	(1,380 – 1,950)	2,370	(2,290 – 2,620)	4,060†	(2,900 – 8,390)	42
60 years and older	2,520	(2,260 – 2,820)	1,740†	(1,640 – 1,910)	2,440	(2,150 – 2,980)	3,290†	(3,000 – 4,330)	43
Females									
Total, 20 years and older	2,450	(2,300 – 2,620)	1,800	(1,690 – 1,870)	2,330	(2,230 – 2,570)	3,380	(3,210 – 3,680)	167
20–39 years	2,370	(2,170 – 2,580)	1,700†	(1,390 – 1,850)	2,230	(2,030 – 2,590)	3,350†	(3,110 – 4,210)	68
40–59 years	2,450	(2,230 – 2,680)	1,780†	(1,260 – 1,940)	2,330	(2,140 – 2,650)	3,370†	(2,930 – 6,230)	56
60 years and older	2,690	(2,520 – 2,870)	2,180†	(1,950 – 2,240)	2,530	(2,400 – 2,790)	3,510†	(3,260 – 4,220)	43

† Estimate is subject to greater uncertainty due to small cell size.

Table 2.15.a.5. Plasma palmitic acid (16:0): Non-Hispanic whites

Geometric mean and selected percentiles of plasma concentrations (in µmol/L) for fasted non-Hispanic whites in the U.S. population aged 20 years and older, National Health and Nutrition Examination Survey, 2003–2004.

	Geometric mean (95% conf. interval)		Selected percentiles (95% conf. interval)						Sample size
			10th		50th		90th		
Males and Females									
Total, 20 years and older	2,720	(2,630 – 2,810)	1,900	(1,800 – 1,950)	2,650	(2,550 – 2,730)	3,960	(3,810 – 4,420)	991
20–39 years	2,550	(2,450 – 2,640)	1,720	(1,600 – 1,810)	2,450	(2,370 – 2,590)	3,790	(3,510 – 4,490)	300
40–59 years	2,750	(2,630 – 2,870)	1,950	(1,900 – 1,990)	2,640	(2,500 – 2,800)	4,040	(3,790 – 4,700)	279
60 years and older	2,910	(2,790 – 3,030)	2,040	(1,950 – 2,140)	2,840	(2,730 – 2,990)	4,150	(3,840 – 4,520)	412
Males									
Total, 20 years and older	2,700	(2,580 – 2,840)	1,890	(1,750 – 1,940)	2,630	(2,500 – 2,740)	3,960	(3,770 – 4,500)	471
20–39 years	2,530	(2,360 – 2,720)	1,680	(1,540 – 1,800)	2,460	(2,350 – 2,620)	3,630	(3,260 – 5,810)	128
40–59 years	2,810	(2,630 – 2,990)	1,950	(1,890 – 2,010)	2,700	(2,460 – 2,930)	4,280	(3,850 – 4,740)	139
60 years and older	2,780	(2,640 – 2,920)	1,950	(1,760 – 2,070)	2,750	(2,600 – 2,930)	3,830	(3,530 – 4,690)	204
Females									
Total, 20 years and older	2,730	(2,640 – 2,820)	1,920	(1,810 – 1,970)	2,650	(2,550 – 2,770)	3,970	(3,810 – 4,500)	520
20–39 years	2,560	(2,410 – 2,710)	1,740	(1,600 – 1,870)	2,440	(2,280 – 2,690)	3,890	(3,490 – 4,960)	172
40–59 years	2,690	(2,570 – 2,830)	1,940	(1,720 – 2,110)	2,580	(2,530 – 2,710)	3,780	(3,510 – 4,690)	140
60 years and older	3,020	(2,860 – 3,200)	2,140	(2,010 – 2,250)	2,960	(2,750 – 3,210)	4,440	(4,030 – 4,660)	208

Table 2.16.a.1. Plasma stearic acid (18:0): Concentrations

Geometric mean and selected percentiles of plasma concentrations (in μmol/L) for the fasted U.S. population aged 20 years and older, National Health and Nutrition Examination Survey, 2003–2004.

| | Geometric mean (95% conf. interval) | Selected percentiles (95% conf. interval) | | | | | Sample size |
		2.5th	5th	50th	95th	97.5th	
Total, 20 years and older	692 (678 – 706)	432 (411 – 444)	471 (440 – 484)	684 (663 – 705)	1,040 (1,020 – 1,100)	1,180 (1,130 – 1,270)	1,806
Age group							
20–39 years	649 (635 – 664)	420 (362 – 437)	444 (422 – 468)	638 (624 – 659)	998 (922 – 1,120)	1,150 (1,030 – 1,470)	609
40–59 years	718 (698 – 738)	430 (383 – 473)	481 (426 – 524)	711 (682 – 733)	1,100 (1,040 – 1,160)	1,210 (1,130 – 1,350)	515
60 years and older	724 (703 – 746)	471 (430 – 489)	511 (473 – 534)	731 (697 – 763)	1,030 (976 – 1,120)	1,130 (1,040 – 1,310)	682
Gender							
Males	690 (671 – 710)	433 (408 – 469)	472 (440 – 483)	673 (644 – 711)	1,090 (1,030 – 1,200)	1,280 (1,170 – 1,360)	864
Females	694 (677 – 712)	421 (399 – 441)	462 (433 – 489)	689 (667 – 712)	1,030 (975 – 1,080)	1,140 (1,080 – 1,190)	942
Race/ethnicity							
Mexican Americans	710 (677 – 745)	440† (411 – 467)	475 (434 – 492)	710 (666 – 748)	1,150 (1,030 – 1,320)	1,210† (1,170 – 1,330)	374
Non-Hispanic Blacks	676 (655 – 697)	440† (356 – 471)	473 (435 – 495)	669 (645 – 693)	961 (901 – 1,130)	1,130† (998 – 2,010)	310
Non-Hispanic Whites	692 (676 – 709)	421 (408 – 441)	465 (430 – 485)	686 (663 – 709)	1,040 (1,020 – 1,090)	1,170 (1,090 – 1,270)	992

† Estimate is subject to greater uncertainty due to small cell size.

Figure 2.16.a. Plasma stearic acid (18:0): Concentrations by age group

Geometric mean (95% confidence interval), National Health and Nutrition Examination Survey, 2003–2004

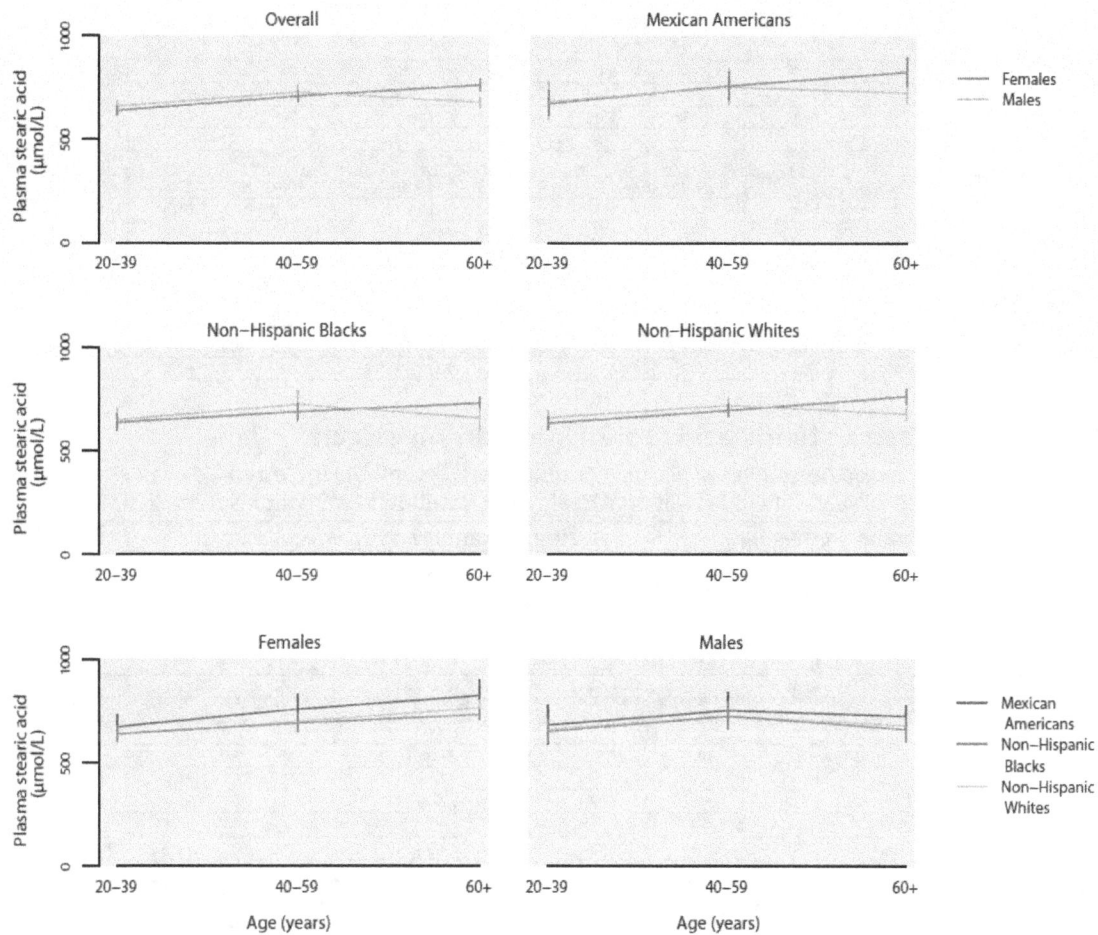

Table 2.16.a.2. Plasma stearic acid (18:0): Total population

Geometric mean and selected percentiles of plasma concentrations (in µmol/L) for the fasted U.S. population aged 20 years and older, National Health and Nutrition Examination Survey, 2003–2004.

	Geometric mean (95% conf. interval)		Selected percentiles (95% conf. interval)						Sample size
			10th		50th		90th		
Males and Females									
Total, 20 years and older	692	(678 – 706)	515	(489 – 531)	684	(663 – 705)	939	(914 – 963)	1,806
20–39 years	649	(635 – 664)	484	(468 – 498)	638	(624 – 659)	870	(831 – 932)	609
40–59 years	718	(698 – 738)	545	(520 – 557)	711	(682 – 733)	989	(955 – 1,030)	515
60 years and older	724	(703 – 746)	552	(538 – 567)	731	(697 – 763)	930	(893 – 976)	682
Males									
Total, 20 years and older	690	(671 – 710)	509	(483 – 527)	673	(644 – 711)	967	(930 – 1,010)	864
20–39 years	660	(636 – 686)	484	(469 – 504)	643	(615 – 672)	888	(831 – 1,010)	282
40–59 years	728	(697 – 761)	548	(520 – 571)	711	(646 – 752)	1,020	(997 – 1,040)	248
60 years and older	679	(656 – 703)	514	(472 – 546)	679	(659 – 718)	874	(825 – 960)	334
Females									
Total, 20 years and older	694	(677 – 712)	522	(484 – 543)	689	(667 – 712)	916	(892 – 951)	942
20–39 years	639	(620 – 658)	483	(454 – 504)	635	(622 – 658)	849	(817 – 919)	327
40–59 years	709	(685 – 733)	532	(478 – 566)	710	(687 – 733)	934	(900 – 990)	267
60 years and older	763	(736 – 790)	617	(573 – 628)	763	(735 – 786)	971	(914 – 1,020)	348

Table 2.16.a.3. Plasma stearic acid (18:0): Mexican Americans

Geometric mean and selected percentiles of plasma concentrations (in µmol/L) for fasted Mexican Americans in the U.S. population aged 20 years and older, National Health and Nutrition Examination Survey, 2003–2004.

	Geometric mean (95% conf. interval)		Selected percentiles (95% conf. interval)						Sample size
			10th		50th		90th		
Males and Females									
Total, 20 years and older	710	(677 – 745)	503	(485 – 528)	710	(666 – 748)	997	(921 – 1,160)	374
20–39 years	678	(632 – 727)	492	(464 – 510)	664	(594 – 755)	971	(801 – 1,330)	131
40–59 years	756	(710 – 806)	534†	(457 – 587)	746	(714 – 770)	1,060†	(915 – 1,470)	93
60 years and older	776	(735 – 820)	602	(491 – 646)	767	(720 – 815)	1,060	(961 – 1,180)	150
Males									
Total, 20 years and older	705	(651 – 764)	501	(480 – 522)	690	(611 – 766)	1,030	(919 – 1,210)	188
20–39 years	682	(596 – 779)	492†	(456 – 508)	647	(540 – 805)	1,040†	(830 – 1,330)	67
40–59 years	753	(675 – 841)	529†	(469 – 595)	725	(656 – 815)	1,010†	(911 – 1,490)	48
60 years and older	726	(678 – 776)	593†	(457 – 610)	720	(658 – 783)	896†	(832 – 1,300)	73
Females									
Total, 20 years and older	716	(677 – 758)	514	(443 – 559)	730	(669 – 777)	996	(885 – 1,140)	186
20–39 years	673	(620 – 732)	481†	(340 – 555)	678	(629 – 751)	835†	(791 – 1,140)	64
40–59 years	759	(696 – 828)	519†	(439 – 624)	756	(700 – 819)	1,070†	(859 – 1,410)	45
60 years and older	826	(760 – 897)	624†	(541 – 652)	810	(736 – 903)	1,100†	(1,050 – 1,250)	77

† Estimate is subject to greater uncertainty due to small cell size.

Table 2.16.a.4. Plasma stearic acid (18:0): Non-Hispanic blacks

Geometric mean and selected percentiles of plasma concentrations (in µmol/L) for fasted non-Hispanic blacks in the U.S. population aged 20 years and older, National Health and Nutrition Examination Survey, 2003–2004.

	Geometric mean (95% conf. interval)		Selected percentiles (95% conf. interval)						Sample size
			10th		50th		90th		
Males and Females									
Total, 20 years and older	676	(655 – 697)	509	(458 – 540)	669	(645 – 693)	886	(835 – 941)	310
20–39 years	645	(610 – 682)	483	(435 – 514)	641	(587 – 672)	887	(808 – 945)	126
40–59 years	706	(675 – 738)	542†	(477 – 567)	693	(664 – 710)	908†	(833 – 1,120)	98
60 years and older	705	(681 – 729)	561†	(511 – 615)	711	(692 – 753)	834†	(806 – 886)	86
Males									
Total, 20 years and older	678	(645 – 713)	483	(455 – 524)	663	(618 – 696)	925	(854 – 1,110)	143
20–39 years	651	(602 – 704)	461†	(422 – 517)	619	(569 – 687)	897†	(803 – 2,540)	58
40–59 years	726	(665 – 792)	544†	(475 – 557)	676	(621 – 738)	1,010†	(877 – 1,670)	42
60 years and older	662	(608 – 720)	503†	(334 – 555)	673	(615 – 738)	830†	(782 – 974)	43
Females									
Total, 20 years and older	674	(649 – 699)	514	(354 – 567)	674	(644 – 702)	834	(789 – 1,030)	167
20–39 years	639	(604 – 677)	496†	(446 – 515)	645	(594 – 667)	833†	(715 – 1,090)	68
40–59 years	691	(651 – 733)	526†	(353 – 589)	693	(643 – 710)	826†	(774 – 2,490)	56
60 years and older	733	(710 – 757)	638†	(558 – 668)	718	(696 – 779)	842†	(800 – 885)	43

† Estimate is subject to greater uncertainty due to small cell size.

Table 2.16.a.5. Plasma stearic acid (18:0): Non-Hispanic whites

Geometric mean and selected percentiles of plasma concentrations (in µmol/L) for fasted non-Hispanic whites in the U.S. population aged 20 years and older, National Health and Nutrition Examination Survey, 2003–2004.

	Geometric mean (95% conf. interval)		Selected percentiles (95% conf. interval)						Sample size
			10th		50th		90th		
Males and Females									
Total, 20 years and older	692	(676 – 709)	515	(484 – 533)	686	(663 – 709)	940	(913 – 973)	992
20–39 years	648	(627 – 669)	481	(441 – 507)	635	(614 – 661)	853	(823 – 953)	300
40–59 years	710	(689 – 733)	540	(494 – 565)	705	(675 – 727)	969	(946 – 1,020)	280
60 years and older	726	(700 – 753)	546	(524 – 566)	733	(695 – 770)	940	(900 – 1,020)	412
Males									
Total, 20 years and older	691	(669 – 715)	512	(480 – 533)	678	(644 – 720)	959	(919 – 1,010)	472
20–39 years	662	(629 – 696)	484	(433 – 513)	654	(615 – 675)	844	(810 – 1,250)	128
40–59 years	723	(691 – 757)	558	(513 – 576)	709	(640 – 749)	1,020	(975 – 1,040)	140
60 years and older	681	(653 – 711)	508	(471 – 545)	687	(652 – 726)	880	(819 – 1,030)	204
Females									
Total, 20 years and older	693	(673 – 713)	516	(481 – 537)	689	(664 – 713)	923	(899 – 954)	520
20–39 years	636	(607 – 666)	460	(427 – 510)	627	(608 – 658)	874	(818 – 1,000)	172
40–59 years	698	(672 – 725)	519	(441 – 554)	699	(675 – 730)	934	(902 – 966)	140
60 years and older	766	(733 – 801)	611	(543 – 630)	767	(735 – 801)	981	(911 – 1,050)	208

Table 2.17.a.1. Plasma arachidic acid (20:0): Concentrations

Geometric mean and selected percentiles of plasma concentrations (in µmol/L) for the fasted U.S. population aged 20 years and older, National Health and Nutrition Examination Survey, 2003–2004.

	Geometric mean (95% conf. interval)	Selected percentiles (95% conf. interval)						Sample size
		2.5th	5th	50th	95th	97.5th		
Total, 20 years and older	23.4 (23.0 – 23.9)	15.1 (14.4 – 15.5)	16.2 (15.4 – 16.7)	23.2 (22.9 – 23.6)	33.6 (32.5 – 35.9)	36.7 (35.0 – 39.1)		1,757
Age group								
20–39 years	22.2 (21.6 – 22.9)	14.8 (13.3 – 15.2)	15.6 (15.0 – 16.2)	22.1 (21.4 – 23.0)	31.6 (30.3 – 34.0)	33.9 (32.4 – 36.6)		592
40–59 years	23.9 (23.3 – 24.5)	15.4 (14.4 – 16.3)	16.8 (15.6 – 17.5)	23.5 (22.9 – 24.2)	34.0 (32.4 – 36.8)	36.9 (34.2 – 43.6)		500
60 years and older	24.8 (24.1 – 25.4)	15.6 (13.7 – 16.3)	16.7 (15.6 – 18.0)	24.9 (23.8 – 25.7)	36.1 (33.8 – 38.6)	38.6 (36.5 – 42.2)		665
Gender								
Males	22.3 (21.8 – 22.8)	14.4 (12.7 – 15.2)	15.5 (14.5 – 16.3)	22.0 (21.7 – 22.3)	32.0 (31.4 – 32.8)	33.8 (32.5 – 36.4)		843
Females	24.5 (23.9 – 25.1)	15.9 (15.0 – 16.5)	16.9 (16.1 – 17.7)	24.3 (23.7 – 25.1)	35.7 (33.6 – 38.4)	38.5 (36.4 – 42.2)		914
Race/ethnicity								
Mexican Americans	22.5 (21.3 – 23.8)	13.5† (11.4 – 15.6)	15.6 (12.7 – 16.8)	22.4 (21.1 – 23.7)	32.7 (31.2 – 35.5)	35.1† (33.2 – 41.0)		367
Non-Hispanic Blacks	23.2 (22.1 – 24.3)	14.6† (9.41 – 15.3)	15.4 (13.6 – 16.7)	22.7 (21.9 – 23.5)	33.4 (31.2 – 40.8)	35.9† (33.6 – 76.6)		307
Non-Hispanic Whites	23.6 (23.0 – 24.2)	15.3 (14.1 – 15.8)	16.3 (15.3 – 16.8)	23.5 (22.9 – 24.0)	34.1 (32.6 – 36.9)	37.5 (35.6 – 39.5)		962

† Estimate is subject to greater uncertainty due to small cell size.

Figure 2.17.a. Plasma arachidic acid (20:0): Concentrations by age group

Geometric mean (95% confidence interval), National Health and Nutrition Examination Survey, 2003–2004

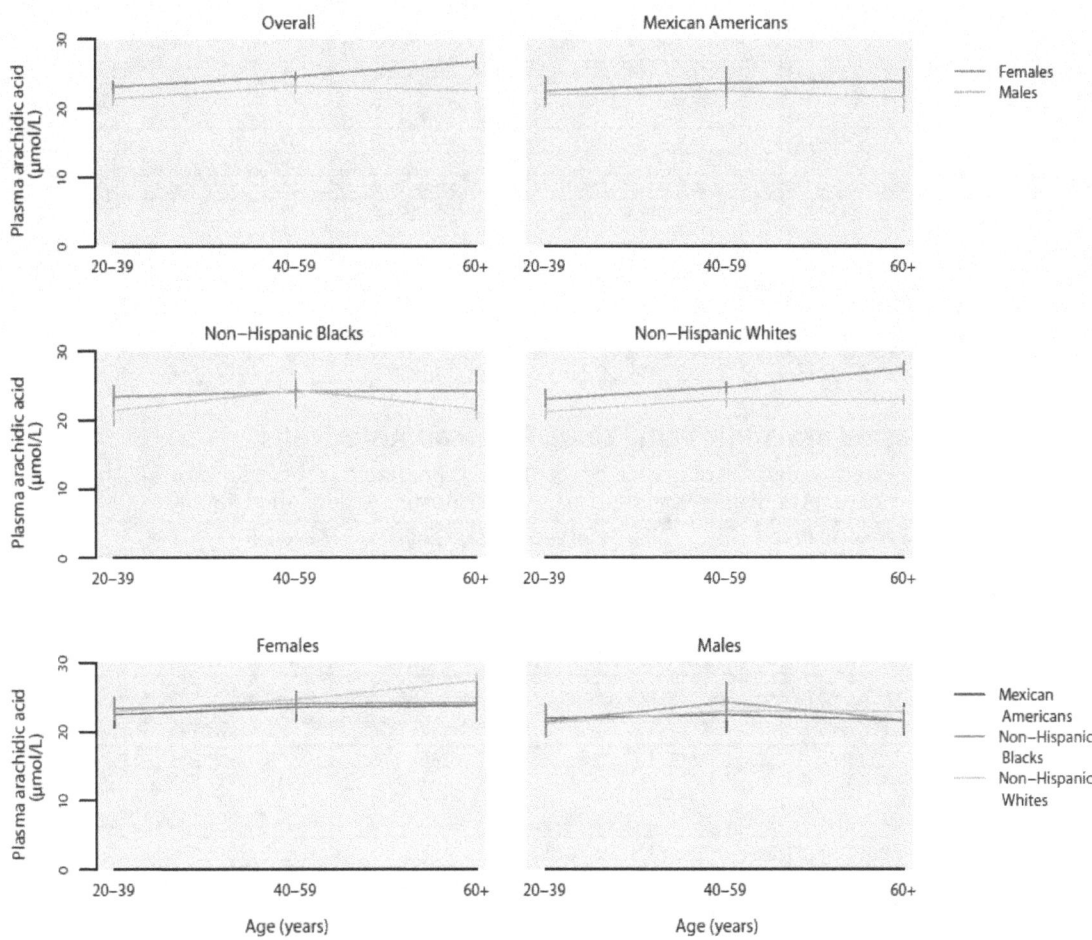

Table 2.17.a.2. Plasma arachidic acid (20:0): Total population

Geometric mean and selected percentiles of plasma concentrations (in μmol/L) for the fasted U.S. population aged 20 years and older, National Health and Nutrition Examination Survey, 2003–2004.

	Geometric mean (95% conf. interval)	Selected percentiles (95% conf. interval)						Sample size
		10th		50th		90th		
Males and Females								
Total, 20 years and older	23.4	(23.0 – 23.9)	17.6	(16.9 – 18.1)	23.2	(22.9 – 23.6)	31.2	(30.4 – 32.1)	1,757
20–39 years	22.2	(21.6 – 22.9)	16.6	(16.0 – 17.2)	22.1	(21.4 – 23.0)	29.5	(28.7 – 30.6)	592
40–59 years	23.9	(23.3 – 24.5)	18.3	(17.5 – 18.8)	23.5	(22.9 – 24.2)	31.4	(30.2 – 32.9)	500
60 years and older	24.8	(24.1 – 25.4)	18.5	(18.0 – 19.1)	24.9	(23.8 – 25.7)	32.9	(31.9 – 34.2)	665
Males								
Total, 20 years and older	22.3	(21.8 – 22.8)	16.8	(16.0 – 17.5)	22.0	(21.7 – 22.3)	29.6	(29.0 – 31.0)	843
20–39 years	21.4	(20.6 – 22.3)	16.4	(15.2 – 17.1)	21.0	(20.5 – 21.8)	28.1	(26.1 – 31.6)	275
40–59 years	23.1	(22.2 – 23.9)	17.4	(16.6 – 18.0)	22.7	(22.0 – 23.8)	31.1	(29.2 – 32.1)	241
60 years and older	22.6	(22.1 – 23.0)	16.8	(15.8 – 18.1)	22.4	(21.8 – 23.0)	29.4	(28.9 – 30.4)	327
Females								
Total, 20 years and older	24.5	(23.9 – 25.1)	18.7	(18.0 – 19.0)	24.3	(23.7 – 25.1)	32.3	(31.2 – 33.6)	914
20–39 years	23.1	(22.3 – 23.9)	16.9	(16.2 – 18.5)	23.4	(22.6 – 23.8)	30.1	(29.2 – 31.2)	317
40–59 years	24.6	(24.1 – 25.2)	18.9	(18.3 – 19.3)	24.2	(23.5 – 25.3)	32.6	(30.7 – 34.4)	259
60 years and older	26.7	(25.8 – 27.7)	20.1	(18.8 – 21.2)	26.9	(25.7 – 28.1)	35.4	(33.2 – 38.1)	338

Table 2.17.a.3. Plasma arachidic acid (20:0): Mexican Americans

Geometric mean and selected percentiles of plasma concentrations (in μmol/L) for fasted Mexican Americans in the U.S. population aged 20 years and older, National Health and Nutrition Examination Survey, 2003–2004.

	Geometric mean (95% conf. interval)	Selected percentiles (95% conf. interval)						Sample size
		10th		50th		90th		
Males and Females								
Total, 20 years and older	22.5	(21.3 – 23.8)	16.9	(15.3 – 18.2)	22.4	(21.1 – 23.7)	29.6	(27.9 – 33.1)	367
20–39 years	22.2	(20.8 – 23.6)	16.5	(12.4 – 18.3)	21.8	(20.6 – 23.6)	29.5	(27.1 – 36.1)	130
40–59 years	23.0	(21.1 – 25.0)	16.9†	(13.9 – 18.7)	23.0	(21.4 – 25.2)	30.6†	(27.4 – 41.6)	91
60 years and older	22.7	(21.2 – 24.4)	17.4	(14.6 – 18.7)	22.9	(21.8 – 24.2)	29.3	(27.4 – 34.1)	146
Males								
Total, 20 years and older	22.1	(20.6 – 23.7)	16.8	(9.37 – 18.3)	22.4	(20.5 – 23.8)	28.3	(26.9 – 32.7)	185
20–39 years	21.9	(20.2 – 23.9)	16.6†	(11.7 – 19.0)	21.7	(19.6 – 23.9)	27.6†	(24.5 – 36.3)	66
40–59 years	22.4	(19.9 – 25.3)	15.9†	(12.5 – 19.1)	23.0	(19.4 – 25.4)	29.3†	(26.8 – 31.9)	47
60 years and older	21.6	(19.5 – 24.0)	15.8†	(9.37 – 18.7)	21.9	(20.2 – 24.7)	27.8†	(25.5 – 32.7)	72
Females								
Total, 20 years and older	23.0	(21.6 – 24.5)	16.8	(15.9 – 18.5)	22.5	(21.3 – 24.0)	31.0	(28.3 – 43.0)	182
20–39 years	22.5	(20.6 – 24.5)	16.4†	(12.9 – 18.5)	21.8	(20.2 – 23.9)	29.7†	(27.3 – 43.7)	64
40–59 years	23.6	(21.6 – 25.8)	17.3†	(15.6 – 19.2)	22.8	(21.3 – 25.3)	31.8†	(27.5 – 41.6)	44
60 years and older	23.8	(21.9 – 25.9)	18.5†	(13.1 – 20.6)	23.9	(22.2 – 24.5)	30.2†	(27.2 – 40.1)	74

† Estimate is subject to greater uncertainty due to small cell size.

Table 2.17.a.4. Plasma arachidic acid (20:0): Non-Hispanic blacks

Geometric mean and selected percentiles of plasma concentrations (in μmol/L) for fasted non-Hispanic blacks in the U.S. population aged 20 years and older, National Health and Nutrition Examination Survey, 2003–2004.

	Geometric mean (95% conf. interval)	Selected percentiles (95% conf. interval)						Sample size
		10th		50th		90th		
Males and Females								
Total, 20 years and older	23.2 (22.1 – 24.3)	17.4	(15.9 – 18.4)	22.7	(21.9 – 23.5)	31.0	(29.3 – 33.1)	307
20–39 years	22.5 (21.3 – 23.8)	17.0	(13.7 – 18.5)	22.0	(21.4 – 22.8)	30.5	(28.0 – 34.0)	124
40–59 years	24.2 (22.6 – 25.8)	17.0†	(15.3 – 19.1)	23.5	(22.5 – 25.2)	31.9†	(29.4 – 35.9)	98
60 years and older	23.2 (21.7 – 24.7)	18.3†	(15.4 – 18.8)	22.9	(21.1 – 25.6)	29.5†	(28.3 – 35.6)	85
Males								
Total, 20 years and older	22.4 (21.2 – 23.7)	15.9	(11.7 – 18.2)	21.5	(20.7 – 22.8)	31.2	(29.0 – 35.8)	142
20–39 years	21.4 (19.2 – 23.9)	14.9†	(11.3 – 18.3)	20.7	(18.6 – 22.4)	31.2†	(23.2 – 71.3)	57
40–59 years	24.3 (21.7 – 27.1)	16.1†	(14.7 – 19.7)	23.1	(21.3 – 26.5)	31.7†	(29.4 – 48.6)	42
60 years and older	21.6 (20.2 – 23.1)	15.5†	(8.59 – 18.4)	21.2	(20.3 – 24.1)	27.9†	(25.6 – 33.8)	43
Females								
Total, 20 years and older	23.8 (22.6 – 25.1)	18.4	(16.2 – 19.9)	23.4	(22.2 – 25.1)	30.3	(28.7 – 34.8)	165
20–39 years	23.4 (22.0 – 25.0)	18.7†	(14.9 – 20.5)	22.8	(21.9 – 23.5)	29.5†	(27.8 – 32.5)	67
40–59 years	24.1 (22.7 – 25.6)	17.0†	(14.8 – 20.5)	23.6	(21.8 – 25.8)	31.8†	(27.7 – 54.9)	56
60 years and older	24.2 (21.5 – 27.1)	18.6†	(14.3 – 20.6)	23.9	(19.8 – 29.5)	29.9†	(29.3 – 37.1)	42

† Estimate is subject to greater uncertainty due to small cell size.

Table 2.17.a.5. Plasma arachidic acid (20:0): Non-Hispanic whites

Geometric mean and selected percentiles of plasma concentrations (in μmol/L) for fasted non-Hispanic whites in the U.S. population aged 20 years and older, National Health and Nutrition Examination Survey, 2003–2004.

	Geometric mean (95% conf. interval)	Selected percentiles (95% conf. interval)						Sample size
		10th		50th		90th		
Males and Females								
Total, 20 years and older	23.6 (23.0 – 24.2)	17.6	(16.7 – 18.4)	23.5	(22.9 – 24.0)	31.6	(30.6 – 32.6)	962
20–39 years	22.2 (21.3 – 23.1)	16.5	(15.4 – 17.0)	22.0	(20.9 – 23.5)	29.6	(28.3 – 31.3)	290
40–59 years	23.8 (23.1 – 24.6)	18.4	(17.4 – 19.3)	23.4	(22.9 – 24.1)	31.5	(29.9 – 34.3)	270
60 years and older	25.2 (24.6 – 25.9)	19.0	(18.0 – 19.4)	25.3	(24.4 – 26.4)	33.5	(32.2 – 35.6)	402
Males								
Total, 20 years and older	22.4 (21.7 – 23.0)	16.7	(16.1 – 17.6)	22.0	(21.7 – 22.4)	29.8	(29.0 – 31.2)	460
20–39 years	21.2 (20.1 – 22.4)	16.3	(13.6 – 17.0)	20.8	(19.9 – 22.0)	28.5	(25.8 – 32.1)	125
40–59 years	23.0 (21.9 – 24.2)	17.6	(15.6 – 18.6)	22.5	(21.9 – 23.8)	31.1	(28.9 – 32.4)	136
60 years and older	22.9 (22.3 – 23.5)	16.9	(16.1 – 18.3)	22.8	(22.1 – 23.5)	29.6	(29.0 – 31.6)	199
Females								
Total, 20 years and older	24.8 (24.0 – 25.7)	18.7	(17.7 – 19.1)	24.8	(23.8 – 25.7)	32.9	(31.4 – 35.6)	502
20–39 years	23.0 (21.9 – 24.3)	16.7	(15.9 – 17.7)	23.6	(22.3 – 24.4)	30.1	(29.3 – 31.3)	165
40–59 years	24.7 (24.0 – 25.5)	18.9	(18.2 – 19.7)	24.2	(23.3 – 25.5)	32.7	(30.5 – 37.1)	134
60 years and older	27.4 (26.4 – 28.4)	20.9	(19.1 – 21.7)	27.6	(26.5 – 28.8)	36.0	(33.6 – 38.6)	203

Table 2.18.a.1. Plasma docosanoic acid (22:0): Concentrations

Geometric mean and selected percentiles of plasma concentrations (in µmol/L) for the fasted U.S. population aged 20 years and older, National Health and Nutrition Examination Survey, 2003–2004.

	Geometric mean (95% conf. interval)	Selected percentiles (95% conf. interval)					Sample size
		2.5th	5th	50th	95th	97.5th	
Total, 20 years and older	69.3 (67.7 – 71.0)	41.5 (38.1 – 43.2)	45.2 (42.9 – 47.6)	69.5 (68.0 – 71.4)	102 (99.0 – 108)	110 (106 – 117)	1,739
Age group							
20–39 years	66.5 (65.1 – 67.9)	42.6 (38.0 – 44.3)	46.1 (43.0 – 48.1)	66.5 (65.0 – 68.5)	97.4 (94.4 – 98.7)	99.9 (98.3 – 104)	589
40–59 years	71.8 (68.5 – 75.2)	41.6 (20.1 – 45.2)	46.4 (40.2 – 49.5)	74.0 (68.3 – 76.6)	105 (99.0 – 111)	111 (106 – 134)	496
60 years and older	70.2 (68.2 – 72.4)	39.2 (31.7 – 42.9)	43.0 (40.1 – 46.2)	70.9 (68.1 – 73.4)	109 (105 – 114)	115 (111 – 128)	654
Gender							
Males	65.8 (64.0 – 67.7)	39.3 (34.2 – 42.4)	43.0 (39.7 – 45.1)	66.2 (64.2 – 68.3)	96.4 (94.9 – 98.2)	105 (98.2 – 111)	834
Females	72.8 (70.4 – 75.2)	43.4 (40.5 – 47.0)	48.4 (45.1 – 50.3)	73.7 (70.7 – 75.6)	106 (102 – 111)	113 (108 – 128)	905
Race/ethnicity							
Mexican Americans	64.4 (61.3 – 67.7)	39.0† (35.4 – 41.8)	42.0 (37.4 – 46.5)	64.4 (60.9 – 67.4)	95.3 (87.1 – 129)	97.9† (94.9 – 129)	367
Non-Hispanic Blacks	69.6 (66.5 – 73.0)	41.1† (20.8 – 47.2)	46.3 (34.5 – 51.1)	69.4 (64.3 – 74.7)	106 (104 – 107)	115† (107 – 123)	306
Non-Hispanic Whites	70.4 (68.9 – 72.0)	42.6 (39.4 – 43.7)	46.9 (43.4 – 48.5)	70.9 (69.4 – 72.8)	104 (99.2 – 110)	111 (108 – 121)	947

† Estimate is subject to greater uncertainty due to small cell size.

Figure 2.18.a. Plasma docosanoic acid (22:0): Concentrations by age group

Geometric mean (95% confidence interval), National Health and Nutrition Examination Survey, 2003–2004

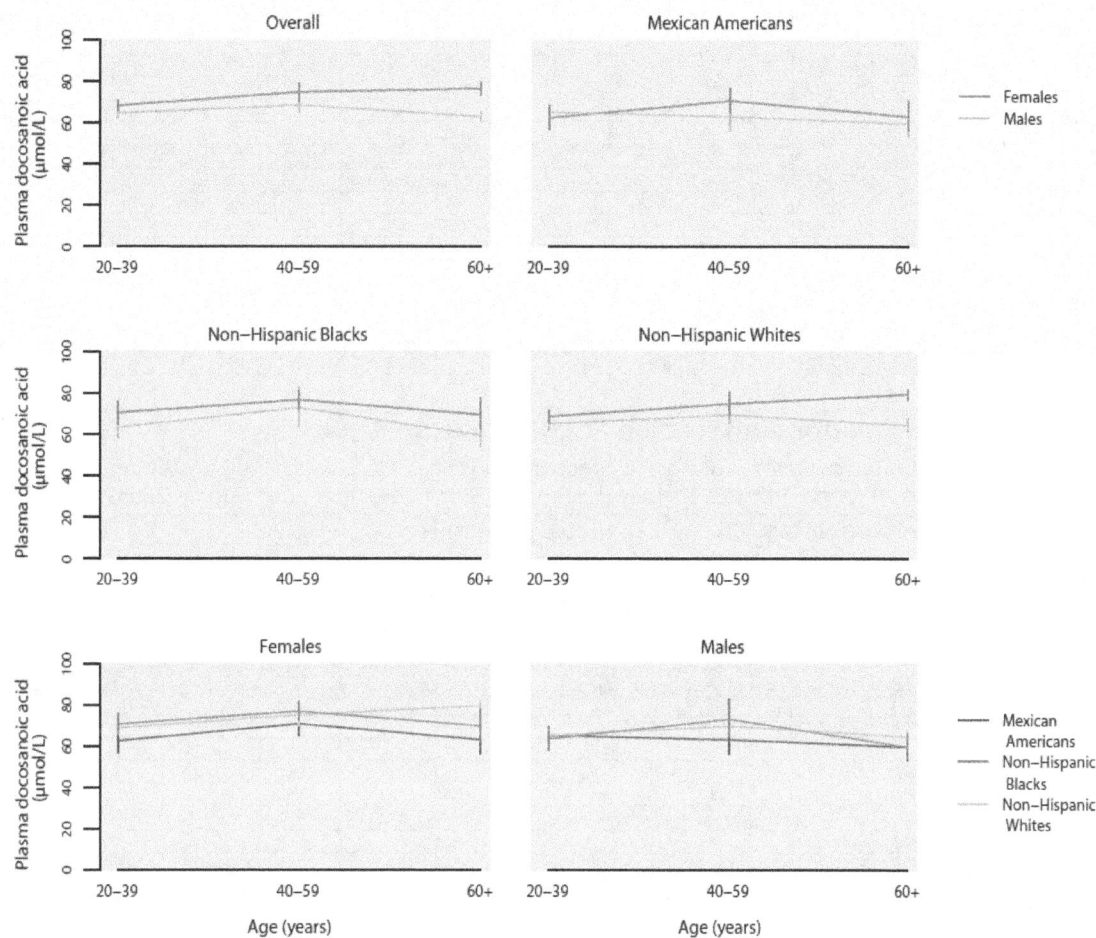

Table 2.18.a.2. Plasma docosanoic acid (22:0): Total population

Geometric mean and selected percentiles of plasma concentrations (in μmol/L) for the fasted U.S. population aged 20 years and older, National Health and Nutrition Examination Survey, 2003–2004.

	Geometric mean (95% conf. interval)	Selected percentiles (95% conf. interval)			Sample size
		10th	50th	90th	
Males and Females					
Total, 20 years and older	69.3 (67.7 – 71.0)	50.1 (48.7 – 51.5)	69.5 (68.0 – 71.4)	95.3 (93.0 – 97.7)	1,739
20–39 years	66.5 (65.1 – 67.9)	49.7 (48.9 – 51.0)	66.5 (65.0 – 68.5)	89.5 (86.7 – 93.6)	589
40–59 years	71.8 (68.5 – 75.2)	51.9 (47.5 – 55.9)	74.0 (68.3 – 76.6)	96.4 (93.8 – 100)	496
60 years and older	70.2 (68.2 – 72.4)	49.1 (46.2 – 50.7)	70.9 (68.1 – 73.4)	100 (96.1 – 105)	654
Males					
Total, 20 years and older	65.8 (64.0 – 67.7)	48.1 (45.1 – 49.7)	66.2 (64.2 – 68.3)	90.5 (88.2 – 92.5)	834
20–39 years	64.7 (62.6 – 66.8)	49.3 (46.8 – 51.2)	63.7 (61.0 – 66.2)	88.7 (82.6 – 93.6)	274
40–59 years	68.7 (65.3 – 72.2)	48.3 (43.0 – 51.4)	70.9 (66.0 – 74.5)	92.2 (89.0 – 96.9)	238
60 years and older	63.1 (60.8 – 65.5)	43.6 (40.8 – 47.0)	64.3 (60.6 – 67.9)	88.2 (85.2 – 91.7)	322
Females					
Total, 20 years and older	72.8 (70.4 – 75.2)	52.4 (50.4 – 55.1)	73.7 (70.7 – 75.6)	98.7 (96.1 – 102)	905
20–39 years	68.3 (66.2 – 70.6)	50.9 (48.4 – 51.7)	69.4 (66.8 – 71.6)	91.4 (86.0 – 97.4)	315
40–59 years	74.9 (70.9 – 79.1)	56.6 (48.1 – 58.3)	76.5 (70.1 – 80.6)	99.0 (94.7 – 108)	258
60 years and older	76.6 (73.8 – 79.6)	54.1 (49.1 – 58.5)	75.7 (73.2 – 80.1)	107 (103 – 112)	332

Table 2.18.a.3. Plasma docosanoic acid (22:0): Mexican Americans

Geometric mean and selected percentiles of plasma concentrations (in μmol/L) for fasted Mexican Americans in the U.S. population aged 20 years and older, National Health and Nutrition Examination Survey, 2003–2004.

	Geometric mean (95% conf. interval)	Selected percentiles (95% conf. interval)			Sample size
		10th	50th	90th	
Males and Females					
Total, 20 years and older	64.4 (61.3 – 67.7)	47.8 (41.7 – 51.6)	64.4 (60.9 – 67.4)	87.1 (81.5 – 95.4)	367
20–39 years	64.0 (60.8 – 67.4)	48.4 (42.0 – 50.6)	63.1 (59.7 – 66.8)	85.7 (80.1 – 95.4)	129
40–59 years	66.5 (61.6 – 71.8)	48.1† (35.5 – 55.5)	67.7 (64.3 – 71.7)	87.9† (80.6 – 106)	91
60 years and older	61.4 (56.4 – 66.9)	42.7 (38.6 – 47.2)	61.4 (59.8 – 64.2)	85.0 (74.6 – 120)	147
Males					
Total, 20 years and older	64.0 (60.5 – 67.7)	48.2 (38.9 – 52.7)	64.4 (60.8 – 67.1)	85.2 (80.7 – 90.4)	185
20–39 years	65.2 (62.2 – 68.3)	49.6† (31.7 – 55.2)	63.8 (60.7 – 66.9)	86.8† (77.5 – 116)	65
40–59 years	63.1 (56.3 – 70.6)	44.8† (35.5 – 55.6)	65.0 (55.7 – 72.0)	81.4† (74.8 – 97.7)	47
60 years and older	59.6 (53.5 – 66.3)	38.8† (35.0 – 43.0)	61.3 (55.7 – 65.1)	87.6† (68.0 – 112)	73
Females					
Total, 20 years and older	64.9 (60.6 – 69.6)	46.5 (41.2 – 50.7)	64.5 (59.9 – 71.3)	92.9 (79.5 – 120)	182
20–39 years	62.5 (57.1 – 68.4)	42.2† (38.2 – 50.3)	61.3 (55.1 – 70.9)	83.6† (76.3 – 97.3)	64
40–59 years	70.7 (65.1 – 76.6)	53.4† (37.4 – 57.1)	68.7 (65.7 – 76.7)	93.5† (85.0 – 106)	44
60 years and older	63.1 (56.5 – 70.6)	47.0† (34.0 – 54.2)	62.0 (57.9 – 66.5)	82.9† (75.2 – 116)	74

† Estimate is subject to greater uncertainty due to small cell size.

Table 2.18.a.4. Plasma docosanoic acid (22:0): Non-Hispanic blacks

Geometric mean and selected percentiles of plasma concentrations (in µmol/L) for fasted non-Hispanic blacks in the U.S. population aged 20 years and older, National Health and Nutrition Examination Survey, 2003–2004.

	Geometric mean (95% conf. interval)	Selected percentiles (95% conf. interval)						Sample size
		10th		50th		90th		
Males and Females								
Total, 20 years and older	69.6	(66.5 – 73.0)	52.1	(46.8 – 53.9)	69.4	(64.3 – 74.7)	94.2	(91.4 – 101)	306
20–39 years	67.3	(63.9 – 70.8)	52.3	(42.4 – 54.1)	65.0	(62.8 – 71.2)	89.8	(86.7 – 97.6)	124
40–59 years	75.2	(70.9 – 79.7)	53.1†	(42.9 – 59.2)	78.6	(71.7 – 82.9)	104†	(91.6 – 118)	98
60 years and older	65.6	(61.9 – 69.5)	47.9†	(27.8 – 53.2)	65.4	(61.9 – 68.1)	91.3†	(81.1 – 118)	84
Males								
Total, 20 years and older	66.1	(62.1 – 70.3)	47.6	(33.1 – 53.2)	64.6	(61.6 – 68.4)	90.2	(87.9 – 98.0)	141
20–39 years	63.5	(58.3 – 69.1)	49.2†	(34.5 – 53.7)	61.5	(57.0 – 66.1)	86.6†	(76.7 – 119)	57
40–59 years	73.0	(64.3 – 83.0)	44.8†	(39.5 – 59.2)	74.5	(62.0 – 85.4)	93.5†	(86.7 – 171)	42
60 years and older	59.6	(54.0 – 65.7)	41.2†	(20.8 – 47.8)	60.2	(53.4 – 67.0)	81.3†	(73.0 – 95.8)	42
Females								
Total, 20 years and older	72.5	(69.2 – 76.0)	53.8	(50.3 – 56.1)	73.9	(66.3 – 78.4)	99.7	(91.4 – 106)	165
20–39 years	70.6	(65.5 – 76.0)	53.0†	(40.9 – 57.0)	71.3	(63.1 – 79.9)	91.5†	(85.6 – 96.2)	67
40–59 years	76.8	(72.5 – 81.4)	55.8†	(43.3 – 61.0)	80.4	(72.4 – 84.5)	105†	(91.6 – 117)	56
60 years and older	69.7	(62.7 – 77.4)	53.1†	(41.5 – 55.8)	67.8	(59.0 – 76.7)	100†	(79.0 – 123)	42

† Estimate is subject to greater uncertainty due to small cell size.

Table 2.18.a.5. Plasma docosanoic acid (22:0): Non-Hispanic whites

Geometric mean and selected percentiles of plasma concentrations (in µmol/L) for fasted non-Hispanic whites in the U.S. population aged 20 years and older, National Health and Nutrition Examination Survey, 2003–2004.

	Geometric mean (95% conf. interval)	Selected percentiles (95% conf. interval)						Sample size
		10th		50th		90th		
Males and Females								
Total, 20 years and older	70.4	(68.9 – 72.0)	50.8	(49.4 – 51.7)	70.9	(69.4 – 72.8)	96.4	(94.6 – 98.5)	947
20–39 years	67.1	(65.4 – 68.8)	49.9	(48.6 – 51.2)	68.1	(65.9 – 69.5)	90.6	(85.6 – 96.6)	288
40–59 years	72.3	(68.7 – 76.0)	52.1	(48.5 – 56.3)	74.3	(68.3 – 76.9)	96.5	(93.4 – 103)	267
60 years and older	72.3	(70.5 – 74.1)	50.1	(47.1 – 53.0)	72.5	(70.4 – 74.6)	102	(98.0 – 108)	392
Males								
Total, 20 years and older	66.9	(64.8 – 69.0)	49.2	(46.5 – 51.0)	67.8	(65.4 – 69.6)	92.0	(88.7 – 94.5)	453
20–39 years	65.3	(62.5 – 68.2)	49.5	(44.6 – 51.7)	64.4	(61.8 – 68.6)	89.1	(80.8 – 97.3)	125
40–59 years	69.6	(66.0 – 73.4)	49.9	(41.9 – 55.0)	72.3	(66.0 – 75.2)	93.1	(90.8 – 96.8)	134
60 years and older	64.6	(61.6 – 67.7)	46.9	(43.1 – 49.4)	65.3	(62.4 – 69.7)	88.4	(85.6 – 92.0)	194
Females								
Total, 20 years and older	73.9	(71.2 – 76.8)	52.8	(49.8 – 56.8)	74.4	(71.7 – 76.5)	99.3	(96.1 – 108)	494
20–39 years	68.8	(66.0 – 71.7)	51.0	(47.5 – 52.1)	69.4	(67.8 – 72.6)	92.8	(85.6 – 98.1)	163
40–59 years	75.0	(69.9 – 80.4)	56.4	(44.8 – 59.1)	76.5	(67.5 – 81.7)	98.6	(94.6 – 110)	133
60 years and older	79.5	(77.1 – 81.9)	57.0	(49.9 – 62.1)	78.5	(75.6 – 83.3)	109	(105 – 113)	198

Table 2.19.a.1. Plasma lignoceric acid (24:0): Concentrations

Geometric mean and selected percentiles of plasma concentrations (in µmol/L) for the fasted U.S. population aged 20 years and older, National Health and Nutrition Examination Survey, 2003–2004.

| | Geometric mean (95% conf. interval) | Selected percentiles (95% conf. interval) | | | | | Sample size |
		2.5th	5th	50th	95th	97.5th	
Total, 20 years and older	54.0 (52.8 – 55.3)	31.2 (29.5 – 33.0)	35.3 (32.7 – 36.8)	53.8 (52.6 – 55.6)	80.9 (79.0 – 83.6)	87.0 (84.9 – 90.2)	1,743
Age group							
20–39 years	51.6 (50.3 – 53.0)	31.8 (26.8 – 35.2)	35.6 (32.4 – 36.6)	51.3 (49.8 – 52.9)	73.6 (71.8 – 78.6)	82.0 (76.0 – 88.3)	583
40–59 years	56.4 (54.2 – 58.7)	33.2 (28.7 – 37.6)	37.8 (32.9 – 39.6)	56.6 (54.1 – 59.6)	81.1 (77.4 – 88.0)	86.8 (83.6 – 94.4)	495
60 years and older	54.3 (52.7 – 56.0)	29.1 (21.7 – 31.0)	31.6 (30.0 – 34.2)	54.8 (52.4 – 57.5)	86.9 (81.9 – 91.9)	92.3 (89.1 – 97.5)	665
Gender							
Males	53.7 (52.2 – 55.2)	30.6 (28.5 – 33.0)	34.6 (30.7 – 37.7)	53.7 (51.6 – 55.8)	80.8 (76.4 – 84.9)	86.1 (84.5 – 93.1)	836
Females	54.4 (52.6 – 56.2)	32.4 (29.8 – 35.0)	35.8 (32.6 – 37.0)	53.8 (52.7 – 56.1)	80.7 (78.7 – 84.5)	87.3 (83.8 – 91.9)	907
Race/ethnicity							
Mexican Americans	50.4 (47.3 – 53.7)	29.9† (19.2 – 32.6)	32.4 (28.7 – 36.0)	50.1 (47.2 – 53.8)	76.4 (71.1 – 83.0)	80.7† (76.9 – 117)	355
Non-Hispanic Blacks	53.3 (50.5 – 56.2)	30.8† (24.0 – 35.4)	34.8 (27.0 – 38.0)	53.1 (49.6 – 57.0)	79.0 (73.3 – 84.2)	83.9† (79.0 – 112)	302
Non-Hispanic Whites	54.7 (53.4 – 56.0)	31.5 (28.7 – 33.6)	35.8 (33.1 – 37.2)	54.8 (53.0 – 56.5)	81.4 (79.1 – 85.0)	87.2 (85.1 – 92.1)	966

† Estimate is subject to greater uncertainty due to small cell size.

Figure 2.19.a. Plasma lignoceric acid (24:0): Concentrations by age group
Geometric mean (95% confidence interval), National Health and Nutrition Examination Survey, 2003–2004

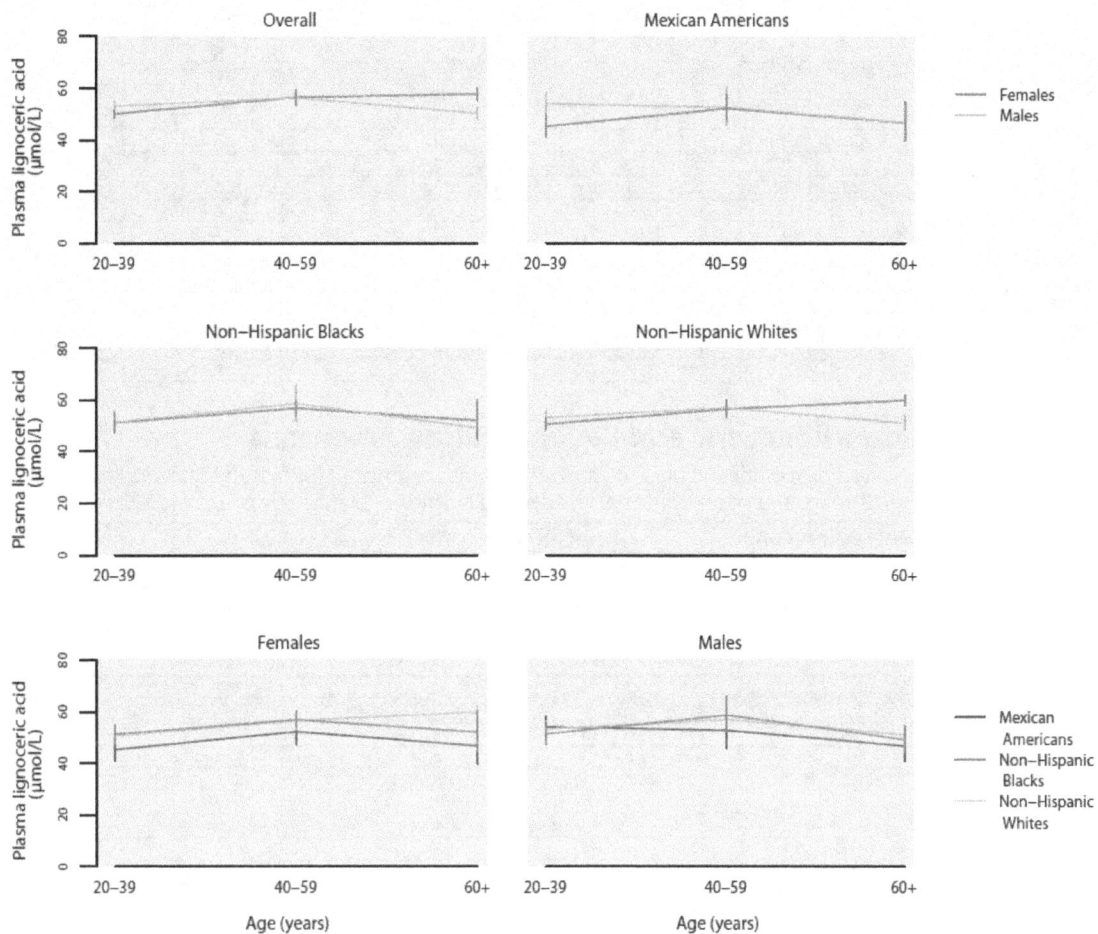

Table 2.19.a.2. Plasma lignoceric acid (24:0): Total population

Geometric mean and selected percentiles of plasma concentrations (in µmol/L) for the fasted U.S. population aged 20 years and older, National Health and Nutrition Examination Survey, 2003–2004.

	Geometric mean (95% conf. interval)		Selected percentiles (95% conf. interval)						Sample size
			10th		50th		90th		
Males and Females									
Total, 20 years and older	54.0	(52.8 – 55.3)	39.0	(37.4 – 40.6)	53.8	(52.6 – 55.6)	74.2	(72.2 – 76.4)	1,743
20–39 years	51.6	(50.3 – 53.0)	37.9	(36.6 – 39.6)	51.3	(49.8 – 52.9)	69.0	(66.5 – 71.8)	583
40–59 years	56.4	(54.2 – 58.7)	41.4	(37.9 – 43.7)	56.6	(54.1 – 59.6)	76.0	(72.9 – 79.2)	495
60 years and older	54.3	(52.7 – 56.0)	37.1	(33.6 – 39.5)	54.8	(52.4 – 57.5)	77.9	(76.4 – 81.4)	665
Males									
Total, 20 years and older	53.7	(52.2 – 55.2)	39.1	(37.1 – 41.0)	53.7	(51.6 – 55.8)	72.6	(70.8 – 74.8)	836
20–39 years	53.1	(51.2 – 55.1)	39.5	(37.9 – 42.3)	52.1	(50.1 – 55.5)	70.9	(67.6 – 74.9)	272
40–59 years	56.3	(53.6 – 59.0)	41.1	(34.7 – 44.2)	56.1	(53.5 – 60.5)	75.1	(71.7 – 83.1)	238
60 years and older	50.3	(48.3 – 52.4)	33.6	(30.2 – 37.8)	50.4	(47.1 – 55.0)	70.2	(68.5 – 74.4)	326
Females									
Total, 20 years and older	54.4	(52.6 – 56.2)	39.0	(36.5 – 41.6)	53.8	(52.7 – 56.1)	76.1	(72.5 – 78.4)	907
20–39 years	50.1	(48.7 – 51.6)	36.6	(34.8 – 37.9)	50.2	(48.9 – 51.9)	67.3	(64.9 – 69.6)	311
40–59 years	56.5	(53.9 – 59.3)	42.2	(39.0 – 43.6)	57.0	(53.5 – 60.0)	76.0	(72.2 – 79.6)	257
60 years and older	57.8	(55.5 – 60.2)	39.9	(35.3 – 42.3)	58.5	(55.2 – 61.3)	82.8	(78.9 – 89.0)	339

Table 2.19.a.3. Plasma lignoceric acid (24:0): Mexican Americans

Geometric mean and selected percentiles of plasma concentrations (in µmol/L) for fasted Mexican Americans in the U.S. population aged 20 years and older, National Health and Nutrition Examination Survey, 2003–2004.

	Geometric mean (95% conf. interval)		Selected percentiles (95% conf. interval)						Sample size
			10th		50th		90th		
Males and Females									
Total, 20 years and older	50.4	(47.3 – 53.7)	37.1	(31.5 – 39.5)	50.1	(47.2 – 53.8)	69.4	(66.9 – 73.7)	355
20–39 years	50.1	(46.5 – 53.9)	37.1	(30.6 – 38.8)	49.2	(44.7 – 56.1)	68.7	(63.7 – 76.3)	120
40–59 years	52.5	(47.5 – 58.0)	38.8†	(21.0 – 44.5)	53.3	(47.1 – 59.6)	71.6†	(65.8 – 81.4)	89
60 years and older	46.7	(41.5 – 52.7)	33.0	(19.2 – 36.9)	47.1	(40.1 – 53.9)	66.4	(58.7 – 97.3)	146
Males									
Total, 20 years and older	52.9	(49.2 – 56.9)	39.3	(33.0 – 43.1)	52.4	(48.7 – 56.2)	72.2	(67.8 – 77.5)	176
20–39 years	54.0	(50.3 – 58.1)	40.7†	(37.8 – 44.4)	52.3	(48.1 – 57.7)	69.7†	(63.8 – 84.8)	61
40–59 years	52.7	(45.9 – 60.5)	36.7†	(28.8 – 45.9)	53.2	(46.0 – 60.5)	72.4†	(65.3 – 81.2)	45
60 years and older	46.7	(40.9 – 53.4)	32.2†	(19.2 – 36.7)	48.2	(38.4 – 54.3)	69.1†	(55.8 – 89.1)	70
Females									
Total, 20 years and older	47.6	(44.6 – 50.7)	32.6	(30.3 – 36.7)	46.5	(43.4 – 51.0)	67.8	(61.8 – 71.1)	179
20–39 years	45.3	(41.0 – 50.0)	32.0†	(29.8 – 36.6)	43.2	(37.9 – 52.6)	64.6†	(57.6 – 78.7)	59
40–59 years	52.2	(47.3 – 57.7)	39.2†	(21.0 – 43.4)	53.3	(44.8 – 60.2)	69.6†	(61.1 – 83.2)	44
60 years and older	46.7	(39.8 – 54.8)	34.7†	(25.4 – 38.0)	45.3	(39.4 – 54.7)	63.8†	(54.4 – 97.3)	76

† Estimate is subject to greater uncertainty due to small cell size.

Table 2.19.a.4. Plasma lignoceric acid (24:0): Non-Hispanic blacks

Geometric mean and selected percentiles of plasma concentrations (in µmol/L) for fasted non-Hispanic blacks in the U.S. population aged 20 years and older, National Health and Nutrition Examination Survey, 2003–2004.

	Geometric mean (95% conf. interval)	Selected percentiles (95% conf. interval)					Sample size
		10th		50th		90th	
Males and Females							
Total, 20 years and older	53.3 (50.5 – 56.2)	38.6	(35.4 – 40.9)	53.1	(49.6 – 57.0)	71.8 (70.3 – 74.3)	302
20–39 years	51.2 (48.2 – 54.5)	37.2	(29.9 – 41.6)	49.9	(48.0 – 55.7)	67.9 (65.1 – 74.2)	123
40–59 years	57.6 (54.6 – 60.8)	40.9†	(33.9 – 46.2)	58.1	(54.2 – 63.3)	73.0† (71.0 – 85.7)	95
60 years and older	50.9 (46.1 – 56.2)	37.3†	(29.8 – 40.2)	50.8	(43.5 – 55.2)	74.1† (63.0 – 94.8)	84
Males							
Total, 20 years and older	53.4 (50.0 – 56.9)	38.8	(27.0 – 43.3)	52.8	(49.1 – 58.6)	71.8 (68.1 – 80.6)	140
20–39 years	51.3 (47.2 – 55.7)	38.8†	(26.2 – 43.5)	49.9	(46.3 – 55.9)	66.5† (63.1 – 83.8)	57
40–59 years	58.6 (52.1 – 65.9)	40.9†	(32.2 – 48.9)	60.1	(50.6 – 70.1)	73.8† (70.1 – 112)	41
60 years and older	49.2 (44.5 – 54.4)	30.6†	(24.0 – 40.9)	49.5	(44.5 – 54.7)	70.7† (62.3 – 79.1)	42
Females							
Total, 20 years and older	53.2 (50.1 – 56.6)	38.2	(35.3 – 40.8)	53.3	(49.2 – 57.7)	72.0 (69.6 – 78.2)	162
20–39 years	51.2 (47.7 – 54.8)	36.8†	(28.1 – 41.1)	49.7	(46.0 – 57.4)	69.3† (65.3 – 72.9)	66
40–59 years	56.8 (53.8 – 60.1)	39.9†	(34.9 – 46.2)	56.6	(51.9 – 61.3)	72.2† (70.3 – 85.2)	54
60 years and older	52.0 (45.0 – 60.1)	39.7†	(31.4 – 40.4)	52.4	(40.8 – 62.0)	78.2† (62.0 – 95.2)	42

† Estimate is subject to greater uncertainty due to small cell size.

Table 2.19.a.5. Plasma lignoceric acid (24:0): Non-Hispanic whites

Geometric mean and selected percentiles of plasma concentrations (in µmol/L) for fasted non-Hispanic whites in the U.S. population aged 20 years and older, National Health and Nutrition Examination Survey, 2003–2004.

	Geometric mean (95% conf. interval)	Selected percentiles (95% conf. interval)					Sample size
		10th		50th		90th	
Males and Females							
Total, 20 years and older	54.7 (53.4 – 56.0)	39.6	(37.7 – 41.6)	54.8	(53.0 – 56.5)	75.3 (73.0 – 77.3)	966
20–39 years	51.8 (50.1 – 53.6)	37.9	(35.9 – 41.2)	51.5	(49.4 – 53.9)	68.9 (66.0 – 72.6)	293
40–59 years	56.7 (54.2 – 59.3)	42.0	(38.6 – 43.2)	57.0	(53.6 – 60.8)	76.4 (72.8 – 80.8)	270
60 years and older	55.7 (54.1 – 57.3)	38.2	(33.4 – 41.0)	56.3	(54.0 – 58.6)	78.7 (76.9 – 82.3)	403
Males							
Total, 20 years and older	54.1 (52.5 – 55.8)	39.4	(36.1 – 41.8)	54.7	(51.8 – 56.5)	72.8 (70.5 – 77.2)	461
20–39 years	53.2 (50.5 – 56.0)	39.4	(35.8 – 42.8)	52.5	(49.5 – 56.8)	70.5 (66.0 – 82.9)	126
40–59 years	56.9 (53.9 – 60.0)	42.1	(35.0 – 44.7)	57.1	(53.1 – 61.8)	76.6 (71.7 – 85.9)	135
60 years and older	51.1 (48.6 – 53.8)	34.8	(29.7 – 39.0)	51.4	(47.1 – 56.4)	70.2 (68.4 – 75.8)	200
Females							
Total, 20 years and older	55.2 (53.1 – 57.4)	39.7	(36.6 – 42.5)	55.1	(53.0 – 57.3)	76.6 (74.2 – 79.2)	505
20–39 years	50.6 (48.5 – 52.8)	36.7	(32.4 – 41.2)	51.3	(48.6 – 53.2)	67.3 (64.8 – 69.9)	167
40–59 years	56.5 (53.2 – 59.9)	41.8	(38.2 – 43.1)	56.9	(53.0 – 62.0)	76.4 (71.8 – 81.2)	135
60 years and older	59.9 (57.8 – 62.0)	40.9	(36.7 – 44.9)	60.4	(58.3 – 62.5)	85.4 (79.9 – 91.5)	203

Table 2.20.a.1. Plasma myristoleic acid (14:1n-5): Concentrations

Geometric mean and selected percentiles of plasma concentrations (in µmol/L) for the fasted U.S. population aged 20 years and older, National Health and Nutrition Examination Survey, 2003–2004.

	Geometric mean (95% conf. interval)	Selected percentiles (95% conf. interval)					Sample size
		2.5th	5th	50th	95th	97.5th	
Total, 20 years and older	6.57 (6.08 – 7.09)	1.45 (1.31 – 1.56)	1.79 (1.68 – 1.96)	6.50 (5.90 – 6.99)	23.9 (21.4 – 29.3)	32.1 (27.0 – 40.2)	1,808
Age group							
20–39 years	6.21 (5.67 – 6.80)	1.47 (1.17 – 1.64)	1.76 (1.64 – 2.01)	6.05 (5.34 – 6.75)	24.0 (19.3 – 32.6)	31.9 (24.8 – 67.0)	610
40–59 years	7.06 (6.30 – 7.90)	1.44 (1.11 – 1.69)	1.86 (1.63 – 2.02)	6.87 (6.20 – 7.62)	25.8 (21.4 – 34.6)	34.6 (27.0 – 52.9)	515
60 years and older	6.39 (5.61 – 7.26)	1.40 (1.17 – 1.67)	1.73 (1.56 – 1.99)	6.40 (5.53 – 7.45)	23.3 (19.3 – 30.9)	26.9 (23.4 – 40.7)	683
Gender							
Males	6.35 (5.70 – 7.07)	1.25 (1.05 – 1.39)	1.70 (1.41 – 1.82)	6.47 (5.47 – 7.28)	24.9 (22.8 – 29.7)	33.0 (29.4 – 40.6)	865
Females	6.77 (6.26 – 7.32)	1.59 (1.46 – 1.75)	1.94 (1.71 – 2.32)	6.51 (5.96 – 6.96)	23.4 (19.9 – 31.2)	30.7 (23.9 – 48.1)	943
Race/ethnicity							
Mexican Americans	6.95 (5.89 – 8.20)	1.53† (1.02 – 1.80)	1.82 (1.51 – 2.05)	6.83 (5.44 – 8.30)	26.1 (21.1 – 35.6)	33.1† (27.4 – 68.4)	376
Non-Hispanic Blacks	3.91 (3.50 – 4.38)	1.06† (.703 – 1.17)	1.18 (1.06 – 1.42)	3.78 (3.17 – 4.49)	12.8 (11.5 – 21.4)	20.3† (13.7 – 31.3)	310
Non-Hispanic Whites	7.07 (6.45 – 7.74)	1.65 (1.42 – 1.79)	2.06 (1.80 – 2.33)	6.84 (6.22 – 7.46)	24.9 (22.3 – 31.8)	32.7 (27.0 – 43.6)	992

† Estimate is subject to greater uncertainty due to small cell size.

Figure 2.20.a. Plasma myristoleic acid (14:1n–5): Concentrations by age group

Geometric mean (95% confidence interval), National Health and Nutrition Examination Survey, 2003–2004

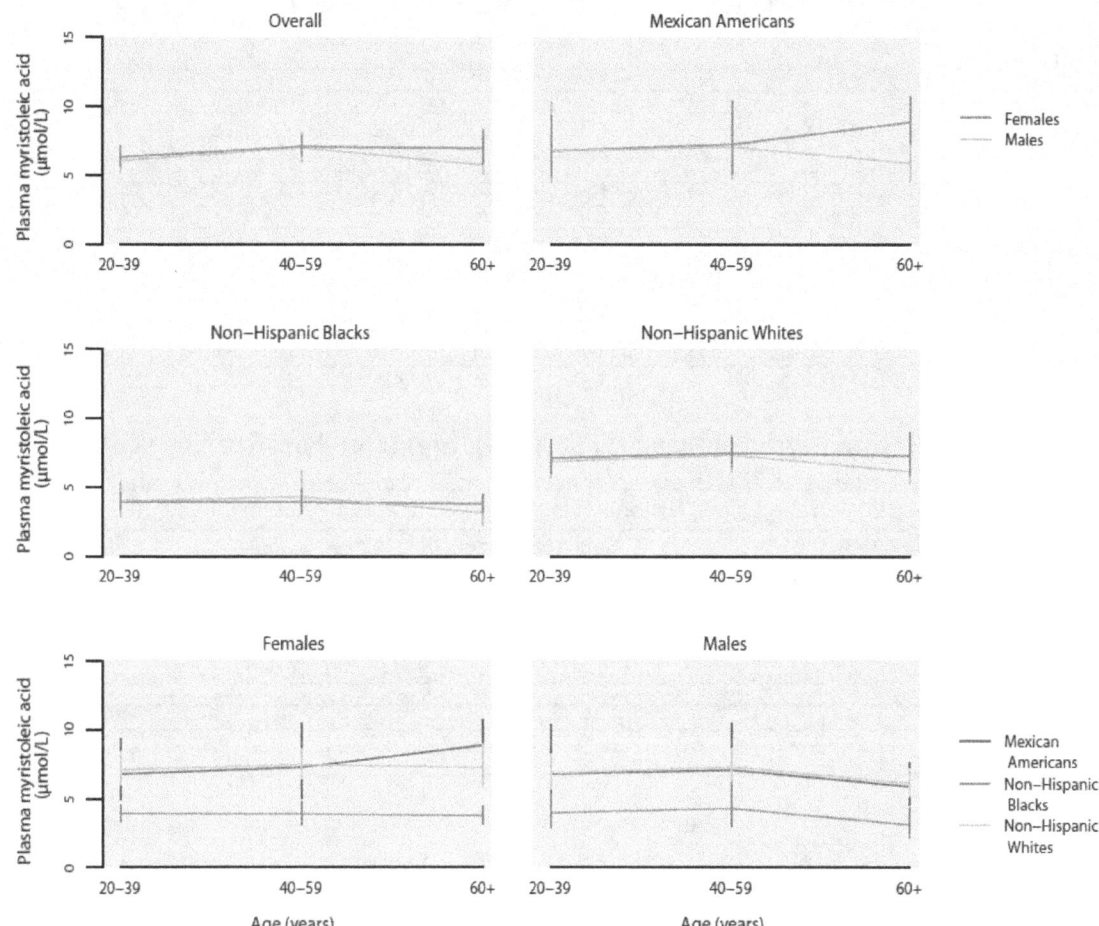

Table 2.20.a.2. Plasma myristoleic acid (14:1n-5): Total population

Geometric mean and selected percentiles of plasma concentrations (in μmol/L) for the fasted U.S. population aged 20 years and older, National Health and Nutrition Examination Survey, 2003–2004.

| | Geometric mean (95% conf. interval) | Selected percentiles (95% conf. interval) | | | Sample size |
		10th	50th	90th	
Males and Females					
Total, 20 years and older	6.57 (6.08 – 7.09)	2.41 (2.26 – 2.59)	6.50 (5.90 – 6.99)	18.5 (16.7 – 20.5)	1,808
20–39 years	6.21 (5.67 – 6.80)	2.33 (2.08 – 2.52)	6.05 (5.34 – 6.75)	16.9 (14.8 – 20.4)	610
40–59 years	7.06 (6.30 – 7.90)	2.53 (2.20 – 2.94)	6.87 (6.20 – 7.62)	19.6 (18.0 – 22.2)	515
60 years and older	6.39 (5.61 – 7.26)	2.43 (2.04 – 2.89)	6.40 (5.53 – 7.45)	17.3 (13.1 – 23.4)	683
Males					
Total, 20 years and older	6.35 (5.70 – 7.07)	2.20 (2.01 – 2.35)	6.47 (5.47 – 7.28)	18.5 (16.5 – 21.2)	865
20–39 years	6.08 (5.23 – 7.08)	2.10 (2.03 – 2.33)	6.09 (5.00 – 7.32)	16.9 (14.5 – 23.9)	282
40–59 years	7.02 (6.06 – 8.12)	2.27 (1.80 – 2.81)	6.98 (5.49 – 8.66)	21.0 (18.5 – 26.2)	248
60 years and older	5.74 (5.08 – 6.48)	2.26 (1.68 – 2.61)	5.82 (5.44 – 6.42)	13.7 (10.9 – 20.0)	335
Females					
Total, 20 years and older	6.77 (6.26 – 7.32)	2.73 (2.52 – 2.96)	6.51 (5.96 – 6.96)	18.4 (15.3 – 21.6)	943
20–39 years	6.34 (5.67 – 7.08)	2.62 (2.06 – 2.94)	5.91 (5.31 – 6.92)	17.2 (13.9 – 22.4)	328
40–59 years	7.09 (6.37 – 7.90)	2.87 (2.39 – 3.40)	6.81 (6.29 – 7.17)	18.7 (13.8 – 23.3)	267
60 years and older	6.97 (5.87 – 8.26)	2.91 (1.76 – 3.22)	6.89 (5.55 – 8.06)	20.0 (16.1 – 23.8)	348

Table 2.20.a.3. Plasma myristoleic acid (14:1n-5): Mexican Americans

Geometric mean and selected percentiles of plasma concentrations (in μmol/L) for fasted Mexican Americans in the U.S. population aged 20 years and older, National Health and Nutrition Examination Survey, 2003–2004.

| | Geometric mean (95% conf. interval) | Selected percentiles (95% conf. interval) | | | Sample size |
		10th	50th	90th	
Males and Females					
Total, 20 years and older	6.95 (5.89 – 8.20)	2.26 (1.82 – 2.82)	6.83 (5.44 – 8.30)	19.4 (17.2 – 22.5)	376
20–39 years	6.79 (5.03 – 9.17)	2.11 (1.71 – 2.75)	6.39 (4.79 – 9.10)	18.7 (15.2 – 32.7)	132
40–59 years	7.17 (5.73 – 8.97)	2.48† (1.66 – 2.92)	6.96 (5.46 – 9.72)	20.0† (16.1 – 32.0)	93
60 years and older	7.30 (6.27 – 8.49)	3.03 (2.65 – 3.26)	7.48 (5.22 – 9.67)	16.7 (14.6 – 24.9)	151
Males					
Total, 20 years and older	6.79 (5.24 – 8.79)	2.27 (1.79 – 2.93)	6.58 (4.63 – 8.66)	20.0 (15.8 – 24.9)	189
20–39 years	6.79 (4.48 – 10.3)	2.15† (1.85 – 2.42)	6.56 (3.74 – 11.8)	20.2† (15.3 – 42.7)	67
40–59 years	7.08 (4.81 – 10.4)	2.69† (1.87 – 3.06)	6.77 (3.71 – 12.3)	18.8† (14.0 – 52.0)	48
60 years and older	5.90 (4.57 – 7.62)	2.72† (1.76 – 3.30)	5.60 (3.54 – 8.59)	13.6† (9.90 – 18.3)	74
Females					
Total, 20 years and older	7.16 (6.00 – 8.55)	2.03 (1.53 – 3.55)	6.86 (5.60 – 9.13)	18.7 (16.3 – 23.9)	187
20–39 years	6.78 (4.95 – 9.30)	1.96† (1.51 – 3.90)	6.02 (4.64 – 9.28)	16.3† (12.9 – 156)	65
40–59 years	7.27 (5.08 – 10.4)	1.93† (1.62 – 2.55)	7.32 (3.75 – 13.4)	22.2† (16.4 – 30.1)	45
60 years and older	8.88 (7.36 – 10.7)	3.63† (2.33 – 4.14)	9.24 (7.46 – 12.9)	17.4† (14.8 – 43.2)	77

† Estimate is subject to greater uncertainty due to small cell size.

Table 2.20.a.4. Plasma myristoleic acid (14:1n-5): Non-Hispanic blacks

Geometric mean and selected percentiles of plasma concentrations (in µmol/L) for fasted non-Hispanic blacks in the U.S. population aged 20 years and older, National Health and Nutrition Examination Survey, 2003–2004.

	Geometric mean (95% conf. interval)	Selected percentiles (95% conf. interval)			Sample size
		10th	50th	90th	
Males and Females					
Total, 20 years and older	3.91 (3.50 – 4.38)	1.48 (1.28 – 1.69)	3.78 (3.17 – 4.49)	10.4 (8.24 – 12.7)	310
20–39 years	3.95 (3.33 – 4.70)	1.68 (1.29 – 1.90)	3.54 (3.05 – 4.70)	10.2 (7.80 – 12.7)	126
40–59 years	4.07 (3.55 – 4.66)	1.44† (1.07 – 1.66)	4.21 (2.82 – 4.90)	11.7† (8.28 – 21.4)	98
60 years and older	3.51 (3.15 – 3.92)	1.30† (1.07 – 1.63)	3.37 (2.94 – 4.54)	9.13† (7.34 – 11.4)	86
Males					
Total, 20 years and older	3.95 (3.24 – 4.80)	1.23 (1.06 – 1.46)	4.23 (2.79 – 4.93)	11.3 (8.12 – 21.6)	143
20–39 years	3.99 (2.96 – 5.36)	1.37† (.992 – 1.92)	3.41 (2.61 – 5.34)	10.7† (7.65 – 61.3)	58
40–59 years	4.30 (3.03 – 6.10)	1.08† (.703 – 1.28)	4.74 (4.11 – 6.89)	12.4† (8.22 – 24.7)	42
60 years and older	3.13 (2.27 – 4.32)	1.30† (1.16 – 1.49)	2.53 (1.60 – 5.17)	8.55† (6.21 – 14.2)	43
Females					
Total, 20 years and older	3.89 (3.46 – 4.37)	1.70 (1.43 – 2.07)	3.60 (3.10 – 4.46)	8.84 (7.45 – 12.7)	167
20–39 years	3.93 (3.38 – 4.56)	1.77† (1.45 – 1.94)	3.65 (3.11 – 4.77)	8.32† (6.65 – 12.6)	68
40–59 years	3.90 (3.15 – 4.82)	1.66† (1.44 – 2.21)	3.42 (2.47 – 4.70)	8.90† (7.34 – 19.3)	56
60 years and older	3.78 (3.23 – 4.42)	1.25† (.999 – 2.33)	3.54 (3.09 – 4.69)	9.24† (5.98 – 19.5)	43

† Estimate is subject to greater uncertainty due to small cell size.

Table 2.20.a.5. Plasma myristoleic acid (14:1n-5): Non-Hispanic whites

Geometric mean and selected percentiles of plasma concentrations (in µmol/L) for fasted non-Hispanic whites in the U.S. population aged 20 years and older, National Health and Nutrition Examination Survey, 2003–2004.

	Geometric mean (95% conf. interval)	Selected percentiles (95% conf. interval)			Sample size
		10th	50th	90th	
Males and Females					
Total, 20 years and older	7.07 (6.45 – 7.74)	2.83 (2.49 – 3.02)	6.84 (6.22 – 7.46)	19.5 (16.9 – 23.0)	992
20–39 years	6.97 (6.26 – 7.77)	2.79 (2.35 – 3.08)	6.61 (5.91 – 7.53)	18.5 (15.1 – 24.6)	300
40–59 years	7.39 (6.43 – 8.48)	2.87 (2.24 – 3.54)	6.97 (6.17 – 7.94)	19.8 (17.0 – 26.7)	280
60 years and older	6.72 (5.80 – 7.78)	2.63 (2.26 – 3.01)	6.72 (5.74 – 7.72)	17.9 (13.8 – 23.5)	412
Males					
Total, 20 years and older	6.84 (6.01 – 7.79)	2.47 (2.07 – 2.86)	6.77 (5.68 – 7.91)	18.7 (16.9 – 22.7)	472
20–39 years	6.84 (5.71 – 8.20)	2.39 (2.03 – 2.95)	6.53 (5.25 – 8.27)	17.0 (14.4 – 31.7)	128
40–59 years	7.31 (6.16 – 8.67)	2.49 (1.82 – 2.96)	7.03 (4.70 – 10.4)	21.0 (18.1 – 27.6)	140
60 years and older	6.13 (5.25 – 7.15)	2.43 (1.75 – 2.89)	6.36 (5.73 – 6.86)	15.9 (11.0 – 23.9)	204
Females					
Total, 20 years and older	7.28 (6.68 – 7.93)	3.16 (2.81 – 3.49)	6.86 (6.52 – 7.22)	19.6 (15.9 – 23.8)	520
20–39 years	7.09 (5.99 – 8.39)	2.94 (2.37 – 3.49)	6.67 (5.66 – 8.11)	19.0 (14.7 – 28.0)	172
40–59 years	7.46 (6.48 – 8.59)	3.56 (2.06 – 4.04)	6.84 (6.33 – 7.23)	18.9 (13.4 – 43.3)	140
60 years and older	7.27 (5.90 – 8.94)	3.01 (1.59 – 3.69)	7.09 (5.55 – 8.67)	20.7 (17.0 – 25.2)	208

Table 2.21.a.1. Plasma palmitoleic acid (16:1n-7): Concentrations

Geometric mean and selected percentiles of plasma concentrations (in μmol/L) for the fasted U.S. population aged 20 years and older, National Health and Nutrition Examination Survey, 2003–2004.

	Geometric mean	Selected percentiles (95% conf. interval)					Sample size
	(95% conf. interval)	2.5th	5th	50th	95th	97.5th	
Total, 20 years and older	217 (205 – 229)	73.3 (65.1 – 78.1)	84.0 (79.0 – 89.6)	213 (196 – 230)	563 (526 – 664)	727 (657 – 806)	1,805
Age group							
20–39 years	195 (185 – 205)	72.5 (60.4 – 78.7)	82.0 (75.0 – 84.1)	185 (173 – 194)	539 (450 – 674)	685 (611 – 840)	610
40–59 years	228 (210 – 248)	69.3 (45.2 – 78.1)	82.4 (71.3 – 96.8)	228 (206 – 251)	572 (525 – 772)	770 (671 – 837)	514
60 years and older	238 (220 – 259)	84.8 (65.4 – 94.1)	100 (87.9 – 113)	241 (216 – 263)	559 (528 – 649)	676 (589 – 763)	681
Gender							
Males	207 (190 – 225)	69.0 (53.4 – 74.7)	77.7 (68.8 – 84.0)	203 (182 – 225)	562 (495 – 683)	682 (578 – 926)	863
Females	226 (214 – 239)	83.2 (71.2 – 88.4)	93.4 (89.1 – 104)	226 (204 – 243)	567 (528 – 679)	729 (630 – 846)	942
Race/ethnicity							
Mexican Americans	240 (209 – 277)	78.6† (60.0 – 86.2)	87.0 (64.2 – 95.4)	239 (204 – 281)	692 (594 – 780)	769† (699 – 1,110)	375
Non-Hispanic Blacks	157 (148 – 167)	64.8† (47.2 – 68.9)	70.3 (64.2 – 73.2)	151 (142 – 162)	429 (352 – 529)	523† (433 – 755)	310
Non-Hispanic Whites	221 (208 – 236)	74.9 (53.0 – 83.5)	88.9 (79.3 – 96.5)	221 (201 – 237)	554 (522 – 661)	722 (615 – 831)	990

† Estimate is subject to greater uncertainty due to small cell size.

Figure 2.21.a. Plasma palmitoleic acid (16:1n–7): Concentrations by age group
Geometric mean (95% confidence interval), National Health and Nutrition Examination Survey, 2003–2004

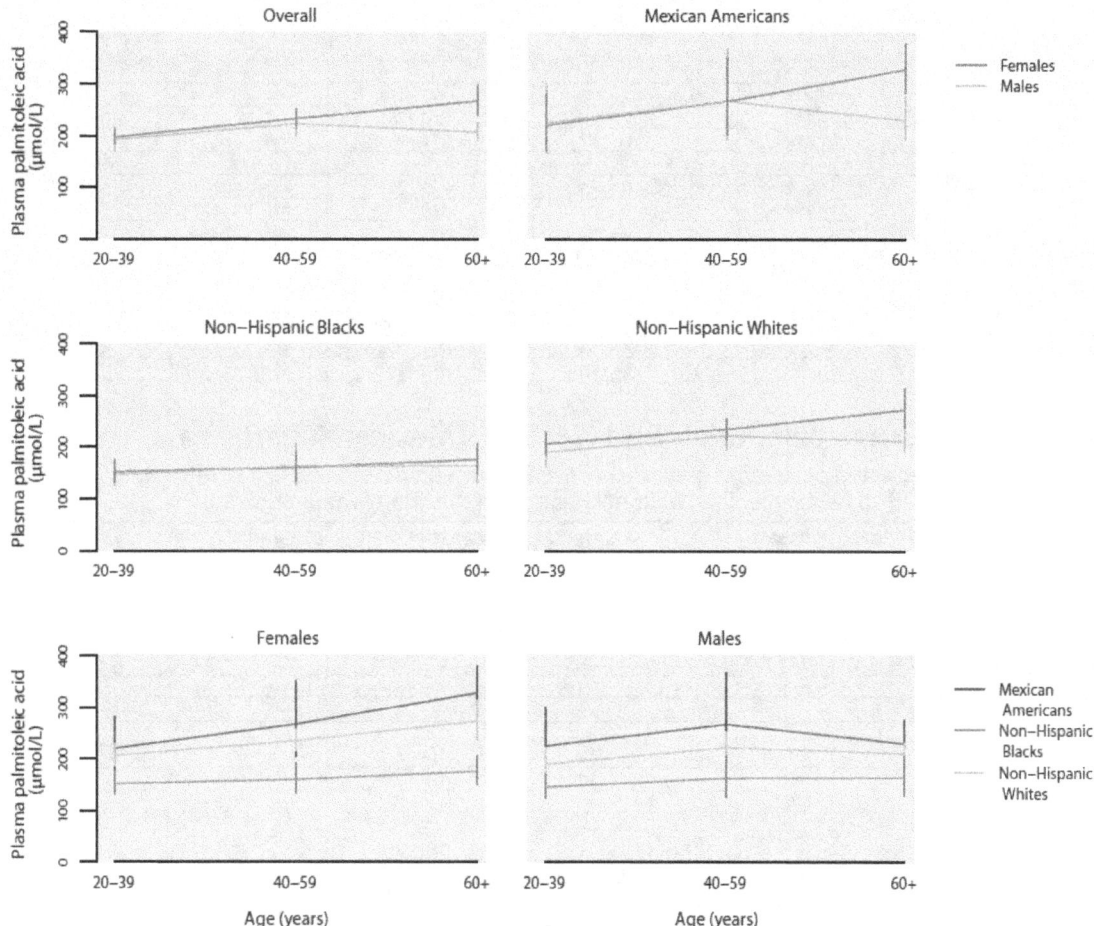

Table 2.21.a.2. Plasma palmitoleic acid (16:1n-7): Total population

Geometric mean and selected percentiles of plasma concentrations (in µmol/L) for the fasted U.S. population aged 20 years and older, National Health and Nutrition Examination Survey, 2003–2004.

	Geometric mean (95% conf. interval)		Selected percentiles (95% conf. interval)						Sample size
			10th		50th		90th		
Males and Females									
Total, 20 years and older	217	(205 – 229)	105	(97.7 – 109)	213	(196 – 230)	454	(424 – 497)	1,805
20–39 years	195	(185 – 205)	92.3	(86.5 – 98.3)	185	(173 – 194)	411	(357 – 472)	610
40–59 years	228	(210 – 248)	106	(92.9 – 118)	228	(206 – 251)	475	(444 – 549)	514
60 years and older	238	(220 – 259)	122	(111 – 135)	241	(216 – 263)	467	(429 – 540)	681
Males									
Total, 20 years and older	207	(190 – 225)	92.6	(84.0 – 98.9)	203	(182 – 225)	456	(400 – 525)	863
20–39 years	192	(171 – 215)	83.9	(76.9 – 93.8)	185	(169 – 211)	410	(344 – 542)	282
40–59 years	223	(198 – 251)	97.4	(78.0 – 108)	218	(184 – 273)	501	(450 – 594)	248
60 years and older	207	(191 – 224)	112	(92.6 – 121)	206	(186 – 228)	386	(339 – 450)	333
Females									
Total, 20 years and older	226	(214 – 239)	114	(108 – 123)	226	(204 – 243)	453	(421 – 525)	942
20–39 years	197	(185 – 211)	108	(92.2 – 111)	184	(170 – 199)	406	(352 – 495)	328
40–59 years	233	(217 – 250)	126	(99.4 – 133)	231	(213 – 256)	455	(395 – 534)	266
60 years and older	267	(240 – 298)	137	(115 – 150)	271	(242 – 297)	537	(493 – 585)	348

Table 2.21.a.3. Plasma palmitoleic acid (16:1n-7): Mexican Americans

Geometric mean and selected percentiles of plasma concentrations (in µmol/L) for fasted Mexican Americans in the U.S. population aged 20 years and older, National Health and Nutrition Examination Survey, 2003–2004.

	Geometric mean (95% conf. interval)		Selected percentiles (95% conf. interval)						Sample size
			10th		50th		90th		
Males and Females									
Total, 20 years and older	240	(209 – 277)	101	(64.3 – 131)	239	(204 – 281)	571	(498 – 645)	375
20–39 years	223	(181 – 274)	95.2	(60.0 – 129)	221	(175 – 274)	498	(386 – 737)	132
40–59 years	267	(232 – 307)	117†	(79.8 – 143)	250	(233 – 272)	639†	(545 – 804)	93
60 years and older	277	(262 – 292)	144	(136 – 158)	281	(250 – 308)	510	(446 – 587)	150
Males									
Total, 20 years and older	237	(192 – 292)	96.0	(61.6 – 134)	226	(178 – 290)	578	(489 – 687)	188
20–39 years	225	(169 – 300)	92.8†	(61.6 – 130)	215	(153 – 314)	519†	(406 – 844)	67
40–59 years	267	(194 – 367)	111†	(79.8 – 150)	240	(190 – 353)	715†	(438 – 942)	48
60 years and older	230	(192 – 276)	131†	(64.1 – 158)	223	(180 – 280)	375†	(309 – 876)	73
Females									
Total, 20 years and older	245	(207 – 291)	110	(61.1 – 132)	248	(188 – 316)	558	(421 – 749)	187
20–39 years	220	(172 – 281)	98.4†	(60.0 – 130)	225	(161 – 293)	449†	(352 – 1,110)	65
40–59 years	267	(204 – 350)	119†	(88.5 – 144)	252	(148 – 396)	613†	(517 – 766)	45
60 years and older	328	(284 – 378)	166†	(120 – 215)	353	(281 – 398)	528†	(469 – 739)	77

† Estimate is subject to greater uncertainty due to small cell size.

Table 2.21.a.4. Plasma palmitoleic acid (16:1n-7): Non-Hispanic blacks

Geometric mean and selected percentiles of plasma concentrations (in µmol/L) for fasted non-Hispanic blacks in the U.S. population aged 20 years and older, National Health and Nutrition Examination Survey, 2003–2004.

	Geometric mean (95% conf. interval)		Selected percentiles (95% conf. interval)						Sample size
			10th		50th		90th		
Males and Females									
Total, 20 years and older	157	(148 – 167)	78.0	(72.0 – 84.1)	151	(142 – 162)	326	(270 – 421)	310
20–39 years	149	(136 – 164)	78.7	(71.8 – 85.0)	148	(126 – 164)	309	(221 – 430)	126
40–59 years	161	(144 – 180)	72.4†	(65.0 – 82.5)	149	(135 – 175)	333†	(288 – 508)	98
60 years and older	171	(155 – 189)	89.5†	(61.4 – 102)	171	(152 – 193)	316†	(265 – 397)	86
Males									
Total, 20 years and older	154	(138 – 172)	74.0	(53.3 – 82.4)	157	(132 – 174)	323	(267 – 437)	143
20–39 years	146	(126 – 169)	71.0†	(47.0 – 79.4)	145	(122 – 168)	305†	(220 – 863)	58
40–59 years	163	(128 – 206)	72.7†	(42.6 – 81.3)	168	(115 – 204)	371†	(231 – 814)	42
60 years and older	164	(130 – 205)	98.3†	(60.8 – 114)	152	(123 – 206)	280†	(222 – 430)	43
Females									
Total, 20 years and older	159	(142 – 178)	84.4	(71.0 – 90.6)	149	(134 – 172)	331	(254 – 494)	167
20–39 years	152	(132 – 175)	85.4†	(75.5 – 94.4)	147	(121 – 167)	314†	(190 – 543)	68
40–59 years	160	(134 – 190)	71.3†	(58.4 – 86.2)	144	(112 – 205)	317†	(255 – 1,360)	56
60 years and older	176	(150 – 205)	89.4†	(49.9 – 104)	178	(142 – 235)	322†	(251 – 548)	43

† Estimate is subject to greater uncertainty due to small cell size.

Table 2.21.a.5. Plasma palmitoleic acid (16:1n-7): Non-Hispanic whites

Geometric mean and selected percentiles of plasma concentrations (in µmol/L) for fasted non-Hispanic whites in the U.S. population aged 20 years and older, National Health and Nutrition Examination Survey, 2003–2004.

	Geometric mean (95% conf. interval)		Selected percentiles (95% conf. interval)						Sample size
			10th		50th		90th		
Males and Females									
Total, 20 years and older	221	(208 – 236)	109	(99.2 – 116)	221	(201 – 237)	453	(411 – 498)	990
20–39 years	199	(184 – 215)	95.5	(84.0 – 109)	191	(174 – 207)	406	(348 – 496)	300
40–59 years	229	(208 – 251)	107	(96.8 – 126)	230	(214 – 253)	462	(409 – 525)	279
60 years and older	243	(221 – 267)	125	(114 – 136)	247	(219 – 272)	484	(415 – 556)	411
Males									
Total, 20 years and older	208	(189 – 229)	95.8	(81.2 – 108)	202	(182 – 231)	447	(386 – 520)	471
20–39 years	190	(164 – 221)	83.9	(69.1 – 97.2)	185	(159 – 215)	359	(319 – 554)	128
40–59 years	222	(196 – 252)	98.2	(74.3 – 111)	223	(175 – 277)	470	(410 – 582)	140
60 years and older	211	(192 – 232)	113	(92.1 – 124)	201	(182 – 241)	392	(343 – 481)	203
Females									
Total, 20 years and older	234	(219 – 249)	122	(108 – 133)	232	(220 – 250)	455	(408 – 538)	519
20–39 years	206	(187 – 228)	109	(91.9 – 118)	194	(173 – 221)	414	(346 – 644)	172
40–59 years	235	(216 – 256)	130	(99.9 – 146)	239	(220 – 257)	452	(362 – 532)	139
60 years and older	273	(238 – 314)	138	(108 – 165)	274	(243 – 303)	550	(460 – 661)	208

Table 2.22.a.1. Plasma cis-vaccenic acid (18:1n-7): Concentrations

Geometric mean and selected percentiles of plasma concentrations (in μmol/L) for the fasted U.S. population aged 20 years and older, National Health and Nutrition Examination Survey, 2003–2004.

	Geometric mean (95% conf. interval)	Selected percentiles (95% conf. interval) 2.5th	5th	50th	95th	97.5th	Sample size
Total, 20 years and older	146 (141–150)	75.3 (65.1–81.0)	83.6 (76.2–89.7)	143 (139–148)	262 (251–274)	303 (283–344)	1,762
Age group							
20–39 years	131 (126–138)	65.6 (58.6–75.3)	76.9 (63.3–82.7)	129 (122–137)	235 (214–259)	269 (248–344)	589
40–59 years	148 (143–154)	76.4 (64.4–85.5)	86.6 (75.1–95.5)	144 (139–150)	282 (251–309)	333 (298–533)	501
60 years and older	168 (162–173)	94.1 (85.3–102)	103 (93.4–109)	166 (162–172)	266 (258–297)	301 (278–344)	672
Gender							
Males	145 (139–151)	71.5 (62.4–81.2)	83.4 (70.4–90.3)	141 (135–148)	265 (242–301)	325 (277–390)	845
Females	147 (141–153)	77.7 (61.8–81.7)	85.8 (75.4–92.0)	145 (139–151)	260 (240–282)	301 (273–345)	917
Race/ethnicity							
Mexican Americans	152 (138–166)	65.9† (55.7–82.7)	80.9 (58.0–93.1)	146 (136–164)	304 (258–378)	336† (326–384)	373
Non-Hispanic Blacks	129 (120–138)	69.5† (54.5–74.7)	74.8 (68.0–80.3)	125 (117–134)	237 (206–354)	295† (251–429)	305
Non-Hispanic Whites	146 (140–152)	77.0 (62.1–85.4)	86.7 (75.1–93.1)	144 (139–149)	260 (242–275)	298 (275–337)	958

† Estimate is subject to greater uncertainty due to small cell size.

Figure 2.22.a. Plasma cis–vaccenic acid (18:1n–7): Concentrations by age group
Geometric mean (95% confidence interval), National Health and Nutrition Examination Survey, 2003–2004

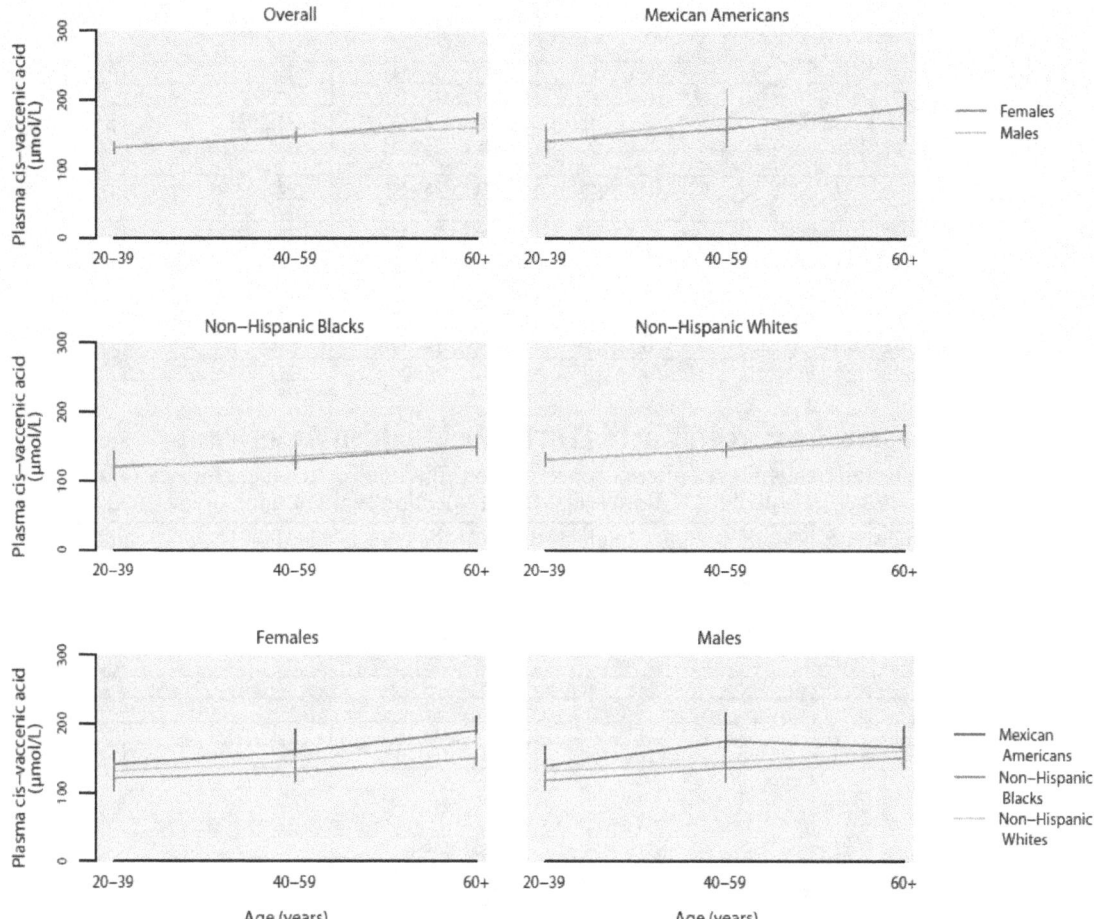

Table 2.22.a.2. Plasma cis-vaccenic acid (18:1n-7): Total population

Geometric mean and selected percentiles of plasma concentrations (in μmol/L) for the fasted U.S. population aged 20 years and older, National Health and Nutrition Examination Survey, 2003–2004.

	Geometric mean (95% conf. interval)	Selected percentiles (95% conf. interval)						Sample size
		10th		50th		90th		
Males and Females								
Total, 20 years and older	146 (141 – 150)	95.1	(89.2 – 99.8)	143	(139 – 148)	225	(216 – 234)	1,762
20–39 years	131 (126 – 138)	87.0	(78.0 – 93.7)	129	(122 – 137)	200	(190 – 215)	589
40–59 years	148 (143 – 154)	99.9	(92.1 – 104)	144	(139 – 150)	229	(211 – 262)	501
60 years and older	168 (162 – 173)	113	(107 – 119)	166	(162 – 172)	242	(231 – 259)	672
Males								
Total, 20 years and older	145 (139 – 151)	95.1	(87.8 – 102)	141	(135 – 148)	222	(210 – 241)	845
20–39 years	132 (126 – 139)	87.9	(73.4 – 94.8)	129	(123 – 138)	197	(184 – 222)	273
40–59 years	149 (139 – 160)	99.8	(85.5 – 105)	146	(133 – 159)	240	(208 – 301)	242
60 years and older	160 (153 – 167)	109	(97.2 – 117)	161	(150 – 168)	226	(215 – 258)	330
Females								
Total, 20 years and older	147 (141 – 153)	95.0	(88.5 – 99.8)	145	(139 – 151)	227	(213 – 238)	917
20–39 years	131 (123 – 139)	85.8	(78.0 – 92.8)	129	(119 – 138)	203	(190 – 222)	316
40–59 years	147 (140 – 154)	99.8	(87.5 – 105)	144	(139 – 147)	219	(187 – 301)	259
60 years and older	174 (166 – 181)	117	(107 – 127)	172	(163 – 182)	248	(237 – 273)	342

Table 2.22.a.3. Plasma cis-vaccenic acid (18:1n-7): Mexican Americans

Geometric mean and selected percentiles of plasma concentrations (in μmol/L) for fasted Mexican Americans in the U.S. population aged 20 years and older, National Health and Nutrition Examination Survey, 2003–2004.

	Geometric mean (95% conf. interval)	Selected percentiles (95% conf. interval)						Sample size
		10th		50th		90th		
Males and Females								
Total, 20 years and older	152 (138 – 166)	97.2	(66.3 – 108)	146	(136 – 164)	240	(222 – 324)	373
20–39 years	140 (125 – 157)	83.4	(55.7 – 108)	140	(125 – 154)	226	(188 – 347)	130
40–59 years	168 (146 – 192)	102†	(90.0 – 110)	157	(145 – 183)	270†	(240 – 375)	92
60 years and older	179 (171 – 187)	123	(73.1 – 139)	177	(169 – 184)	277	(247 – 310)	151
Males								
Total, 20 years and older	151 (130 – 176)	94.6	(58.1 – 111)	144	(127 – 178)	255	(217 – 331)	187
20–39 years	139 (117 – 166)	83.3†	(58.1 – 108)	136	(117 – 168)	224†	(179 – 350)	66
40–59 years	175 (142 – 216)	103†	(88.8 – 127)	159	(139 – 212)	321†	(229 – 454)	47
60 years and older	167 (142 – 197)	101†	(68.8 – 140)	155	(140 – 209)	263†	(217 – 634)	74
Females								
Total, 20 years and older	152 (142 – 162)	97.2	(72.8 – 104)	153	(137 – 167)	235	(222 – 261)	186
20–39 years	141 (124 – 160)	87.7†	(57.9 – 102)	144	(113 – 169)	221†	(186 – 410)	64
40–59 years	159 (133 – 191)	98.6†	(81.2 – 109)	151	(125 – 188)	246†	(197 – 421)	45
60 years and older	190 (173 – 210)	130†	(110 – 142)	187	(165 – 214)	284†	(228 – 375)	77

† Estimate is subject to greater uncertainty due to small cell size.

Table 2.22.a.4. Plasma cis-vaccenic acid (18:1n-7): Non-Hispanic blacks

Geometric mean and selected percentiles of plasma concentrations (in µmol/L) for fasted non-Hispanic blacks in the U.S. population aged 20 years and older, National Health and Nutrition Examination Survey, 2003–2004.

	Geometric mean (95% conf. interval)		Selected percentiles (95% conf. interval)						Sample size
			10th		50th		90th		
Males and Females									
Total, 20 years and older	129	(120 – 138)	82.6	(74.8 – 88.4)	125	(117 – 134)	202	(186 – 225)	305
20–39 years	119	(107 – 134)	80.5	(63.7 – 84.9)	112	(99.8 – 134)	184	(155 – 395)	124
40–59 years	133	(121 – 146)	80.1†	(69.5 – 89.8)	124	(118 – 135)	204†	(187 – 266)	96
60 years and older	151	(145 – 157)	108†	(99.6 – 115)	143	(141 – 147)	218†	(191 – 303)	85
Males									
Total, 20 years and older	129	(119 – 139)	79.8	(71.9 – 84.8)	124	(117 – 134)	205	(185 – 235)	141
20–39 years	118	(104 – 133)	72.2†	(54.1 – 82.8)	114	(89.0 – 136)	185†	(136 – 435)	57
40–59 years	136	(117 – 158)	80.3†	(69.7 – 90.3)	121	(117 – 132)	221†	(188 – 409)	41
60 years and older	151	(136 – 168)	108†	(89.1 – 116)	147	(136 – 168)	217†	(179 – 250)	43
Females									
Total, 20 years and older	129	(116 – 143)	84.9	(67.1 – 94.9)	126	(111 – 139)	197	(165 – 284)	164
20–39 years	121	(102 – 142)	82.6†	(56.8 – 94.3)	111	(99.1 – 140)	177†	(153 – 284)	67
40–59 years	130	(117 – 145)	76.7†	(66.9 – 92.1)	128	(115 – 136)	197†	(163 – 575)	55
60 years and older	150	(139 – 162)	108†	(102 – 124)	141	(136 – 148)	214†	(180 – 323)	42

† Estimate is subject to greater uncertainty due to small cell size.

Table 2.22.a.5. Plasma cis-vaccenic acid (18:1n-7): Non-Hispanic whites

Geometric mean and selected percentiles of plasma concentrations (in µmol/L) for fasted non-Hispanic whites in the U.S. population aged 20 years and older, National Health and Nutrition Examination Survey, 2003–2004.

	Geometric mean (95% conf. interval)		Selected percentiles (95% conf. interval)						Sample size
			10th		50th		90th		
Males and Females									
Total, 20 years and older	146	(140 – 152)	95.8	(89.8 – 102)	144	(139 – 149)	222	(211 – 234)	958
20–39 years	131	(123 – 139)	88.8	(70.0 – 95.5)	127	(120 – 138)	200	(183 – 218)	285
40–59 years	145	(139 – 153)	100	(89.1 – 104)	144	(137 – 149)	219	(199 – 244)	270
60 years and older	168	(162 – 174)	113	(106 – 117)	167	(162 – 172)	247	(231 – 261)	403
Males									
Total, 20 years and older	144	(138 – 150)	96.3	(89.6 – 103)	141	(132 – 149)	217	(205 – 240)	456
20–39 years	131	(122 – 140)	92.8	(67.7 – 97.1)	125	(117 – 139)	185	(173 – 229)	121
40–59 years	145	(135 – 156)	99.8	(84.1 – 105)	144	(127 – 158)	224	(203 – 276)	136
60 years and older	161	(153 – 169)	109	(95.0 – 116)	163	(151 – 170)	229	(216 – 260)	199
Females									
Total, 20 years and older	148	(141 – 154)	95.6	(87.9 – 103)	147	(141 – 152)	226	(209 – 240)	502
20–39 years	131	(122 – 141)	87.7	(61.8 – 95.4)	130	(121 – 139)	204	(187 – 234)	164
40–59 years	146	(137 – 155)	100	(86.2 – 105)	144	(139 – 148)	212	(180 – 322)	134
60 years and older	174	(166 – 183)	116	(103 – 128)	171	(162 – 183)	253	(235 – 279)	204

Table 2.23.a.1. Plasma oleic acid (18:1n-9): Concentrations

Geometric mean and selected percentiles of plasma concentrations (in μmol/L) for the fasted U.S. population aged 20 years and older, National Health and Nutrition Examination Survey, 2003–2004.

| | Geometric mean (95% conf. interval) | | Selected percentiles (95% conf. interval) | | | | | | | | | | Sample size |
			2.5th		5th		50th		95th		97.5th		
Total, 20 years and older	2,100	(2,050 – 2,150)	1,110	(1,030 – 1,170)	1,220	(1,170 – 1,270)	2,070	(2,000 – 2,150)	3,850	(3,590 – 4,220)	4,480	(4,230 – 4,940)	1,798
Age group													
20–39 years	1,910	(1,840 – 1,980)	1,020	(955 – 1,080)	1,130	(1,080 – 1,170)	1,840	(1,750 – 1,970)	3,710	(3,120 – 4,140)	4,190	(3,770 – 8,650)	608
40–59 years	2,160	(2,100 – 2,230)	1,160	(993 – 1,220)	1,280	(1,180 – 1,350)	2,120	(2,010 – 2,190)	4,150	(3,610 – 4,800)	4,790	(4,290 – 5,320)	512
60 years and older	2,360	(2,290 – 2,440)	1,330	(1,290 – 1,400)	1,430	(1,340 – 1,550)	2,380	(2,290 – 2,450)	3,850	(3,490 – 4,410)	4,410	(4,120 – 4,930)	678
Gender													
Males	2,140	(2,060 – 2,220)	1,140	(1,040 – 1,210)	1,230	(1,160 – 1,300)	2,100	(2,010 – 2,200)	4,110	(3,560 – 4,930)	4,930	(4,500 – 5,530)	858
Females	2,070	(2,000 – 2,140)	1,090	(972 – 1,140)	1,200	(1,130 – 1,270)	2,020	(1,940 – 2,140)	3,810	(3,490 – 4,020)	4,240	(4,030 – 4,400)	940
Race/ethnicity													
Mexican Americans	2,240	(2,060 – 2,430)	1,110†	(871 – 1,240)	1,270	(987 – 1,340)	2,170	(1,990 – 2,470)	4,280	(3,850 – 5,240)	4,940†	(4,400 – 6,640)	375
Non-Hispanic Blacks	1,810	(1,730 – 1,890)	1,020†	(892 – 1,080)	1,150	(1,010 – 1,180)	1,710	(1,620 – 1,830)	3,180	(2,890 – 3,760)	3,760†	(3,350 – 8,200)	308
Non-Hispanic Whites	2,130	(2,060 – 2,200)	1,120	(990 – 1,210)	1,230	(1,140 – 1,320)	2,120	(2,020 – 2,180)	3,840	(3,580 – 4,190)	4,380	(4,160 – 4,930)	986

† Estimate is subject to greater uncertainty due to small cell size.

Figure 2.23.a. Plasma oleic acid (18:1n–9): Concentrations by age group

Geometric mean (95% confidence interval), National Health and Nutrition Examination Survey, 2003–2004

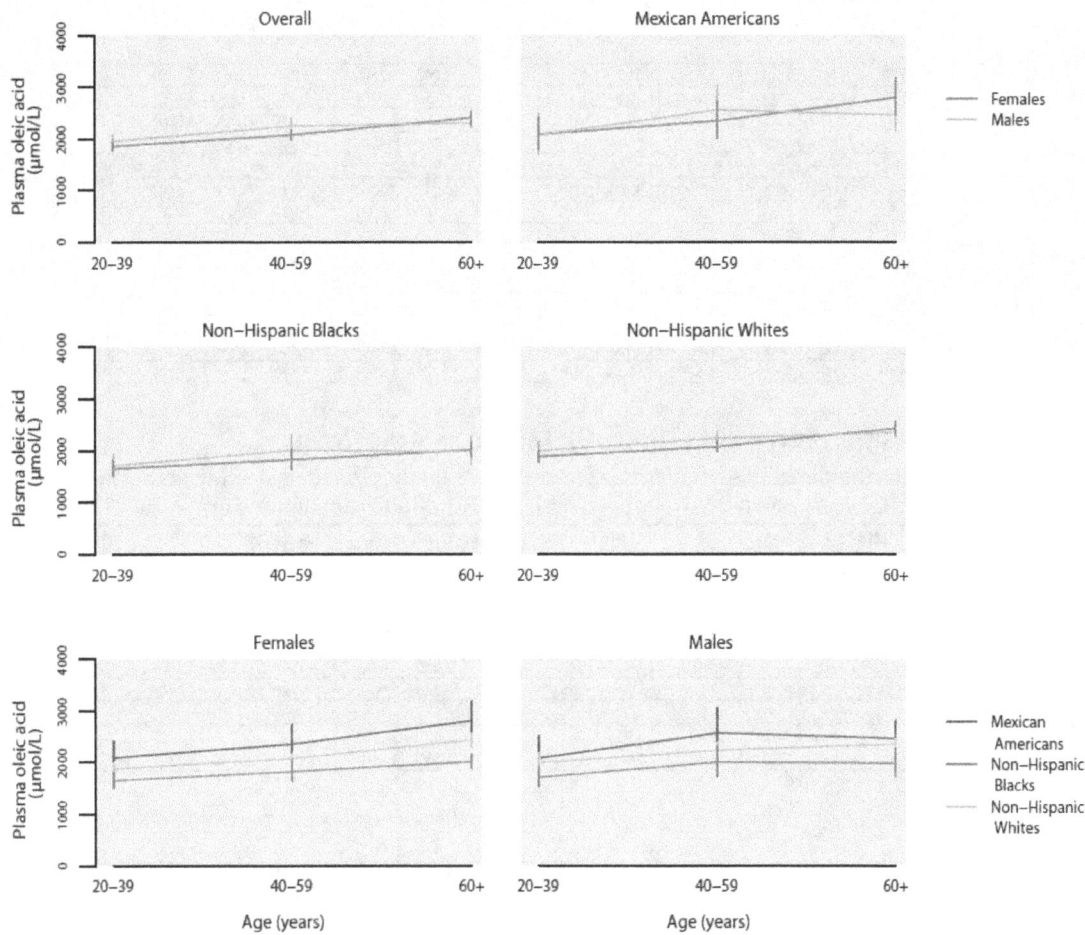

Table 2.23.a.2. Plasma oleic acid (18:1n-9): Total population

Geometric mean and selected percentiles of plasma concentrations (in µmol/L) for the fasted U.S. population aged 20 years and older, National Health and Nutrition Examination Survey, 2003–2004.

	Geometric mean (95% conf. interval)		Selected percentiles (95% conf. interval)						Sample size
			10th		50th		90th		
Males and Females									
Total, 20 years and older	2,100	(2,050 – 2,150)	1,360	(1,310 – 1,400)	2,070	(2,000 – 2,150)	3,230	(3,090 – 3,440)	1,798
20–39 years	1,910	(1,840 – 1,980)	1,240	(1,200 – 1,300)	1,840	(1,750 – 1,970)	2,900	(2,710 – 3,160)	608
40–59 years	2,160	(2,100 – 2,230)	1,410	(1,350 – 1,530)	2,120	(2,010 – 2,190)	3,380	(3,100 – 3,660)	512
60 years and older	2,360	(2,290 – 2,440)	1,630	(1,550 – 1,690)	2,380	(2,290 – 2,450)	3,360	(3,200 – 3,640)	678
Males									
Total, 20 years and older	2,140	(2,060 – 2,220)	1,360	(1,310 – 1,410)	2,100	(2,010 – 2,200)	3,340	(3,060 – 3,660)	858
20–39 years	1,960	(1,850 – 2,080)	1,240	(1,220 – 1,310)	1,890	(1,770 – 2,060)	2,950	(2,640 – 3,700)	281
40–59 years	2,250	(2,120 – 2,400)	1,410	(1,310 – 1,550)	2,200	(1,970 – 2,350)	3,580	(3,180 – 4,480)	247
60 years and older	2,310	(2,220 – 2,400)	1,600	(1,400 – 1,730)	2,340	(2,170 – 2,420)	3,310	(3,040 – 3,850)	330
Females									
Total, 20 years and older	2,070	(2,000 – 2,140)	1,380	(1,300 – 1,410)	2,020	(1,940 – 2,140)	3,180	(2,960 – 3,370)	940
20–39 years	1,860	(1,790 – 1,940)	1,220	(1,140 – 1,300)	1,780	(1,700 – 1,940)	2,820	(2,570 – 3,620)	327
40–59 years	2,080	(2,000 – 2,160)	1,400	(1,330 – 1,520)	2,000	(1,920 – 2,140)	3,100	(2,830 – 3,700)	265
60 years and older	2,410	(2,280 – 2,530)	1,660	(1,480 – 1,740)	2,430	(2,270 – 2,530)	3,410	(3,260 – 3,820)	348

Table 2.23.a.3. Plasma oleic acid (18:1n-9): Mexican Americans

Geometric mean and selected percentiles of plasma concentrations (in µmol/L) for fasted Mexican Americans in the U.S. population aged 20 years and older, National Health and Nutrition Examination Survey, 2003–2004.

	Geometric mean (95% conf. interval)		Selected percentiles (95% conf. interval)						Sample size
			10th		50th		90th		
Males and Females									
Total, 20 years and older	2,240	(2,060 – 2,430)	1,410	(1,250 – 1,500)	2,170	(1,990 – 2,470)	3,680	(3,330 – 4,270)	375
20–39 years	2,080	(1,850 – 2,350)	1,320	(882 – 1,470)	2,020	(1,710 – 2,390)	3,330	(2,900 – 4,590)	132
40–59 years	2,460	(2,220 – 2,730)	1,610†	(1,140 – 1,790)	2,330	(2,090 – 2,670)	4,210†	(3,520 – 5,160)	93
60 years and older	2,630	(2,460 – 2,820)	1,800	(1,740 – 1,820)	2,650	(2,320 – 2,900)	3,730	(3,570 – 4,720)	150
Males									
Total, 20 years and older	2,240	(1,970 – 2,540)	1,410	(1,150 – 1,510)	2,160	(1,820 – 2,570)	3,940	(3,120 – 4,880)	188
20–39 years	2,080	(1,720 – 2,500)	1,340†	(989 – 1,480)	1,930	(1,530 – 2,550)	3,390†	(2,640 – 5,270)	67
40–59 years	2,560	(2,160 – 3,040)	1,550†	(1,280 – 1,980)	2,490	(2,000 – 3,090)	4,270†	(3,570 – 5,640)	48
60 years and older	2,460	(2,160 – 2,800)	1,790†	(1,030 – 1,830)	2,350	(1,900 – 3,040)	3,440†	(3,270 – 4,860)	73
Females									
Total, 20 years and older	2,240	(2,060 – 2,450)	1,400	(859 – 1,680)	2,160	(2,020 – 2,500)	3,500	(3,280 – 3,970)	187
20–39 years	2,090	(1,810 – 2,410)	1,240†	(831 – 1,570)	2,020	(1,750 – 2,330)	3,210†	(2,850 – 4,200)	65
40–59 years	2,350	(2,020 – 2,730)	1,590†	(1,080 – 1,770)	2,200	(1,990 – 2,730)	3,760†	(2,920 – 5,280)	45
60 years and older	2,800	(2,470 – 3,180)	1,890†	(1,600 – 2,040)	2,730	(2,320 – 3,420)	4,260†	(3,660 – 5,490)	77

† Estimate is subject to greater uncertainty due to small cell size.

Table 2.23.a.4. Plasma oleic acid (18:1n-9): Non-Hispanic blacks

Geometric mean and selected percentiles of plasma concentrations (in µmol/L) for fasted non-Hispanic blacks in the U.S. population aged 20 years and older, National Health and Nutrition Examination Survey, 2003–2004.

	Geometric mean (95% conf. interval)		Selected percentiles (95% conf. interval)						Sample size
			10th		50th		90th		
Males and Females									
Total, 20 years and older	1,810	(1,730 – 1,890)	1,210	(1,170 – 1,260)	1,710	(1,620 – 1,830)	2,750	(2,610 – 2,990)	308
20–39 years	1,680	(1,560 – 1,810)	1,170	(1,050 – 1,210)	1,540	(1,470 – 1,760)	2,470	(2,310 – 3,740)	125
40–59 years	1,900	(1,750 – 2,050)	1,240†	(1,060 – 1,310)	1,790	(1,640 – 1,970)	2,840†	(2,610 – 3,590)	97
60 years and older	2,000	(1,870 – 2,150)	1,400†	(1,190 – 1,570)	1,960	(1,800 – 2,190)	2,800†	(2,670 – 3,020)	86
Males									
Total, 20 years and older	1,850	(1,720 – 1,990)	1,200	(1,140 – 1,240)	1,720	(1,570 – 1,920)	2,930	(2,470 – 4,190)	142
20–39 years	1,710	(1,540 – 1,910)	1,140†	(887 – 1,230)	1,560	(1,380 – 1,830)	2,480†	(2,400 – 6,770)	57
40–59 years	2,000	(1,730 – 2,310)	1,290†	(1,010 – 1,410)	1,850	(1,600 – 2,060)	3,160†	(2,570 – 8,560)	42
60 years and older	1,980	(1,730 – 2,270)	1,350†	(1,080 – 1,620)	1,960	(1,700 – 2,140)	2,870†	(2,440 – 4,520)	43
Females									
Total, 20 years and older	1,770	(1,670 – 1,890)	1,210	(1,150 – 1,280)	1,700	(1,600 – 1,840)	2,660	(2,460 – 2,960)	166
20–39 years	1,650	(1,510 – 1,810)	1,160†	(1,080 – 1,250)	1,540	(1,470 – 1,710)	2,430†	(2,130 – 3,240)	68
40–59 years	1,820	(1,640 – 2,030)	1,200†	(863 – 1,280)	1,760	(1,620 – 2,010)	2,620†	(2,360 – 6,740)	55
60 years and older	2,010	(1,880 – 2,160)	1,410†	(1,280 – 1,590)	1,930	(1,700 – 2,400)	2,780†	(2,640 – 3,030)	43

† Estimate is subject to greater uncertainty due to small cell size.

Table 2.23.a.5. Plasma oleic acid (18:1n-9): Non-Hispanic whites

Geometric mean and selected percentiles of plasma concentrations (in µmol/L) for fasted non-Hispanic whites in the U.S. population aged 20 years and older, National Health and Nutrition Examination Survey, 2003–2004.

	Geometric mean (95% conf. interval)		Selected percentiles (95% conf. interval)						Sample size
			10th		50th		90th		
Males and Females									
Total, 20 years and older	2,130	(2,060 – 2,200)	1,390	(1,320 – 1,480)	2,120	(2,020 – 2,180)	3,240	(3,100 – 3,430)	986
20–39 years	1,940	(1,820 – 2,050)	1,260	(1,140 – 1,360)	1,870	(1,750 – 2,040)	2,820	(2,630 – 3,710)	299
40–59 years	2,150	(2,070 – 2,220)	1,400	(1,320 – 1,550)	2,140	(2,030 – 2,180)	3,320	(3,020 – 3,600)	279
60 years and older	2,390	(2,310 – 2,470)	1,650	(1,530 – 1,730)	2,420	(2,330 – 2,480)	3,410	(3,250 – 3,700)	408
Males									
Total, 20 years and older	2,170	(2,070 – 2,280)	1,380	(1,290 – 1,520)	2,150	(2,040 – 2,240)	3,300	(3,030 – 3,630)	468
20–39 years	1,990	(1,830 – 2,170)	1,250	(1,070 – 1,380)	1,960	(1,760 – 2,130)	2,830	(2,610 – 4,110)	128
40–59 years	2,230	(2,080 – 2,380)	1,390	(1,220 – 1,570)	2,200	(1,950 – 2,370)	3,460	(3,020 – 4,000)	140
60 years and older	2,350	(2,240 – 2,460)	1,600	(1,390 – 1,730)	2,400	(2,320 – 2,470)	3,340	(3,070 – 4,100)	200
Females									
Total, 20 years and older	2,090	(2,010 – 2,180)	1,390	(1,320 – 1,470)	2,080	(1,970 – 2,160)	3,200	(2,910 – 3,660)	518
20–39 years	1,880	(1,770 – 2,000)	1,260	(1,120 – 1,360)	1,790	(1,670 – 2,010)	2,810	(2,530 – 3,860)	171
40–59 years	2,070	(1,980 – 2,170)	1,410	(1,100 – 1,560)	2,010	(1,890 – 2,160)	3,100	(2,720 – 3,910)	139
60 years and older	2,430	(2,300 – 2,560)	1,670	(1,470 – 1,810)	2,430	(2,250 – 2,540)	3,470	(3,220 – 4,060)	208

Table 2.24.a.1. Plasma eicosenoic acid (20:1n-9): Concentrations

Geometric mean and selected percentiles of plasma concentrations (in μmol/L) for the fasted U.S. population aged 20 years and older, National Health and Nutrition Examination Survey, 2003–2004.

	Geometric mean (95% conf. interval)	Selected percentiles (95% conf. interval)						Sample size
		2.5th	5th	50th	95th	97.5th	
Total, 20 years and older	13.6 (13.2 – 14.1)	6.69 (6.33 – 7.03)	7.56 (6.83 – 7.98)	13.3 (12.8 – 13.8)	25.9 (24.2 – 30.5)	33.1 (29.9 – 38.3)	1,805
Age group							
20–39 years	12.6 (12.0 – 13.3)	6.35 (5.53 – 6.66)	6.82 (6.35 – 7.49)	12.1 (11.4 – 12.9)	25.8 (22.7 – 37.3)	34.7 (26.3 – 45.2)	608
40–59 years	13.5 (13.0 – 14.1)	6.96 (4.20 – 7.54)	7.59 (7.00 – 8.25)	13.2 (12.3 – 13.8)	25.7 (23.6 – 31.7)	31.8 (27.6 – 47.0)	514
60 years and older	15.6 (15.1 – 16.1)	8.94 (7.50 – 9.41)	9.74 (8.98 – 10.3)	15.1 (14.7 – 15.8)	26.0 (24.4 – 30.4)	31.1 (28.1 – 39.5)	683
Gender							
Males	13.9 (13.3 – 14.5)	6.70 (6.12 – 7.50)	7.68 (6.72 – 8.27)	13.5 (12.9 – 14.2)	28.7 (24.6 – 33.4)	37.1 (31.8 – 42.5)	865
Females	13.4 (12.8 – 14.0)	6.66 (5.98 – 7.01)	7.48 (6.83 – 7.84)	13.0 (12.6 – 13.6)	24.9 (23.2 – 26.6)	30.1 (26.1 – 35.3)	940
Race/ethnicity							
Mexican Americans	15.4 (14.4 – 16.5)	6.86† (6.00 – 8.62)	8.65 (6.33 – 9.25)	14.7 (13.7 – 16.4)	33.1 (27.9 – 40.8)	38.7† (33.2 – 45.9)	376
Non-Hispanic Blacks	11.7 (11.0 – 12.4)	6.11† (5.11 – 6.37)	6.39 (6.08 – 6.85)	11.1 (10.2 – 12.1)	23.4 (21.3 – 28.1)	29.4† (25.1 – 51.3)	310
Non-Hispanic Whites	13.6 (13.1 – 14.2)	6.83 (5.83 – 7.46)	7.63 (6.70 – 8.15)	13.4 (12.9 – 13.8)	24.9 (23.5 – 30.1)	31.7 (26.5 – 39.3)	989

† Estimate is subject to greater uncertainty due to small cell size.

Figure 2.24.a. Plasma eicosenoic acid (20:1n–9): Concentrations by age group
Geometric mean (95% confidence interval), National Health and Nutrition Examination Survey, 2003–2004

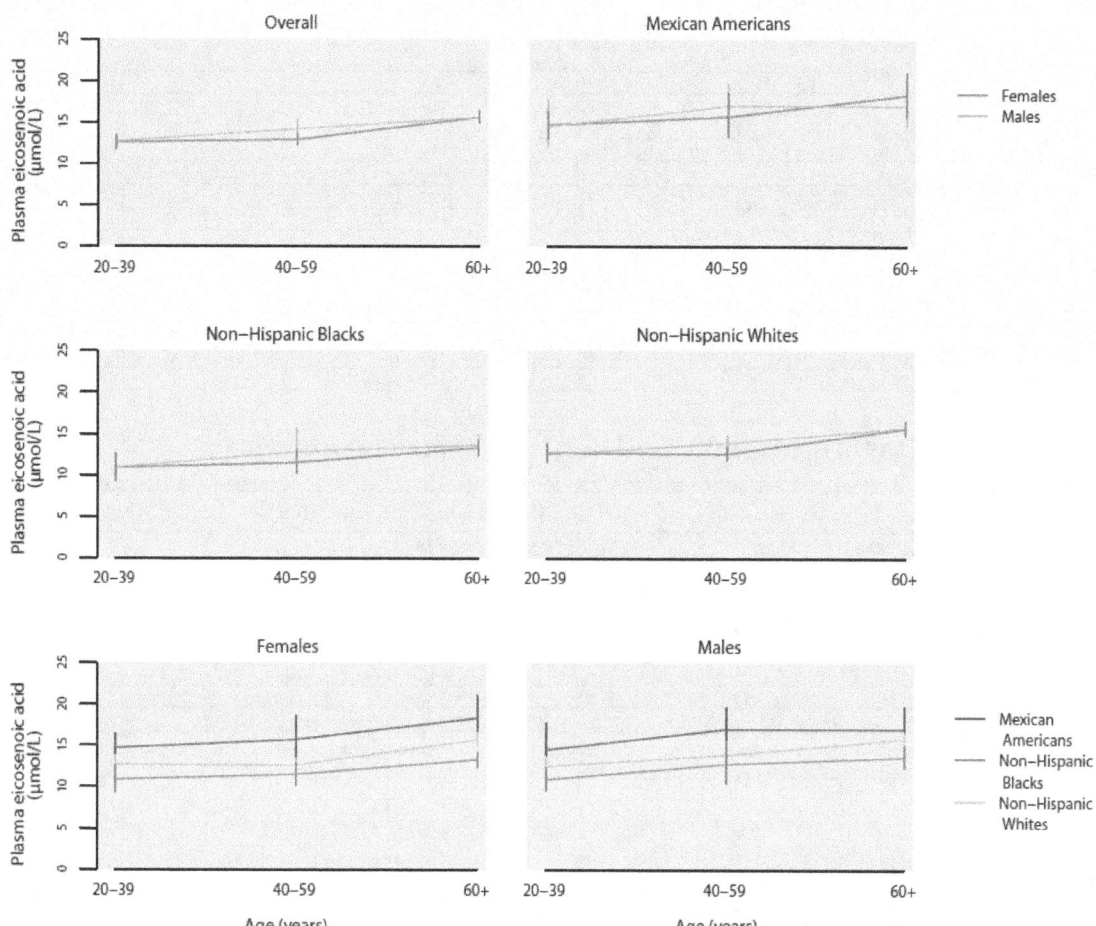

Table 2.24.a.2. Plasma eicosenoic acid (20:1n-9): Total population

Geometric mean and selected percentiles of plasma concentrations (in µmol/L) for the fasted U.S. population aged 20 years and older, National Health and Nutrition Examination Survey, 2003–2004.

	Geometric mean (95% conf. interval)		Selected percentiles (95% conf. interval)						Sample size
			10th		50th		90th		
Males and Females									
Total, 20 years and older	13.6	(13.2 – 14.1)	8.46	(7.94 – 8.95)	13.3	(12.8 – 13.8)	22.2	(21.4 – 23.2)	1,805
20–39 years	12.6	(12.0 – 13.3)	7.85	(6.91 – 8.20)	12.1	(11.4 – 12.9)	21.6	(20.3 – 23.2)	608
40–59 years	13.5	(13.0 – 14.1)	8.71	(7.75 – 9.34)	13.2	(12.3 – 13.8)	22.3	(20.3 – 24.2)	514
60 years and older	15.6	(15.1 – 16.1)	10.7	(10.3 – 10.9)	15.1	(14.7 – 15.8)	23.1	(21.8 – 24.6)	683
Males									
Total, 20 years and older	13.9	(13.3 – 14.5)	8.77	(8.41 – 8.97)	13.5	(12.9 – 14.2)	22.8	(21.2 – 24.7)	865
20–39 years	12.7	(11.9 – 13.5)	7.88	(6.97 – 8.43)	12.2	(11.6 – 13.0)	21.2	(17.8 – 25.8)	282
40–59 years	14.2	(13.3 – 15.3)	8.96	(8.39 – 9.70)	13.9	(12.7 – 14.7)	23.2	(20.5 – 31.5)	248
60 years and older	15.6	(15.0 – 16.2)	10.5	(10.2 – 10.9)	14.9	(14.4 – 16.1)	23.5	(21.8 – 24.8)	335
Females									
Total, 20 years and older	13.4	(12.8 – 14.0)	8.18	(7.55 – 8.94)	13.0	(12.6 – 13.6)	21.8	(21.0 – 22.9)	940
20–39 years	12.6	(11.8 – 13.4)	7.74	(6.79 – 8.08)	12.0	(10.8 – 13.2)	21.7	(20.6 – 23.4)	326
40–59 years	12.9	(12.3 – 13.6)	8.31	(7.29 – 9.14)	12.5	(11.9 – 13.1)	19.9	(18.5 – 23.0)	266
60 years and older	15.6	(14.9 – 16.4)	10.8	(9.70 – 11.4)	15.1	(14.6 – 15.9)	22.6	(21.6 – 25.1)	348

Table 2.24.a.3. Plasma eicosenoic acid (20:1n-9): Mexican Americans

Geometric mean and selected percentiles of plasma concentrations (in µmol/L) for fasted Mexican Americans in the U.S. population aged 20 years and older, National Health and Nutrition Examination Survey, 2003–2004.

	Geometric mean (95% conf. interval)		Selected percentiles (95% conf. interval)						Sample size
			10th		50th		90th		
Males and Females									
Total, 20 years and older	15.4	(14.4 – 16.5)	9.39	(8.68 – 10.3)	14.7	(13.7 – 16.4)	26.9	(22.7 – 33.2)	376
20–39 years	14.6	(13.2 – 16.2)	8.93	(7.04 – 9.80)	14.1	(12.1 – 16.5)	23.5	(20.3 – 40.8)	132
40–59 years	16.4	(14.8 – 18.2)	10.2†	(7.11 – 11.7)	15.2	(14.6 – 16.8)	28.4†	(25.1 – 32.9)	93
60 years and older	17.6	(16.3 – 19.1)	12.0	(10.4 – 12.6)	16.7	(14.6 – 19.8)	27.7	(24.8 – 37.1)	151
Males									
Total, 20 years and older	15.4	(13.7 – 17.3)	9.18	(8.78 – 10.6)	14.7	(13.3 – 16.8)	26.1	(21.8 – 39.8)	189
20–39 years	14.5	(12.0 – 17.7)	8.87†	(7.99 – 9.35)	14.2	(11.5 – 16.7)	22.7†	(17.5 – 40.9)	67
40–59 years	17.0	(14.8 – 19.6)	10.5†	(7.01 – 12.6)	15.3	(14.5 – 17.7)	30.7†	(24.6 – 44.8)	48
60 years and older	17.0	(14.6 – 19.7)	11.7†	(5.88 – 13.3)	16.4	(12.8 – 21.4)	25.3†	(21.4 – 59.6)	74
Females									
Total, 20 years and older	15.4	(14.4 – 16.5)	9.59	(6.32 – 10.4)	15.0	(13.6 – 16.6)	27.1	(22.6 – 35.3)	187
20–39 years	14.7	(13.2 – 16.4)	9.04†	(6.32 – 10.1)	14.0	(11.6 – 16.6)	23.8†	(21.5 – 38.7)	65
40–59 years	15.7	(13.3 – 18.6)	9.79†	(6.66 – 11.9)	14.9	(12.8 – 18.8)	26.4†	(19.1 – 38.4)	45
60 years and older	18.3	(15.9 – 21.0)	11.9†	(9.58 – 13.0)	16.8	(14.6 – 21.4)	32.3†	(24.3 – 38.0)	77

† Estimate is subject to greater uncertainty due to small cell size.

Table 2.24.a.4. Plasma eicosenoic acid (20:1n-9): Non-Hispanic blacks

Geometric mean and selected percentiles of plasma concentrations (in µmol/L) for fasted non-Hispanic blacks in the U.S. population aged 20 years and older, National Health and Nutrition Examination Survey, 2003–2004.

	Geometric mean (95% conf. interval)	Selected percentiles (95% conf. interval)			Sample size
		10th	50th	90th	
Males and Females					
Total, 20 years and older	11.7 (11.0 – 12.4)	7.28 (6.35 – 7.86)	11.1 (10.2 – 12.1)	20.0 (17.7 – 22.1)	310
20–39 years	10.9 (9.78 – 12.1)	6.75 (6.07 – 7.51)	9.90 (9.05 – 11.4)	19.7 (15.0 – 25.9)	126
40–59 years	12.1 (10.9 – 13.3)	7.40† (5.83 – 8.31)	11.4 (10.1 – 12.4)	20.0† (16.8 – 33.4)	98
60 years and older	13.4 (12.7 – 14.1)	9.43† (8.18 – 9.88)	13.1 (12.2 – 14.6)	19.7† (17.7 – 24.3)	86
Males					
Total, 20 years and older	11.9 (11.1 – 12.8)	7.12 (6.18 – 7.71)	11.0 (9.88 – 12.3)	21.2 (17.6 – 35.8)	143
20–39 years	10.9 (9.62 – 12.4)	6.33† (5.90 – 7.47)	9.97 (8.73 – 12.2)	17.2† (14.7 – 35.2)	58
40–59 years	12.8 (10.5 – 15.6)	7.86† (5.24 – 8.80)	11.1 (9.28 – 14.0)	21.3† (16.6 – 61.1)	42
60 years and older	13.6 (12.4 – 15.0)	9.07† (6.71 – 10.5)	12.3 (11.2 – 15.0)	22.3† (18.9 – 25.7)	43
Females					
Total, 20 years and older	11.5 (10.4 – 12.7)	7.29 (6.37 – 7.99)	11.3 (9.96 – 12.5)	19.0 (15.8 – 25.1)	167
20–39 years	10.9 (9.36 – 12.6)	6.88† (5.96 – 7.70)	9.60 (8.86 – 11.9)	20.2† (14.6 – 26.0)	68
40–59 years	11.5 (10.2 – 12.9)	7.20† (5.09 – 7.95)	11.6 (9.98 – 12.5)	17.6† (14.1 – 40.8)	56
60 years and older	13.3 (12.4 – 14.2)	9.42† (8.21 – 9.77)	13.3 (12.6 – 14.6)	18.0† (15.3 – 24.3)	43

† Estimate is subject to greater uncertainty due to small cell size.

Table 2.24.a.5. Plasma eicosenoic acid (20:1n-9): Non-Hispanic whites

Geometric mean and selected percentiles of plasma concentrations (in µmol/L) for fasted non-Hispanic whites in the U.S. population aged 20 years and older, National Health and Nutrition Examination Survey, 2003–2004.

	Geometric mean (95% conf. interval)	Selected percentiles (95% conf. interval)			Sample size
		10th	50th	90th	
Males and Females					
Total, 20 years and older	13.6 (13.1 – 14.2)	8.60 (7.88 – 9.22)	13.4 (12.9 – 13.8)	22.0 (20.7 – 23.3)	989
20–39 years	12.6 (11.8 – 13.6)	7.88 (6.83 – 8.26)	12.1 (11.4 – 13.0)	21.6 (19.4 – 24.2)	298
40–59 years	13.3 (12.7 – 13.9)	8.71 (7.53 – 9.56)	13.0 (11.9 – 13.7)	21.7 (19.0 – 23.1)	279
60 years and older	15.8 (15.2 – 16.3)	10.8 (10.4 – 11.1)	15.2 (14.7 – 15.9)	23.1 (21.7 – 25.4)	412
Males					
Total, 20 years and older	13.9 (13.2 – 14.5)	8.91 (8.24 – 9.44)	13.6 (12.9 – 14.2)	22.2 (20.4 – 24.2)	472
20–39 years	12.5 (11.5 – 13.7)	7.92 (6.33 – 8.95)	11.9 (11.4 – 13.0)	18.2 (15.7 – 42.2)	128
40–59 years	13.9 (12.9 – 15.0)	8.97 (7.92 – 9.80)	13.8 (11.9 – 14.7)	22.2 (19.9 – 25.5)	140
60 years and older	15.8 (15.1 – 16.6)	10.6 (10.2 – 11.2)	15.3 (14.7 – 16.4)	23.4 (21.7 – 26.6)	204
Females					
Total, 20 years and older	13.4 (12.8 – 14.1)	8.17 (7.57 – 9.08)	13.1 (12.6 – 13.7)	21.8 (20.5 – 23.4)	517
20–39 years	12.7 (11.7 – 13.8)	7.83 (5.75 – 8.15)	12.3 (10.7 – 13.7)	21.7 (20.6 – 25.6)	170
40–59 years	12.6 (11.9 – 13.4)	8.42 (6.89 – 9.47)	12.1 (11.7 – 13.0)	19.0 (17.2 – 22.9)	139
60 years and older	15.7 (14.9 – 16.5)	10.9 (10.5 – 11.4)	15.1 (14.5 – 15.9)	22.8 (21.2 – 26.1)	208

Table 2.25.a.1. Plasma docosenoic acid (22:1n-9): Concentrations

Geometric mean and selected percentiles of plasma concentrations (in µmol/L) for the fasted U.S. population aged 20 years and older, National Health and Nutrition Examination Survey, 2003–2004.

	Geometric mean (95% conf. interval)	Selected percentiles (95% conf. interval)					Sample size
		2.5th	5th	50th	95th	97.5th	
Total, 20 years and older	3.44 (2.97–3.99)	<LOD	.712 (<LOD–1.25)	3.62 (3.30–4.07)	10.3 (9.50–12.2)	13.6 (11.8–16.6)	1,604
Age group							
20–39 years	3.36 (2.75–4.11)	<LOD	.612 (<LOD–1.38)	3.46 (3.10–4.06)	11.6 (9.32–16.7)	14.7 (12.4–20.1)	533
40–59 years	3.39 (2.89–3.97)	.310 (<LOD–.677)	.729 (<LOD–1.15)	3.51 (3.16–4.23)	9.45 (8.62–13.4)	12.6 (10.8–16.6)	454
60 years and older	3.67 (3.18–4.24)	.421 (<LOD–.890)	.831 (<LOD–1.46)	3.93 (3.55–4.47)	9.69 (8.60–10.9)	11.2 (9.74–15.5)	617
Gender							
Males	3.34 (2.85–3.92)	<LOD	.620 (<LOD–1.11)	3.54 (3.24–4.04)	10.1 (9.39–11.9)	12.9 (10.9–14.0)	767
Females	3.54 (3.04–4.12)	.334 (<LOD–.936)	.941 (<LOD–1.41)	3.66 (3.33–4.23)	11.0 (8.65–14.7)	14.7 (11.9–17.7)	837
Race/ethnicity							
Mexican Americans	3.38 (2.83–4.03)	<LOD†	.692 (<LOD–1.46)	3.69 (3.32–4.29)	10.5 (7.40–23.0)	13.3† (8.78–23.8)	345
Non-Hispanic Blacks	3.81 (3.39–4.29)	.673† (<LOD–1.47)	1.43 (<LOD–1.72)	3.83 (3.46–4.50)	10.8 (9.41–15.0)	13.4† (11.0–20.1)	280
Non-Hispanic Whites	3.36 (2.79–4.05)	<LOD	.613 (<LOD–1.15)	3.54 (3.16–4.23)	10.1 (9.13–12.6)	13.6 (11.4–16.8)	863

< LOD means less than the limit of detection, which may vary for some compounds by year. See Appendix D for LOD.

† Estimate is subject to greater uncertainty due to small cell size.

Figure 2.25.a. Plasma docosenoic acid (22:1n–9): Concentrations by age group

Geometric mean (95% confidence interval), National Health and Nutrition Examination Survey, 2003–2004

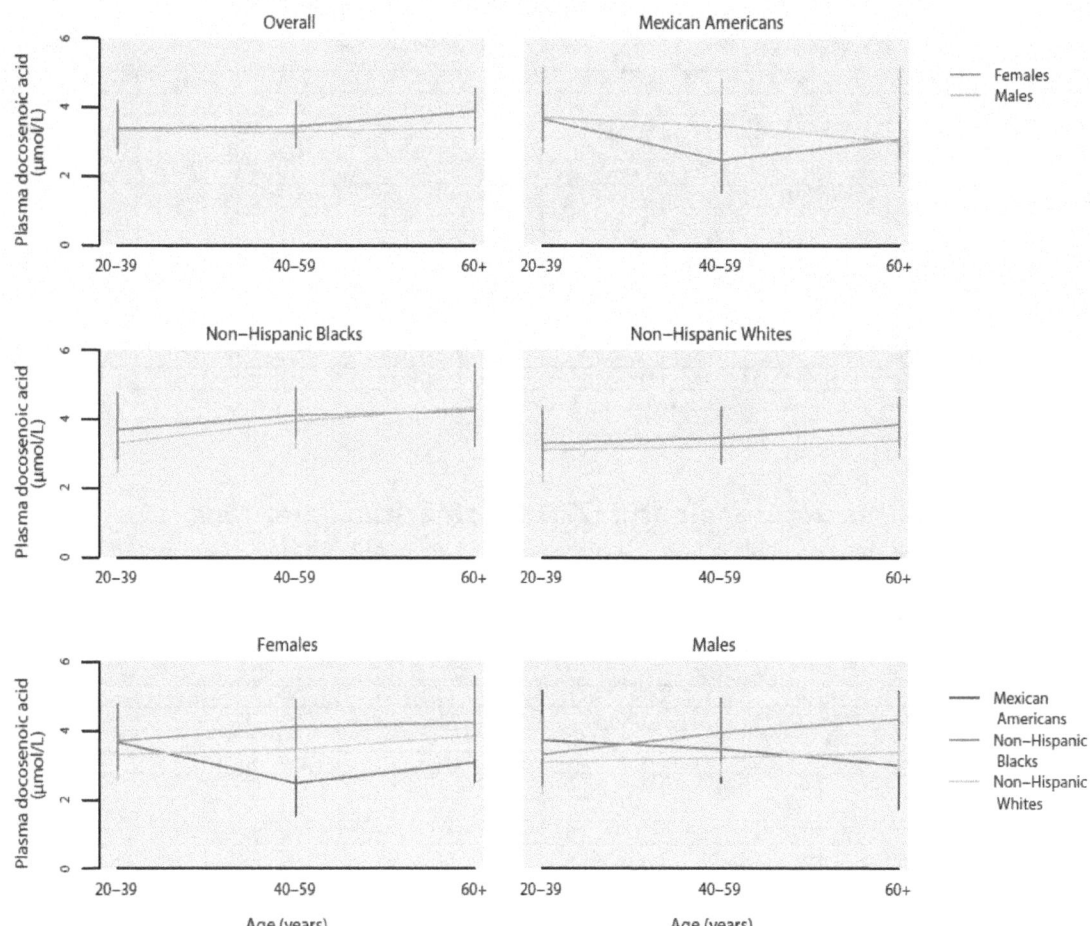

Table 2.25.a.2. Plasma docosenoic acid (22:1n-9): Total population

Geometric mean and selected percentiles of plasma concentrations (in µmol/L) for the fasted U.S. population aged 20 years and older, National Health and Nutrition Examination Survey, 2003–2004.

	Geometric mean (95% conf. interval)	Selected percentiles (95% conf. interval)						Sample size
		10th		50th		90th		
Males and Females								
Total, 20 years and older	3.44	(2.97 – 3.99)	1.38	(.670 – 1.82)	3.62	(3.30 – 4.07)	8.15	(7.41 – 9.51)	1,604
20–39 years	3.36	(2.75 – 4.11)	1.38	(< LOD – 1.87)	3.46	(3.10 – 4.06)	8.64	(7.27 – 11.3)	533
40–59 years	3.39	(2.89 – 3.97)	1.21	(.624 – 1.79)	3.51	(3.16 – 4.23)	8.03	(7.04 – 9.44)	454
60 years and older	3.67	(3.18 – 4.24)	1.55	(.813 – 1.94)	3.93	(3.55 – 4.47)	7.86	(7.43 – 8.68)	617
Males								
Total, 20 years and older	3.34	(2.85 – 3.92)	1.22	(.372 – 1.85)	3.54	(3.24 – 4.04)	8.37	(7.59 – 9.60)	767
20–39 years	3.33	(2.63 – 4.20)	1.11	(< LOD – 1.89)	3.38	(2.94 – 4.18)	9.18	(7.58 – 12.3)	249
40–59 years	3.32	(2.85 – 3.86)	1.21	(.324 – 1.87)	3.68	(3.16 – 4.39)	8.06	(6.79 – 9.60)	219
60 years and older	3.42	(2.95 – 3.95)	1.33	(.641 – 1.75)	3.65	(3.35 – 3.95)	7.93	(7.45 – 9.69)	299
Females								
Total, 20 years and older	3.54	(3.04 – 4.12)	1.47	(.937 – 1.84)	3.66	(3.33 – 4.23)	7.82	(7.24 – 9.41)	837
20–39 years	3.40	(2.83 – 4.08)	1.44	(.483 – 1.70)	3.58	(2.95 – 4.23)	7.58	(6.98 – 14.6)	284
40–59 years	3.46	(2.85 – 4.19)	1.16	(.666 – 1.76)	3.44	(3.03 – 4.43)	7.92	(7.18 – 11.5)	235
60 years and older	3.89	(3.33 – 4.54)	1.77	(.727 – 2.27)	4.25	(3.69 – 5.32)	7.69	(7.38 – 8.54)	318

< LOD means less than the limit of detection, which may vary for some compounds by year. See Appendix D for LOD.

Table 2.25.a.3. Plasma docosenoic acid (22:1n-9): Mexican Americans

Geometric mean and selected percentiles of plasma concentrations (in µmol/L) for fasted Mexican Americans in the U.S. population aged 20 years and older, National Health and Nutrition Examination Survey, 2003–2004.

	Geometric mean (95% conf. interval)	Selected percentiles (95% conf. interval)						Sample size
		10th		50th		90th		
Males and Females								
Total, 20 years and older	3.38	(2.83 – 4.03)	1.47	(.698 – 1.86)	3.69	(3.32 – 4.29)	7.40	(6.31 – 12.3)	345
20–39 years	3.70	(2.96 – 4.62)	1.58	(< LOD – 2.35)	3.97	(3.54 – 4.50)	7.41	(6.18 – 16.2)	117
40–59 years	2.97	(2.04 – 4.31)	1.20†	(< LOD – 1.85)	3.45	(2.09 – 4.69)	7.48†	(5.26 – 12.2)	91
60 years and older	3.04	(2.44 – 3.79)	1.48	(< LOD – 1.90)	3.41	(2.89 – 3.83)	6.86	(5.67 – 12.0)	137
Males								
Total, 20 years and older	3.57	(2.84 – 4.49)	1.51	(< LOD – 1.96)	3.93	(3.52 – 4.30)	8.15	(6.07 – 23.8)	170
20–39 years	3.72	(2.68 – 5.16)	1.38†	(< LOD – 2.15)	4.00	(3.27 – 4.92)	7.88†	(6.00 – 23.8)	58
40–59 years	3.47	(2.50 – 4.81)	1.47†	(< LOD – 2.04)	3.82	(2.77 – 4.66)	8.18†	(5.28 – 11.5)	47
60 years and older	3.00	(1.75 – 5.14)	1.47†	(< LOD – 2.17)	3.41	(1.76 – 5.76)	7.10†	(5.04 – 13.1)	65
Females								
Total, 20 years and older	3.16	(2.54 – 3.92)	1.43	(< LOD – 1.87)	3.55	(2.85 – 4.70)	6.83	(5.85 – 7.88)	175
20–39 years	3.67	(3.03 – 4.43)	1.68†	(< LOD – 2.49)	3.76	(3.30 – 4.88)	7.10†	(5.69 – 18.2)	59
40–59 years	2.48	(1.54 – 3.98)	.740†	(< LOD – 1.71)	2.87	(1.88 – 4.31)	6.29†	(4.79 – 12.2)	44
60 years and older	3.08	(2.53 – 3.75)	1.48†	(< LOD – 2.10)	3.39	(2.65 – 3.84)	6.46†	(4.82 – 10.8)	72

< LOD means less than the limit of detection, which may vary for some compounds by year. See Appendix D for LOD.
† Estimate is subject to greater uncertainty due to small cell size.

Table 2.25.a.4. Plasma docosenoic acid (22:1n-9): Non-Hispanic blacks

Geometric mean and selected percentiles of plasma concentrations (in µmol/L) for fasted non-Hispanic blacks in the U.S. population aged 20 years and older, National Health and Nutrition Examination Survey, 2003–2004.

	Geometric mean (95% conf. interval)	Selected percentiles (95% conf. interval)						Sample size
		10th		50th		90th		
Males and Females								
Total, 20 years and older	3.81 (3.39 – 4.29)	1.76	(.712 – 2.22)	3.83	(3.46 – 4.50)	8.37	(7.02 – 13.4)	280
20–39 years	3.52 (2.85 – 4.34)	1.68	(< LOD – 2.11)	3.54	(3.15 – 4.17)	8.10	(5.61 – 23.4)	116
40–59 years	4.04 (3.53 – 4.64)	1.64†	(< LOD – 2.46)	4.52	(3.73 – 5.02)	8.15†	(7.20 – 11.6)	82
60 years and older	4.28 (3.65 – 5.01)	2.24†	(.542 – 2.55)	4.19	(3.30 – 5.58)	8.49†	(7.12 – 19.0)	82
Males								
Total, 20 years and older	3.66 (3.11 – 4.30)	1.82	(< LOD – 2.26)	3.63	(3.08 – 4.53)	9.58	(7.05 – 13.4)	130
20–39 years	3.31 (2.46 – 4.44)	1.50†	(< LOD – 2.27)	3.28	(2.35 – 4.53)	7.50†	(5.46 – 23.8)	54
40–59 years	3.95 (3.14 – 4.96)	1.76†	(< LOD – 2.60)	4.00	(3.07 – 5.03)	9.73†	(6.86 – 14.6)	35
60 years and older	4.34 (3.73 – 5.05)	1.86†	(< LOD – 2.52)	3.87	(3.28 – 6.41)	9.45†	(8.02 – 19.0)	41
Females								
Total, 20 years and older	3.94 (3.40 – 4.56)	1.75	(1.28 – 2.16)	4.14	(3.39 – 4.92)	8.10	(6.84 – 16.2)	150
20–39 years	3.70 (2.87 – 4.77)	1.68†	(< LOD – 2.25)	3.57	(3.18 – 4.43)	8.27†	(5.30 – 19.7)	62
40–59 years	4.12 (3.48 – 4.89)	1.57†	(.381 – 2.46)	4.86	(3.40 – 6.24)	8.08†	(6.93 – 11.9)	47
60 years and older	4.24 (3.22 – 5.58)	2.30†	(1.77 – 2.61)	4.23	(2.58 – 6.59)	7.56†	(6.37 – 11.8)	41

< LOD means less than the limit of detection, which may vary for some compounds by year. See Appendix D for LOD.
† Estimate is subject to greater uncertainty due to small cell size.

Table 2.25.a.5. Plasma docosenoic acid (22:1n-9): Non-Hispanic whites

Geometric mean and selected percentiles of plasma concentrations (in µmol/L) for fasted non-Hispanic whites in the U.S. population aged 20 years and older, National Health and Nutrition Examination Survey, 2003–2004.

	Geometric mean (95% conf. interval)	Selected percentiles (95% conf. interval)						Sample size
		10th		50th		90th		
Males and Females								
Total, 20 years and older	3.36 (2.79 – 4.05)	1.18	(.420 – 1.78)	3.54	(3.16 – 4.23)	8.12	(7.40 – 9.59)	863
20–39 years	3.21 (2.41 – 4.27)	1.09	(< LOD – 1.87)	3.37	(2.71 – 4.30)	8.51	(7.27 – 11.9)	255
40–59 years	3.33 (2.77 – 4.01)	1.11	(.402 – 1.71)	3.44	(2.98 – 4.49)	8.10	(6.96 – 11.0)	242
60 years and older	3.63 (3.07 – 4.29)	1.49	(.647 – 1.90)	3.93	(3.52 – 4.55)	7.77	(7.44 – 8.50)	366
Males								
Total, 20 years and older	3.21 (2.64 – 3.91)	1.09	(< LOD – 1.85)	3.48	(3.05 – 4.20)	8.14	(7.22 – 9.56)	412
20–39 years	3.10 (2.19 – 4.39)	.749†	(< LOD – 1.86)	3.20	(2.56 – 4.88)	8.97†	(7.37 – 12.8)	110
40–59 years	3.21 (2.69 – 3.82)	1.08	(< LOD – 1.91)	3.52	(3.01 – 4.49)	7.62	(5.91 – 9.68)	122
60 years and older	3.38 (2.85 – 4.02)	1.37	(.534 – 1.82)	3.63	(3.33 – 4.15)	7.79	(6.98 – 9.24)	180
Females								
Total, 20 years and older	3.51 (2.89 – 4.25)	1.36	(.604 – 1.76)	3.66	(3.21 – 4.30)	7.92	(7.38 – 10.4)	451
20–39 years	3.31 (2.57 – 4.24)	1.37	(< LOD – 1.89)	3.61	(2.73 – 4.30)	7.62	(6.64 – 16.9)	145
40–59 years	3.46 (2.74 – 4.36)	1.09	(.381 – 1.71)	3.43	(2.89 – 5.00)	8.43	(7.34 – 13.9)	120
60 years and older	3.85 (3.20 – 4.63)	1.54	(.484 – 2.18)	4.22	(3.61 – 5.48)	7.71	(7.39 – 8.61)	186

< LOD means less than the limit of detection, which may vary for some compounds by year. See Appendix D for LOD.
† Estimate is subject to greater uncertainty due to small cell size.

Table 2.26.a.1. Plasma nervonic acid (24:1n-9): Concentrations

Geometric mean and selected percentiles of plasma concentrations (in μmol/L) for the fasted U.S. population aged 20 years and older, National Health and Nutrition Examination Survey, 2003–2004.

	Geometric mean (95% conf. interval)		Selected percentiles (95% conf. interval)								Sample size
			2.5th	5th	50th	95th	97.5th				
Total, 20 years and older	74.9	(72.4–77.4)	45.6 (42.9–47.8)	49.8 (45.9–52.0)	75.0 (72.0–77.7)	116 (112–121)	126 (122–134)				1,696
Age group											
20–39 years	72.2	(68.7–75.8)	44.5 (40.1–45.9)	47.8 (44.5–51.6)	72.1 (67.8–77.2)	109 (103–115)	118 (112–126)				573
40–59 years	74.3	(71.5–77.1)	46.4 (34.9–50.4)	51.2 (46.2–53.2)	74.1 (71.4–77.6)	109 (105–121)	123 (113–140)				492
60 years and older	81.0	(77.7–84.6)	44.1 (41.8–49.9)	50.7 (44.6–53.2)	79.9 (77.2–84.8)	128 (121–138)	137 (129–161)				631
Gender											
Males	72.0	(69.5–74.5)	44.3 (40.3–45.9)	47.0 (44.5–50.9)	71.9 (69.8–74.4)	109 (105–114)	118 (113–127)				816
Females	77.7	(74.8–80.7)	47.9 (44.6–50.0)	51.6 (47.0–55.3)	77.6 (74.3–80.0)	121 (116–126)	131 (124–141)				880
Race/ethnicity											
Mexican Americans	74.4	(71.0–78.0)	46.4† (32.6–52.8)	51.4 (43.8–54.3)	76.0 (71.1–77.9)	108 (101–121)	115† (108–157)				373
Non-Hispanic Blacks	77.3	(72.1–82.8)	44.4† (23.7–49.2)	49.3 (38.9–53.8)	77.5 (72.6–81.8)	123 (115–131)	129† (124–161)				288
Non-Hispanic Whites	74.1	(71.3–77.0)	45.0 (42.5–46.4)	49.2 (45.4–51.8)	74.0 (71.0–77.4)	117 (111–122)	127 (122–135)				914

† Estimate is subject to greater uncertainty due to small cell size.

Figure 2.26.a. Plasma nervonic acid (24:1n–9): Concentrations by age group

Geometric mean (95% confidence interval), National Health and Nutrition Examination Survey, 2003–2004

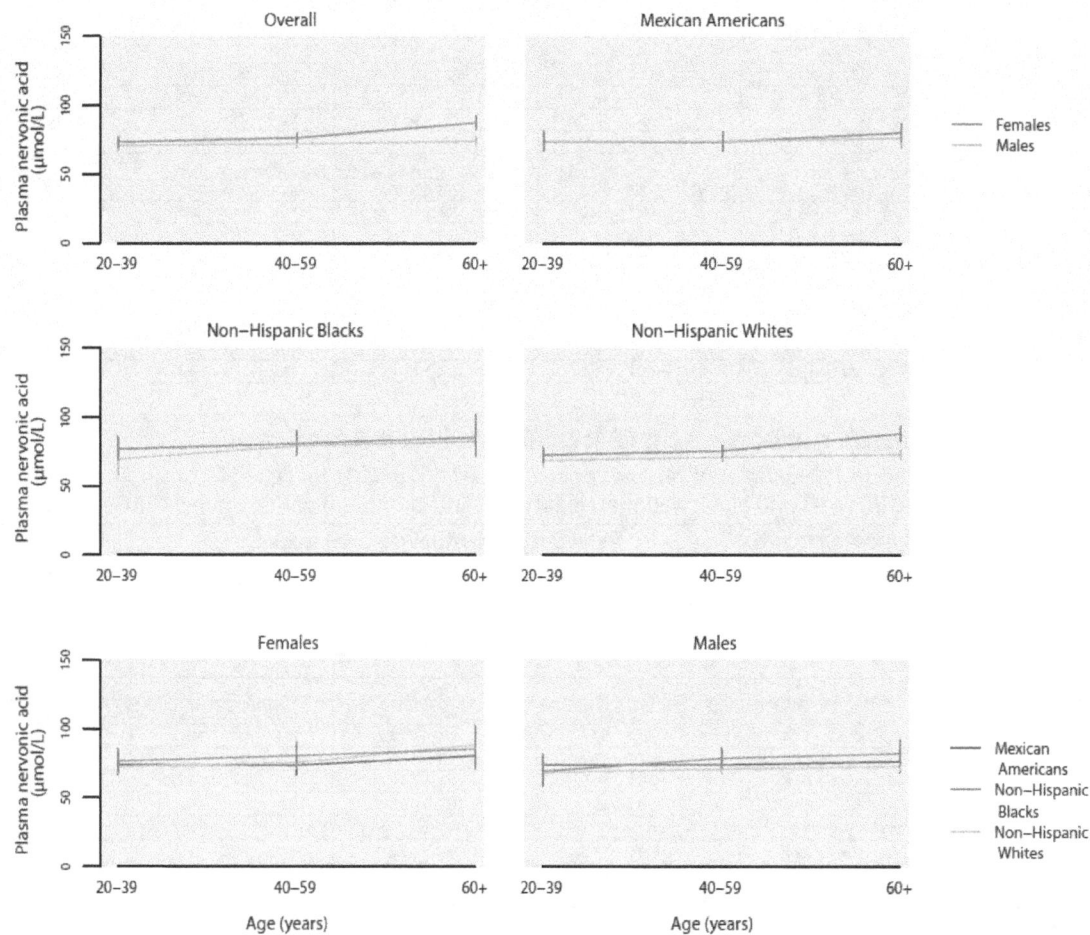

Table 2.26.a.2. Plasma nervonic acid (24:1n-9): Total population

Geometric mean and selected percentiles of plasma concentrations (in µmol/L) for the fasted U.S. population aged 20 years and older, National Health and Nutrition Examination Survey, 2003–2004.

	Geometric mean (95% conf. interval)	Selected percentiles (95% conf. interval)						Sample size
		10th		50th		90th		
Males and Females								
Total, 20 years and older	74.9	(72.4 – 77.4)	54.4	(51.9 – 56.6)	75.0	(72.0 – 77.7)	103	(99.6 – 108)	1,696
20–39 years	72.2	(68.7 – 75.8)	53.0	(48.3 – 56.2)	72.1	(67.8 – 77.2)	97.3	(94.2 – 103)	573
40–59 years	74.3	(71.5 – 77.1)	55.0	(52.8 – 57.6)	74.1	(71.4 – 77.6)	98.7	(94.9 – 105)	492
60 years and older	81.0	(77.7 – 84.6)	55.9	(51.8 – 60.0)	79.9	(77.2 – 84.8)	118	(110 – 124)	631
Males								
Total, 20 years and older	72.0	(69.5 – 74.5)	52.8	(49.8 – 54.8)	71.9	(69.8 – 74.4)	98.6	(95.6 – 102)	816
20–39 years	70.9	(67.0 – 75.0)	52.5	(46.1 – 55.4)	69.2	(64.8 – 76.3)	99.1	(94.0 – 106)	267
40–59 years	72.1	(69.4 – 74.9)	53.1	(47.3 – 57.2)	72.6	(71.1 – 74.6)	96.2	(88.9 – 104)	240
60 years and older	73.9	(70.9 – 77.0)	51.4	(46.3 – 55.2)	74.2	(71.1 – 78.3)	103	(98.0 – 112)	309
Females								
Total, 20 years and older	77.7	(74.8 – 80.7)	56.9	(52.7 – 59.5)	77.6	(74.3 – 80.0)	107	(101 – 115)	880
20–39 years	73.4	(70.0 – 77.0)	53.9	(48.4 – 58.2)	74.9	(71.5 – 77.6)	96.9	(92.9 – 104)	306
40–59 years	76.4	(73.2 – 79.8)	57.4	(51.9 – 59.8)	76.8	(70.4 – 81.2)	101	(97.7 – 109)	252
60 years and older	87.3	(82.8 – 92.0)	62.0	(55.7 – 65.4)	86.3	(80.7 – 92.6)	123	(119 – 135)	322

Table 2.26.a.3. Plasma nervonic acid (24:1n-9): Mexican Americans

Geometric mean and selected percentiles of plasma concentrations (in µmol/L) for fasted Mexican Americans in the U.S. population aged 20 years and older, National Health and Nutrition Examination Survey, 2003–2004.

	Geometric mean (95% conf. interval)	Selected percentiles (95% conf. interval)						Sample size
		10th		50th		90th		
Males and Females								
Total, 20 years and older	74.4	(71.0 – 78.0)	55.3	(50.7 – 58.6)	76.0	(71.1 – 77.9)	99.1	(93.7 – 107)	373
20–39 years	73.9	(69.6 – 78.6)	55.3	(43.9 – 58.9)	75.8	(70.4 – 77.8)	96.1	(93.3 – 108)	129
40–59 years	73.9	(69.3 – 78.6)	54.3†	(46.6 – 58.8)	74.0	(69.0 – 81.3)	96.6†	(89.4 – 122)	93
60 years and older	78.6	(74.8 – 82.7)	58.7	(50.2 – 62.1)	80.2	(76.6 – 82.5)	105	(98.7 – 115)	151
Males								
Total, 20 years and older	74.2	(71.0 – 77.6)	55.5	(52.7 – 57.7)	73.5	(70.5 – 77.7)	99.6	(93.4 – 107)	187
20–39 years	74.0	(70.5 – 77.6)	54.5†	(46.3 – 58.7)	72.2	(69.5 – 78.7)	94.9†	(91.2 – 107)	65
40–59 years	74.1	(68.4 – 80.2)	55.7†	(46.0 – 59.9)	70.1	(66.9 – 80.6)	102†	(89.0 – 127)	48
60 years and older	76.6	(69.3 – 84.7)	53.2†	(39.5 – 63.4)	78.0	(66.3 – 88.3)	104†	(97.5 – 157)	74
Females								
Total, 20 years and older	74.6	(69.7 – 79.9)	55.2	(45.9 – 59.3)	77.2	(67.2 – 82.0)	96.6	(90.8 – 116)	186
20–39 years	73.9	(67.3 – 81.2)	55.3†	(43.1 – 59.1)	77.1	(63.6 – 79.7)	98.6†	(89.2 – 129)	64
40–59 years	73.6	(67.1 – 80.8)	50.9†	(44.5 – 59.4)	78.4	(63.4 – 85.5)	92.1†	(86.2 – 121)	45
60 years and older	80.5	(74.5 – 87.0)	60.5†	(32.6 – 67.0)	80.6	(73.5 – 88.3)	104†	(92.5 – 159)	77

† Estimate is subject to greater uncertainty due to small cell size.

Table 2.26.a.4. Plasma nervonic acid (24:1n-9): Non-Hispanic blacks

Geometric mean and selected percentiles of plasma concentrations (in μmol/L) for fasted non-Hispanic blacks in the U.S. population aged 20 years and older, National Health and Nutrition Examination Survey, 2003–2004.

	Geometric mean (95% conf. interval)	Selected percentiles (95% conf. interval)						Sample size
		10th		50th		90th		
Males and Females								
Total, 20 years and older	77.3 (72.1 – 82.8)	54.4	(49.3 – 57.4)	77.5	(72.6 – 81.8)	110	(102 – 121)	288
20–39 years	73.1 (67.2 – 79.6)	50.9	(44.3 – 55.8)	74.1	(67.5 – 79.8)	101	(93.6 – 128)	116
40–59 years	79.9 (74.1 – 86.2)	56.3†	(50.0 – 61.9)	78.7	(72.8 – 81.6)	112†	(99.6 – 137)	93
60 years and older	84.1 (74.8 – 94.6)	55.3†	(43.3 – 59.2)	87.7	(77.2 – 94.2)	122†	(114 – 131)	79
Males								
Total, 20 years and older	74.4 (67.7 – 81.8)	53.3	(45.2 – 55.5)	74.4	(67.4 – 81.1)	111	(97.0 – 128)	133
20–39 years	69.3 (58.5 – 82.0)	45.2†	(23.7 – 53.9)	67.4	(60.3 – 80.6)	104†	(81.7 – 129)	54
40–59 years	78.9 (72.2 – 86.3)	56.7†	(53.9 – 66.2)	76.6	(68.8 – 81.4)	109†	(94.2 – 133)	40
60 years and older	82.3 (73.6 – 92.0)	54.7†	(49.6 – 62.2)	84.5	(59.7 – 104)	117†	(104 – 129)	39
Females								
Total, 20 years and older	79.6 (73.4 – 86.4)	55.7	(50.1 – 60.1)	79.3	(73.1 – 88.6)	109	(101 – 123)	155
20–39 years	76.6 (68.7 – 85.4)	55.6†	(48.6 – 61.3)	75.4	(70.3 – 86.2)	98.9†	(92.0 – 123)	62
40–59 years	80.6 (72.3 – 90.0)	55.5†	(43.4 – 62.9)	79.2	(71.0 – 89.5)	112†	(101 – 160)	53
60 years and older	85.3 (71.6 – 102)	51.8†	(39.7 – 62.8)	89.2	(75.8 – 95.2)	123†	(101 – 167)	40

† Estimate is subject to greater uncertainty due to small cell size.

Table 2.26.a.5. Plasma nervonic acid (24:1n-9): Non-Hispanic whites

Geometric mean and selected percentiles of plasma concentrations (in μmol/L) for fasted non-Hispanic whites in the U.S. population aged 20 years and older, National Health and Nutrition Examination Survey, 2003–2004.

	Geometric mean (95% conf. interval)	Selected percentiles (95% conf. interval)						Sample size
		10th		50th		90th		
Males and Females								
Total, 20 years and older	74.1 (71.3 – 77.0)	53.5	(51.3 – 56.2)	74.0	(71.0 – 77.4)	102	(98.6 – 109)	914
20–39 years	70.5 (66.5 – 74.8)	51.9	(45.2 – 56.2)	70.7	(64.8 – 76.2)	94.0	(88.1 – 109)	281
40–59 years	73.2 (70.1 – 76.5)	53.9	(51.0 – 57.6)	73.6	(69.8 – 77.6)	97.6	(91.9 – 108)	265
60 years and older	81.0 (77.1 – 85.1)	55.4	(51.8 – 58.7)	79.9	(75.7 – 85.4)	118	(109 – 132)	368
Males								
Total, 20 years and older	70.6 (68.1 – 73.1)	52.1	(48.1 – 54.1)	71.0	(68.4 – 73.4)	97.2	(90.7 – 101)	437
20–39 years	68.4 (64.3 – 72.7)	52.0	(43.7 – 55.7)	66.3	(61.7 – 73.0)	92.2	(84.4 – 109)	120
40–59 years	71.0 (67.8 – 74.5)	52.8	(46.3 – 54.4)	72.3	(70.9 – 74.2)	93.2	(86.4 – 107)	135
60 years and older	73.0 (70.0 – 76.1)	50.9	(43.5 – 54.8)	73.7	(68.5 – 78.8)	102	(93.9 – 113)	182
Females								
Total, 20 years and older	77.5 (73.8 – 81.3)	56.2	(51.9 – 59.2)	77.4	(72.4 – 81.0)	108	(101 – 119)	477
20–39 years	72.5 (67.9 – 77.5)	51.9	(45.2 – 57.6)	74.1	(68.9 – 78.3)	96.1	(90.0 – 115)	161
40–59 years	75.5 (71.7 – 79.4)	57.2	(51.9 – 59.3)	74.7	(68.4 – 80.7)	100	(94.7 – 109)	130
60 years and older	88.4 (83.1 – 94.1)	61.8	(53.5 – 68.4)	88.3	(79.8 – 96.5)	126	(119 – 137)	186

Table 2.27.a.1. Plasma linoleic acid (18:2n-6): Concentrations

Geometric mean and selected percentiles of plasma concentrations (in µmol/L) for the fasted U.S. population aged 20 years and older, National Health and Nutrition Examination Survey, 2003–2004.

	Geometric mean (95% conf. interval)	Selected percentiles (95% conf. interval)					Sample size
		2.5th	5th	50th	95th	97.5th	
Total, 20 years and older	3,450 (3,390 – 3,510)	2,210 (2,070 – 2,300)	2,370 (2,310 – 2,450)	3,430 (3,370 – 3,520)	4,980 (4,810 – 5,190)	5,410 (5,140 – 5,840)	1,806
Age group							
20–39 years	3,340 (3,260 – 3,410)	2,150 (1,830 – 2,290)	2,340 (2,200 – 2,460)	3,310 (3,240 – 3,370)	4,810 (4,630 – 5,230)	5,250 (4,910 – 6,260)	610
40–59 years	3,520 (3,440 – 3,600)	2,230 (1,740 – 2,360)	2,420 (2,250 – 2,570)	3,500 (3,410 – 3,620)	5,060 (4,830 – 5,610)	5,550 (5,110 – 5,880)	515
60 years and older	3,520 (3,430 – 3,600)	2,250 (1,960 – 2,320)	2,360 (2,280 – 2,490)	3,570 (3,480 – 3,640)	5,090 (4,870 – 5,220)	5,440 (5,160 – 5,890)	681
Gender							
Males	3,380 (3,300 – 3,470)	2,240 (2,120 – 2,310)	2,340 (2,310 – 2,410)	3,360 (3,240 – 3,450)	4,900 (4,640 – 5,360)	5,240 (5,090 – 5,810)	863
Females	3,500 (3,430 – 3,580)	2,170 (1,910 – 2,340)	2,420 (2,300 – 2,540)	3,530 (3,450 – 3,600)	5,040 (4,880 – 5,280)	5,500 (5,100 – 5,900)	943
Race/ethnicity							
Mexican Americans	3,730 (3,570 – 3,900)	2,320† (1,840 – 2,480)	2,490 (2,330 – 2,610)	3,660 (3,510 – 3,900)	5,800 (5,270 – 6,570)	6,320† (5,810 – 7,000)	375
Non-Hispanic Blacks	3,210 (3,090 – 3,340)	2,140† (1,850 – 2,200)	2,250 (2,110 – 2,360)	3,130 (3,030 – 3,230)	4,610 (4,460 – 4,810)	4,960† (4,640 – 8,680)	310
Non-Hispanic Whites	3,440 (3,370 – 3,510)	2,210 (2,020 – 2,300)	2,360 (2,270 – 2,500)	3,440 (3,360 – 3,540)	4,950 (4,800 – 5,080)	5,190 (5,050 – 5,780)	991

† Estimate is subject to greater uncertainty due to small cell size.

Figure 2.27.a. Plasma linoleic acid (18:2n–6): Concentrations by age group

Geometric mean (95% confidence interval), National Health and Nutrition Examination Survey, 2003–2004

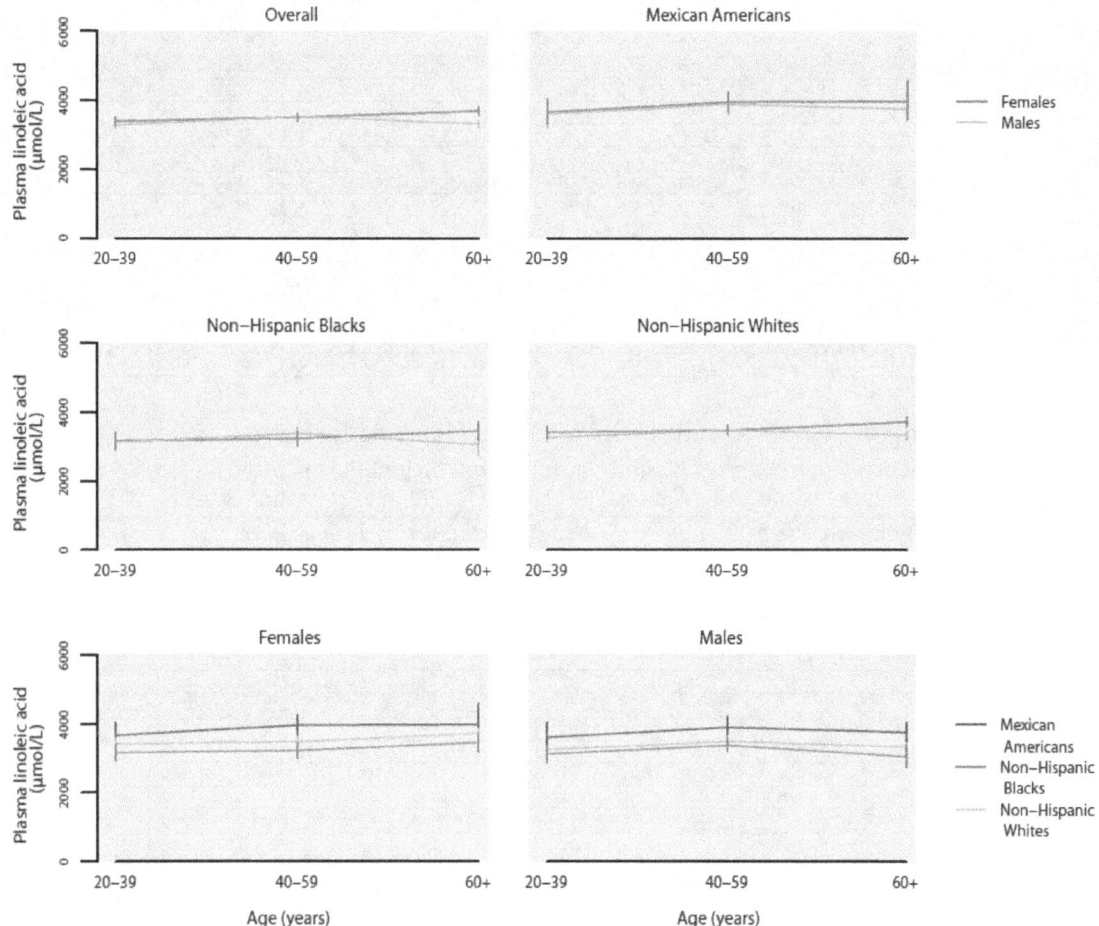

Table 2.27.a.2. Plasma linoleic acid (18:2n-6): Total population

Geometric mean and selected percentiles of plasma concentrations (in µmol/L) for the fasted U.S. population aged 20 years and older, National Health and Nutrition Examination Survey, 2003–2004.

	Geometric mean (95% conf. interval)		Selected percentiles (95% conf. interval)						Sample size
			10th		50th		90th		
Males and Females									
Total, 20 years and older	3,450	(3,390 – 3,510)	2,610	(2,550 – 2,700)	3,430	(3,370 – 3,520)	4,570	(4,410 – 4,730)	1,806
20–39 years	3,340	(3,260 – 3,410)	2,570	(2,470 – 2,610)	3,310	(3,240 – 3,370)	4,410	(4,280 – 4,670)	610
40–59 years	3,520	(3,440 – 3,600)	2,700	(2,520 – 2,780)	3,500	(3,410 – 3,620)	4,700	(4,510 – 4,830)	515
60 years and older	3,520	(3,430 – 3,600)	2,690	(2,480 – 2,790)	3,570	(3,480 – 3,640)	4,580	(4,410 – 4,870)	681
Males									
Total, 20 years and older	3,380	(3,300 – 3,470)	2,590	(2,480 – 2,680)	3,360	(3,240 – 3,450)	4,510	(4,240 – 4,720)	863
20–39 years	3,280	(3,190 – 3,380)	2,510	(2,420 – 2,600)	3,210	(3,150 – 3,320)	4,380	(4,030 – 4,910)	282
40–59 years	3,530	(3,430 – 3,620)	2,710	(2,600 – 2,790)	3,490	(3,350 – 3,640)	4,610	(4,350 – 4,860)	248
60 years and older	3,320	(3,220 – 3,420)	2,420	(2,320 – 2,570)	3,370	(3,180 – 3,510)	4,310	(4,160 – 4,680)	333
Females									
Total, 20 years and older	3,500	(3,430 – 3,580)	2,640	(2,580 – 2,740)	3,530	(3,450 – 3,600)	4,660	(4,490 – 4,820)	943
20–39 years	3,390	(3,270 – 3,510)	2,590	(2,530 – 2,630)	3,390	(3,280 – 3,520)	4,420	(4,270 – 4,860)	328
40–59 years	3,510	(3,390 – 3,630)	2,630	(2,350 – 2,860)	3,530	(3,420 – 3,620)	4,790	(4,380 – 5,030)	267
60 years and older	3,690	(3,580 – 3,800)	2,870	(2,770 – 2,940)	3,700	(3,600 – 3,790)	4,820	(4,540 – 5,080)	348

Table 2.27.a.3. Plasma linoleic acid (18:2n-6): Mexican Americans

Geometric mean and selected percentiles of plasma concentrations (in µmol/L) for fasted Mexican Americans in the U.S. population aged 20 years and older, National Health and Nutrition Examination Survey, 2003–2004.

	Geometric mean (95% conf. interval)		Selected percentiles (95% conf. interval)						Sample size
			10th		50th		90th		
Males and Females									
Total, 20 years and older	3,730	(3,570 – 3,900)	2,700	(2,500 – 2,900)	3,660	(3,510 – 3,900)	5,170	(4,740 – 5,900)	375
20–39 years	3,630	(3,350 – 3,920)	2,620	(2,350 – 2,730)	3,530	(3,280 – 3,960)	5,120	(4,570 – 6,320)	132
40–59 years	3,920	(3,720 – 4,130)	2,900†	(2,410 – 3,150)	3,810	(3,690 – 4,100)	5,370†	(4,730 – 7,050)	93
60 years and older	3,860	(3,540 – 4,210)	2,910	(2,120 – 3,360)	3,840	(3,530 – 4,250)	5,050	(4,590 – 6,170)	150
Males									
Total, 20 years and older	3,700	(3,460 – 3,950)	2,630	(2,330 – 2,910)	3,640	(3,280 – 4,140)	5,100	(4,650 – 6,350)	188
20–39 years	3,600	(3,220 – 4,040)	2,490†	(2,310 – 2,860)	3,500	(3,030 – 4,300)	5,020†	(4,440 – 6,640)	67
40–59 years	3,890	(3,610 – 4,200)	3,010†	(2,020 – 3,250)	3,860	(3,600 – 4,150)	5,050†	(4,530 – 7,450)	48
60 years and older	3,750	(3,490 – 4,030)	2,750†	(2,170 – 3,290)	3,760	(3,580 – 3,990)	4,960†	(4,330 – 5,580)	73
Females									
Total, 20 years and older	3,780	(3,610 – 3,960)	2,710	(2,260 – 3,040)	3,680	(3,530 – 3,920)	5,260	(4,810 – 5,960)	187
20–39 years	3,660	(3,320 – 4,030)	2,710†	(1,840 – 3,050)	3,550	(3,470 – 3,910)	5,130†	(4,350 – 6,500)	65
40–59 years	3,950	(3,680 – 4,250)	2,720†	(2,350 – 3,130)	3,780	(3,580 – 4,330)	5,440†	(4,800 – 6,970)	45
60 years and older	3,970	(3,440 – 4,580)	2,920†	(2,120 – 3,520)	3,930	(3,450 – 4,570)	5,080†	(4,570 – 6,220)	77

† Estimate is subject to greater uncertainty due to small cell size.

Table 2.27.a.4. Plasma linoleic acid (18:2n-6): Non-Hispanic blacks

Geometric mean and selected percentiles of plasma concentrations (in µmol/L) for fasted non-Hispanic blacks in the U.S. population aged 20 years and older, National Health and Nutrition Examination Survey, 2003–2004.

	Geometric mean (95% conf. interval)		Selected percentiles (95% conf. interval)						Sample size
			10th		50th		90th		
Males and Females									
Total, 20 years and older	3,210	(3,090 – 3,340)	2,430	(2,350 – 2,490)	3,130	(3,030 – 3,230)	4,250	(4,120 – 4,540)	310
20–39 years	3,140	(2,940 – 3,340)	2,360	(2,150 – 2,460)	3,050	(2,860 – 3,230)	4,200	(4,030 – 4,570)	126
40–59 years	3,280	(3,110 – 3,470)	2,540†	(2,240 – 2,690)	3,160	(3,040 – 3,260)	4,330†	(4,100 – 5,000)	98
60 years and older	3,290	(3,080 – 3,510)	2,470†	(1,190 – 2,710)	3,410	(3,090 – 3,550)	4,210†	(3,930 – 5,080)	86
Males									
Total, 20 years and older	3,190	(3,070 – 3,320)	2,350	(2,180 – 2,480)	3,070	(2,980 – 3,190)	4,380	(3,940 – 4,840)	143
20–39 years	3,120	(2,900 – 3,350)	2,320†	(1,800 – 2,450)	3,030	(2,790 – 3,290)	4,110†	(3,750 – 7,040)	58
40–59 years	3,370	(3,190 – 3,570)	2,610†	(2,200 – 2,750)	3,160	(2,990 – 3,280)	4,570†	(4,110 – 8,980)	42
60 years and older	3,050	(2,750 – 3,380)	2,300†	(1,190 – 2,500)	3,070	(2,730 – 3,650)	4,010†	(3,800 – 4,250)	43
Females									
Total, 20 years and older	3,230	(3,050 – 3,410)	2,460	(2,390 – 2,560)	3,180	(2,970 – 3,380)	4,210	(4,040 – 5,050)	167
20–39 years	3,160	(2,920 – 3,410)	2,410†	(2,220 – 2,470)	3,100	(2,820 – 3,340)	4,230†	(3,900 – 5,030)	68
40–59 years	3,220	(3,000 – 3,440)	2,490†	(2,160 – 2,630)	3,100	(2,910 – 3,410)	4,120†	(3,720 – 7,490)	56
60 years and older	3,450	(3,190 – 3,720)	2,640†	(2,420 – 2,910)	3,430	(3,050 – 3,750)	4,350†	(4,100 – 5,080)	43

† Estimate is subject to greater uncertainty due to small cell size.

Table 2.27.a.5. Plasma linoleic acid (18:2n-6): Non-Hispanic whites

Geometric mean and selected percentiles of plasma concentrations (in µmol/L) for fasted non-Hispanic whites in the U.S. population aged 20 years and older, National Health and Nutrition Examination Survey, 2003–2004.

	Geometric mean (95% conf. interval)		Selected percentiles (95% conf. interval)						Sample size
			10th		50th		90th		
Males and Females									
Total, 20 years and older	3,440	(3,370 – 3,510)	2,620	(2,530 – 2,710)	3,440	(3,360 – 3,540)	4,520	(4,340 – 4,720)	991
20–39 years	3,330	(3,250 – 3,420)	2,580	(2,520 – 2,620)	3,310	(3,250 – 3,380)	4,360	(4,130 – 4,730)	300
40–59 years	3,470	(3,370 – 3,580)	2,690	(2,360 – 2,830)	3,480	(3,340 – 3,620)	4,560	(4,300 – 4,820)	280
60 years and older	3,530	(3,430 – 3,630)	2,680	(2,420 – 2,800)	3,590	(3,490 – 3,690)	4,600	(4,440 – 4,930)	411
Males									
Total, 20 years and older	3,360	(3,260 – 3,470)	2,580	(2,440 – 2,690)	3,370	(3,210 – 3,500)	4,330	(4,130 – 4,740)	471
20–39 years	3,250	(3,140 – 3,370)	2,530	(2,420 – 2,600)	3,210	(3,130 – 3,330)	4,150	(3,860 – 5,070)	128
40–59 years	3,480	(3,340 – 3,630)	2,710	(2,430 – 2,830)	3,480	(3,290 – 3,650)	4,430	(4,200 – 4,930)	140
60 years and older	3,330	(3,210 – 3,450)	2,420	(2,300 – 2,580)	3,370	(3,090 – 3,600)	4,320	(4,110 – 4,780)	203
Females									
Total, 20 years and older	3,510	(3,430 – 3,590)	2,660	(2,570 – 2,770)	3,530	(3,420 – 3,610)	4,660	(4,480 – 4,820)	520
20–39 years	3,410	(3,240 – 3,580)	2,610	(2,430 – 2,740)	3,390	(3,250 – 3,580)	4,390	(4,180 – 4,970)	172
40–59 years	3,470	(3,330 – 3,610)	2,570	(2,220 – 2,870)	3,480	(3,340 – 3,610)	4,720	(4,290 – 4,940)	140
60 years and older	3,720	(3,580 – 3,860)	2,900	(2,810 – 2,970)	3,760	(3,640 – 3,840)	4,860	(4,530 – 5,140)	208

Table 2.28.a.1. Plasma alpha-linolenic acid (18:3n-3): Concentrations

Geometric mean and selected percentiles of plasma concentrations (in µmol/L) for the fasted U.S. population aged 20 years and older, National Health and Nutrition Examination Survey, 2003–2004.

	Geometric mean (95% conf. interval)	Selected percentiles (95% conf. interval)					Sample size
		2.5th	5th	50th	95th	97.5th	
Total, 20 years and older	63.1 (60.5–65.8)	25.2 (21.4–27.5)	30.0 (26.0–33.1)	61.4 (58.9–63.7)	137 (128–151)	165 (153–192)	1,801
Age group							
20–39 years	58.1 (55.8–60.6)	24.9 (19.9–26.6)	27.3 (25.2–30.3)	57.5 (55.2–59.9)	127 (117–150)	159 (137–221)	610
40–59 years	65.0 (60.7–69.6)	25.1 (14.3–30.3)	30.8 (22.7–35.6)	61.2 (58.2–66.9)	134 (127–162)	174 (157–203)	513
60 years and older	69.0 (65.2–73.0)	29.3 (20.8–33.2)	33.5 (28.4–36.4)	68.3 (64.9–72.3)	143 (138–154)	159 (147–234)	678
Gender							
Males	62.1 (58.8–65.5)	23.0 (17.0–26.2)	27.6 (22.4–31.7)	59.9 (57.3–64.2)	142 (128–172)	173 (155–210)	859
Females	64.1 (61.1–67.2)	27.2 (23.6–30.6)	32.8 (27.5–34.7)	62.4 (59.9–65.5)	131 (123–150)	158 (146–184)	942
Race/ethnicity							
Mexican Americans	69.0 (63.8–74.5)	23.9† (20.1–30.7)	31.8 (24.3–36.1)	66.2 (59.6–73.9)	160 (135–246)	199† (159–421)	375
Non-Hispanic Blacks	53.8 (50.4–57.4)	24.5† (13.3–28.8)	28.8 (23.7–30.8)	50.5 (48.2–53.1)	115 (107–147)	149† (121–362)	310
Non-Hispanic Whites	63.3 (59.9–66.8)	25.2 (20.0–27.5)	29.5 (25.8–33.0)	62.3 (58.9–65.7)	133 (124–153)	157 (143–193)	986

† Estimate is subject to greater uncertainty due to small cell size.

Figure 2.28.a. Plasma alpha–linolenic acid (18:3n–3): Concentrations by age group

Geometric mean (95% confidence interval), National Health and Nutrition Examination Survey, 2003–2004

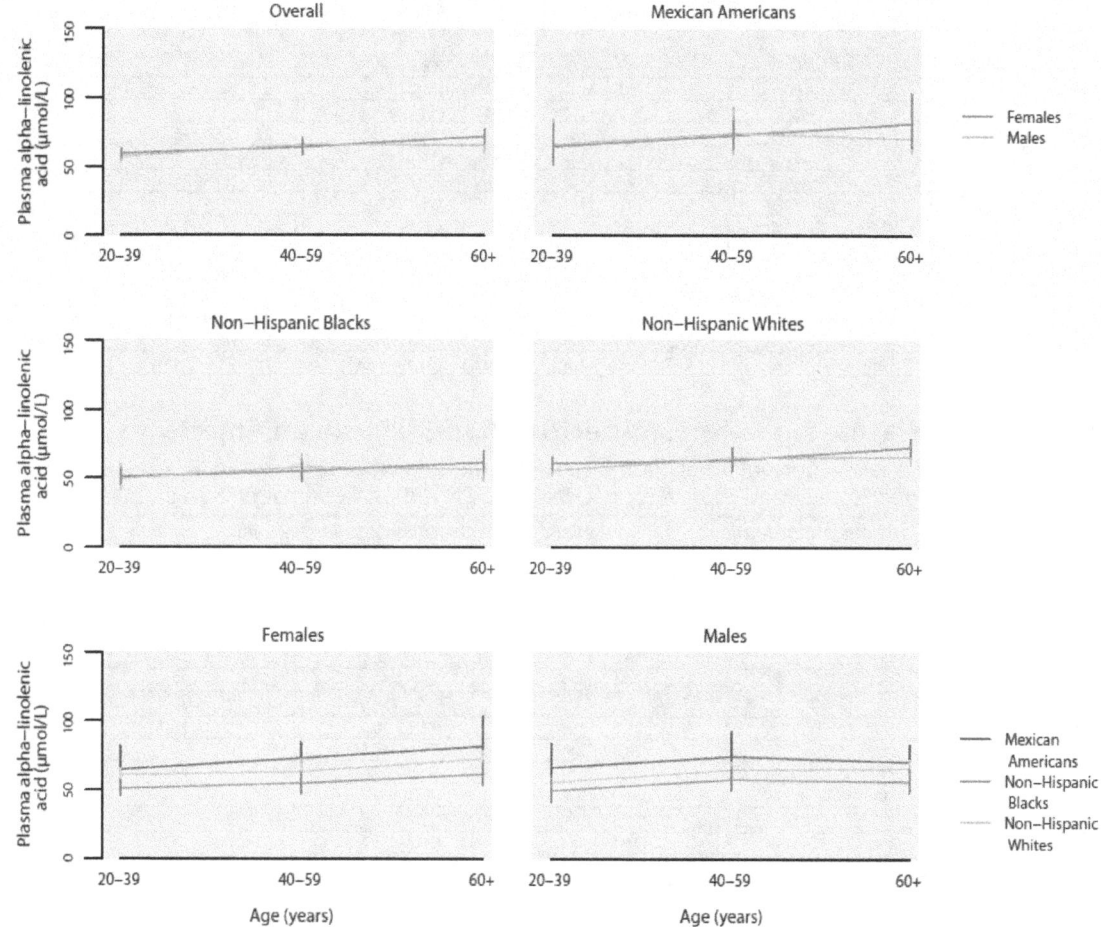

Table 2.28.a.2. Plasma alpha-linolenic acid (18:3n-3): Total population

Geometric mean and selected percentiles of plasma concentrations (in μmol/L) for the fasted U.S. population aged 20 years and older, National Health and Nutrition Examination Survey, 2003–2004.

| | Geometric mean (95% conf. interval) | Selected percentiles (95% conf. interval) | | | | | | Sample size |
		10th		50th		90th		
Males and Females								
Total, 20 years and older	63.1	(60.5 – 65.8)	35.3	(33.1 – 38.0)	61.4	(58.9 – 63.7)	114 (110 – 121)	1,801
20–39 years	58.1	(55.8 – 60.6)	32.9	(30.8 – 34.2)	57.5	(55.2 – 59.9)	107 (98.2 – 116)	610
40–59 years	65.0	(60.7 – 69.6)	37.6	(31.3 – 40.5)	61.2	(58.2 – 66.9)	117 (110 – 128)	513
60 years and older	69.0	(65.2 – 73.0)	39.3	(34.8 – 43.2)	68.3	(64.9 – 72.3)	123 (112 – 137)	678
Males								
Total, 20 years and older	62.1	(58.8 – 65.5)	33.6	(28.6 – 37.0)	59.9	(57.3 – 64.2)	116 (110 – 127)	859
20–39 years	56.9	(53.5 – 60.6)	31.6	(27.5 – 34.3)	55.7	(51.2 – 59.6)	107 (98.1 – 121)	282
40–59 years	65.9	(61.5 – 70.6)	34.5	(23.9 – 43.7)	63.6	(58.1 – 72.9)	125 (112 – 132)	246
60 years and older	65.4	(60.1 – 71.2)	35.3	(31.7 – 39.8)	63.8	(57.2 – 73.8)	120 (107 – 147)	331
Females								
Total, 20 years and older	64.1	(61.1 – 67.2)	38.1	(35.1 – 39.7)	62.4	(59.9 – 65.5)	113 (106 – 122)	942
20–39 years	59.3	(56.1 – 62.7)	34.0	(30.7 – 36.2)	59.1	(56.0 – 62.6)	105 (93.4 – 125)	328
40–59 years	64.2	(58.4 – 70.4)	38.5	(34.1 – 40.6)	58.8	(55.3 – 65.7)	112 (103 – 125)	267
60 years and older	72.0	(67.3 – 77.1)	42.9	(36.5 – 47.5)	71.1	(66.9 – 76.6)	123 (109 – 141)	347

Table 2.28.a.3. Plasma alpha-linolenic acid (18:3n-3): Mexican Americans

Geometric mean and selected percentiles of plasma concentrations (in μmol/L) for fasted Mexican Americans in the U.S. population aged 20 years and older, National Health and Nutrition Examination Survey, 2003–2004.

| | Geometric mean (95% conf. interval) | Selected percentiles (95% conf. interval) | | | | | | Sample size |
		10th		50th		90th		
Males and Females								
Total, 20 years and older	69.0	(63.8 – 74.5)	39.4	(30.2 – 43.0)	66.2	(59.6 – 73.9)	133 (117 – 159)	375
20–39 years	65.6	(56.2 – 76.6)	36.8	(25.2 – 41.3)	61.4	(54.6 – 73.8)	125 (111 – 215)	132
40–59 years	73.8	(65.4 – 83.2)	43.8†	(30.1 – 47.8)	70.5	(59.0 – 88.4)	133† (115 – 146)	93
60 years and older	76.1	(65.5 – 88.5)	43.6	(34.4 – 47.4)	75.9	(67.6 – 82.9)	136 (108 – 292)	150
Males								
Total, 20 years and older	68.9	(61.1 – 77.7)	40.5	(25.8 – 43.5)	65.9	(54.6 – 80.2)	134 (113 – 201)	188
20–39 years	66.2	(52.3 – 83.9)	39.3†	(22.8 – 42.6)	58.5	(44.6 – 86.5)	130† (91.9 – 222)	67
40–59 years	74.4	(59.7 – 92.8)	43.7†	(22.7 – 50.8)	70.4	(55.6 – 95.9)	133† (105 – 421)	48
60 years and older	70.6	(60.3 – 82.5)	39.6†	(31.8 – 47.0)	69.6	(55.1 – 79.4)	125† (94.7 – 292)	73
Females								
Total, 20 years and older	69.1	(62.1 – 76.8)	37.5	(23.1 – 44.8)	66.2	(60.2 – 73.2)	131 (118 – 147)	187
20–39 years	64.7	(51.4 – 81.5)	32.7†	(20.1 – 43.7)	63.6	(55.0 – 73.4)	125† (102 – 278)	65
40–59 years	73.0	(63.4 – 84.1)	41.4†	(23.1 – 52.1)	69.0	(54.1 – 87.9)	132† (110 – 194)	45
60 years and older	81.6	(64.4 – 103)	45.2†	(32.3 – 58.1)	82.0	(64.8 – 94.8)	144† (111 – 197)	77

† Estimate is subject to greater uncertainty due to small cell size.

Table 2.28.a.4. Plasma alpha-linolenic acid (18:3n-3): Non-Hispanic blacks

Geometric mean and selected percentiles of plasma concentrations (in μmol/L) for fasted non-Hispanic blacks in the U.S. population aged 20 years and older, National Health and Nutrition Examination Survey, 2003–2004.

	Geometric mean (95% conf. interval)		Selected percentiles (95% conf. interval)						Sample size
			10th		50th		90th		
Males and Females									
Total, 20 years and older	53.8	(50.4 – 57.4)	31.8	(29.4 – 34.0)	50.5	(48.2 – 53.1)	91.7	(81.0 – 112)	310
20–39 years	50.4	(44.6 – 56.8)	30.7	(26.4 – 33.1)	48.1	(43.0 – 53.0)	76.8	(69.0 – 142)	126
40–59 years	56.2	(52.0 – 60.6)	32.8†	(23.4 – 36.2)	51.5	(47.1 – 55.1)	99.0†	(81.8 – 315)	98
60 years and older	59.4	(53.3 – 66.2)	35.9†	(29.4 – 40.4)	60.0	(53.5 – 63.0)	92.9†	(81.4 – 142)	86
Males									
Total, 20 years and older	53.4	(48.6 – 58.7)	29.4	(24.1 – 32.4)	51.7	(44.9 – 55.3)	93.3	(78.9 – 149)	143
20–39 years	49.6	(41.2 – 59.8)	28.8†	(13.3 – 33.5)	45.5	(42.4 – 57.9)	75.7†	(65.3 – 523)	58
40–59 years	57.9	(49.9 – 67.2)	29.7†	(18.1 – 35.2)	51.6	(40.9 – 63.7)	124†	(97.4 – 284)	42
60 years and older	56.4	(48.8 – 65.1)	30.6†	(25.3 – 39.9)	59.8	(46.2 – 72.5)	90.7†	(79.0 – 105)	43
Females									
Total, 20 years and older	54.1	(50.0 – 58.5)	34.4	(32.1 – 37.0)	50.3	(47.5 – 54.6)	88.9	(77.4 – 120)	167
20–39 years	51.0	(45.7 – 56.9)	32.7†	(28.1 – 35.9)	48.2	(41.2 – 57.7)	80.1†	(67.0 – 134)	68
40–59 years	54.9	(47.8 – 62.9)	35.2†	(23.1 – 39.9)	51.2	(44.3 – 57.6)	84.7†	(75.8 – 332)	56
60 years and older	61.4	(53.7 – 70.1)	38.8†	(32.9 – 43.2)	59.2	(52.0 – 64.8)	101†	(81.5 – 142)	43

† Estimate is subject to greater uncertainty due to small cell size.

Table 2.28.a.5. Plasma alpha-linolenic acid (18:3n-3): Non-Hispanic whites

Geometric mean and selected percentiles of plasma concentrations (in μmol/L) for fasted non-Hispanic whites in the U.S. population aged 20 years and older, National Health and Nutrition Examination Survey, 2003–2004.

	Geometric mean (95% conf. interval)		Selected percentiles (95% conf. interval)						Sample size
			10th		50th		90th		
Males and Females									
Total, 20 years and older	63.3	(59.9 – 66.8)	34.9	(32.3 – 38.0)	62.3	(58.9 – 65.7)	113	(109 – 120)	986
20–39 years	58.3	(55.5 – 61.3)	32.4	(30.2 – 34.1)	58.4	(56.4 – 61.9)	103	(93.8 – 116)	300
40–59 years	64.0	(57.9 – 70.7)	37.5	(28.1 – 40.8)	60.5	(57.3 – 68.0)	114	(108 – 123)	278
60 years and older	69.4	(65.1 – 74.0)	39.4	(34.3 – 44.1)	69.0	(65.1 – 72.7)	125	(111 – 140)	408
Males									
Total, 20 years and older	61.8	(58.1 – 65.7)	33.0	(27.5 – 36.6)	60.6	(57.4 – 65.4)	113	(108 – 124)	467
20–39 years	55.7	(52.2 – 59.5)	30.6	(26.4 – 33.7)	55.1	(47.7 – 60.6)	103	(95.6 – 113)	128
40–59 years	64.8	(59.6 – 70.5)	33.7	(16.1 – 45.7)	63.6	(58.1 – 70.8)	116	(108 – 132)	138
60 years and older	65.8	(60.1 – 72.1)	36.0	(29.2 – 41.6)	63.8	(57.1 – 74.4)	118	(109 – 145)	201
Females									
Total, 20 years and older	64.7	(61.0 – 68.5)	38.2	(34.6 – 40.0)	62.8	(59.8 – 67.0)	113	(106 – 121)	519
20–39 years	60.8	(56.7 – 65.1)	34.0	(30.4 – 37.3)	61.0	(56.4 – 66.1)	103	(88.8 – 128)	172
40–59 years	63.2	(55.2 – 72.3)	38.4	(33.6 – 40.7)	58.4	(52.1 – 68.1)	111	(102 – 120)	140
60 years and older	72.5	(67.0 – 78.5)	41.9	(34.7 – 48.1)	71.2	(67.3 – 76.6)	127	(108 – 154)	207

Table 2.29.a.1. Plasma gamma-linolenic acid (18:3n-6): Concentrations

Geometric mean and selected percentiles of plasma concentrations (in µmol/L) for the fasted U.S. population aged 20 years and older, National Health and Nutrition Examination Survey, 2003–2004.

	Geometric mean (95% conf. interval)	Selected percentiles (95% conf. interval)						Sample size
		2.5th	5th	50th	95th	97.5th	
Total, 20 years and older	46.9 (45.0 – 49.0)	17.1 (13.7 – 19.1)	20.2 (19.0 – 22.0)	49.0 (46.4 – 51.5)	100 (94.2 – 106)	117 (107 – 127)	1,795
Age group							
20–39 years	41.7 (39.4 – 44.1)	15.0 (12.6 – 17.7)	19.3 (15.1 – 21.2)	41.9 (38.7 – 46.5)	85.1 (79.1 – 105)	99.8 (86.2 – 140)	603
40–59 years	51.0 (48.4 – 53.8)	18.4 (15.0 – 19.4)	20.4 (18.3 – 24.0)	53.3 (50.1 – 56.4)	108 (96.5 – 118)	121 (113 – 129)	513
60 years and older	49.6 (45.9 – 53.6)	18.3 (14.4 – 20.3)	22.0 (20.3 – 23.6)	51.2 (46.1 – 57.0)	102 (97.4 – 119)	115 (104 – 142)	679
Gender							
Males	48.0 (45.5 – 50.6)	17.1 (13.1 – 20.3)	22.0 (18.7 – 23.5)	50.0 (48.0 – 52.4)	99.2 (90.5 – 120)	120 (105 – 129)	855
Females	46.0 (43.7 – 48.4)	16.8 (12.8 – 19.1)	19.5 (17.0 – 21.6)	47.2 (44.0 – 50.6)	100 (92.8 – 106)	110 (106 – 128)	940
Race/ethnicity							
Mexican Americans	41.8 (38.1 – 45.8)	12.6† (6.25 – 15.0)	15.1 (9.90 – 18.6)	43.1 (38.4 – 49.9)	94.0 (89.7 – 115)	116† (96.3 – 132)	375
Non-Hispanic Blacks	42.5 (40.4 – 44.7)	16.5† (14.9 – 18.3)	20.6 (15.8 – 23.1)	42.8 (40.0 – 46.4)	84.1 (76.7 – 112)	105† (86.7 – 138)	309
Non-Hispanic Whites	48.8 (46.1 – 51.6)	19.2 (13.9 – 21.3)	22.1 (19.7 – 23.8)	50.5 (47.5 – 53.2)	101 (93.4 – 108)	117 (105 – 128)	981

† Estimate is subject to greater uncertainty due to small cell size.

Figure 2.29.a. Plasma gamma–linolenic acid (18:3n–6): Concentrations by age group

Geometric mean (95% confidence interval), National Health and Nutrition Examination Survey, 2003–2004

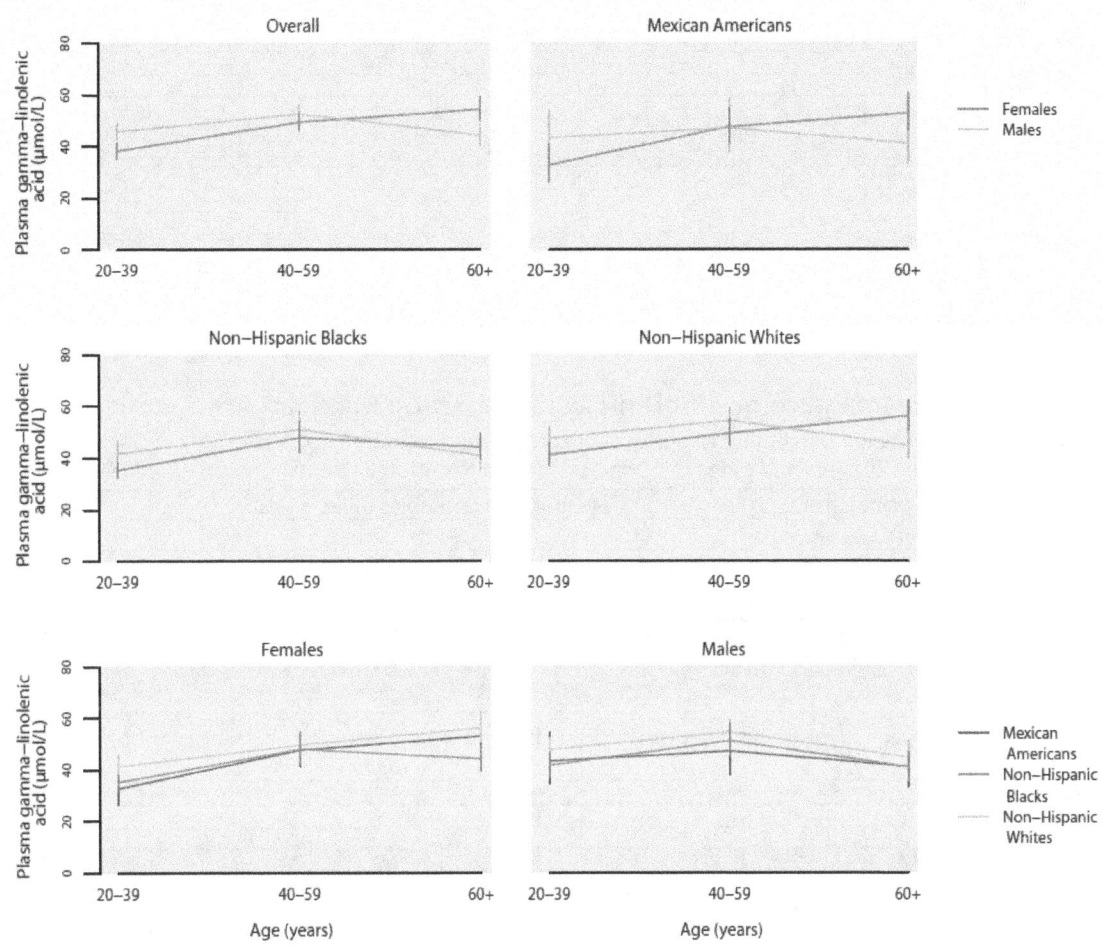

Table 2.29.a.2. Plasma gamma-linolenic acid (18:3n-6): Total population

Geometric mean and selected percentiles of plasma concentrations (in µmol/L) for the fasted U.S. population aged 20 years and older, National Health and Nutrition Examination Survey, 2003–2004.

	Geometric mean (95% conf. interval)	Selected percentiles (95% conf. interval)						Sample size
		10th		50th		90th		
Males and Females								
Total, 20 years and older	46.9 (45.0 – 49.0)	24.4	(22.9 – 25.8)	49.0	(46.4 – 51.5)	85.7	(82.1 – 90.3)	1,795
20–39 years	41.7 (39.4 – 44.1)	22.5	(20.6 – 24.1)	41.9	(38.7 – 46.5)	75.2	(69.9 – 80.9)	603
40–59 years	51.0 (48.4 – 53.8)	25.7	(23.4 – 29.5)	53.3	(50.1 – 56.4)	90.5	(87.1 – 94.7)	513
60 years and older	49.6 (45.9 – 53.6)	26.7	(23.9 – 29.1)	51.2	(46.1 – 57.0)	90.8	(82.8 – 101)	679
Males								
Total, 20 years and older	48.0 (45.5 – 50.6)	25.6	(23.8 – 27.0)	50.0	(48.0 – 52.4)	85.7	(81.2 – 94.4)	855
20–39 years	45.7 (42.7 – 48.8)	25.1	(21.7 – 26.9)	48.8	(44.3 – 52.1)	79.5	(68.4 – 90.5)	277
40–59 years	52.7 (49.5 – 56.2)	26.3	(23.9 – 30.8)	55.7	(51.5 – 59.2)	91.9	(85.6 – 110)	246
60 years and older	44.3 (40.3 – 48.7)	24.7	(19.5 – 27.7)	44.5	(42.4 – 48.4)	79.8	(70.5 – 101)	332
Females								
Total, 20 years and older	46.0 (43.7 – 48.4)	23.0	(21.5 – 24.8)	47.2	(44.0 – 50.6)	85.1	(80.4 – 89.8)	940
20–39 years	38.2 (35.3 – 41.3)	21.5	(16.6 – 23.1)	37.3	(34.7 – 41.3)	73.0	(62.6 – 79.0)	326
40–59 years	49.5 (46.3 – 53.0)	24.5	(20.1 – 27.8)	51.7	(48.2 – 55.8)	89.7	(81.9 – 101)	267
60 years and older	54.4 (50.0 – 59.2)	29.1	(26.2 – 30.6)	57.9	(50.7 – 64.5)	97.2	(88.0 – 105)	347

Table 2.29.a.3. Plasma gamma-linolenic acid (18:3n-6): Mexican Americans

Geometric mean and selected percentiles of plasma concentrations (in µmol/L) for fasted Mexican Americans in the U.S. population aged 20 years and older, National Health and Nutrition Examination Survey, 2003–2004.

	Geometric mean (95% conf. interval)	Selected percentiles (95% conf. interval)						Sample size
		10th		50th		90th		
Males and Females								
Total, 20 years and older	41.8 (38.1 – 45.8)	19.5	(15.2 – 22.8)	43.1	(38.4 – 49.9)	83.5	(77.3 – 89.8)	375
20–39 years	38.5 (33.2 – 44.5)	18.1	(13.0 – 20.2)	40.4	(32.6 – 51.1)	71.2	(67.0 – 87.0)	132
40–59 years	47.4 (42.9 – 52.3)	24.2†	(17.3 – 27.6)	48.3	(39.6 – 55.1)	94.9†	(81.5 – 123)	93
60 years and older	46.9 (40.9 – 53.7)	24.0	(13.3 – 29.1)	48.7	(41.9 – 61.0)	86.0	(79.1 – 89.7)	150
Males								
Total, 20 years and older	44.2 (38.1 – 51.2)	20.6	(14.5 – 26.3)	45.9	(38.4 – 54.8)	87.3	(74.0 – 91.6)	188
20–39 years	43.3 (34.6 – 54.2)	20.1†	(7.22 – 25.2)	46.7	(32.8 – 60.0)	81.3†	(67.1 – 107)	67
40–59 years	47.1 (37.9 – 58.6)	25.8†	(9.42 – 31.7)	44.7	(38.0 – 55.2)	94.2†	(70.9 – 155)	48
60 years and older	41.1 (33.5 – 50.5)	21.3†	(11.1 – 25.6)	42.9	(26.9 – 60.8)	71.0†	(57.5 – 131)	73
Females								
Total, 20 years and older	39.0 (34.4 – 44.1)	16.5	(10.6 – 21.9)	40.1	(33.0 – 50.6)	82.4	(72.2 – 90.6)	187
20–39 years	32.8 (26.5 – 40.6)	14.7†	(6.25 – 19.3)	34.6	(29.0 – 41.4)	61.6†	(50.6 – 89.6)	65
40–59 years	47.6 (41.4 – 54.8)	21.0†	(15.0 – 27.4)	51.3	(35.0 – 61.6)	94.9†	(81.2 – 108)	45
60 years and older	52.9 (46.0 – 60.7)	26.6†	(9.56 – 39.1)	55.3	(50.3 – 62.2)	88.9†	(86.4 – 98.2)	77

† Estimate is subject to greater uncertainty due to small cell size.

Table 2.29.a.4. Plasma gamma-linolenic acid (18:3n-6): Non-Hispanic blacks

Geometric mean and selected percentiles of plasma concentrations (in μmol/L) for fasted non-Hispanic blacks in the U.S. population aged 20 years and older, National Health and Nutrition Examination Survey, 2003–2004.

	Geometric mean (95% conf. interval)		Selected percentiles (95% conf. interval)						Sample size
			10th		50th		90th		
Males and Females									
Total, 20 years and older	42.5	(40.4 – 44.7)	23.7	(22.0 – 25.1)	42.8	(40.0 – 46.4)	73.7	(68.3 – 80.0)	309
20–39 years	38.0	(35.1 – 41.2)	22.1	(18.2 – 24.1)	37.1	(32.7 – 41.8)	67.3	(61.8 – 76.2)	125
40–59 years	49.2	(45.5 – 53.2)	27.0†	(19.9 – 33.0)	50.1	(48.6 – 53.3)	82.2†	(73.0 – 111)	98
60 years and older	42.9	(40.1 – 45.9)	25.3†	(11.9 – 30.0)	45.8	(39.8 – 48.6)	68.5†	(66.3 – 74.0)	86
Males									
Total, 20 years and older	44.7	(41.2 – 48.4)	24.8	(22.5 – 27.5)	44.2	(38.7 – 51.2)	75.4	(72.8 – 88.6)	142
20–39 years	41.7	(37.3 – 46.6)	23.4†	(14.7 – 26.3)	42.5	(32.5 – 52.0)	73.1†	(60.3 – 181)	57
40–59 years	51.1	(45.1 – 57.8)	27.9†	(23.2 – 34.8)	48.8	(39.2 – 58.8)	88.5†	(73.1 – 121)	42
60 years and older	40.9	(35.6 – 46.9)	23.6†	(20.0 – 26.3)	39.8	(33.3 – 51.3)	69.4†	(57.4 – 83.1)	43
Females									
Total, 20 years and older	40.9	(38.9 – 43.0)	22.4	(18.9 – 25.2)	41.7	(37.8 – 46.2)	69.3	(65.9 – 78.6)	167
20–39 years	35.3	(32.6 – 38.2)	21.2†	(15.5 – 24.3)	36.7	(29.9 – 39.1)	60.0†	(50.6 – 82.2)	68
40–59 years	47.9	(42.3 – 54.2)	21.8†	(17.8 – 33.3)	50.8	(46.4 – 54.0)	78.1†	(68.2 – 109)	56
60 years and older	44.2	(39.6 – 49.4)	25.4†	(11.9 – 31.0)	46.8	(36.5 – 54.0)	68.3†	(61.7 – 78.4)	43

† Estimate is subject to greater uncertainty due to small cell size.

Table 2.29.a.5. Plasma gamma-linolenic acid (18:3n-6): Non-Hispanic whites

Geometric mean and selected percentiles of plasma concentrations (in μmol/L) for fasted non-Hispanic whites in the U.S. population aged 20 years and older, National Health and Nutrition Examination Survey, 2003–2004.

	Geometric mean (95% conf. interval)		Selected percentiles (95% conf. interval)						Sample size
			10th		50th		90th		
Males and Females									
Total, 20 years and older	48.8	(46.1 – 51.6)	25.6	(23.9 – 27.8)	50.5	(47.5 – 53.2)	86.9	(82.2 – 93.2)	981
20–39 years	44.1	(40.9 – 47.6)	24.0	(21.8 – 26.7)	45.3	(39.0 – 50.9)	76.3	(69.5 – 84.7)	294
40–59 years	51.9	(48.1 – 56.0)	26.6	(22.8 – 32.2)	54.2	(50.0 – 58.7)	90.3	(86.4 – 94.7)	278
60 years and older	50.6	(46.1 – 55.5)	26.8	(22.8 – 29.6)	52.4	(46.2 – 58.7)	92.5	(83.2 – 104)	409
Males									
Total, 20 years and older	49.6	(46.0 – 53.4)	26.3	(23.9 – 29.6)	51.4	(49.0 – 53.5)	86.1	(79.7 – 101)	464
20–39 years	47.7	(43.6 – 52.1)	26.3	(22.5 – 29.5)	49.8	(46.8 – 52.9)	80.5	(67.7 – 115)	124
40–59 years	54.4	(50.0 – 59.2)	28.5	(24.0 – 33.3)	56.9	(51.7 – 60.7)	92.4	(85.5 – 117)	138
60 years and older	44.7	(39.8 – 50.3)	24.6	(16.3 – 28.7)	44.6	(41.8 – 49.7)	80.9	(67.4 – 119)	202
Females									
Total, 20 years and older	48.1	(45.4 – 50.9)	24.6	(22.4 – 27.7)	49.1	(45.1 – 53.5)	87.3	(82.1 – 92.2)	517
20–39 years	41.3	(37.2 – 45.8)	23.0	(20.1 – 25.2)	39.6	(35.8 – 45.4)	75.5	(64.7 – 81.7)	170
40–59 years	49.5	(44.8 – 54.8)	25.4	(19.2 – 31.5)	50.5	(46.2 – 56.1)	88.9	(77.0 – 103)	140
60 years and older	56.1	(50.6 – 62.2)	29.6	(22.8 – 33.5)	60.6	(52.8 – 66.0)	97.4	(88.3 – 107)	207

Table 2.30.a.1. Plasma eicosadienoic acid (20:2n-6): Concentrations

Geometric mean and selected percentiles of plasma concentrations (in μmol/L) for the fasted U.S. population aged 20 years and older, National Health and Nutrition Examination Survey, 2003–2004.

	Geometric mean (95% conf. interval)	Selected percentiles (95% conf. interval)						Sample size
		2.5th	5th	50th	95th	97.5th	
Total, 20 years and older	21.2 (20.7 – 21.8)	11.2 (10.5 – 11.6)	12.4 (11.9 – 12.8)	20.9 (20.3 – 21.6)	36.9 (35.1 – 39.9)	42.2 (39.9 – 47.3)	1,805
Age group							
20–39 years	20.2 (19.5 – 20.9)	10.4 (9.44 – 11.0)	11.3 (10.7 – 12.0)	19.4 (18.6 – 20.3)	38.5 (35.8 – 43.2)	43.9 (40.7 – 50.1)	607
40–59 years	21.5 (20.6 – 22.3)	11.7 (10.3 – 12.2)	12.8 (11.8 – 13.7)	21.2 (20.3 – 22.4)	35.4 (33.9 – 40.3)	42.0 (38.1 – 47.5)	515
60 years and older	22.8 (22.1 – 23.5)	12.9 (10.6 – 14.0)	14.3 (13.1 – 15.3)	23.1 (22.3 – 23.6)	35.4 (33.7 – 37.4)	38.6 (36.6 – 46.6)	683
Gender							
Males	20.4 (19.7 – 21.2)	11.4 (10.6 – 11.9)	12.6 (11.8 – 13.0)	20.2 (19.3 – 21.1)	32.9 (31.3 – 37.1)	40.0 (35.1 – 44.9)	865
Females	22.0 (21.3 – 22.7)	11.0 (10.4 – 11.4)	12.2 (11.4 – 13.0)	21.7 (21.0 – 22.3)	38.5 (36.4 – 43.8)	46.5 (40.9 – 49.6)	940
Race/ethnicity							
Mexican Americans	25.2 (23.5 – 27.1)	11.4† (8.60 – 13.3)	13.3 (11.3 – 14.4)	24.9 (22.8 – 26.6)	49.5 (43.2 – 69.3)	55.0† (49.5 – 121)	375
Non-Hispanic Blacks	19.2 (18.3 – 20.1)	10.8† (9.00 – 11.2)	11.4 (10.5 – 12.5)	19.0 (18.1 – 19.7)	33.5 (28.4 – 40.5)	36.3† (34.6 – 51.6)	310
Non-Hispanic Whites	20.9 (20.3 – 21.5)	11.2 (9.83 – 11.8)	12.3 (11.7 – 12.9)	20.7 (20.1 – 21.4)	35.0 (33.5 – 38.1)	40.7 (36.9 – 46.5)	990

† Estimate is subject to greater uncertainty due to small cell size.

Figure 2.30.a. Plasma eicosadienoic acid (20:2n–6): Concentrations by age group
Geometric mean (95% confidence interval), National Health and Nutrition Examination Survey, 2003–2004

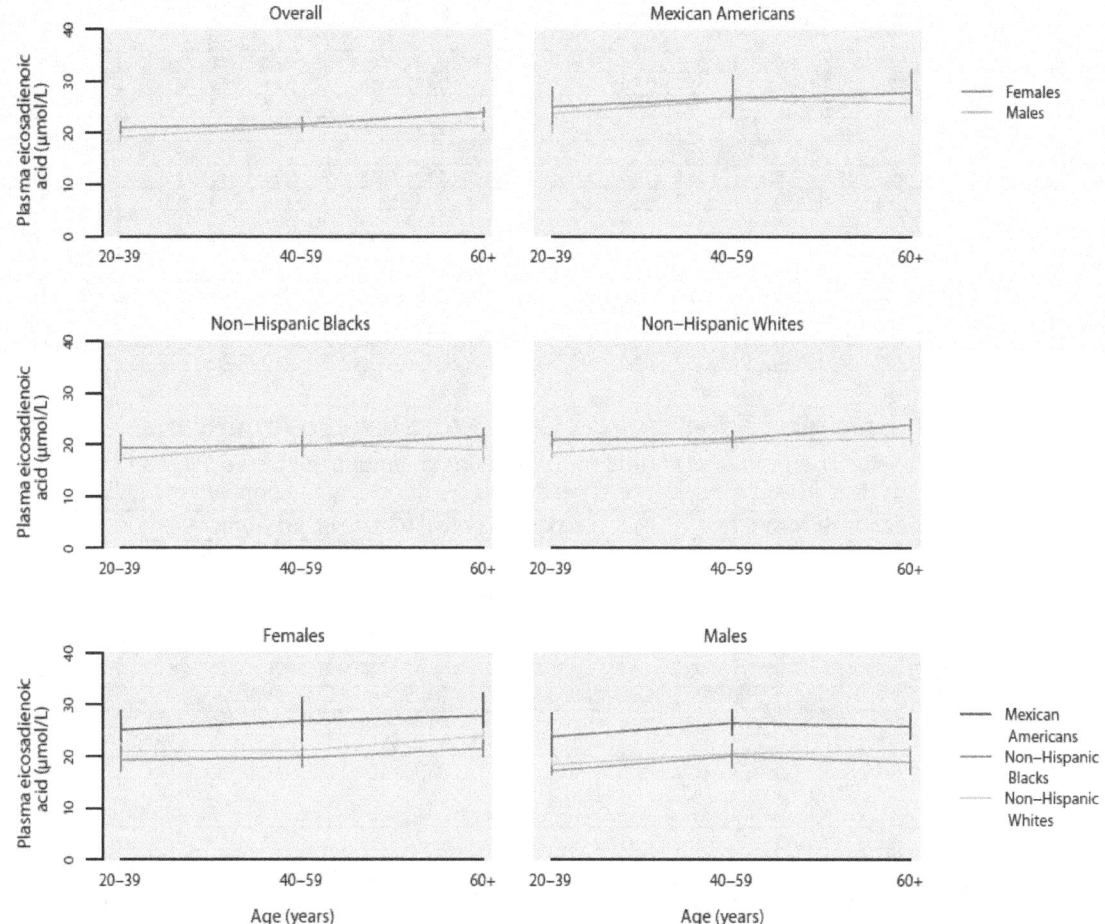

Table 2.30.a.2. Plasma eicosadienoic acid (20:2n-6): Total population

Geometric mean and selected percentiles of plasma concentrations (in μmol/L) for the fasted U.S. population aged 20 years and older, National Health and Nutrition Examination Survey, 2003–2004.

	Geometric mean (95% conf. interval)	Selected percentiles (95% conf. interval)			Sample size
		10th	50th	90th	
Males and Females					
Total, 20 years and older	21.2 (20.7 – 21.8)	14.1 (13.5 – 14.6)	20.9 (20.3 – 21.6)	32.0 (30.8 – 33.8)	1,805
20–39 years	20.2 (19.5 – 20.9)	13.0 (12.0 – 13.7)	19.4 (18.6 – 20.3)	33.1 (30.9 – 36.6)	607
40–59 years	21.5 (20.6 – 22.3)	14.5 (13.2 – 15.3)	21.2 (20.3 – 22.4)	30.8 (30.0 – 33.7)	515
60 years and older	22.8 (22.1 – 23.5)	16.2 (15.2 – 16.8)	23.1 (22.3 – 23.6)	32.2 (31.0 – 33.4)	683
Males					
Total, 20 years and older	20.4 (19.7 – 21.2)	13.9 (13.0 – 14.7)	20.2 (19.3 – 21.1)	29.6 (28.1 – 31.3)	865
20–39 years	19.3 (18.4 – 20.2)	13.1 (11.6 – 13.9)	19.2 (18.1 – 19.9)	28.3 (26.4 – 31.4)	282
40–59 years	21.2 (20.3 – 22.2)	14.5 (12.9 – 15.3)	20.9 (19.6 – 22.8)	30.3 (28.1 – 32.4)	248
60 years and older	21.4 (20.6 – 22.2)	15.3 (13.2 – 16.6)	21.0 (20.3 – 21.9)	29.5 (28.1 – 33.4)	335
Females					
Total, 20 years and older	22.0 (21.3 – 22.7)	14.4 (13.7 – 14.8)	21.7 (21.0 – 22.3)	34.2 (32.5 – 36.2)	940
20–39 years	21.1 (20.1 – 22.3)	12.9 (12.2 – 13.8)	20.0 (19.0 – 21.2)	36.3 (34.3 – 39.4)	325
40–59 years	21.7 (20.6 – 22.9)	14.6 (12.2 – 15.7)	21.4 (20.5 – 22.2)	31.5 (29.9 – 37.8)	267
60 years and older	24.0 (23.1 – 24.9)	16.7 (15.6 – 17.7)	24.0 (23.1 – 25.4)	33.5 (32.4 – 35.7)	348

Table 2.30.a.3. Plasma eicosadienoic acid (20:2n-6): Mexican Americans

Geometric mean and selected percentiles of plasma concentrations (in μmol/L) for fasted Mexican Americans in the U.S. population aged 20 years and older, National Health and Nutrition Examination Survey, 2003–2004.

	Geometric mean (95% conf. interval)	Selected percentiles (95% conf. interval)			Sample size
		10th	50th	90th	
Males and Females					
Total, 20 years and older	25.2 (23.5 – 27.1)	15.7 (13.4 – 17.2)	24.9 (22.8 – 26.6)	42.1 (35.6 – 51.2)	375
20–39 years	24.3 (21.7 – 27.3)	14.1 (12.6 – 16.7)	23.5 (20.5 – 27.8)	43.9 (33.7 – 55.6)	131
40–59 years	26.6 (24.6 – 28.8)	17.7† (12.3 – 20.2)	25.5 (24.5 – 26.5)	42.3† (35.8 – 73.3)	93
60 years and older	26.8 (25.4 – 28.3)	19.9 (18.1 – 20.4)	26.4 (24.7 – 27.6)	37.0 (35.1 – 49.3)	151
Males					
Total, 20 years and older	24.7 (22.2 – 27.5)	14.9 (13.0 – 17.2)	24.7 (22.4 – 26.6)	39.9 (31.9 – 63.7)	189
20–39 years	23.8 (20.1 – 28.2)	13.7† (12.1 – 15.9)	23.9 (19.8 – 28.8)	36.5† (28.8 – 56.4)	67
40–59 years	26.4 (24.2 – 28.9)	17.6† (12.5 – 20.6)	25.2 (23.8 – 26.9)	41.6† (34.7 – 73.3)	48
60 years and older	25.8 (23.6 – 28.2)	18.7† (10.7 – 20.5)	25.6 (22.1 – 27.9)	37.0† (31.3 – 69.2)	74
Females					
Total, 20 years and older	25.9 (24.0 – 28.0)	16.7 (11.4 – 17.4)	25.1 (22.2 – 27.7)	45.8 (37.6 – 55.9)	186
20–39 years	25.1 (21.8 – 28.8)	14.5† (10.8 – 17.2)	22.7 (20.1 – 27.0)	48.8† (37.2 – 56.6)	64
40–59 years	26.8 (23.1 – 31.2)	18.3† (8.60 – 20.6)	25.7 (23.0 – 28.3)	42.2† (32.9 – 58.3)	45
60 years and older	27.8 (24.0 – 32.2)	20.2† (17.8 – 20.8)	26.9 (22.9 – 34.5)	36.1† (34.7 – 51.5)	77

† Estimate is subject to greater uncertainty due to small cell size.

Table 2.30.a.4. Plasma eicosadienoic acid (20:2n-6): Non-Hispanic blacks

Geometric mean and selected percentiles of plasma concentrations (in μmol/L) for fasted non-Hispanic blacks in the U.S. population aged 20 years and older, National Health and Nutrition Examination Survey, 2003–2004.

	Geometric mean (95% conf. interval)	Selected percentiles (95% conf. interval)			Sample size
		10th	50th	90th	
Males and Females					
Total, 20 years and older	19.2 (18.3 – 20.1)	12.8 (11.3 – 13.7)	19.0 (18.1 – 19.7)	27.8 (25.4 – 33.8)	310
20–39 years	18.3 (17.0 – 19.7)	12.2 (10.9 – 13.1)	17.9 (16.3 – 19.1)	26.4 (24.5 – 36.1)	126
40–59 years	19.8 (18.6 – 21.1)	13.3† (10.5 – 14.9)	19.2 (17.8 – 21.1)	28.1† (26.1 – 34.9)	98
60 years and older	20.5 (19.6 – 21.3)	14.2† (12.6 – 15.4)	21.1 (19.7 – 22.4)	27.5† (25.3 – 28.2)	86
Males					
Total, 20 years and older	18.4 (17.3 – 19.5)	12.3 (10.9 – 13.3)	17.9 (16.5 – 19.2)	26.4 (24.3 – 31.6)	143
20–39 years	17.2 (16.4 – 18.1)	11.3† (9.43 – 13.2)	16.4 (16.0 – 18.2)	25.1† (22.0 – 48.7)	58
40–59 years	20.0 (17.8 – 22.3)	13.8† (10.2 – 15.5)	18.2 (16.8 – 20.4)	31.9† (26.2 – 52.2)	42
60 years and older	18.9 (16.7 – 21.3)	12.4† (8.53 – 14.5)	19.6 (17.1 – 21.5)	25.6† (23.5 – 35.0)	43
Females					
Total, 20 years and older	19.8 (18.3 – 21.5)	12.9 (11.2 – 14.7)	19.4 (18.3 – 21.6)	28.2 (24.8 – 40.6)	167
20–39 years	19.3 (17.1 – 21.8)	12.5† (11.2 – 14.1)	18.5 (16.8 – 20.1)	32.1† (24.5 – 47.8)	68
40–59 years	19.7 (18.0 – 21.5)	12.9† (8.30 – 15.4)	19.3 (17.5 – 22.1)	27.0† (23.6 – 96.5)	56
60 years and older	21.5 (20.1 – 23.1)	15.9† (13.1 – 17.7)	21.9 (19.9 – 23.2)	27.7† (24.3 – 40.5)	43

† Estimate is subject to greater uncertainty due to small cell size.

Table 2.30.a.5. Plasma eicosadienoic acid (20:2n-6): Non-Hispanic whites

Geometric mean and selected percentiles of plasma concentrations (in μmol/L) for fasted non-Hispanic whites in the U.S. population aged 20 years and older, National Health and Nutrition Examination Survey, 2003–2004.

	Geometric mean (95% conf. interval)	Selected percentiles (95% conf. interval)			Sample size
		10th	50th	90th	
Males and Females					
Total, 20 years and older	20.9 (20.3 – 21.5)	14.0 (13.1 – 14.7)	20.7 (20.1 – 21.4)	31.0 (29.8 – 33.3)	990
20–39 years	19.7 (18.9 – 20.5)	12.8 (11.7 – 13.6)	19.3 (18.1 – 20.0)	33.1 (29.5 – 37.1)	298
40–59 years	20.8 (19.7 – 21.9)	13.9 (12.7 – 15.1)	20.8 (19.8 – 21.8)	30.2 (28.0 – 32.2)	280
60 years and older	22.7 (21.9 – 23.5)	16.0 (14.5 – 16.8)	23.0 (22.0 – 23.8)	31.9 (29.9 – 33.5)	412
Males					
Total, 20 years and older	20.0 (19.3 – 20.7)	13.7 (12.8 – 14.8)	19.9 (18.9 – 20.8)	28.2 (27.1 – 30.4)	472
20–39 years	18.4 (17.4 – 19.5)	12.7 (10.9 – 13.9)	18.3 (17.3 – 19.4)	25.7 (23.3 – 29.6)	128
40–59 years	20.5 (19.4 – 21.6)	14.1 (12.8 – 15.1)	20.4 (18.7 – 22.5)	28.2 (27.3 – 30.6)	140
60 years and older	21.3 (20.4 – 22.2)	15.4 (12.9 – 16.7)	21.0 (20.1 – 22.1)	29.4 (28.0 – 33.4)	204
Females					
Total, 20 years and older	21.8 (20.9 – 22.7)	14.3 (13.2 – 14.8)	21.5 (20.9 – 22.2)	33.8 (31.8 – 36.2)	518
20–39 years	20.9 (19.5 – 22.5)	12.8 (12.0 – 13.7)	20.0 (18.5 – 21.4)	36.9 (34.1 – 40.4)	170
40–59 years	21.1 (19.7 – 22.7)	13.8 (11.8 – 15.4)	21.1 (20.2 – 22.0)	30.9 (28.2 – 36.5)	140
60 years and older	23.9 (22.8 – 25.1)	16.5 (15.0 – 18.1)	24.1 (23.0 – 25.5)	33.2 (32.2 – 35.2)	208

Table 2.31.a.1. Plasma homo-gamma-linolenic acid (20:3n-6): Concentrations

Geometric mean and selected percentiles of plasma concentrations (in µmol/L) for the fasted U.S. population aged 20 years and older, National Health and Nutrition Examination Survey, 2003–2004.

	Geometric mean (95% conf. interval)	Selected percentiles (95% conf. interval)						Sample size
		2.5th	5th	50th	95th	97.5th		
Total, 20 years and older	151 (147 – 156)	73.2 (67.9 – 79.6)	87.5 (84.6 – 89.9)	151 (145 – 156)	262 (254 – 274)	289 (281 – 320)		1,806
Age group								
20–39 years	145 (140 – 149)	71.5 (57.7 – 78.3)	84.9 (75.9 – 91.3)	139 (135 – 146)	251 (239 – 276)	281 (262 – 317)		609
40–59 years	155 (147 – 163)	72.0 (67.7 – 86.3)	88.3 (83.1 – 94.0)	156 (147 – 164)	265 (258 – 286)	312 (284 – 337)		514
60 years and older	156 (148 – 164)	77.0 (62.8 – 84.0)	86.6 (77.7 – 92.8)	158 (148 – 167)	262 (254 – 285)	288 (275 – 357)		683
Gender								
Males	145 (139 – 153)	72.8 (62.2 – 76.4)	86.1 (76.4 – 90.0)	144 (135 – 153)	252 (237 – 277)	281 (260 – 373)		864
Females	157 (152 – 162)	72.9 (67.9 – 84.9)	88.5 (84.7 – 93.0)	156 (150 – 163)	272 (261 – 287)	304 (287 – 321)		942
Race/ethnicity								
Mexican Americans	166 (154 – 179)	82.2† (58.9 – 89.6)	92.0 (77.8 – 101)	167 (153 – 180)	297 (260 – 363)	330† (295 – 716)		375
Non-Hispanic Blacks	131 (128 – 135)	70.0† (52.8 – 75.7)	76.7 (70.3 – 85.5)	131 (127 – 136)	203 (196 – 230)	223† (206 – 276)		310
Non-Hispanic Whites	152 (146 – 159)	76.0 (67.7 – 84.6)	88.9 (84.9 – 92.9)	152 (144 – 157)	261 (250 – 281)	287 (275 – 324)		991

† Estimate is subject to greater uncertainty due to small cell size.

Figure 2.31.a. Plasma homo–gamma–linolenic acid (20:3n–6): Concentrations by age group

Geometric mean (95% confidence interval), National Health and Nutrition Examination Survey, 2003–2004

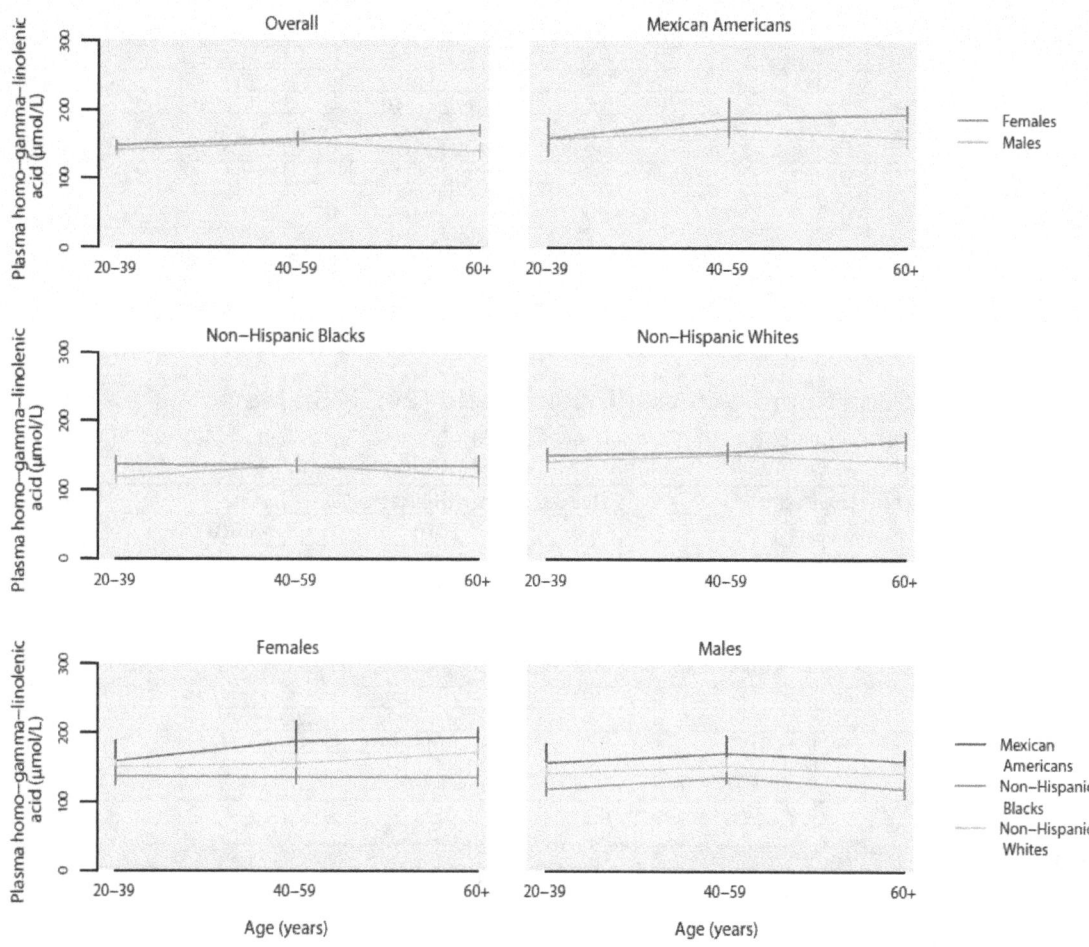

Table 2.31.a.2. Plasma homo-gamma-linolenic acid (20:3n-6): Total population

Geometric mean and selected percentiles of plasma concentrations (in µmol/L) for the fasted U.S. population aged 20 years and older, National Health and Nutrition Examination Survey, 2003–2004.

	Geometric mean (95% conf. interval)	Selected percentiles (95% conf. interval)						Sample size
		10th		50th		90th		
Males and Females								
Total, 20 years and older	151 (147 – 156)	98.4	(95.2 – 102)	151	(145 – 156)	232	(221 – 245)	1,806
20–39 years	145 (140 – 149)	95.6	(92.4 – 99.4)	139	(135 – 146)	223	(213 – 239)	609
40–59 years	155 (147 – 163)	102	(94.2 – 107)	156	(147 – 164)	240	(222 – 258)	514
60 years and older	156 (148 – 164)	100	(94.3 – 104)	158	(148 – 167)	236	(222 – 250)	683
Males								
Total, 20 years and older	145 (139 – 153)	96.7	(93.1 – 100)	144	(135 – 153)	222	(210 – 246)	864
20–39 years	141 (134 – 149)	95.2	(88.2 – 97.7)	137	(131 – 145)	219	(201 – 247)	282
40–59 years	153 (144 – 163)	101	(93.8 – 107)	155	(141 – 161)	232	(217 – 272)	247
60 years and older	140 (131 – 150)	92.2	(84.0 – 97.9)	141	(133 – 153)	203	(185 – 244)	335
Females								
Total, 20 years and older	157 (152 – 162)	102	(96.6 – 105)	156	(150 – 163)	241	(227 – 258)	942
20–39 years	148 (142 – 154)	97.3	(91.9 – 103)	142	(135 – 156)	226	(209 – 270)	327
40–59 years	157 (148 – 167)	104	(93.3 – 107)	157	(151 – 166)	241	(214 – 264)	267
60 years and older	170 (162 – 178)	107	(98.4 – 115)	175	(159 – 185)	258	(236 – 274)	348

Table 2.31.a.3. Plasma homo-gamma-linolenic acid (20:3n-6): Mexican Americans

Geometric mean and selected percentiles of plasma concentrations (in µmol/L) for fasted Mexican Americans in the U.S. population aged 20 years and older, National Health and Nutrition Examination Survey, 2003–2004.

	Geometric mean (95% conf. interval)	Selected percentiles (95% conf. interval)						Sample size
		10th		50th		90th		
Males and Females								
Total, 20 years and older	166 (154 – 179)	103	(90.3 – 109)	167	(153 – 180)	258	(245 – 293)	375
20–39 years	158 (140 – 177)	96.7	(82.8 – 104)	158	(131 – 189)	254	(239 – 295)	131
40–59 years	178 (166 – 192)	110†	(81.4 – 129)	178	(168 – 186)	289†	(241 – 360)	93
60 years and older	177 (169 – 185)	119	(108 – 130)	185	(169 – 199)	245	(237 – 261)	151
Males								
Total, 20 years and older	161 (143 – 181)	103	(85.0 – 114)	161	(138 – 192)	246	(222 – 296)	189
20–39 years	157 (133 – 185)	102†	(65.4 – 113)	148	(121 – 204)	248†	(215 – 329)	67
40–59 years	171 (149 – 196)	111†	(84.1 – 132)	168	(148 – 194)	244†	(213 – 361)	48
60 years and older	160 (146 – 176)	113†	(49.9 – 123)	165	(143 – 181)	228†	(188 – 288)	74
Females								
Total, 20 years and older	172 (155 – 190)	93.0	(65.6 – 109)	175	(159 – 201)	272	(240 – 716)	186
20–39 years	159 (135 – 188)	89.4†	(55.8 – 103)	160	(127 – 200)	269†	(225 – 716)	64
40–59 years	188 (162 – 217)	106†	(65.9 – 149)	190	(171 – 214)	303†	(244 – 372)	45
60 years and older	194 (183 – 207)	128†	(117 – 135)	204	(193 – 214)	258†	(238 – 328)	77

† Estimate is subject to greater uncertainty due to small cell size.

Table 2.31.a.4. Plasma homo-gamma-linolenic acid (20:3n-6): Non-Hispanic blacks

Geometric mean and selected percentiles of plasma concentrations (in µmol/L) for fasted non-Hispanic blacks in the U.S. population aged 20 years and older, National Health and Nutrition Examination Survey, 2003–2004.

	Geometric mean (95% conf. interval)		Selected percentiles (95% conf. interval)						Sample size
			10th		50th		90th		
Males and Females									
Total, 20 years and older	131	(128 – 135)	91.5	(81.3 – 96.1)	131	(127 – 136)	187	(181 – 200)	310
20–39 years	129	(122 – 136)	88.0	(72.5 – 96.0)	128	(117 – 139)	186	(172 – 206)	126
40–59 years	136	(130 – 143)	98.8†	(63.0 – 109)	134	(128 – 141)	198†	(182 – 235)	98
60 years and older	130	(123 – 136)	85.9†	(75.4 – 92.8)	134	(117 – 147)	183†	(173 – 215)	86
Males									
Total, 20 years and older	125	(119 – 131)	82.5	(73.7 – 94.9)	121	(112 – 130)	188	(173 – 203)	143
20–39 years	119	(111 – 128)	77.7†	(53.1 – 94.7)	115	(106 – 130)	174†	(168 – 196)	58
40–59 years	136	(129 – 144)	99.7†	(71.4 – 105)	128	(118 – 147)	197†	(174 – 261)	42
60 years and older	120	(107 – 134)	76.3†	(45.9 – 90.2)	118	(105 – 141)	184†	(156 – 213)	43
Females									
Total, 20 years and older	136	(129 – 144)	93.0	(85.4 – 103)	135	(124 – 150)	186	(180 – 206)	167
20–39 years	137	(125 – 149)	92.6†	(77.6 – 104)	134	(116 – 159)	193†	(174 – 272)	68
40–59 years	136	(126 – 147)	94.2†	(49.0 – 116)	135	(128 – 145)	189†	(156 – 298)	56
60 years and older	136	(124 – 149)	92.6†	(70.7 – 102)	144	(115 – 160)	182†	(171 – 216)	43

† Estimate is subject to greater uncertainty due to small cell size.

Table 2.31.a.5. Plasma homo-gamma-linolenic acid (20:3n-6): Non-Hispanic whites

Geometric mean and selected percentiles of plasma concentrations (in µmol/L) for fasted non-Hispanic whites in the U.S. population aged 20 years and older, National Health and Nutrition Examination Survey, 2003–2004.

	Geometric mean (95% conf. interval)		Selected percentiles (95% conf. interval)						Sample size
			10th		50th		90th		
Males and Females									
Total, 20 years and older	152	(146 – 159)	99.3	(94.2 – 103)	152	(144 – 157)	233	(218 – 250)	991
20–39 years	147	(140 – 154)	97.2	(91.2 – 103)	140	(135 – 148)	226	(215 – 245)	300
40–59 years	154	(143 – 165)	101	(92.9 – 107)	156	(143 – 166)	232	(213 – 261)	279
60 years and older	158	(149 – 167)	100	(91.9 – 107)	160	(148 – 172)	242	(226 – 256)	412
Males									
Total, 20 years and older	146	(137 – 155)	97.0	(90.8 – 101)	144	(134 – 155)	222	(206 – 254)	471
20–39 years	142	(129 – 156)	95.2	(73.6 – 101)	136	(126 – 147)	222	(187 – 279)	128
40–59 years	152	(139 – 165)	100	(90.4 – 107)	155	(134 – 165)	227	(210 – 284)	139
60 years and older	142	(132 – 153)	93.6	(86.9 – 99.4)	141	(133 – 154)	206	(184 – 250)	204
Females									
Total, 20 years and older	159	(152 – 165)	104	(97.0 – 106)	157	(150 – 168)	242	(224 – 261)	520
20–39 years	151	(143 – 160)	99.5	(93.5 – 109)	141	(135 – 160)	232	(210 – 285)	172
40–59 years	156	(144 – 169)	103	(86.2 – 107)	156	(149 – 168)	240	(210 – 264)	140
60 years and older	172	(161 – 184)	107	(88.1 – 124)	177	(161 – 191)	260	(245 – 271)	208

Table 2.32.a.1. Plasma arachidonic acid (20:4n-6): Concentrations

Geometric mean and selected percentiles of plasma concentrations (in μmol/L) for the fasted U.S. population aged 20 years and older, National Health and Nutrition Examination Survey, 2003–2004.

| | Geometric mean (95% conf. interval) | Selected percentiles (95% conf. interval) | | | | | Sample size |
		2.5th	5th	50th	95th	97.5th	
Total, 20 years and older	776 (761 – 791)	445 (418 – 463)	484 (456 – 500)	789 (772 – 805)	1,180 (1,150 – 1,230)	1,320 (1,240 – 1,420)	1,807
Age group							
20-39 years	735 (716 – 755)	429 (386 – 455)	479 (445 – 504)	737 (713 – 761)	1,110 (1,050 – 1,230)	1,230 (1,140 – 1,380)	610
40-59 years	793 (772 – 814)	445 (372 – 470)	480 (450 – 496)	808 (785 – 829)	1,220 (1,160 – 1,360)	1,380 (1,260 – 1,560)	514
60 years and older	819 (798 – 841)	448 (421 – 480)	502 (460 – 535)	841 (814 – 868)	1,200 (1,180 – 1,260)	1,430 (1,310 – 1,490)	683
Gender							
Males	764 (744 – 785)	452 (424 – 473)	480 (455 – 495)	780 (756 – 806)	1,150 (1,090 – 1,220)	1,230 (1,160 – 1,460)	864
Females	787 (769 – 806)	429 (386 – 465)	490 (436 – 520)	792 (769 – 821)	1,220 (1,180 – 1,300)	1,370 (1,320 – 1,460)	943
Race/ethnicity							
Mexican Americans	722 (678 – 768)	419† (376 – 432)	440 (396 – 487)	726 (675 – 768)	1,110 (1,040 – 1,310)	1,290† (1,140 – 1,460)	376
Non-Hispanic Blacks	884 (839 – 932)	526† (226 – 572)	576 (493 – 611)	883 (831 – 941)	1,330 (1,260 – 1,580)	1,520† (1,360 – 1,770)	310
Non-Hispanic Whites	773 (752 – 795)	445 (419 – 463)	485 (446 – 511)	785 (767 – 807)	1,160 (1,120 – 1,220)	1,260 (1,190 – 1,480)	991

† Estimate is subject to greater uncertainty due to small cell size.

Figure 2.32.a. Plasma arachidonic acid (20:4n–6): Concentrations by age group

Geometric mean (95% confidence interval), National Health and Nutrition Examination Survey, 2003–2004

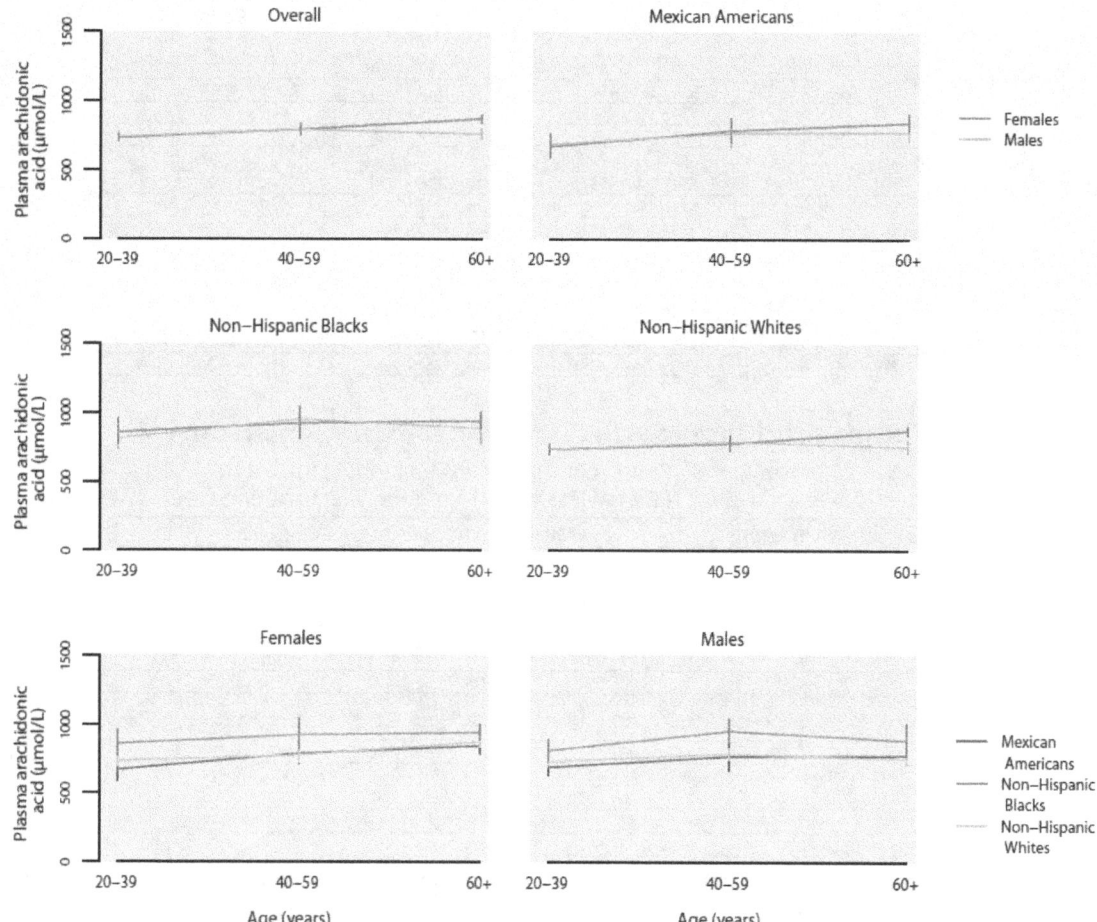

Table 2.32.a.2. Plasma arachidonic acid (20:4n-6): Total population

Geometric mean and selected percentiles of plasma concentrations (in µmol/L) for the fasted U.S. population aged 20 years and older, National Health and Nutrition Examination Survey, 2003–2004.

	Geometric mean (95% conf. interval)		Selected percentiles (95% conf. interval)						Sample size
			10th		50th		90th		
Males and Females									
Total, 20 years and older	776	(761 – 791)	538	(516 – 560)	789	(772 – 805)	1,070	(1,040 – 1,110)	1,807
20–39 years	735	(716 – 755)	529	(510 – 542)	737	(713 – 761)	1,000	(959 – 1,080)	610
40–59 years	793	(772 – 814)	534	(488 – 569)	808	(785 – 829)	1,090	(1,050 – 1,140)	514
60 years and older	819	(798 – 841)	562	(533 – 591)	841	(814 – 868)	1,120	(1,090 – 1,140)	683
Males									
Total, 20 years and older	764	(744 – 785)	534	(502 – 547)	780	(756 – 806)	1,040	(1,000 – 1,090)	864
20–39 years	739	(710 – 769)	533	(505 – 542)	736	(713 – 766)	999	(945 – 1,100)	282
40–59 years	792	(761 – 825)	529	(487 – 566)	823	(795 – 842)	1,070	(1,020 – 1,150)	247
60 years and older	761	(726 – 798)	532	(453 – 570)	796	(740 – 839)	1,030	(986 – 1,100)	335
Females									
Total, 20 years and older	787	(769 – 806)	549	(517 – 575)	792	(769 – 821)	1,100	(1,050 – 1,160)	943
20–39 years	732	(710 – 755)	523	(497 – 552)	738	(705 – 766)	1,010	(956 – 1,120)	328
40–59 years	793	(755 – 833)	534	(464 – 597)	787	(753 – 864)	1,130	(1,020 – 1,230)	267
60 years and older	870	(844 – 896)	620	(551 – 654)	878	(854 – 904)	1,150	(1,120 – 1,200)	348

Table 2.32.a.3. Plasma arachidonic acid (20:4n-6): Mexican Americans

Geometric mean and selected percentiles of plasma concentrations (in µmol/L) for fasted Mexican Americans in the U.S. population aged 20 years and older, National Health and Nutrition Examination Survey, 2003–2004.

	Geometric mean (95% conf. interval)		Selected percentiles (95% conf. interval)						Sample size
			10th		50th		90th		
Males and Females									
Total, 20 years and older	722	(678 – 768)	499	(439 – 536)	726	(675 – 768)	1,030	(975 – 1,080)	376
20–39 years	681	(631 – 735)	483	(413 – 526)	687	(628 – 745)	993	(892 – 1,070)	132
40–59 years	778	(718 – 844)	510†	(420 – 602)	774	(749 – 835)	1,120†	(948 – 1,350)	93
60 years and older	811	(777 – 846)	567	(496 – 592)	826	(769 – 874)	1,170	(1,050 – 1,330)	151
Males									
Total, 20 years and older	719	(669 – 773)	502	(426 – 535)	745	(674 – 788)	1,030	(937 – 1,090)	189
20–39 years	689	(637 – 746)	503†	(380 – 540)	707	(609 – 758)	983†	(851 – 1,110)	67
40–59 years	770	(675 – 878)	489†	(377 – 606)	800	(748 – 843)	1,040†	(881 – 1,460)	48
60 years and older	776	(714 – 842)	527†	(376 – 590)	811	(643 – 924)	1,090†	(1,000 – 1,360)	74
Females									
Total, 20 years and older	724	(659 – 796)	479	(352 – 582)	716	(653 – 782)	1,020	(945 – 1,310)	187
20–39 years	670	(591 – 760)	436†	(352 – 539)	676	(626 – 723)	987†	(856 – 1,310)	65
40–59 years	788	(711 – 874)	567†	(447 – 616)	756	(652 – 885)	1,250†	(964 – 1,430)	45
60 years and older	844	(790 – 902)	586†	(580 – 600)	835	(810 – 873)	1,220†	(987 – 1,940)	77

† Estimate is subject to greater uncertainty due to small cell size.

Table 2.32.a.4. Plasma arachidonic acid (20:4n-6): Non-Hispanic blacks

Geometric mean and selected percentiles of plasma concentrations (in µmol/L) for fasted non-Hispanic blacks in the U.S. population aged 20 years and older, National Health and Nutrition Examination Survey, 2003–2004.

	Geometric mean (95% conf. interval)		Selected percentiles (95% conf. interval)						Sample size
			10th		50th		90th		
Males and Females									
Total, 20 years and older	884	(839 – 932)	630	(588 – 670)	883	(831 – 941)	1,220	(1,160 – 1,330)	310
20–39 years	836	(776 – 901)	602	(542 – 635)	839	(769 – 887)	1,210	(1,040 – 1,380)	126
40–59 years	936	(858 – 1,020)	681†	(513 – 711)	942	(827 – 1,040)	1,230†	(1,170 – 1,760)	98
60 years and older	919	(859 – 983)	714†	(534 – 744)	933	(830 – 1,030)	1,200†	(1,160 – 1,330)	86
Males									
Total, 20 years and older	870	(817 – 925)	591	(512 – 659)	859	(811 – 976)	1,200	(1,130 – 1,330)	143
20–39 years	811	(737 – 892)	580†	(479 – 616)	812	(692 – 891)	1,120†	(1,020 – 1,660)	58
40–59 years	953	(875 – 1,040)	666†	(501 – 727)	984	(780 – 1,070)	1,230†	(1,110 – 2,240)	42
60 years and older	886	(774 – 1,010)	535†	(226 – 722)	940	(833 – 1,050)	1,180†	(1,130 – 1,440)	43
Females									
Total, 20 years and older	895	(829 – 967)	648	(588 – 704)	884	(823 – 958)	1,230	(1,130 – 1,470)	167
20–39 years	858	(773 – 952)	616†	(570 – 661)	857	(746 – 955)	1,230†	(1,010 – 1,390)	68
40–59 years	923	(818 – 1,040)	679†	(468 – 714)	912	(824 – 1,020)	1,230†	(1,100 – 2,020)	56
60 years and older	940	(889 – 995)	740†	(715 – 762)	916	(809 – 1,040)	1,220†	(1,130 – 1,490)	43

† Estimate is subject to greater uncertainty due to small cell size.

Table 2.32.a.5. Plasma arachidonic acid (20:4n-6): Non-Hispanic whites

Geometric mean and selected percentiles of plasma concentrations (in µmol/L) for fasted non-Hispanic whites in the U.S. population aged 20 years and older, National Health and Nutrition Examination Survey, 2003–2004.

	Geometric mean (95% conf. interval)		Selected percentiles (95% conf. interval)						Sample size
			10th		50th		90th		
Males and Females									
Total, 20 years and older	773	(752 – 795)	539	(497 – 569)	785	(767 – 807)	1,050	(1,010 – 1,100)	991
20–39 years	733	(711 – 755)	533	(490 – 569)	736	(706 – 766)	971	(929 – 1,060)	300
40–59 years	782	(749 – 817)	531	(465 – 579)	800	(777 – 830)	1,040	(1,010 – 1,120)	279
60 years and older	815	(788 – 843)	562	(504 – 604)	839	(811 – 870)	1,110	(1,070 – 1,140)	412
Males									
Total, 20 years and older	760	(733 – 788)	534	(488 – 558)	783	(752 – 810)	1,000	(981 – 1,050)	471
20–39 years	731	(702 – 762)	527	(480 – 562)	735	(698 – 771)	957	(899 – 1,160)	128
40–59 years	789	(748 – 832)	539	(476 – 569)	823	(786 – 863)	1,030	(997 – 1,160)	139
60 years and older	752	(711 – 795)	524	(444 – 573)	769	(715 – 833)	998	(962 – 1,110)	204
Females									
Total, 20 years and older	785	(761 – 811)	552	(500 – 583)	786	(769 – 816)	1,080	(1,040 – 1,160)	520
20–39 years	733	(701 – 768)	532	(432 – 583)	738	(699 – 768)	997	(920 – 1,150)	172
40–59 years	776	(722 – 835)	530	(403 – 598)	780	(726 – 858)	1,060	(991 – 1,240)	140
60 years and older	873	(841 – 905)	610	(541 – 665)	889	(857 – 916)	1,150	(1,120 – 1,200)	208

Table 2.33.a.1. Plasma eicosapentaenoic acid (20:5n-3): Concentrations

Geometric mean and selected percentiles of plasma concentrations (in µmol/L) for the fasted U.S. population aged 20 years and older, National Health and Nutrition Examination Survey, 2003–2004.

	Geometric mean	Selected percentiles (95% conf. interval)						Sample size
	(95% conf. interval)	2.5th	5th	50th	95th	97.5th		
Total, 20 years and older	42.1 (39.5 – 45.0)	14.8 (11.8 – 16.1)	17.1 (15.7 – 18.6)	40.9 (37.6 – 43.8)	113 (103 – 138)	151 (136 – 176)		1,806
Age group								
20–39 years	35.9 (33.8 – 38.1)	13.5 (9.10 – 14.9)	15.8 (13.6 – 16.8)	34.2 (32.0 – 36.2)	106 (84.3 – 137)	134 (110 – 193)		609
40–59 years	45.5 (41.8 – 49.5)	17.1 (14.6 – 17.4)	19.0 (17.1 – 20.8)	45.0 (41.0 – 48.3)	114 (102 – 153)	156 (134 – 200)		515
60 years and older	48.5 (43.3 – 54.4)	15.3 (7.79 – 19.9)	20.0 (11.8 – 23.1)	49.4 (43.5 – 53.8)	132 (111 – 162)	175 (139 – 207)		682
Gender								
Males	43.1 (39.8 – 46.6)	15.7 (11.2 – 16.9)	17.1 (15.5 – 20.1)	41.4 (37.6 – 45.1)	121 (103 – 150)	156 (136 – 199)		863
Females	41.3 (38.7 – 44.1)	14.1 (11.2 – 15.7)	16.9 (15.2 – 18.3)	40.1 (37.5 – 43.1)	111 (99.9 – 143)	146 (118 – 177)		943
Race/ethnicity								
Mexican Americans	31.0 (28.7 – 33.5)	8.80† (6.03 – 10.9)	10.9 (7.53 – 15.3)	31.4 (28.4 – 35.4)	77.1 (69.0 – 86.4)	86.5† (79.1 – 98.9)		375
Non-Hispanic Blacks	38.8 (34.7 – 43.4)	14.9† (10.8 – 16.1)	16.7 (14.4 – 18.8)	36.1 (33.0 – 41.6)	113 (95.3 – 169)	141† (114 – 247)		310
Non-Hispanic Whites	43.5 (39.8 – 47.7)	15.8 (11.6 – 17.3)	18.1 (14.9 – 20.8)	42.6 (38.1 – 46.0)	112 (101 – 142)	152 (133 – 177)		991

† Estimate is subject to greater uncertainty due to small cell size.

Figure 2.33.a. Plasma eicosapentaenoic acid (20:5n–3): Concentrations by age group

Geometric mean (95% confidence interval), National Health and Nutrition Examination Survey, 2003–2004

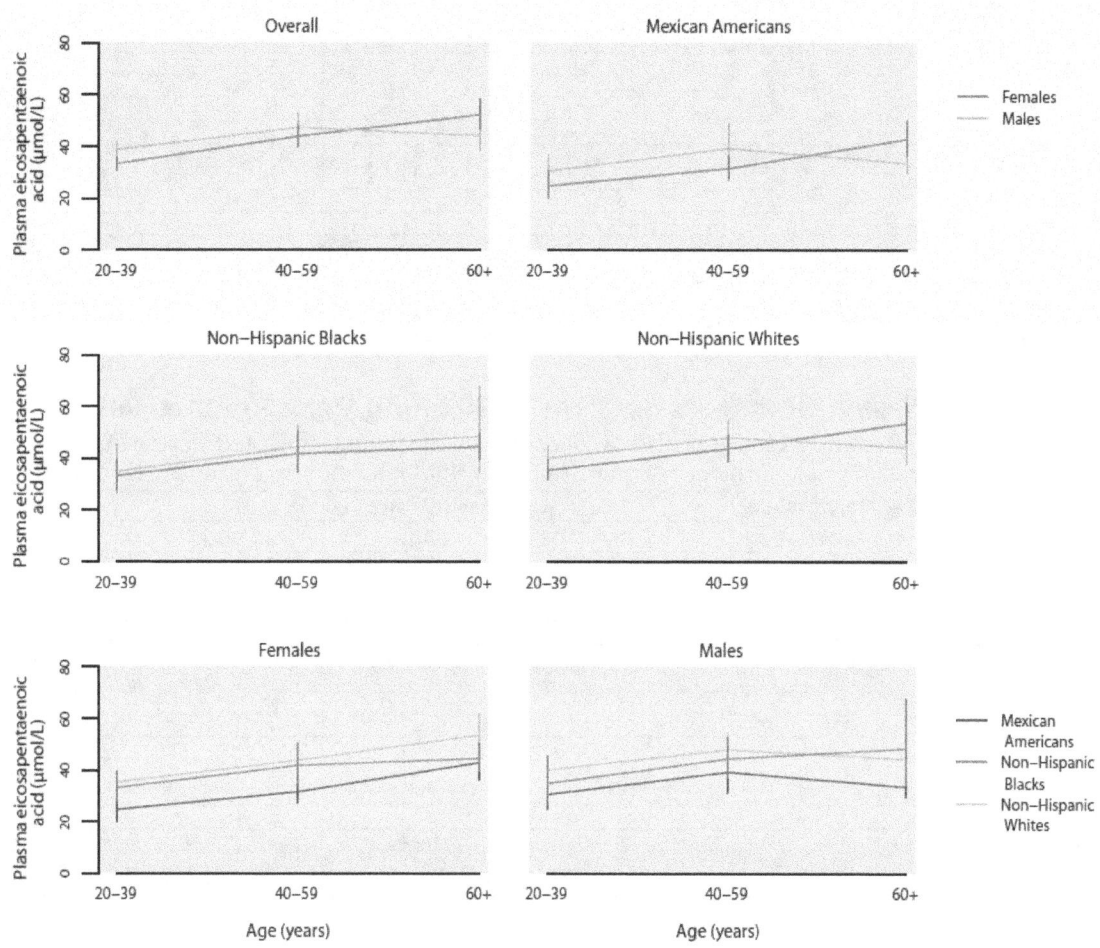

Table 2.33.a.2. Plasma eicosapentaenoic acid (20:5n-3): Total population

Geometric mean and selected percentiles of plasma concentrations (in µmol/L) for the fasted U.S. population aged 20 years and older, National Health and Nutrition Examination Survey, 2003–2004.

	Geometric mean (95% conf. interval)	Selected percentiles (95% conf. interval) 10th		50th		90th		Sample size
Males and Females								
Total, 20 years and older	42.1 (39.5 – 45.0)	20.8	(18.9 – 22.2)	40.9	(37.6 – 43.8)	89.9	(80.0 – 99.9)	1,806
20–39 years	35.9 (33.8 – 38.1)	18.2	(16.7 – 20.2)	34.2	(32.0 – 36.2)	74.5	(64.8 – 94.2)	609
40–59 years	45.5 (41.8 – 49.5)	22.8	(19.4 – 26.2)	45.0	(41.0 – 48.3)	92.8	(81.5 – 103)	515
60 years and older	48.5 (43.3 – 54.4)	24.4	(15.6 – 29.1)	49.4	(43.5 – 53.8)	100	(90.6 – 116)	682
Males								
Total, 20 years and older	43.1 (39.8 – 46.6)	21.0	(18.5 – 23.0)	41.4	(37.6 – 45.1)	92.8	(81.4 – 104)	863
20–39 years	38.7 (35.6 – 42.0)	18.7	(16.8 – 20.6)	36.1	(34.3 – 40.5)	86.1	(70.8 – 108)	281
40–59 years	47.3 (42.5 – 52.7)	23.4	(20.8 – 26.6)	45.7	(40.0 – 48.9)	97.4	(82.2 – 136)	248
60 years and older	44.2 (38.7 – 50.5)	22.1	(10.4 – 27.5)	44.6	(38.7 – 51.3)	88.7	(74.8 – 109)	334
Females								
Total, 20 years and older	41.3 (38.7 – 44.1)	20.4	(18.5 – 22.2)	40.1	(37.5 – 43.1)	86.3	(76.6 – 101)	943
20–39 years	33.3 (30.9 – 36.0)	17.4	(15.8 – 19.8)	31.4	(30.1 – 34.1)	64.6	(56.5 – 80.8)	328
40–59 years	43.9 (40.1 – 48.1)	21.9	(17.2 – 27.5)	43.4	(40.3 – 47.8)	84.6	(76.6 – 100)	267
60 years and older	52.4 (47.2 – 58.1)	25.2	(21.5 – 29.7)	51.7	(49.2 – 57.1)	105	(94.5 – 134)	348

Table 2.33.a.3. Plasma eicosapentaenoic acid (20:5n-3): Mexican Americans

Geometric mean and selected percentiles of plasma concentrations (in µmol/L) for fasted Mexican Americans in the U.S. population aged 20 years and older, National Health and Nutrition Examination Survey, 2003–2004.

	Geometric mean (95% conf. interval)	Selected percentiles (95% conf. interval) 10th		50th		90th		Sample size
Males and Females								
Total, 20 years and older	31.0 (28.7 – 33.5)	15.8	(11.1 – 18.4)	31.4	(28.4 – 35.4)	63.8	(58.1 – 70.0)	375
20–39 years	28.0 (24.9 – 31.4)	15.4	(8.96 – 18.3)	28.3	(21.7 – 35.1)	59.1	(50.9 – 68.1)	132
40–59 years	35.5 (30.7 – 41.0)	17.0†	(12.2 – 19.0)	35.9	(31.0 – 40.8)	76.2†	(56.8 – 91.5)	93
60 years and older	38.2 (35.8 – 40.7)	17.9	(12.9 – 21.6)	40.5	(34.3 – 43.5)	72.9	(61.1 – 95.6)	150
Males								
Total, 20 years and older	33.1 (29.9 – 36.8)	16.4	(15.5 – 18.4)	34.3	(29.0 – 37.9)	68.9	(60.4 – 77.9)	188
20–39 years	30.6 (25.4 – 36.8)	16.1†	(9.95 – 18.9)	29.4	(22.2 – 40.7)	63.9†	(50.2 – 78.0)	67
40–59 years	39.3 (31.6 – 48.8)	16.2†	(11.8 – 22.3)	37.6	(30.0 – 51.3)	82.2†	(66.1 – 180)	48
60 years and older	33.6 (29.9 – 37.8)	16.0†	(12.8 – 18.3)	34.4	(24.2 – 43.5)	56.5†	(48.9 – 161)	73
Females								
Total, 20 years and older	28.6 (24.9 – 32.8)	13.8	(7.13 – 18.3)	29.1	(23.4 – 35.1)	60.2	(49.1 – 76.5)	187
20–39 years	24.8 (20.1 – 30.7)	10.8†	(6.03 – 18.2)	23.5	(19.9 – 31.6)	53.1†	(39.3 – 90.1)	65
40–59 years	31.6 (27.4 – 36.4)	17.1†	(8.81 – 19.8)	31.3	(26.8 – 37.9)	55.9†	(46.3 – 84.0)	45
60 years and older	42.9 (36.7 – 50.1)	22.2†	(8.91 – 26.3)	43.3	(38.1 – 49.3)	85.0†	(63.7 – 147)	77

† Estimate is subject to greater uncertainty due to small cell size.

Table 2.33.a.4. Plasma eicosapentaenoic acid (20:5n-3): Non-Hispanic blacks

Geometric mean and selected percentiles of plasma concentrations (in μmol/L) for fasted non-Hispanic blacks in the U.S. population aged 20 years and older, National Health and Nutrition Examination Survey, 2003–2004.

	Geometric mean (95% conf. interval)		Selected percentiles (95% conf. interval)						Sample size
			10th		50th		90th		
Males and Females									
Total, 20 years and older	38.8	(34.7 – 43.4)	19.9	(17.5 – 21.2)	36.1	(33.0 – 41.6)	80.3	(64.8 – 121)	310
20–39 years	33.9	(28.3 – 40.8)	17.9	(15.0 – 20.1)	32.6	(25.1 – 40.6)	64.8	(53.4 – 253)	126
40–59 years	42.9	(37.2 – 49.6)	20.8†	(16.4 – 24.8)	39.9	(35.3 – 44.2)	96.3†	(72.1 – 147)	98
60 years and older	46.0	(39.2 – 53.9)	27.2†	(19.4 – 30.4)	44.5	(36.2 – 51.1)	88.6†	(64.3 – 209)	86
Males									
Total, 20 years and older	39.9	(34.4 – 46.2)	18.9	(15.3 – 22.2)	35.5	(32.4 – 41.6)	106	(70.6 – 134)	143
20–39 years	34.9	(26.9 – 45.3)	16.6†	(12.9 – 19.5)	33.3	(24.6 – 43.0)	64.8†	(51.9 – 150)	58
40–59 years	44.4	(37.5 – 52.5)	21.0†	(17.3 – 26.5)	36.0	(30.8 – 50.1)	117†	(79.5 – 206)	42
60 years and older	48.4	(34.5 – 67.7)	26.1†	(7.52 – 32.4)	44.4	(35.0 – 59.2)	102†	(61.1 – 209)	43
Females									
Total, 20 years and older	38.0	(34.0 – 42.4)	20.1	(18.5 – 21.4)	36.2	(30.4 – 43.9)	71.2	(61.3 – 105)	167
20–39 years	33.2	(27.9 – 39.5)	18.6†	(13.2 – 20.4)	29.7	(25.6 – 35.7)	64.3†	(44.7 – 253)	68
40–59 years	41.8	(34.9 – 50.2)	19.8†	(12.6 – 25.5)	41.3	(35.8 – 46.4)	71.2†	(64.0 – 193)	56
60 years and older	44.5	(39.7 – 50.0)	25.5†	(20.0 – 30.5)	44.1	(35.2 – 51.1)	75.9†	(62.8 – 104)	43

† Estimate is subject to greater uncertainty due to small cell size.

Table 2.33.a.5. Plasma eicosapentaenoic acid (20:5n-3): Non-Hispanic whites

Geometric mean and selected percentiles of plasma concentrations (in μmol/L) for fasted non-Hispanic whites in the U.S. population aged 20 years and older, National Health and Nutrition Examination Survey, 2003–2004.

	Geometric mean (95% conf. interval)		Selected percentiles (95% conf. interval)						Sample size
			10th		50th		90th		
Males and Females									
Total, 20 years and older	43.5	(39.8 – 47.7)	21.9	(18.6 – 24.7)	42.6	(38.1 – 46.0)	90.5	(78.4 – 102)	991
20–39 years	37.5	(34.3 – 41.0)	20.4	(16.3 – 21.9)	35.3	(32.0 – 38.3)	74.7	(63.8 – 110)	299
40–59 years	45.8	(41.5 – 50.6)	23.9	(18.8 – 27.7)	45.2	(40.5 – 48.7)	89.0	(78.7 – 101)	280
60 years and older	49.0	(42.5 – 56.5)	23.5	(11.7 – 29.6)	49.9	(44.2 – 54.8)	101	(91.7 – 117)	412
Males									
Total, 20 years and older	44.3	(40.1 – 48.9)	21.9	(17.3 – 25.8)	43.1	(37.6 – 47.6)	89.8	(78.2 – 105)	471
20–39 years	40.1	(35.9 – 44.7)	20.6	(16.9 – 22.7)	37.8	(34.8 – 42.9)	89.0	(67.8 – 119)	127
40–59 years	48.0	(42.2 – 54.6)	25.1	(20.7 – 27.5)	47.3	(40.0 – 50.2)	92.4	(80.9 – 140)	140
60 years and older	44.3	(38.0 – 51.6)	21.8	(10.3 – 28.6)	44.8	(37.6 – 52.3)	87.2	(75.6 – 105)	204
Females									
Total, 20 years and older	42.9	(39.0 – 47.2)	21.8	(18.3 – 24.6)	42.0	(37.9 – 45.6)	91.3	(76.7 – 104)	520
20–39 years	35.4	(31.7 – 39.4)	18.2	(15.8 – 21.9)	31.9	(30.2 – 37.0)	68.2	(54.3 – 112)	172
40–59 years	43.8	(39.1 – 48.9)	22.3	(12.3 – 30.0)	43.3	(37.8 – 48.4)	81.0	(74.2 – 100)	140
60 years and older	53.5	(46.4 – 61.6)	24.6	(18.7 – 30.9)	53.5	(49.3 – 59.7)	110	(96.5 – 138)	208

Table 2.34.a.1. Plasma docosatetraenoic acid (22:4n-6): Concentrations

Geometric mean and selected percentiles of plasma concentrations (in µmol/L) for the fasted U.S. population aged 20 years and older, National Health and Nutrition Examination Survey, 2003–2004.

| | Geometric mean | | Selected percentiles (95% conf. interval) | | | | | | | | | | Sample |
	(95% conf. interval)		2.5th		5th		50th		95th		97.5th		size
Total, 20 years and older	25.0	(24.4 – 25.6)	12.1	(10.4 – 13.1)	14.4	(13.3 – 14.9)	24.7	(24.1 – 25.6)	43.0	(41.6 – 44.7)	47.7	(45.4 – 53.5)	1,808
Age group													
20–39 years	24.4	(23.4 – 25.4)	12.2	(10.4 – 13.8)	14.3	(13.1 – 15.0)	23.9	(23.1 – 24.9)	41.1	(38.8 – 46.0)	47.1	(42.8 – 58.0)	610
40–59 years	25.5	(24.5 – 26.4)	11.2	(9.62 – 12.9)	14.3	(12.0 – 15.4)	25.0	(24.3 – 26.6)	44.5	(42.1 – 46.2)	50.0	(45.0 – 63.4)	515
60 years and older	25.3	(24.6 – 26.0)	12.6	(9.34 – 14.4)	14.8	(12.9 – 15.8)	25.7	(24.5 – 26.6)	42.2	(39.6 – 45.3)	47.1	(44.7 – 49.5)	683
Gender													
Males	25.3	(24.4 – 26.2)	11.8	(9.72 – 13.1)	14.5	(13.5 – 14.9)	25.0	(24.3 – 26.1)	42.4	(41.0 – 44.9)	46.8	(44.6 – 58.2)	865
Females	24.7	(24.0 – 25.5)	12.2	(9.93 – 13.9)	14.3	(13.0 – 15.1)	24.5	(23.6 – 25.6)	43.7	(41.4 – 45.9)	48.0	(44.8 – 56.3)	943
Race/ethnicity													
Mexican Americans	27.5	(25.6 – 29.5)	13.1†	(11.2 – 15.6)	15.8	(12.9 – 16.6)	27.4	(25.1 – 29.6)	47.3	(45.9 – 53.3)	58.5†	(48.0 – 66.9)	376
Non-Hispanic Blacks	26.0	(25.1 – 26.8)	13.4†	(9.11 – 15.0)	15.0	(13.2 – 16.7)	25.8	(24.3 – 26.8)	45.0	(42.0 – 46.7)	50.4†	(46.1 – 72.9)	310
Non-Hispanic Whites	24.8	(23.9 – 25.6)	12.1	(10.0 – 13.5)	14.5	(13.0 – 15.1)	24.6	(23.9 – 25.6)	41.9	(39.6 – 44.7)	47.2	(44.5 – 56.1)	992

† Estimate is subject to greater uncertainty due to small cell size.

Figure 2.34.a. Plasma docosatetraenoic acid (22:4n–6): Concentrations by age group

Geometric mean (95% confidence interval), National Health and Nutrition Examination Survey, 2003–2004

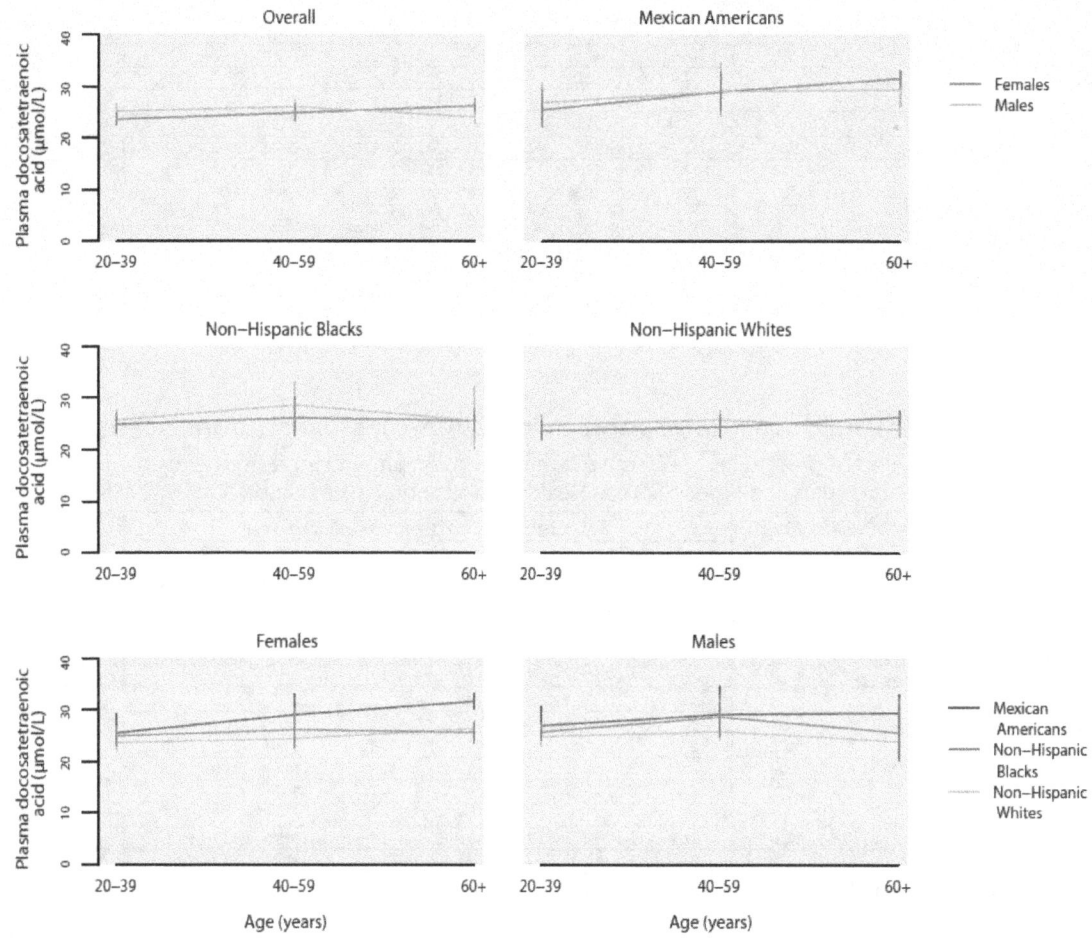

Table 2.34.a.2. Plasma docosatetraenoic acid (22:4n-6): Total population

Geometric mean and selected percentiles of plasma concentrations (in µmol/L) for the fasted U.S. population aged 20 years and older, National Health and Nutrition Examination Survey, 2003–2004.

	Geometric mean (95% conf. interval)	Selected percentiles (95% conf. interval)						Sample size
		10th		50th		90th		
Males and Females								
Total, 20 years and older	25.0 (24.4 – 25.6)	16.8	(15.7 – 17.4)	24.7	(24.1 – 25.6)	37.7	(36.7 – 39.4)	1,808
20–39 years	24.4 (23.4 – 25.4)	16.7	(15.0 – 17.5)	23.9	(23.1 – 24.9)	37.1	(34.7 – 39.1)	610
40–59 years	25.5 (24.5 – 26.4)	17.0	(14.8 – 18.0)	25.0	(24.3 – 26.6)	39.4	(37.4 – 41.6)	515
60 years and older	25.3 (24.6 – 26.0)	16.7	(16.0 – 17.5)	25.7	(24.5 – 26.6)	37.0	(36.3 – 38.3)	683
Males								
Total, 20 years and older	25.3 (24.4 – 26.2)	16.9	(15.8 – 18.0)	25.0	(24.3 – 26.1)	38.2	(36.5 – 40.0)	865
20–39 years	25.2 (23.8 – 26.6)	17.1	(14.8 – 18.7)	24.5	(23.6 – 26.1)	38.3	(35.5 – 40.8)	282
40–59 years	26.1 (24.9 – 27.3)	17.3	(14.7 – 19.5)	25.9	(24.5 – 27.9)	39.8	(36.8 – 43.7)	248
60 years and older	24.1 (22.9 – 25.3)	16.0	(14.8 – 16.8)	24.3	(22.5 – 26.5)	35.9	(34.2 – 37.6)	335
Females								
Total, 20 years and older	24.7 (24.0 – 25.5)	16.5	(15.4 – 17.4)	24.5	(23.6 – 25.6)	37.5	(36.0 – 40.6)	943
20–39 years	23.6 (22.5 – 24.8)	15.8	(14.4 – 17.1)	23.1	(21.3 – 24.7)	35.9	(32.7 – 38.8)	328
40–59 years	24.9 (23.4 – 26.5)	15.6	(14.5 – 17.5)	24.6	(23.4 – 26.4)	38.3	(35.3 – 43.3)	267
60 years and older	26.3 (25.1 – 27.6)	17.6	(16.4 – 18.5)	26.2	(24.9 – 27.8)	38.3	(36.3 – 43.9)	348

Table 2.34.a.3. Plasma docosatetraenoic acid (22:4n-6): Mexican Americans

Geometric mean and selected percentiles of plasma concentrations (in µmol/L) for fasted Mexican Americans in the U.S. population aged 20 years and older, National Health and Nutrition Examination Survey, 2003–2004.

	Geometric mean (95% conf. interval)	Selected percentiles (95% conf. interval)						Sample size
		10th		50th		90th		
Males and Females								
Total, 20 years and older	27.5 (25.6 – 29.5)	17.9	(15.5 – 19.6)	27.4	(25.1 – 29.6)	43.1	(40.6 – 46.6)	376
20–39 years	26.3 (24.0 – 28.8)	16.4	(12.1 – 19.5)	26.1	(21.9 – 29.9)	41.1	(36.6 – 47.8)	132
40–59 years	29.1 (26.8 – 31.6)	18.2†	(13.2 – 20.2)	28.4	(26.2 – 31.2)	45.6†	(42.2 – 59.9)	93
60 years and older	30.5 (29.3 – 31.8)	20.6	(17.6 – 22.4)	30.2	(28.3 – 32.1)	43.6	(40.4 – 48.5)	151
Males								
Total, 20 years and older	27.7 (25.0 – 30.8)	18.4	(13.6 – 20.3)	27.3	(24.4 – 31.1)	41.5	(39.1 – 48.7)	189
20–39 years	26.9 (23.6 – 30.6)	18.5†	(12.6 – 20.7)	26.2	(22.5 – 29.9)	40.4†	(36.1 – 58.6)	67
40–59 years	29.1 (24.5 – 34.6)	17.9†	(13.8 – 21.3)	28.3	(25.3 – 33.8)	44.6†	(37.0 – 63.5)	48
60 years and older	29.4 (26.2 – 32.9)	18.8†	(17.0 – 21.2)	28.5	(24.6 – 34.1)	45.0†	(37.4 – 67.2)	74
Females								
Total, 20 years and older	27.2 (24.6 – 30.1)	16.9	(11.4 – 19.7)	27.6	(23.8 – 30.3)	43.5	(40.3 – 50.5)	187
20–39 years	25.5 (22.2 – 29.2)	15.6†	(11.2 – 18.0)	25.1	(20.0 – 32.3)	42.9†	(34.4 – 58.4)	65
40–59 years	29.0 (25.6 – 32.9)	18.5†	(13.2 – 21.6)	27.2	(23.7 – 31.6)	45.8†	(42.0 – 61.3)	45
60 years and older	31.6 (30.2 – 33.1)	20.8†	(17.8 – 25.8)	31.1	(29.8 – 33.2)	41.7†	(36.9 – 66.9)	77

† Estimate is subject to greater uncertainty due to small cell size.

Table 2.34.a.4. Plasma docosatetraenoic acid (22:4n-6): Non-Hispanic blacks

Geometric mean and selected percentiles of plasma concentrations (in µmol/L) for fasted non-Hispanic blacks in the U.S. population aged 20 years and older, National Health and Nutrition Examination Survey, 2003–2004.

	Geometric mean (95% conf. interval)		Selected percentiles (95% conf. interval)						Sample size
			10th		50th		90th		
Males and Females									
Total, 20 years and older	26.0	(25.1 – 26.8)	17.4	(15.5 – 18.7)	25.8	(24.3 – 26.8)	38.6	(37.0 – 41.1)	310
20–39 years	25.3	(24.1 – 26.4)	17.5	(14.8 – 18.9)	24.0	(22.6 – 26.3)	37.8	(34.6 – 44.2)	126
40–59 years	27.2	(25.0 – 29.5)	17.4†	(14.3 – 19.8)	26.7	(24.7 – 28.2)	41.1†	(38.8 – 46.3)	98
60 years and older	25.6	(22.9 – 28.6)	16.8†	(9.11 – 20.5)	25.8	(24.0 – 29.4)	35.7†	(33.3 – 40.3)	86
Males									
Total, 20 years and older	26.7	(24.6 – 28.9)	17.5	(13.0 – 19.5)	25.8	(23.0 – 29.1)	41.6	(38.0 – 46.0)	143
20–39 years	25.7	(24.1 – 27.5)	17.5†	(11.3 – 19.7)	23.8	(21.7 – 27.5)	39.9†	(34.0 – 75.9)	58
40–59 years	28.6	(24.8 – 33.0)	18.0†	(12.7 – 20.7)	26.9	(23.7 – 30.4)	41.9†	(36.6 – 96.8)	42
60 years and older	25.6	(20.3 – 32.3)	15.3†	(9.11 – 23.9)	26.0	(24.1 – 31.6)	37.0†	(32.0 – 47.5)	43
Females									
Total, 20 years and older	25.4	(24.0 – 27.0)	17.3	(15.1 – 18.7)	25.6	(23.6 – 27.2)	36.4	(34.4 – 40.4)	167
20–39 years	24.9	(23.1 – 26.8)	17.5†	(13.4 – 19.2)	24.5	(22.3 – 27.7)	35.9†	(30.8 – 46.3)	68
40–59 years	26.1	(22.7 – 30.1)	15.6†	(13.4 – 20.0)	26.6	(22.7 – 27.9)	39.1†	(31.1 – 118)	56
60 years and older	25.6	(23.6 – 27.6)	17.5†	(13.4 – 21.3)	25.1	(23.5 – 27.4)	35.5†	(32.5 – 36.6)	43

† Estimate is subject to greater uncertainty due to small cell size.

Table 2.34.a.5. Plasma docosatetraenoic acid (22:4n-6): Non-Hispanic whites

Geometric mean and selected percentiles of plasma concentrations (in µmol/L) for fasted non-Hispanic whites in the U.S. population aged 20 years and older, National Health and Nutrition Examination Survey, 2003–2004.

	Geometric mean (95% conf. interval)		Selected percentiles (95% conf. interval)						Sample size
			10th		50th		90th		
Males and Females									
Total, 20 years and older	24.8	(23.9 – 25.6)	16.8	(15.6 – 17.5)	24.6	(23.9 – 25.6)	36.8	(35.3 – 37.9)	992
20–39 years	24.1	(22.8 – 25.6)	16.4	(14.6 – 17.6)	23.8	(22.9 – 24.9)	35.5	(32.1 – 39.6)	300
40–59 years	25.0	(23.5 – 26.6)	17.2	(14.5 – 18.6)	24.7	(23.6 – 26.5)	36.8	(34.8 – 41.3)	280
60 years and older	25.2	(24.3 – 26.0)	16.6	(15.6 – 17.4)	25.6	(24.1 – 27.0)	36.9	(36.3 – 38.2)	412
Males									
Total, 20 years and older	24.9	(23.8 – 26.1)	16.9	(15.0 – 18.1)	24.7	(24.0 – 26.1)	36.7	(35.1 – 38.3)	472
20–39 years	24.8	(22.9 – 26.7)	17.0	(12.5 – 18.9)	24.3	(23.3 – 26.1)	36.3	(33.0 – 39.7)	128
40–59 years	25.8	(24.1 – 27.5)	17.8	(10.9 – 19.8)	25.2	(24.4 – 27.9)	36.9	(35.2 – 44.0)	140
60 years and older	23.9	(22.5 – 25.4)	15.9	(14.5 – 16.8)	24.1	(22.1 – 26.6)	34.9	(33.5 – 37.2)	204
Females									
Total, 20 years and older	24.6	(23.7 – 25.6)	16.6	(15.4 – 17.4)	24.4	(23.5 – 25.6)	36.9	(34.4 – 41.0)	520
20–39 years	23.6	(21.9 – 25.4)	15.8	(14.3 – 17.2)	23.0	(21.0 – 25.1)	34.6	(31.9 – 45.6)	172
40–59 years	24.4	(22.4 – 26.6)	15.9	(13.7 – 18.0)	24.3	(22.5 – 25.9)	35.5	(32.9 – 44.5)	140
60 years and older	26.3	(25.0 – 27.6)	17.3	(16.5 – 18.0)	26.2	(24.7 – 28.1)	38.7	(36.3 – 44.4)	208

Table 2.35.a.1. Plasma docosapentaenoic-3 acid (22:5n-3): Concentrations

Geometric mean and selected percentiles of plasma concentrations (in μmol/L) for the fasted U.S. population aged 20 years and older, National Health and Nutrition Examination Survey, 2003–2004.

	Geometric mean (95% conf. interval)	Selected percentiles (95% conf. interval)					Sample size
		2.5th	5th	50th	95th	97.5th	
Total, 20 years and older	41.6 (40.2 – 43.1)	22.1 (17.2 – 23.8)	24.5 (22.8 – 25.8)	41.4 (40.0 – 42.8)	72.7 (69.7 – 76.7)	82.9 (78.5 – 92.2)	1,808
Age group							
20–39 years	38.1 (37.1 – 39.0)	20.0 (15.1 – 22.7)	23.2 (20.9 – 24.4)	38.0 (36.8 – 39.3)	63.0 (58.0 – 73.3)	73.0 (65.5 – 95.1)	610
40–59 years	43.1 (41.1 – 45.3)	22.2 (13.5 – 24.3)	24.9 (20.6 – 26.9)	43.2 (40.6 – 46.0)	77.0 (72.6 – 81.0)	84.9 (79.4 – 105)	515
60 years and older	45.5 (42.3 – 48.8)	24.5 (11.7 – 26.7)	26.5 (23.6 – 28.5)	45.7 (42.8 – 49.1)	74.0 (70.7 – 81.9)	82.0 (76.6 – 97.8)	683
Gender							
Males	42.8 (41.0 – 44.8)	24.2 (15.0 – 25.6)	26.2 (24.7 – 27.1)	42.5 (40.6 – 44.1)	72.7 (68.1 – 81.6)	87.2 (78.7 – 97.2)	865
Females	40.5 (39.1 – 42.0)	20.5 (13.6 – 22.8)	23.1 (20.7 – 24.5)	40.6 (38.8 – 42.0)	72.7 (67.8 – 78.6)	80.4 (75.5 – 89.8)	943
Race/ethnicity							
Mexican Americans	39.9 (37.2 – 42.9)	16.9† (12.1 – 22.3)	22.4 (14.1 – 25.0)	40.0 (36.4 – 44.1)	71.5 (67.8 – 79.3)	80.9† (72.5 – 112)	376
Non-Hispanic Blacks	38.9 (36.8 – 41.0)	20.1† (17.5 – 21.5)	22.3 (20.6 – 23.8)	38.1 (36.2 – 40.0)	64.5 (62.0 – 80.1)	85.0† (67.0 – 108)	310
Non-Hispanic Whites	42.1 (40.1 – 44.1)	22.8 (15.6 – 24.2)	24.7 (22.5 – 26.7)	42.2 (40.4 – 43.8)	71.7 (67.9 – 78.5)	81.2 (75.5 – 92.7)	992

† Estimate is subject to greater uncertainty due to small cell size.

Figure 2.35.a. Plasma docosapentaenoic–3 acid (22:5n–3): Concentrations by age group

Geometric mean (95% confidence interval), National Health and Nutrition Examination Survey, 2003–2004

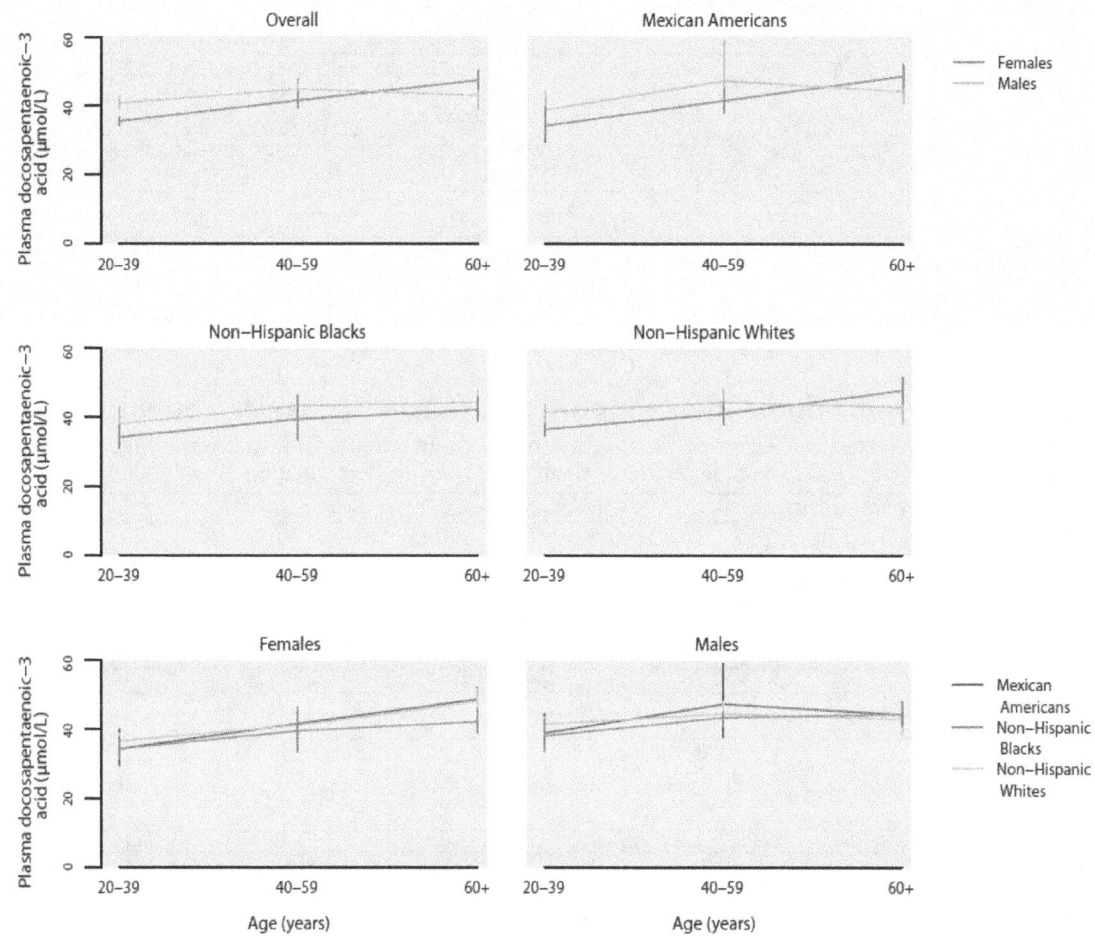

Table 2.35.a.2. Plasma docosapentaenoic-3 acid (22:5n-3): Total population

Geometric mean and selected percentiles of plasma concentrations (in µmol/L) for the fasted U.S. population aged 20 years and older, National Health and Nutrition Examination Survey, 2003–2004.

| | Geometric mean (95% conf. interval) | Selected percentiles (95% conf. interval) | | | Sample size |
		10th	50th	90th	
Males and Females					
Total, 20 years and older	41.6 (40.2 – 43.1)	27.4 (26.2 – 28.4)	41.4 (40.0 – 42.8)	62.3 (60.4 – 65.4)	1,808
20–39 years	38.1 (37.1 – 39.0)	26.1 (24.8 – 26.7)	38.0 (36.8 – 39.3)	54.8 (52.4 – 59.9)	610
40–59 years	43.1 (41.1 – 45.3)	27.6 (26.0 – 29.8)	43.2 (40.6 – 46.0)	65.2 (61.6 – 69.7)	515
60 years and older	45.5 (42.3 – 48.8)	29.6 (25.8 – 33.7)	45.7 (42.8 – 49.1)	67.6 (63.0 – 72.4)	683
Males					
Total, 20 years and older	42.8 (41.0 – 44.8)	28.8 (26.9 – 30.4)	42.5 (40.6 – 44.1)	63.7 (60.0 – 68.0)	865
20–39 years	40.8 (39.1 – 42.6)	27.3 (25.6 – 29.1)	40.5 (38.5 – 42.9)	59.1 (54.0 – 66.2)	282
40–59 years	44.9 (41.9 – 48.0)	30.2 (28.4 – 31.6)	44.2 (40.7 – 47.8)	68.0 (63.3 – 77.9)	248
60 years and older	43.1 (39.2 – 47.4)	28.7 (23.4 – 33.1)	42.9 (40.9 – 47.2)	60.3 (58.1 – 66.1)	335
Females					
Total, 20 years and older	40.5 (39.1 – 42.0)	26.2 (24.8 – 27.4)	40.6 (38.8 – 42.0)	61.4 (59.9 – 65.0)	943
20–39 years	35.6 (34.4 – 36.7)	23.9 (22.8 – 25.7)	35.8 (34.2 – 37.7)	50.4 (48.4 – 56.6)	328
40–59 years	41.6 (39.3 – 44.1)	26.1 (23.1 – 27.7)	41.9 (39.3 – 44.7)	61.2 (58.6 – 71.2)	267
60 years and older	47.5 (44.8 – 50.3)	30.0 (26.8 – 34.2)	48.0 (44.5 – 50.6)	70.1 (67.7 – 74.5)	348

Table 2.35.a.3. Plasma docosapentaenoic-3 acid (22:5n-3): Mexican Americans

Geometric mean and selected percentiles of plasma concentrations (in µmol/L) for fasted Mexican Americans in the U.S. population aged 20 years and older, National Health and Nutrition Examination Survey, 2003–2004.

| | Geometric mean (95% conf. interval) | Selected percentiles (95% conf. interval) | | | Sample size |
		10th	50th	90th	
Males and Females					
Total, 20 years and older	39.9 (37.2 – 42.9)	25.9 (20.2 – 29.5)	40.0 (36.4 – 44.1)	61.2 (57.8 – 67.9)	376
20–39 years	36.9 (33.4 – 40.7)	24.4 (15.2 – 27.2)	36.8 (34.2 – 39.9)	54.9 (50.1 – 75.1)	132
40–59 years	44.5 (39.4 – 50.3)	27.8† (25.5 – 30.9)	44.9 (39.4 – 48.2)	69.4† (58.3 – 127)	93
60 years and older	46.5 (45.2 – 47.9)	30.5 (25.7 – 35.6)	46.6 (44.5 – 50.8)	67.4 (57.5 – 80.9)	151
Males					
Total, 20 years and older	41.6 (37.6 – 46.0)	26.8 (22.1 – 30.9)	40.5 (36.3 – 46.4)	67.4 (59.1 – 74.5)	189
20–39 years	38.9 (34.0 – 44.4)	25.4† (15.2 – 30.7)	37.2 (35.5 – 40.8)	60.5† (52.3 – 73.1)	67
40–59 years	47.3 (37.9 – 59.0)	29.4† (26.2 – 31.9)	46.6 (33.3 – 60.1)	76.8† (55.8 – 127)	48
60 years and older	44.3 (40.8 – 48.0)	27.9† (20.5 – 32.2)	46.4 (40.6 – 50.0)	63.3† (55.2 – 83.1)	74
Females					
Total, 20 years and older	38.0 (34.6 – 41.6)	24.3 (13.1 – 29.6)	39.2 (34.1 – 44.9)	57.5 (52.2 – 60.8)	187
20–39 years	34.3 (29.6 – 39.9)	20.0† (12.1 – 28.3)	35.3 (30.6 – 41.1)	50.6† (47.1 – 85.4)	65
40–59 years	41.6 (38.4 – 45.0)	25.9† (17.2 – 32.5)	41.5 (36.9 – 47.2)	60.2† (55.9 – 74.8)	45
60 years and older	48.7 (45.6 – 52.0)	31.5† (27.6 – 39.2)	50.2 (44.4 – 52.9)	69.2† (57.4 – 90.2)	77

† Estimate is subject to greater uncertainty due to small cell size.

Table 2.35.a.4. Plasma docosapentaenoic-3 acid (22:5n-3): Non-Hispanic blacks

Geometric mean and selected percentiles of plasma concentrations (in µmol/L) for fasted non-Hispanic blacks in the U.S. population aged 20 years and older, National Health and Nutrition Examination Survey, 2003–2004.

	Geometric mean (95% conf. interval)		Selected percentiles (95% conf. interval)						Sample size
			10th		50th		90th		
Males and Females									
Total, 20 years and older	38.9	(36.8 – 41.0)	25.6	(24.6 – 26.5)	38.1	(36.2 – 40.0)	59.3	(55.1 – 62.4)	310
20–39 years	36.0	(32.7 – 39.5)	24.3	(21.5 – 25.8)	35.2	(32.0 – 38.1)	54.6	(48.6 – 63.5)	126
40–59 years	41.1	(37.4 – 45.2)	26.6†	(24.3 – 28.0)	40.0	(35.2 – 44.2)	60.3†	(57.2 – 84.5)	98
60 years and older	43.0	(40.4 – 45.8)	30.5†	(21.3 – 34.2)	43.0	(39.5 – 47.7)	60.6†	(54.6 – 63.6)	86
Males									
Total, 20 years and older	40.8	(38.5 – 43.2)	26.1	(24.7 – 29.2)	38.7	(37.7 – 41.4)	60.2	(58.8 – 69.2)	143
20–39 years	38.1	(33.8 – 43.0)	25.3†	(20.3 – 28.5)	37.7	(32.3 – 39.9)	59.8†	(44.2 – 131)	58
40–59 years	43.4	(41.7 – 45.1)	28.4†	(24.7 – 30.5)	40.3	(38.6 – 42.1)	68.5†	(57.2 – 108)	42
60 years and older	44.4	(41.1 – 48.0)	31.7†	(17.8 – 36.7)	44.9	(40.9 – 50.5)	60.5†	(58.2 – 64.6)	43
Females									
Total, 20 years and older	37.4	(35.0 – 40.1)	24.4	(22.4 – 26.2)	36.8	(34.3 – 40.1)	54.4	(51.8 – 62.5)	167
20–39 years	34.3	(31.2 – 37.7)	21.9†	(18.8 – 25.8)	33.5	(28.9 – 38.8)	53.0†	(45.4 – 64.5)	68
40–59 years	39.5	(33.5 – 46.5)	23.9†	(20.6 – 27.1)	39.3	(33.9 – 44.8)	58.0†	(48.6 – 148)	56
60 years and older	42.2	(39.0 – 45.7)	29.5†	(25.6 – 34.3)	41.7	(37.8 – 47.7)	56.6†	(52.5 – 70.1)	43

† Estimate is subject to greater uncertainty due to small cell size.

Table 2.35.a.5. Plasma docosapentaenoic-3 acid (22:5n-3): Non-Hispanic whites

Geometric mean and selected percentiles of plasma concentrations (in µmol/L) for fasted non-Hispanic whites in the U.S. population aged 20 years and older, National Health and Nutrition Examination Survey, 2003–2004.

	Geometric mean (95% conf. interval)		Selected percentiles (95% conf. interval)						Sample size
			10th		50th		90th		
Males and Females									
Total, 20 years and older	42.1	(40.1 – 44.1)	27.7	(26.1 – 29.0)	42.2	(40.4 – 43.8)	62.8	(60.0 – 67.4)	992
20–39 years	38.8	(37.5 – 40.2)	26.7	(24.8 – 28.1)	38.8	(36.8 – 41.0)	54.7	(52.1 – 61.5)	300
40–59 years	42.8	(40.1 – 45.7)	27.6	(24.8 – 30.1)	43.3	(39.7 – 47.0)	63.6	(60.8 – 68.0)	280
60 years and older	45.6	(41.8 – 49.8)	29.5	(25.0 – 33.7)	45.8	(42.5 – 50.1)	68.0	(64.1 – 73.0)	412
Males									
Total, 20 years and older	43.1	(40.7 – 45.6)	29.2	(26.9 – 31.2)	43.1	(40.6 – 45.3)	63.0	(59.6 – 66.9)	472
20–39 years	41.5	(39.4 – 43.6)	27.5	(26.4 – 29.3)	42.3	(39.1 – 44.4)	56.4	(53.0 – 72.1)	128
40–59 years	44.5	(41.1 – 48.2)	30.8	(27.1 – 32.2)	44.2	(39.7 – 48.3)	66.1	(61.6 – 75.0)	140
60 years and older	43.0	(38.4 – 48.1)	29.5	(14.9 – 33.9)	42.7	(39.7 – 47.5)	60.2	(57.3 – 70.0)	204
Females									
Total, 20 years and older	41.2	(39.3 – 43.1)	26.5	(24.5 – 28.2)	41.3	(38.8 – 43.0)	62.4	(59.2 – 71.1)	520
20–39 years	36.6	(34.7 – 38.6)	24.8	(22.8 – 28.3)	36.8	(34.2 – 38.5)	50.0	(46.5 – 61.2)	172
40–59 years	41.1	(38.0 – 44.6)	26.0	(22.3 – 27.7)	42.0	(38.8 – 46.6)	60.1	(57.1 – 73.0)	140
60 years and older	48.0	(44.4 – 51.8)	29.5	(24.8 – 34.5)	48.4	(44.1 – 52.6)	72.4	(68.4 – 75.1)	208

Table 2.36.a.1. Plasma docosapentaenoic-6 acid (22:5n-6): Concentrations

Geometric mean and selected percentiles of plasma concentrations (in µmol/L) for the fasted U.S. population aged 20 years and older, National Health and Nutrition Examination Survey, 2003–2004.

	Geometric mean	Selected percentiles (95% conf. interval)						Sample size
	(95% conf. interval)	2.5th	5th	50th	95th	97.5th		
Total, 20 years and older	19.6 (18.9 – 20.4)	8.56 (7.60 – 9.46)	9.80 (9.30 – 10.5)	19.3 (18.6 – 20.1)	39.0 (36.1 – 42.4)	46.5 (42.9 – 52.2)		1,808
Age group								
20-39 years	19.5 (18.6 – 20.5)	9.15 (8.17 – 9.51)	9.88 (9.25 – 11.1)	18.8 (17.9 – 20.0)	41.4 (35.5 – 46.3)	47.8 (45.1 – 54.4)		610
40-59 years	19.4 (18.4 – 20.4)	8.37 (4.40 – 9.67)	9.80 (7.79 – 11.1)	19.0 (18.3 – 20.5)	36.0 (34.5 – 39.1)	41.6 (37.2 – 50.8)		515
60 years and older	20.3 (19.5 – 21.2)	8.00 (5.88 – 8.84)	9.63 (8.26 – 10.8)	20.5 (19.5 – 21.5)	41.4 (37.9 – 48.4)	52.1 (46.8 – 58.0)		683
Gender								
Males	18.6 (17.7 – 19.7)	8.11 (6.96 – 9.23)	9.66 (8.83 – 10.4)	18.6 (17.8 – 19.3)	34.6 (32.2 – 40.5)	42.8 (38.6 – 45.2)		865
Females	20.6 (19.8 – 21.4)	8.92 (7.74 – 9.55)	9.95 (9.30 – 11.2)	20.5 (19.2 – 21.7)	41.9 (38.5 – 47.8)	50.6 (46.4 – 59.0)		943
Race/ethnicity								
Mexican Americans	23.5 (21.0 – 26.2)	10.4† (6.86 – 11.5)	11.6 (8.94 – 13.5)	22.8 (19.7 – 27.1)	47.6 (44.2 – 56.0)	53.6† (48.5 – 60.2)		376
Non-Hispanic Blacks	21.3 (20.3 – 22.4)	9.27† (5.89 – 10.3)	10.2 (9.35 – 11.6)	20.8 (19.7 – 22.4)	43.0 (40.4 – 50.4)	50.6† (45.0 – 63.2)		310
Non-Hispanic Whites	19.1 (18.3 – 19.9)	8.15 (7.49 – 9.20)	9.67 (8.52 – 10.6)	18.9 (18.3 – 19.8)	36.0 (34.0 – 40.9)	45.2 (40.7 – 51.4)		992

† Estimate is subject to greater uncertainty due to small cell size.

Figure 2.36.a. Plasma docosapentaenoic–6 acid (22:5n–6): Concentrations by age group

Geometric mean (95% confidence interval), National Health and Nutrition Examination Survey, 2003–2004

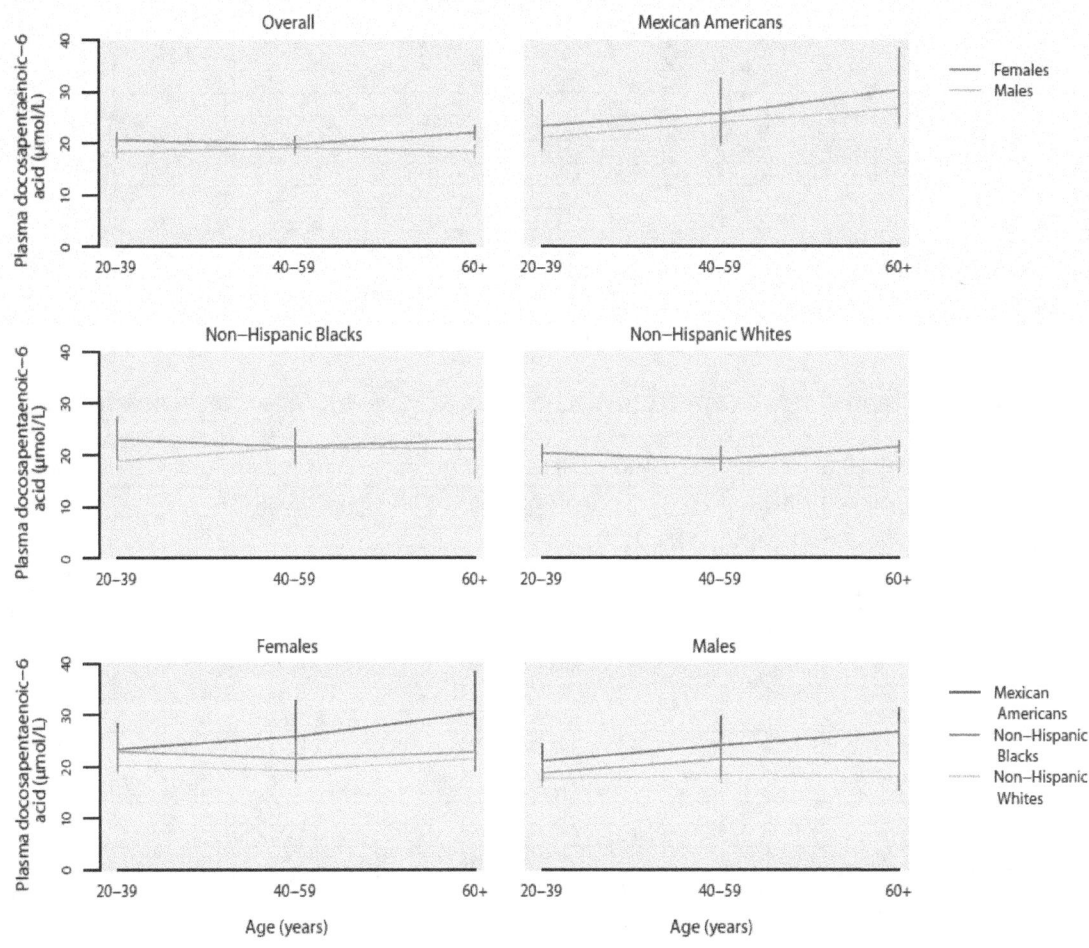

Table 2.36.a.2. Plasma docosapentaenoic-6 acid (22:5n-6): Total population

Geometric mean and selected percentiles of plasma concentrations (in μmol/L) for the fasted U.S. population aged 20 years and older, National Health and Nutrition Examination Survey, 2003–2004.

| | Geometric mean (95% conf. interval) | Selected percentiles (95% conf. interval) | | | Sample size |
		10th	50th	90th	
Males and Females					
Total, 20 years and older	19.6 (18.9 – 20.4)	11.8 (11.4 – 12.3)	19.3 (18.6 – 20.1)	32.5 (31.4 – 33.9)	1,808
20–39 years	19.5 (18.6 – 20.5)	11.8 (11.2 – 12.9)	18.8 (17.9 – 20.0)	32.4 (31.3 – 34.8)	610
40–59 years	19.4 (18.4 – 20.4)	11.5 (11.2 – 12.1)	19.0 (18.3 – 20.5)	31.8 (29.8 – 34.2)	515
60 years and older	20.3 (19.5 – 21.2)	12.2 (10.6 – 12.8)	20.5 (19.5 – 21.5)	33.2 (31.2 – 38.6)	683
Males					
Total, 20 years and older	18.6 (17.7 – 19.7)	11.7 (11.0 – 12.3)	18.6 (17.8 – 19.3)	29.8 (28.8 – 32.1)	865
20–39 years	18.4 (17.3 – 19.6)	12.1 (10.8 – 13.1)	18.0 (17.1 – 18.7)	29.6 (27.2 – 33.4)	282
40–59 years	19.0 (17.7 – 20.3)	11.8 (10.6 – 12.4)	19.0 (17.6 – 20.7)	29.4 (28.1 – 33.3)	248
60 years and older	18.4 (17.2 – 19.7)	10.4 (9.64 – 11.7)	18.7 (17.7 – 20.0)	31.2 (27.9 – 35.6)	335
Females					
Total, 20 years and older	20.6 (19.8 – 21.4)	12.0 (11.3 – 12.7)	20.5 (19.2 – 21.7)	34.5 (33.0 – 36.6)	943
20–39 years	20.6 (19.4 – 21.9)	11.6 (9.88 – 13.0)	20.5 (18.7 – 22.2)	35.0 (32.4 – 41.2)	328
40–59 years	19.8 (18.3 – 21.3)	11.3 (10.7 – 12.1)	19.1 (17.8 – 21.7)	34.3 (31.1 – 36.4)	267
60 years and older	22.0 (20.7 – 23.3)	13.7 (12.4 – 14.4)	22.0 (20.7 – 23.1)	35.5 (31.4 – 48.5)	348

Table 2.36.a.3. Plasma docosapentaenoic-6 acid (22:5n-6): Mexican Americans

Geometric mean and selected percentiles of plasma concentrations (in μmol/L) for fasted Mexican Americans in the U.S. population aged 20 years and older, National Health and Nutrition Examination Survey, 2003–2004.

| | Geometric mean (95% conf. interval) | Selected percentiles (95% conf. interval) | | | Sample size |
		10th	50th	90th	
Males and Females					
Total, 20 years and older	23.5 (21.0 – 26.2)	14.1 (11.5 – 15.0)	22.8 (19.7 – 27.1)	42.8 (38.9 – 46.1)	376
20–39 years	22.0 (19.6 – 24.8)	13.2 (9.09 – 14.9)	21.0 (18.0 – 25.7)	40.8 (33.5 – 45.8)	132
40–59 years	24.9 (21.6 – 28.7)	14.2† (8.50 – 16.5)	24.7 (20.6 – 29.6)	43.8† (38.4 – 52.6)	93
60 years and older	28.5 (24.4 – 33.3)	17.8 (15.1 – 19.7)	28.2 (23.4 – 33.9)	45.1 (36.8 – 71.9)	151
Males					
Total, 20 years and older	22.4 (19.8 – 25.4)	13.7 (10.4 – 15.7)	21.2 (19.1 – 26.0)	38.7 (34.0 – 44.6)	189
20–39 years	21.1 (18.5 – 24.1)	13.3† (9.51 – 15.4)	19.8 (17.6 – 23.2)	33.4† (29.0 – 51.2)	67
40–59 years	24.1 (19.7 – 29.6)	13.8† (6.48 – 17.7)	24.5 (18.1 – 33.3)	42.5† (31.7 – 52.7)	48
60 years and older	26.7 (22.9 – 31.2)	16.4† (12.7 – 19.2)	26.1 (20.7 – 33.2)	41.8† (35.3 – 56.1)	74
Females					
Total, 20 years and older	24.8 (21.5 – 28.7)	14.1 (9.21 – 15.0)	24.5 (20.1 – 31.4)	44.7 (41.4 – 53.8)	187
20–39 years	23.4 (19.3 – 28.2)	12.0† (8.52 – 14.8)	22.1 (15.0 – 32.1)	45.5† (35.2 – 104)	65
40–59 years	25.8 (20.4 – 32.6)	14.4† (10.5 – 16.8)	24.6 (18.0 – 35.8)	43.5† (37.4 – 70.9)	45
60 years and older	30.3 (23.9 – 38.3)	19.5† (14.3 – 21.0)	28.8 (22.4 – 41.5)	48.8† (37.9 – 71.9)	77

† Estimate is subject to greater uncertainty due to small cell size.

Table 2.36.a.4. Plasma docosapentaenoic-6 acid (22:5n-6): Non-Hispanic blacks

Geometric mean and selected percentiles of plasma concentrations (in µmol/L) for fasted non-Hispanic blacks in the U.S. population aged 20 years and older, National Health and Nutrition Examination Survey, 2003–2004.

	Geometric mean (95% conf. interval)		Selected percentiles (95% conf. interval)						Sample size
			10th		50th		90th		
Males and Females									
Total, 20 years and older	21.3	(20.3 – 22.4)	12.4	(10.4 – 13.5)	20.8	(19.7 – 22.4)	35.3	(33.3 – 41.5)	310
20–39 years	21.0	(19.2 – 22.8)	12.8	(11.7 – 13.4)	19.9	(18.3 – 23.5)	34.8	(31.5 – 50.8)	126
40–59 years	21.5	(19.4 – 23.7)	12.1†	(9.42 – 13.5)	21.7	(19.7 – 22.6)	34.9†	(30.5 – 44.0)	98
60 years and older	22.1	(18.4 – 26.6)	12.8†	(5.89 – 14.9)	22.9	(17.6 – 28.4)	37.7†	(32.6 – 45.7)	86
Males									
Total, 20 years and older	20.0	(18.1 – 22.2)	11.7	(9.26 – 13.2)	19.8	(18.3 – 21.6)	34.8	(30.9 – 43.6)	143
20–39 years	18.8	(17.2 – 20.6)	11.4†	(5.94 – 13.4)	18.9	(15.9 – 19.9)	32.8†	(27.6 – 47.8)	58
40–59 years	21.4	(18.2 – 25.1)	12.2†	(9.72 – 13.8)	21.7	(18.1 – 23.2)	32.9†	(27.0 – 89.5)	42
60 years and older	21.1	(15.6 – 28.7)	9.26†	(5.89 – 15.5)	21.5	(16.0 – 31.7)	39.9†	(32.2 – 50.3)	43
Females									
Total, 20 years and older	22.4	(20.3 – 24.7)	13.0	(10.3 – 14.6)	22.0	(19.5 – 25.3)	35.3	(33.0 – 45.2)	167
20–39 years	22.9	(19.3 – 27.2)	14.0†	(9.93 – 16.1)	22.2	(18.4 – 27.0)	35.3†	(31.8 – 100)	68
40–59 years	21.6	(18.7 – 24.9)	11.1†	(8.75 – 13.5)	21.3	(18.9 – 26.4)	35.1†	(28.2 – 99.4)	56
60 years and older	22.8	(19.3 – 26.9)	13.0†	(7.21 – 15.0)	23.2	(17.4 – 29.7)	33.7†	(32.4 – 47.7)	43

† Estimate is subject to greater uncertainty due to small cell size.

Table 2.36.a.5. Plasma docosapentaenoic-6 acid (22:5n-6): Non-Hispanic whites

Geometric mean and selected percentiles of plasma concentrations (in µmol/L) for fasted non-Hispanic whites in the U.S. population aged 20 years and older, National Health and Nutrition Examination Survey, 2003–2004.

	Geometric mean (95% conf. interval)		Selected percentiles (95% conf. interval)						Sample size
			10th		50th		90th		
Males and Females									
Total, 20 years and older	19.1	(18.3 – 19.9)	11.7	(11.0 – 12.3)	18.9	(18.3 – 19.8)	31.1	(29.4 – 32.6)	992
20–39 years	19.0	(17.9 – 20.2)	11.6	(9.68 – 12.9)	18.5	(17.3 – 20.3)	31.3	(29.1 – 33.0)	300
40–59 years	18.7	(17.3 – 20.3)	11.4	(10.1 – 12.6)	18.6	(17.6 – 19.6)	29.6	(27.6 – 33.3)	280
60 years and older	19.9	(19.2 – 20.6)	11.9	(10.4 – 12.8)	20.1	(19.3 – 21.3)	31.9	(30.5 – 35.2)	412
Males									
Total, 20 years and older	18.0	(17.0 – 19.1)	11.4	(10.1 – 12.3)	18.3	(17.6 – 19.0)	28.3	(26.7 – 30.8)	472
20–39 years	17.7	(16.3 – 19.2)	11.5	(8.97 – 13.1)	17.5	(16.8 – 18.5)	27.4	(22.5 – 39.7)	128
40–59 years	18.3	(16.9 – 19.8)	11.6	(8.23 – 13.7)	18.8	(16.9 – 20.2)	28.7	(25.9 – 31.6)	140
60 years and older	18.1	(16.8 – 19.5)	10.4	(9.64 – 11.7)	18.6	(16.9 – 20.4)	29.9	(26.7 – 33.1)	204
Females									
Total, 20 years and older	20.2	(19.3 – 21.1)	12.1	(11.2 – 12.8)	20.2	(18.6 – 21.6)	32.9	(31.3 – 35.6)	520
20–39 years	20.3	(18.9 – 21.9)	11.5	(9.55 – 13.2)	20.5	(18.0 – 22.5)	32.6	(30.9 – 42.8)	172
40–59 years	19.2	(17.1 – 21.4)	11.4	(10.0 – 12.5)	18.4	(16.8 – 21.9)	32.3	(27.4 – 37.2)	140
60 years and older	21.5	(20.4 – 22.7)	13.5	(12.0 – 14.1)	21.6	(20.5 – 22.9)	33.6	(30.5 – 49.5)	208

Table 2.37.a.1. Plasma docosahexaenoic acid (22:6n-3): Concentrations

Geometric mean and selected percentiles of plasma concentrations (in μmol/L) for the fasted U.S. population aged 20 years and older, National Health and Nutrition Examination Survey, 2003–2004.

| | Geometric mean (95% conf. interval) | Selected percentiles (95% conf. interval) | | | | | Sample size |
		2.5th	5th	50th	95th	97.5th	
Total, 20 years and older	125 (118 – 133)	54.9 (52.4 – 57.8)	61.1 (56.2 – 65.2)	121 (114 – 128)	277 (248 – 310)	323 (302 – 372)	1,808
Age group							
20–39 years	115 (108 – 122)	54.3 (45.5 – 57.3)	58.1 (53.6 – 62.5)	111 (102 – 119)	254 (228 – 316)	316 (275 – 484)	610
40–59 years	125 (115 – 136)	54.1 (50.2 – 58.3)	60.6 (53.8 – 65.6)	121 (111 – 136)	272 (237 – 303)	305 (290 – 400)	515
60 years and older	145 (135 – 156)	64.5 (54.8 – 70.4)	73.5 (56.2 – 81.9)	142 (132 – 154)	305 (268 – 358)	373 (330 – 398)	683
Gender							
Males	117 (110 – 125)	53.9 (49.3 – 55.7)	57.9 (54.0 – 62.4)	114 (107 – 123)	253 (229 – 299)	303 (277 – 368)	865
Females	133 (125 – 141)	57.8 (48.3 – 63.0)	65.2 (56.1 – 72.0)	127 (121 – 135)	293 (258 – 323)	337 (315 – 385)	943
Race/ethnicity							
Mexican Americans	111 (105 – 119)	54.4† (46.4 – 58.0)	58.8 (55.2 – 60.2)	111 (99.8 – 123)	211 (191 – 251)	250† (218 – 342)	376
Non-Hispanic Blacks	140 (124 – 157)	64.9† (47.5 – 72.4)	72.5 (59.4 – 80.3)	133 (118 – 152)	304 (254 – 425)	348† (321 – 416)	310
Non-Hispanic Whites	122 (113 – 130)	54.7 (51.3 – 56.2)	59.5 (55.0 – 64.6)	117 (110 – 127)	259 (241 – 294)	315 (283 – 375)	992

† Estimate is subject to greater uncertainty due to small cell size.

Figure 2.37.a. Plasma docosahexaenoic acid (22:6n–3): Concentrations by age group

Geometric mean (95% confidence interval), National Health and Nutrition Examination Survey, 2003–2004

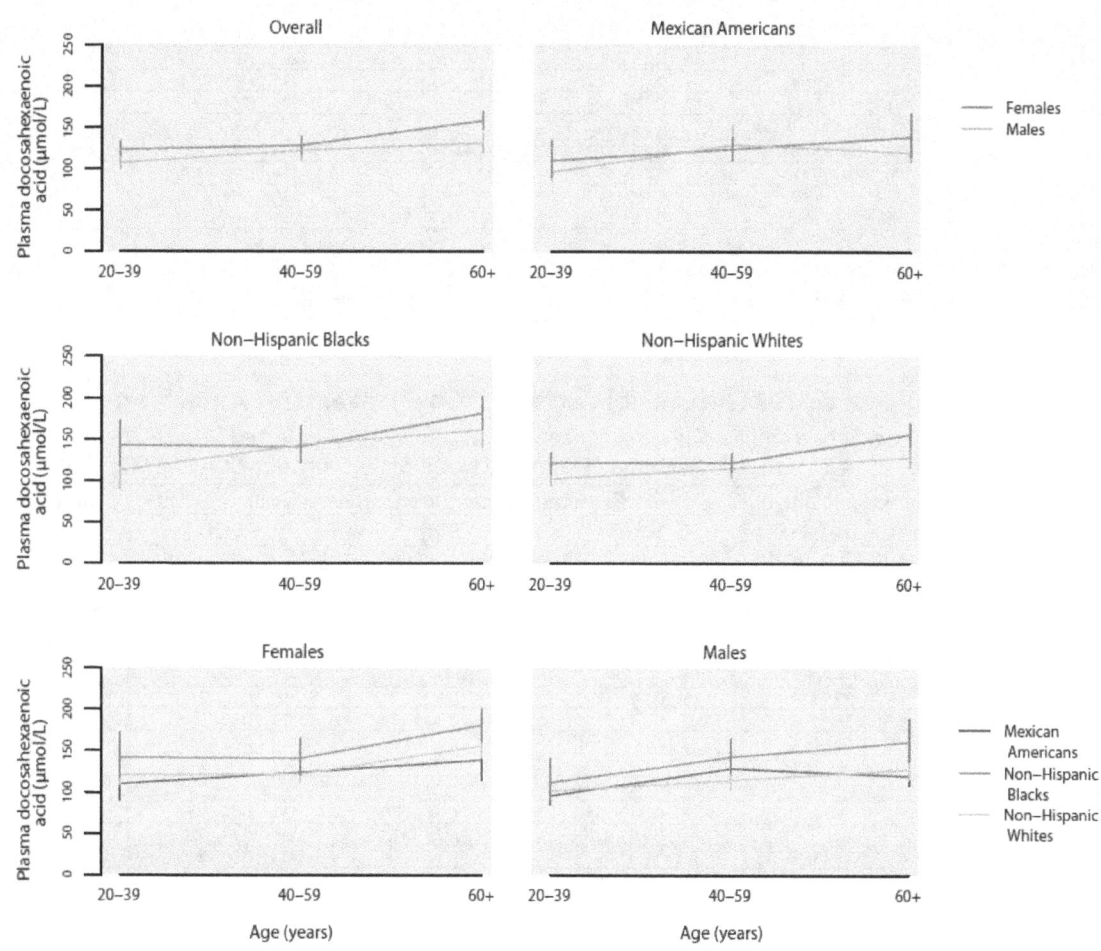

Table 2.37.a.2. Plasma docosahexaenoic acid (22:6n-3): Total population

Geometric mean and selected percentiles of plasma concentrations (in µmol/L) for the fasted U.S. population aged 20 years and older, National Health and Nutrition Examination Survey, 2003–2004.

	Geometric mean (95% conf. interval)	Selected percentiles (95% conf. interval)						Sample size
		10th		50th		90th		
Males and Females								
Total, 20 years and older	125	(118 – 133)	71.7	(67.1 – 74.9)	121	(114 – 128)	227	(208 – 244)	1,808
20–39 years	115	(108 – 122)	67.0	(62.3 – 71.6)	111	(102 – 119)	204	(187 – 234)	610
40–59 years	125	(115 – 136)	70.1	(62.3 – 77.7)	121	(111 – 136)	217	(201 – 244)	515
60 years and older	145	(135 – 156)	84.2	(73.5 – 94.3)	142	(132 – 154)	247	(234 – 268)	683
Males								
Total, 20 years and older	117	(110 – 125)	67.9	(62.5 – 71.7)	114	(107 – 123)	206	(189 – 235)	865
20–39 years	107	(99.5 – 115)	62.3	(57.6 – 68.1)	102	(93.2 – 113)	186	(170 – 209)	282
40–59 years	122	(110 – 135)	68.7	(61.4 – 74.4)	118	(106 – 135)	219	(189 – 296)	248
60 years and older	131	(119 – 143)	77.8	(53.6 – 92.8)	125	(117 – 142)	219	(194 – 256)	335
Females								
Total, 20 years and older	133	(125 – 141)	75.6	(68.7 – 80.0)	127	(121 – 135)	238	(223 – 256)	943
20–39 years	123	(115 – 133)	72.4	(61.8 – 78.6)	117	(110 – 127)	220	(194 – 283)	328
40–59 years	128	(117 – 138)	72.3	(59.3 – 79.4)	124	(112 – 143)	210	(201 – 256)	267
60 years and older	158	(148 – 169)	91.4	(82.5 – 99.1)	154	(144 – 168)	272	(249 – 307)	348

Table 2.37.a.3. Plasma docosahexaenoic acid (22:6n-3): Mexican Americans

Geometric mean and selected percentiles of plasma concentrations (in µmol/L) for fasted Mexican Americans in the U.S. population aged 20 years and older, National Health and Nutrition Examination Survey, 2003–2004.

	Geometric mean (95% conf. interval)	Selected percentiles (95% conf. interval)						Sample size
		10th		50th		90th		
Males and Females								
Total, 20 years and older	111	(105 – 119)	67.1	(57.8 – 73.0)	111	(99.8 – 123)	185	(165 – 199)	376
20–39 years	102	(91.1 – 114)	60.0	(55.3 – 67.6)	100	(80.6 – 122)	161	(150 – 204)	132
40–59 years	127	(117 – 137)	84.9†	(56.6 – 94.3)	125	(112 – 139)	189†	(163 – 266)	93
60 years and older	129	(118 – 142)	81.2	(61.1 – 92.2)	131	(114 – 144)	202	(185 – 246)	151
Males								
Total, 20 years and older	107	(99.7 – 114)	64.8	(55.1 – 69.2)	104	(95.3 – 124)	165	(158 – 188)	189
20–39 years	96.1	(85.8 – 108)	59.4†	(52.4 – 67.1)	99.4	(78.2 – 119)	147†	(136 – 158)	67
40–59 years	129	(110 – 152)	83.3†	(66.8 – 93.9)	127	(101 – 153)	194†	(155 – 355)	48
60 years and older	120	(109 – 132)	69.0†	(46.1 – 90.1)	121	(105 – 143)	190†	(159 – 272)	74
Females								
Total, 20 years and older	118	(105 – 131)	68.8	(52.3 – 83.3)	116	(102 – 133)	191	(166 – 250)	187
20–39 years	110	(90.5 – 134)	60.4†	(54.0 – 73.7)	109	(75.7 – 150)	191†	(158 – 325)	65
40–59 years	124	(111 – 139)	87.9†	(52.3 – 99.1)	119	(110 – 139)	173†	(150 – 268)	45
60 years and older	139	(115 – 168)	88.9†	(77.0 – 107)	133	(109 – 164)	229†	(183 – 334)	77

† Estimate is subject to greater uncertainty due to small cell size.

Table 2.37.a.4. Plasma docosahexaenoic acid (22:6n-3): Non-Hispanic blacks

Geometric mean and selected percentiles of plasma concentrations (in μmol/L) for fasted non-Hispanic blacks in the U.S. population aged 20 years and older, National Health and Nutrition Examination Survey, 2003–2004.

	Geometric mean (95% conf. interval)		Selected percentiles (95% conf. interval)						Sample size
			10th		50th		90th		
Males and Females									
Total, 20 years and older	140	(124 – 157)	83.4	(72.4 – 90.8)	133	(118 – 152)	251	(207 – 333)	310
20–39 years	128	(107 – 153)	77.2	(66.4 – 89.0)	119	(103 – 140)	237	(177 – 367)	126
40–59 years	142	(127 – 159)	84.1†	(69.9 – 95.8)	133	(119 – 157)	234†	(204 – 374)	98
60 years and older	173	(155 – 193)	117†	(56.2 – 135)	173	(149 – 197)	258†	(216 – 368)	86
Males									
Total, 20 years and older	129	(114 – 147)	72.4	(60.4 – 82.2)	124	(110 – 145)	233	(198 – 361)	143
20–39 years	112	(89.9 – 141)	67.9†	(52.5 – 76.1)	107	(84.5 – 140)	193†	(143 – 367)	58
40–59 years	143	(124 – 165)	77.8†	(62.1 – 89.4)	131	(113 – 171)	283†	(217 – 404)	42
60 years and older	161	(138 – 189)	113†	(47.5 – 127)	159	(144 – 175)	251†	(195 – 368)	43
Females									
Total, 20 years and older	148	(129 – 171)	96.2	(80.8 – 104)	136	(120 – 176)	254	(203 – 442)	167
20–39 years	142	(118 – 172)	93.1†	(80.7 – 98.8)	127	(106 – 186)	254†	(191 – 340)	68
40–59 years	141	(121 – 165)	90.3†	(47.6 – 110)	132	(119 – 163)	208†	(184 – 442)	56
60 years and older	181	(162 – 201)	121†	(63.8 – 136)	182	(149 – 213)	258†	(222 – 351)	43

† Estimate is subject to greater uncertainty due to small cell size.

Table 2.37.a.5. Plasma docosahexaenoic acid (22:6n-3): Non-Hispanic whites

Geometric mean and selected percentiles of plasma concentrations (in μmol/L) for fasted non-Hispanic whites in the U.S. population aged 20 years and older, National Health and Nutrition Examination Survey, 2003–2004.

	Geometric mean (95% conf. interval)		Selected percentiles (95% conf. interval)						Sample size
			10th		50th		90th		
Males and Females									
Total, 20 years and older	122	(113 – 130)	69.8	(64.4 – 74.5)	117	(110 – 127)	215	(202 – 235)	992
20–39 years	111	(102 – 121)	65.2	(58.4 – 72.4)	110	(97.8 – 118)	201	(170 – 258)	300
40–59 years	118	(108 – 130)	65.9	(55.3 – 75.7)	114	(106 – 128)	206	(181 – 252)	280
60 years and older	142	(131 – 155)	84.2	(67.8 – 95.3)	136	(125 – 154)	244	(233 – 266)	412
Males									
Total, 20 years and older	113	(105 – 122)	65.3	(59.6 – 71.8)	112	(102 – 121)	198	(178 – 229)	472
20–39 years	102	(94.4 – 110)	60.8	(54.8 – 68.1)	96.1	(84.4 – 113)	180	(157 – 212)	128
40–59 years	115	(103 – 128)	64.9	(53.7 – 73.5)	113	(97.8 – 127)	194	(167 – 303)	140
60 years and older	128	(116 – 142)	77.0	(49.3 – 93.0)	121	(113 – 141)	213	(188 – 254)	204
Females									
Total, 20 years and older	130	(120 – 140)	74.4	(65.3 – 79.0)	124	(116 – 133)	229	(209 – 259)	520
20–39 years	121	(109 – 134)	72.4	(54.3 – 79.2)	114	(104 – 127)	204	(178 – 315)	172
40–59 years	122	(111 – 133)	68.0	(52.5 – 78.9)	120	(106 – 139)	207	(188 – 244)	140
60 years and older	156	(142 – 170)	89.5	(81.0 – 97.4)	150	(132 – 174)	274	(243 – 330)	208

References

Astrup A, Dyerberg J, Elwood P, Hermansen K, Hu FB, Jakobsen MU, *et al.* The role of reducing intakes of saturated fat in the prevention of cardiovascular disease: where does the evidence stand in 2010? Am J Clin Nutr. 2011;93:684–688.

Cleeman JI, Grundy SM, Becker D, Clark LT, Cooper RS, Denke MA, *et al.* Executive summary of the Third Report of the National Cholesterol Education Program (NCEP) expert panel on detection, evaluation, and treatment of high blood cholesterol in adults (Adult Treatment Panel III). JAMA. 2001;285(19):2486–2497

Harris WS, Mozaffarian D, Rimm E, Kris-Etherton P, Rudel LL, Appel LJ, *et al.* Omega-6 fatty acids and risk for cardiovascular disease a science advisory from the American Heart Association Nutrition Subcommittee of the Council on Nutrition, Physical Activity, and Metabolism; Council on Cardiovascular Nursing; and Council on Epidemiology and Prevention. Circulation. 2009;119:902–907.

Hodson L, Skeaff CM, Fielding BA. Fatty acid composition of adipose tissue and blood in humans and its use as a biomarker of dietary intake. Progress in Lipid Research. 2008;47:348–80.

Hu FB. Are refined carbohydrates worse than saturated fat? Am J Clin Nutr. 2010;91:1541-2.

Institute of Medicine, Food and Nutrition Board. Dietary reference intakes for energy, carbohydrate, fiber, fat, fatty acids, cholesterol, protein, and amino acids. Washington, D.C.: National Academy Press; 2005.

International Life Sciences Institute. 8th edition. Present Knowledge in Nutrition. Washington, D.C.: ILSI Press; 2001.

Jakobsen MU, O'Reilly EJ, Heitmann BL, Pereira MA, Bälter K, Fraser GE, *et al.* Major types of dietary fat and risk of coronary heart disease: a pooled analysis of 11 cohort studies. Am J Clin Nutr. 2009;89:1425–1432.

Jakobsen MU, Dethlefsen C, Joensen AM, Stegger J, Tjonneland A, Schmidt EB, Overvad K. Intake of carbohydrates compared with intake of saturated fatty acids and risk of myocardial infarction: importance of the glycemic index. Am J Clin Nutr. 2010; 91:1764–1768.

Kris-Etherton PM, Harris WS, Appel LJ, for the Nutrition Committee. Fish consumption, fish oil, omega-3 fatty acids, and cardiovascular disease. Circulation. 2002;106:2747–2757.

Lagerstedt SA, Hinrichs DR, Batt SM, Magera MJ, Rinaldo P, McConnell JP. Quantitative determination of plasma C8-C26 total fatty acids for the biochemical diagnosis of nutritional and metabolic disorders. Mol Genet Metab. 2001;73:38–45.

Lichtenstein AH. Fats and oils. In: Benjamin C, ed. Encyclopedia of Human Nutrition. Oxford: Elsevier 2005. pp.177–186.

Micha R, Mozaffarian D. Saturated fat and cardiometabolic risk factors, coronary heart disease, stroke, and diabetes: a fresh look at the evidence. Lipids. 2010;45:893–905.

Sun Q, Ma J, Campos H, Hankinson SE, Hu FB. Comparison between plasma and erythrocyte fatty acid content as biomarkers of fatty acid intake in US women. Am J Clin Nutr. 2007;86:74–81.

U.S. Department of Agriculture and U.S. Department of Health and Human Services. *Dietary Guidelines for Americans, 2010.* 7th Edition, Washington, DC: U.S. Government Printing Office, December 2010 [cited 2011]. Available at: http://www.cnpp.usda.gov/DGAs2010-PolicyDocument.htm.

U.S. National Institutes of Health. National Cancer Institute. Sources of Saturated Fat, Stearic Acid, & Cholesterol Raising Fat among the US Population, 2005–06. Risk Factor Monitoring and Methods Branch Web site. Applied Research Program. Updated December 21, 2010a. Available at: http://riskfactor.cancer.gov/diet/foodsources/sat_fat/.

U.S. National Institutes of Health. National Cancer Institute. Sources of Selected Fatty Acids among the US Population, 2005–06. Risk Factor Monitoring and Methods Branch Web site. Applied Research Program. Updated December 21, 2010b. Available at: http://riskfactor.cancer.gov/diet/foodsources/fatty_acids/.

Zelman K. The great fat debate: A closer look at the controversy - Questioning the validity of age-old dietary guidance. J Am Diet Assoc. 2011;111(5):655–658.

3. Trace Elements

Iron-Status Indicators

- Ferritin
- Soluble transferrin receptor
- Body iron

Iodine

Iron-Status Indicators

Background Information

Sources and Physiological Functions. Iron functions as a component of proteins and enzymes. Almost two-thirds of the iron in the body (approximately 2.5 grams of iron) is found in hemoglobin, the protein in red blood cells that carries oxygen to tissues, and about 15% is in the myoglobin of muscle tissue. The average American diet provides 10–15 milligrams (mg) of iron daily in the form of heme and nonheme iron. Heme iron is found in animal foods that originally contained hemoglobin and myoglobin, such as red meat, fish, and poultry. Nonheme iron is found in plant foods, such as lentils and beans, and also is provided in iron-enriched and iron-fortified foods. Although heme iron is absorbed better than nonheme iron, most dietary iron is nonheme iron (Miret 2003). Each day the body absorbs approximately 1–2 mg of iron to compensate for the 1 to 2 mg of iron that the (nonmenstruating) body loses (Institute of Medicine 2001). The current Dietary Guidelines for Americans list iron as a nutrient of concern for specific population groups. The guidelines recommend that pregnant women take an iron supplement, as recommended by an obstetrician or other health care provider (U.S. Department of Agriculture 2010).

Health Effects. Transporting iron from one organ to another is accomplished by the reversible binding of iron to the transport protein, transferrin, which will then form a complex with a highly specific transferrin receptor (TfR) located on the plasma membrane surfaces of cells. Intracellular iron availability is regulated through the increased expression of cellular TfR concentration by iron-deficient cells. Ferritin is the major iron-storage compound: its production increases in cells as iron supplies increase. The major function of ferritin is to provide a store of iron which may be used for haem synthesis when required. Although all cells are capable of storing iron, the liver, spleen, and bone marrow cells are primary iron-storage sites in people (Institute of Medicine 2001).

Iron deficiency and iron overload are the two major disorders of iron metabolism. Iron-deficiency anemia is the most severe form of iron deficiency. It is linked to many adverse consequences of iron deficiency, such as reduced physical capacity (Haas 2001) and poor pregnancy outcomes (Schorr 1994). Iron deficiency with and without anemia, however, has been linked to negative effects on cognitive development among infants and adolescents (Beard 1999; Grantham-McGregor 2001). Iron overload is the accumulation of excess iron in body tissues, and it usually occurs as a result of a genetic predisposition to absorb iron in excess of normal. However, it can also be caused by excessive ingestion of iron supplements or multiple blood transfusions (Pietrangelo 2004). In advanced stages of iron overload disease (hemochromatosis), the iron accumulates in the parenchymal cells of several organs, but particularly the liver, followed by the heart and pancreas; this condition can lead to organ dysfunction and even death (Pietrangelo 2004).

Intake Recommendations. The Recommended Dietary Allowance (RDA) for all age groups of men and postmenopausal women is 8 mg per day; the RDA for premenopausal women is 18 mg per day. The Tolerable Upper Uptake Level for adults is 45 mg per day of iron, a level based on gastrointestinal distress as an adverse effect (Institute of Medicine 2001).

Biochemical Indicators and Methods. Ferritin is present in the blood in very low concentrations. Serum ferritin is in equilibrium with tissue stores, and its concentration declines early in the development of iron deficiency. Low serum ferritin concentration thus is a sensitive indicator of iron deficiency, but it does not necessarily reflect the severity of the depletion as it progresses (World Health Organization 2011). Ferritin is also an acute-phase protein; acute and chronic diseases can result in increased ferritin concentration, potentially masking an iron-deficiency diagnosis. A review article on serum ferritin written as part of a 2004 WHO/CDC Technical Consultation on the Assessment of Iron Status at the Population Level provides comprehensive information on this topic (Worwood 2007). The generally accepted cutoff value for serum ferritin below which iron stores are considered to be depleted is 15 nanogram per milliliter (ng/mL) for people aged 5 years and older and 12 ng/mL for people younger than 5 years of age (World Health Organization 2001; World Health Organization 2011). Serum ferritin concentrations above 200 ng/mL for adult males and 150 ng/mL for adult females are considered to represent severe risk of iron overload (World Health Organization 2001; World Health Organization 2011).

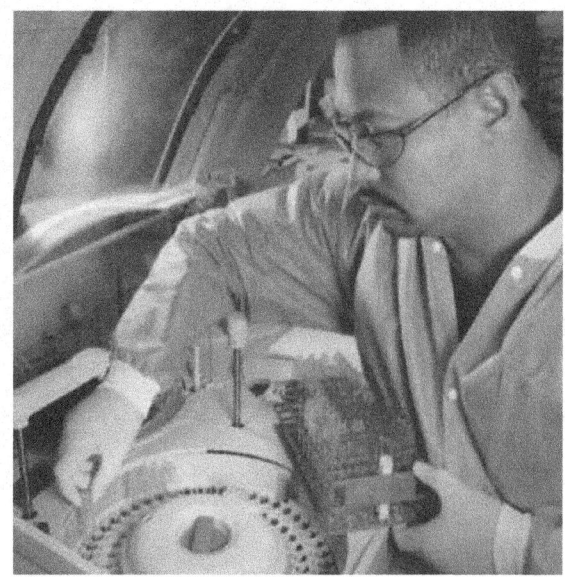

Soluble TfR (sTfR) is the truncated form of the membrane-bound TfR that is cleaved and released into the serum. The amount of sTfR is proportional to the number of membrane-bound TfR. sTfR circulates bound to transferrin, and its concentration is not strongly affected by concurrent inflammation or infection (Beard 2007). Serum sTfR concentration increases when the iron functional pool is depleted and during activated erythropoiesis (Kuiper-Kramer 1998). It continues to do so as the severity of iron-deficient erythropoiesis increases, reflecting the increasing number of receptors on the erythroid cells of the bone marrow. The measurement of sTfR is therefore a powerful tool for the diagnosis of iron deficiency or for monitoring erythropoiesis.

Serum ferritin is the most sensitive index of iron status when there are residual iron stores, whereas serum sTfR is more sensitive when there is functional iron deficiency (Skikne 1990). There is a close, linear relationship between the logarithm of the sTfR to serum ferritin ratio and stored iron (body iron) expressed as mg per kg body weight (Skikne 1990). Recently Cook et al. demonstrated that in healthy persons body iron may be estimated from the ratio of sTfR to serum ferritin (reported in microgram [µg]/mL for both assays) (2003). Body iron is in a positive balance (≥ 0 mg/kg) when there is residual storage iron or in a negative balance (< 0 mg/kg) when there is functional iron deficiency. The latter represents a deficit in iron required to maintain a normal hemoglobin concentration. The body iron methodology allows the full range of iron status of populations to be evaluated. Other iron status indicators, such as serum iron, total iron binding capacity, transferrin saturation, and erythrocyte protoporphyrin, were described in the previous report of this series. They are not included in the current report.

Clinical laboratories typically use conventional units for iron-status indicators: ferritin is calculated in nanograms per milliliter (ng/mL) and sTfR in milligrams per liter (mg/L). Conversion factors to international system (SI) units are as follows: 1 ng/mL = 2.247 picomole (pmol)/L for ferritin and 1 mg/L = 0.085 nanomole (nmol)/L for sTfR.

The most widely used methods to measure both serum ferritin and sTfR are immunoassay-based (ELISA, immuno-turbidimetry, immunonephelometry) (Worwood 2002a; Worwood 2002b). A WHO-supported international reference material from the United Kingdom National Institute for Biological Standards and Control (NIBSC) has been available for ferritin for several years (94/572); it has helped to improve the comparability of commercial kit assays. On the other hand, commercial kit assays for sTfR produce different results, making the use of assay-specific reference intervals and cutoff values necessary (Beard 2007). Recently, the WHO supported the development of a reference reagent for sTfR by the NIBSC, and material 07-202 was released in 2010. It is hoped that this material will be used by manufacturers to standardize sTfR assays and promote the establishment of cutoff values used to assess the iron status of populations (Thorpe 2010).

Data in NHANES. Monitoring the iron status of the U.S. population has been an important component since the inception of NHANES in 1971, and each NHANES has included a battery of hematologic and biochemical indicators of iron status (Looker 1995). Since NHANES II (1976–1980), models that employ multiple biochemical iron-status indicators have been used to define iron deficiency in the population (Pilch 1984). The ferritin model (also known as the three-indicator model), using serum ferritin, transferrin saturation, and erythrocyte protoporphyrin, was developed in 1980 and applied to NHANES III (1988–1994) as well as to the first few years of the continuous NHANES survey beginning in 1999. Prevalence estimates of iron deficiency using the three-indicator model were similar in NHANES III (Looker 1997) and in NHANES 1999–2000 (Looker 2002).

Starting in 2003, NHANES limited the population of interest to children (1–5 years) and women of childbearing age (12–49 years). Furthermore, the measurement of serum sTfR was introduced, which allows the evaluation of iron status by the body iron model developed by Cook et al. (2003). Using data for children and non-pregnant women from NHANES 2003–2006, Cogswell et al. compared the new body iron model to the previously used ferritin model (2009). The agreement between the two models was fair to good. Among non-pregnant women, the body iron model produced lower estimates of iron deficiency prevalence and better predicted anemia. The body iron model appeared to be less affected by inflammation than the ferritin model.

Two national health objectives that relate to iron deficiency reduction are part of the objectives for Healthy People 2020: Objective NWS HP2020-21 (reduce iron deficiency among young children and females of childbearing age) and Objective NWS HP2020-22 (reduce iron deficiency among pregnant females) (http://www.healthypeople.gov/HP2020/). To provide data for these objectives, NHANES continues with periodic monitoring of iron status in the population groups of interest.

Ferritin and sTfR data presented in this report were generated by use of commercial assay kits. Serum ferritin was first measured by use of the BioRad QuantImune immunoradiometric assay (1999–2003), then by use of the Roche TinaQuant immunoturbidimetric assay on the Hitachi 912 clinical analyzer (2004–2006). The public release data file for 2003–2004 has already been adjusted to the new assay. We used adjustment equations provided in the analytical note for data from 1999–2002 to make the data comparable to the new assay (http://www.cdc.gov/nchs/nhanes/nhanes2003-2004/L06TFR_C.htm#Analytic_Notes). Serum sTfR was measured with the Roche immunoturbidimetric assay on the Hitachi 912 clinical analyzer (2003–2006). We calculated body iron by using the following formula (Cook 2003): body iron (mg/kg) = -[log10 (sTfR * 1000 / ferritin) – 2.8229] / 0.1207. The sTfR concentration in this formula represents an adjusted concentration to make the Roche sTfR concentrations equivalent to the Flowers assay (1989) used in the development of the body iron model: Flowers sTfR = 1.5 * Roche sTfR + 0.35 mg/L (Pfeiffer 2007).

To estimate the prevalence of low serum ferritin concentrations, we used the generally accepted cutoff values mentioned above: 12 ng/mL for children 1-5 years of age and 15 ng/mL for women of childbearing age and males 6 years and older. To estimate the prevalence of high serum ferritin concentrations, we also used the cutoff values mentioned above: 150 ng/mL for women 12-49 years of age and 200 ng/mL for men 12 years and older. Due to the lack of generally accepted cutoff values for serum sTfR, we used the manufacturer provided assay-specific cutoff value of 4.4 mg/L to estimate the prevalence of high sTfR concentrations in women of childbearing age. The prevalence of low body iron (< 0 mg/kg) is indicative of the extent of iron deficiency in the population.

For more information about iron, see the Institute of Medicine's Dietary Reference Intake reports (Institute of Medicine 2001) and fact sheets from the National Institutes of Health, Office of Dietary Supplements (http://ods.od.nih.gov/Health_Information/Information_About_Individual_Dietary_Supplements.aspx).

Highlights

Serum concentrations of ferritin and sTfR in the U.S. population showed the following demographic patterns and characteristics:

- Children had the lowest ferritin concentrations and highest sTfR concentrations compared to other age groups.

- Regardless of the indicator selected (serum ferritin, sTfR, or body iron), the likelihood of being iron deficient varied by race/ethnic group.

- While children and women of childbearing age were at risk for iron deficiency, men were at risk for iron excess.

New data from NHANES 2003–2006 allow for the first time assessment of the iron status of children and women of childbearing age by way of a new indicator, body iron. Using the ferritin model in NHANES 1999–2000, Looker and colleagues (2002) showed that the prevalence of iron deficiency was higher in Mexican-American (22%) and non-Hispanic black (19%) women aged 12–49 years than for non-Hispanic white women (10%). We saw the same pattern in NHANES 2003–2006 for women of childbearing age by using low body iron < 0 mg/kg) as an indicator of iron deficiency (Figure H.3.a). We saw a higher prevalence of low body iron in Mexican-American children (1–5 years) than in non-Hispanic black and non-Hispanic white children (Figure H.3.a).

The prevalence estimates of iron deficiency may vary depending on which indicator or set of indicators is used. Furthermore, the prevalence may be overestimated by using only a single indicator. In women of childbearing age, we found the lowest prevalence by using body iron (10%), intermediate prevalence by using low ferritin concentrations (13%), and the highest prevalence by using high sTfR concentrations (19%) (Figure H.3.b).

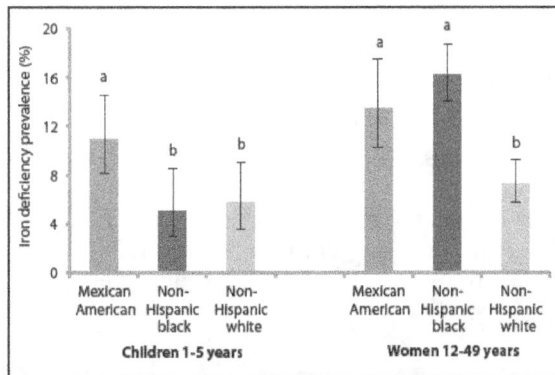

Figure H.3.a. *Age-adjusted prevalence estimates of low body iron stores (< 0 mg/kg) in U.S. children and women by race/ethnicity, National Health and Nutrition Examination Survey, 2003–2006.*

Error bars represent 95% confidence intervals. Bars not sharing a common letter differ within children and women (p < 0.05). Age adjustment was done using direct standardization.

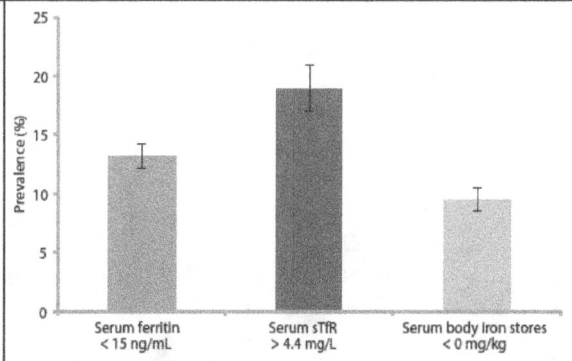

Figure H.3.b. *Prevalence estimates of low serum ferritin, high serum soluble transferrin receptor, and low serum body iron in U.S. women 12–49 years of age, National Health and Nutrition Examination Survey, 2003–2006.*

Error bars represent 95% confidence intervals.

Women were at risk for iron deficiency, while men were at risk for iron excess, as can be seen from the large differences in the prevalence of low and high serum ferritin concentrations between men and women (Figure H.3.c). During NHANES 1999–2002, the prevalence of low serum ferritin concentrations (< 15 ng/mL) was much lower in 12–49 year-old men (1%) than in 12–49 year-old women (13%). Conversely, the prevalence of high serum ferritin concentrations (> 200 ng/mL for men and > 150 ng/mL for women) was much higher in men (29%) than in women (6%). NHANES 2003–2006 showed similar prevalence estimates for women as were seen in 1999–2002. No data are available for men in 2003–2006.

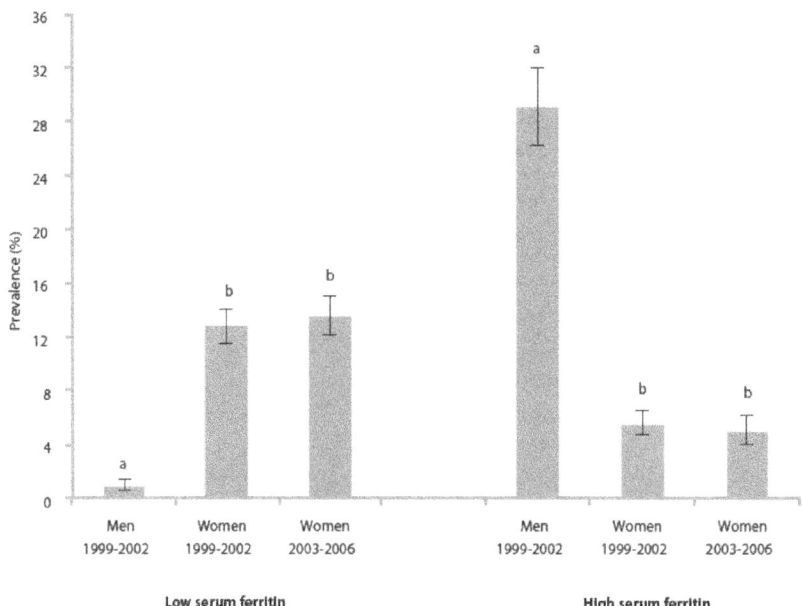

Figure H.3.c. *Age-adjusted prevalence estimates of low (< 15 ng/mL) and high serum ferritin (> 200 ng/mL for men and > 150 ng/mL for women) in U.S. men and women aged 12–49 years, National Health and Nutrition Examination Survey, 1999–2006.*

Error bars represent 95% confidence intervals. Within each ferritin status category, bars not sharing a common letter differ (p < 0.05). Age adjustment was done using direct standardization.

Serum ferritin has been assessed as part of NHANES for many years, allowing for the evaluation of temporal changes in concentrations. Overall, there were only minor changes in serum ferritin concentrations in women of childbearing age over a period of almost two decades (Figure H.3.d). Age-adjusted mean serum ferritin concentrations in women of childbearing age were slightly lower (< 10%) in 1999–2002 and 2003–2006 than in 1988–1994. We observed the same pattern for non-Hispanic white women, while serum ferritin concentrations decreased further during 2003–2006 for non-Hispanic black women. Mexican-American women had lower serum ferritin concentrations in 1999–2002 than in 1988–1994, but concentrations in 2003–2006 did not differ from concentrations in the two previous time periods.

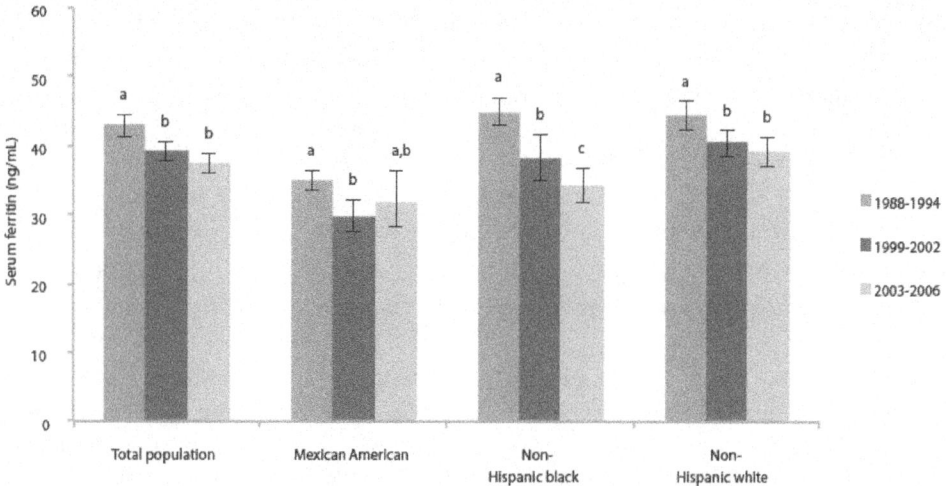

Figure H.3.d. *Age-adjusted geometric mean concentrations of serum ferritin in U.S. women aged 12–49 years by race/ethnicity, National Health and Nutrition Examination Survey, 1988–2006.*

Error bars represent 95% confidence intervals. Within a demographic group, bars not sharing a common letter differ (p < 0.05). Age adjustment was done using direct standardization.

Detailed Observations

The selected observations mentioned below are derived from the tables and figures presented next. Statements about categorical differences between demographic groups noted below are based on non-overlapping confidence limits from univariate analysis without adjusting for demographic variables (e.g., age, sex, race/ethnicity) or other determinants of these blood concentrations (e.g., dietary intake, supplement usage, smoking, BMI). A multivariate analysis may alter the size and statistical significance of these categorical differences. Furthermore, additional significant differences of smaller magnitude may be present despite their lack of mention here (e.g., if confidence limits slightly overlap or if differences are not statistically significant before covariate adjustment has occurred). For a selection of citations of descriptive NHANES papers related to these biochemical indicators of diet and nutrition, see **Appendix G**.

Geometric/arithmetic mean concentrations (NHANES 2003–2006):

- The distribution of body iron was reasonably symmetric and for that reason we present arithmetic means.

- Serum ferritin concentrations increased with age (Table 3.1.a.1 and Figure 3.1.a).

- sTfR concentrations were highest in children than for both adolescent and adult women (Table 3.2.a.1 and Figure 3.2.a).

- Body iron was lowest in children, intermediate in adolescent women, and highest in adult women (Table 3.3.a.1 and Figure 3.3.a).

- Non-Hispanic whites had higher serum ferritin concentrations than Mexican Americans, and non-Hispanic blacks had intermediate concentrations (Table 3.1.a.1).

- Non-Hispanic whites had lower sTfR concentrations than Mexican Americans, who had lower concentrations still than non-Hispanic blacks (Table 3.2.a.1).

- Non-Hispanic whites had higher body iron than the other two race/ethnic groups (Table 3.3.a.1).

Changes in geometric/arithmetic mean concentrations across survey cycles:

- All three iron status indicators remained stable across the survey cycles measured: serum ferritin geometric mean concentrations (Table 3.1.b) between 1999 and 2006; sTfR geometric mean concentrations (Table 3.2.b) and body iron arithmetic means (Table 3.3.b) between 2003 and 2006.

Prevalence estimates of low or high biochemical indicator concentrations:

- In 2003–2006, approximately 9% of children (1–5 years) (Table 3.1.c.1) had serum ferritin concentrations < 12 ng/mL and 14% of women (12–49 years) had serum ferritin concentrations < 15 ng/mL (Table 3.1.c.2). Approximately 5% of women (12–49 years) (Table 3.1.c.3) had high serum ferritin concentrations (> 150 ng/mL), indicating severe risk of iron overload.

- The prevalence of low serum ferritin concentrations did not change between 1999 and 2006 in children (Table 3.1.d.1) and women of childbearing age (Table 3.1.d.2), nor between 1999 and 2002 in males 6 years and older (Table 3.1.d.3). The prevalence of high serum ferritin concentrations also remained constant between 1999 and 2006 in women of childbearing age (Table 3.1.d.4) and between 1999–2002 in men 12 years and older (Table 3.1.d.5).

- In 2003–2006, approximately 19% of women (12–49 years) had serum sTfR concentrations > 4.4 mg/L (Table 3.2.c), and the prevalence was the same in both survey cycles (Table 3.2.d).

- Less than 10% of children (8% of boys and 5% of girls 1–5 years) and 10% of women (12–49 years) had negative body iron balance, indicative of iron deficiency (Tables 3.3.c.1 and 3.3.c.2), and the prevalence was the same in both survey cycles (Tables 3.3.d.1 and 3.3.d.2).

Table 3.1.a.1. Serum ferritin: Concentrations

Geometric mean and selected percentiles of serum concentrations (in ng/mL) for children aged 1–5 years and women aged 12–49 years in the U.S. population, National Health and Nutrition Examination Survey, 2003–2006.

	Geometric mean (95% conf. interval)	Selected percentiles (95% conf. interval)					Sample size
		2.5th	5th	50th	95th	97.5th	
Total							
(Children 1–5 years women 12–49 years)	35.7 (34.4 – 37.1)	4.65 (4.52 – 4.78)	6.99 (6.15 – 7.71)	36.2 (34.7 – 38.1)	143 (133 – 157)	194 (177 – 210)	6,012
Age group							
1–5 years (Children)	26.2 (25.2 – 27.3)	6.68 (5.19 – 7.72)	9.14 (7.87 – 9.82)	26.7 (25.5 – 27.9)	65.6 (59.6 – 68.1)	77.5 (70.2 – 91.4)	1,482
12–19 years (Women)	29.3 (27.7 – 30.9)	4.64 (4.31 – 4.98)	6.83 (5.19 – 7.77)	31.9 (29.9 – 33.3)	81.4 (76.7 – 92.2)	103 (91.8 – 134)	1,991
20–39 years (Women)	38.1 (36.1 – 40.2)	4.67 (4.45 – 4.88)	7.19 (5.66 – 8.21)	40.5 (38.3 – 43.3)	135 (114 – 159)	176 (153 – 206)	1,780
40–49 years (Women)	43.2 (39.0 – 47.7)	4.38 (4.06 – 4.69)	5.81 (4.73 – 7.10)	45.9 (40.5 – 50.7)	211 (184 – 262)	264 (231 – 317)	759
Gender							
Males (1–5 years)	26.2 (24.9 – 27.7)	6.90 (4.61 – 7.90)	8.90 (8.01 – 9.68)	26.9 (25.1 – 28.5)	63.6 (56.9 – 70.7)	77.9 (67.7 – 111)	757
Females (1–5, 12–49 years)	36.6 (35.2 – 38.1)	4.62 (4.48 – 4.75)	6.80 (5.96 – 7.56)	38.1 (36.0 – 39.4)	145 (136 – 165)	198 (180 – 219)	5,255
Race/ethnicity							
(Children 1–5 years, women 12–49 years)							
Mexican Americans	30.2 (27.5 – 33.1)	4.18 (3.78 – 4.43)	4.87 (4.62 – 5.46)	31.7 (28.7 – 34.0)	121 (101 – 161)	166 (140 – 231)	1,704
Non-Hispanic Blacks	33.5 (31.4 – 35.7)	4.13 (3.31 – 4.70)	5.49 (4.69 – 6.46)	33.7 (31.8 – 35.8)	165 (133 – 201)	212 (182 – 261)	1,676
Non-Hispanic Whites	37.5 (35.5 – 39.6)	4.89 (4.66 – 5.44)	8.07 (6.52 – 8.85)	38.2 (35.9 – 39.8)	143 (131 – 159)	194 (172 – 233)	2,089

Figure 3.1. a . Serum ferritin: Concentrations by age group

Geometric mean (95% confidence interval), National Health and Nutrition Examination Survey, 2003–2006

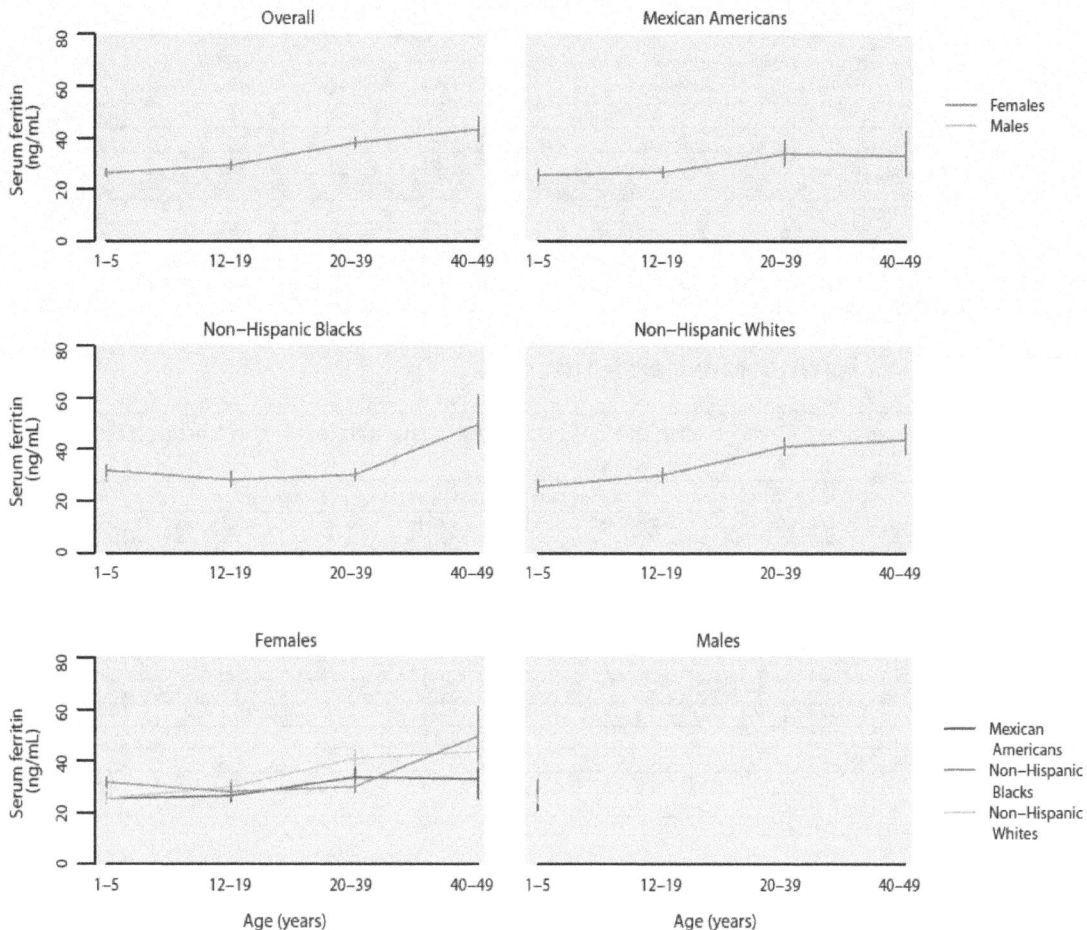

Table 3.1.a.2. Serum ferritin: Total population

Geometric mean and selected percentiles of serum concentrations (in ng/mL) for children aged 1–5 years and women aged 12–49 years in the U.S. population, National Health and Nutrition Examination Survey, 2003–2006.

| | Geometric mean (95% conf. interval) | Selected percentiles (95% conf. interval) | | | Sample size |
		5th	50th	95th	
Males and Females					
Total, Children 1–5 years, women 12–49 years	35.7 (34.4 – 37.1)	6.99 (6.15 – 7.71)	36.2 (34.7 – 38.1)	143 (133 – 157)	6,012
1–5 years	26.2 (25.2 – 27.3)	9.14 (7.87 – 9.82)	26.7 (25.5 – 27.9)	65.6 (59.6 – 68.1)	1,482
Males					
1–5 years	26.2 (24.9 – 27.7)	8.90 (8.01 – 9.68)	26.9 (25.1 – 28.5)	63.6 (56.9 – 70.7)	757
Females					
Total, 1–5, 12–49 years	36.6 (35.2 – 38.1)	6.80 (5.96 – 7.56)	38.1 (36.0 – 39.4)	145 (136 – 165)	5,255
1–5 years	26.3 (24.9 – 27.7)	9.29 (6.81 – 10.1)	26.5 (24.8 – 28.0)	67.0 (59.2 – 74.3)	725
12–19 years	29.3 (27.7 – 30.9)	6.83 (5.19 – 7.77)	31.9 (29.9 – 33.3)	81.4 (76.7 – 92.2)	1,991
20–39 years	38.1 (36.1 – 40.2)	7.19 (5.66 – 8.21)	40.5 (38.3 – 43.3)	135 (114 – 159)	1,780
40–49 years	43.2 (39.0 – 47.7)	5.81 (4.73 – 7.10)	45.9 (40.5 – 50.7)	211 (184 – 262)	759

Table 3.1.a.3. Serum ferritin: Mexican Americans

Geometric mean and selected percentiles of serum concentrations (in ng/mL) for Mexican-American children aged 1–5 years and women aged 12–49 years in the U.S. population, National Health and Nutrition Examination Survey, 2003–2006.

| | Geometric mean (95% conf. interval) | Selected percentiles (95% conf. interval) | | | Sample size |
		5th	50th	95th	
Males and Females					
Total, Children 1–5 years, women 12–49 years	30.2 (27.5 – 33.1)	4.87 (4.62 – 5.46)	31.7 (28.7 – 34.0)	121 (101 – 161)	1,704
1–5 years	24.5 (22.8 – 26.3)	6.44 (4.69 – 7.69)	25.5 (23.5 – 27.6)	68.9 (57.7 – 83.3)	468
Males					
1–5 years	23.5 (21.3 – 25.9)	6.04 (4.33 – 7.21)	24.6 (23.1 – 27.0)	63.8 (52.5 – 118)	225
Females					
Total, 1–5, 12–49 years	31.0 (28.0 – 34.5)	4.84 (4.59 – 5.33)	33.2 (29.3 – 36.1)	126 (104 – 167)	1,479
1–5 years	25.5 (23.6 – 27.6)	6.81 (4.56 – 9.78)	26.7 (23.2 – 29.8)	69.6 (60.7 – 88.6)	243
12–19 years	26.6 (24.8 – 28.5)	6.35 (4.85 – 7.38)	27.3 (25.5 – 29.2)	89.6 (80.6 – 97.3)	647
20–39 years	33.7 (29.2 – 38.9)	4.89 (4.62 – 5.51)	37.1 (31.6 – 43.9)	139 (106 – 213)	434
40–49 years	33.1 (25.7 – 42.7)	4.27† (3.48 – 4.66)	34.3 (28.3 – 42.9)	170† (134 – 262)	155

† Estimate is subject to greater uncertainty due to small cell size.

Table 3.1.a.4. Serum ferritin: Non-Hispanic blacks

Geometric mean and selected percentiles of serum concentrations (in ng/mL) for non-Hispanic black children aged 1–5 years and women aged 12–49 years in the U.S. population, National Health and Nutrition Examination Survey, 2003–2006.

	Geometric mean (95% conf. interval)	Selected percentiles (95% conf. interval)						Sample size
		5th		50th		95th		
Males and Females								
Total, Children 1–5 years, women 12–49 years	33.5 (31.4 – 35.7)	5.49	(4.69 – 6.46)	33.7	(31.8 – 35.8)	165	(133 – 201)	1,676
1–5 years	30.8 (28.9 – 32.8)	11.4	(9.51 – 14.2)	30.7	(28.7 – 32.7)	72.5	(65.8 – 88.9)	429
Males								
1–5 years	30.0 (27.3 – 32.9)	10.6†	(5.39 – 14.4)	29.6	(26.6 – 33.4)	66.2†	(58.1 – 96.6)	218
Females								
Total, 1–5, 12–49 years	33.8 (31.5 – 36.2)	5.26	(4.56 – 6.25)	34.1	(32.1 – 36.9)	171	(139 – 207)	1,458
1–5 years	31.7 (29.8 – 33.7)	12.4†	(9.78 – 14.6)	31.6	(29.1 – 33.6)	75.8†	(67.6 – 89.4)	211
12–19 years	28.2 (25.5 – 31.2)	6.61	(4.97 – 7.55)	31.1	(27.4 – 33.7)	88.7	(79.4 – 104)	674
20–39 years	30.1 (27.9 – 32.4)	5.02	(4.22 – 6.08)	31.1	(28.4 – 34.1)	132	(122 – 173)	375
40–49 years	49.6 (40.4 – 61.0)	4.31†	(< LOD – 8.31)	53.5	(42.2 – 63.9)	257†	(207 – 531)	198

< LOD means less than the limit of detection, which may vary for some compounds by year. See Appendix D for LOD.

† Estimate is subject to greater uncertainty due to small cell size.

Table 3.1.a.5. Serum ferritin: Non-Hispanic whites

Geometric mean and selected percentiles of serum concentrations (in ng/mL) for non-Hispanic white children aged 1–5 years and women aged 12–49 years in the U.S. population, National Health and Nutrition Examination Survey, 2003–2006.

	Geometric mean (95% conf. interval)	Selected percentiles (95% conf. interval)						Sample size
		5th		50th		95th		
Males and Females								
Total, Children 1–5 years, women 12–49 years	37.5 (35.5 – 39.6)	8.07	(6.52 – 8.85)	38.2	(35.9 – 39.8)	143	(131 – 159)	2,089
1–5 years	25.9 (24.2 – 27.7)	9.30	(8.13 – 10.0)	26.3	(24.4 – 28.1)	61.4	(55.7 – 67.8)	416
Males								
1–5 years	26.1 (23.8 – 28.6)	9.13	(4.71 – 10.5)	27.1	(24.3 – 29.7)	56.9	(53.5 – 89.4)	229
Females								
Total, 1–5, 12–49 years	38.5 (36.3 – 40.7)	7.96	(6.36 – 8.78)	39.4	(37.2 – 41.0)	144	(135 – 167)	1,860
1–5 years	25.6 (23.4 – 27.9)	9.40†	(5.96 – 10.3)	25.5	(23.4 – 27.8)	63.7†	(53.8 – 87.4)	187
12–19 years	30.0 (27.7 – 32.6)	6.88	(4.67 – 8.55)	33.0	(31.1 – 34.9)	78.2	(70.9 – 93.0)	520
20–39 years	41.0 (37.8 – 44.5)	8.75	(7.16 – 10.1)	42.3	(39.2 – 47.0)	134	(112 – 171)	812
40–49 years	43.6 (38.3 – 49.6)	6.61	(4.82 – 8.43)	46.1	(39.7 – 51.2)	212	(164 – 266)	341

† Estimate is subject to greater uncertainty due to small cell size.

Table 3.1.b. Serum ferritin: Concentrations by survey cycle

Geometric mean and selected percentiles of serum concentrations (in ng/mL) for children aged 1–5 and women aged 12–49 years in the U.S. population, National Health and Nutrition Examination Survey, 1999–2006.

	Geometric mean (95% conf. interval)	Selected percentiles (95% conf. interval) 5th		Selected percentiles (95% conf. interval) 50th		Selected percentiles (95% conf. interval) 95th		Sample size
Total (Children 1–5 years, women 12–49 years)								
1999–2000	38.8 (36.7 – 41.0)	8.06	(5.23 – 9.99)	38.3	(34.7 – 42.5)	139	(129 – 173)	2,919
2001–2002	36.1 (34.2 – 38.0)	5.23	**	35.2	(33.2 – 37.2)	149	(136 – 175)	3,365
2003–2004	36.4 (34.7 – 38.3)	7.70	(5.80 – 8.58)	36.1	(34.6 – 38.6)	151	(141 – 173)	2,981
2005–2006	35.0 (32.9 – 37.2)	6.46	(5.69 – 7.19)	36.2	(33.6 – 38.7)	135	(113 – 167)	3,031
Age group								
1–5 years (Children)								
1999–2000	28.7 (26.9 – 30.7)	10.6	(5.95 – 13.5)	28.2	(26.0 – 31.6)	74.6	(57.9 – 94.2)	680
2001–2002	27.9 (25.6 – 30.5)	6.43	(5.23 – 9.79)	28.2	(26.2 – 30.4)	78.6	(68.5 – 105)	843
2003–2004	25.2 (23.7 – 26.8)	9.27	(8.08 – 9.76)	24.9	(23.2 – 26.7)	64.0	(57.0 – 67.8)	796
2005–2006	27.6 (26.0 – 29.2)	8.95	(7.95 – 9.78)	28.5	(27.4 – 30.1)	66.7	(63.2 – 77.2)	686
12–19 years (Women)								
1999–2000	32.5 (29.6 – 35.8)	9.26	(5.23 – 10.4)	32.8	(29.6 – 37.1)	83.3	(79.4 – 99.7)	1,048
2001–2002	30.1 (28.5 – 31.9)	6.55	(5.23 – 8.62)	32.5	(29.9 – 33.7)	84.5	(79.3 – 95.6)	1,120
2003–2004	28.0 (25.5 – 30.7)	6.11	(4.43 – 7.97)	30.1	(27.9 – 32.7)	86.4	(75.6 – 102)	998
2005–2006	30.6 (28.6 – 32.8)	7.21	(5.52 – 8.79)	33.4	(30.9 – 35.7)	79.0	(75.0 – 94.0)	993
20–39 years (Women)								
1999–2000	40.0 (36.0 – 44.4)	5.23	**	43.5	(36.3 – 52.2)	137	(118 – 187)	838
2001–2002	37.8 (35.2 – 40.5)	5.23	**	38.3	(34.5 – 41.7)	142	(119 – 192)	992
2003–2004	39.8 (37.1 – 42.7)	8.40	(7.52 – 9.20)	41.1	(39.2 – 44.6)	132	(111 – 172)	822
2005–2006	36.5 (33.5 – 39.9)	5.60	(4.70 – 7.17)	39.2	(34.1 – 44.6)	135	(110 – 179)	958
40–49 years (Women)								
1999–2000	50.3 (43.6 – 57.9)	9.15	(5.23 – 12.1)	50.0	(42.8 – 59.8)	227	(202 – 275)	353
2001–2002	43.7 (39.3 – 48.6)	5.23	**	46.5	(39.2 – 53.9)	221	(195 – 249)	410
2003–2004	46.6 (39.9 – 54.4)	5.16	(4.21 – 8.44)	47.1	(43.5 – 53.6)	227	(197 – 317)	365
2005–2006	40.0 (34.5 – 46.3)	6.26	(4.89 – 6.96)	41.6	(34.0 – 51.7)	169	(144 – 264)	394
Gender								
Males (1–5 years)								
1999–2000	27.4 (25.4 – 29.6)	10.8	(6.11 – 13.1)	26.6	(24.7 – 28.4)	73.7	(55.4 – 95.7)	377
2001–2002	26.1 (23.4 – 29.0)	5.23	**	27.4	(24.4 – 30.3)	77.9	(67.2 – 112)	428
2003–2004	25.0 (23.1 – 27.1)	9.19	(6.68 – 10.2)	24.8	(22.5 – 27.0)	57.3	(55.3 – 67.6)	415
2005–2006	27.8 (25.8 – 29.9)	8.71	(8.18 – 9.54)	29.3	(26.9 – 31.0)	70.4	(55.8 – 105)	342
Females (1–5, 12–49 years)								
1999–2000	40.0 (37.7 – 42.5)	7.86	(5.23 – 9.85)	40.8	(37.0 – 45.1)	146	(132 – 179)	2,542
2001–2002	37.0 (35.2 – 38.9)	5.23	**	36.3	(34.5 – 38.3)	157	(141 – 186)	2,937
2003–2004	37.7 (35.6 – 39.8)	7.60	(5.49 – 8.51)	38.7	(36.0 – 40.1)	158	(143 – 186)	2,566
2005–2006	35.6 (33.4 – 37.9)	6.31	(5.46 – 7.04)	37.2	(34.2 – 40.0)	137	(115 – 176)	2,689
Race/ethnicity (Children 1–5 years, women 12–49 years)								
Mexican Americans								
1999–2000	29.0 (26.6 – 31.6)	5.23	**	30.2	(27.9 – 32.7)	117	(81.2 – 179)	1,077
2001–2002	27.9 (25.6 – 30.4)	5.23	**	28.9	(26.8 – 31.3)	102	(82.4 – 162)	967
2003–2004	32.0 (27.4 – 37.4)	6.36	(4.30 – 7.98)	33.2	(28.1 – 36.8)	140	(98.8 – 203)	793
2005–2006	28.4 (25.7 – 31.4)	4.57	(4.01 – 5.22)	29.7	(27.6 – 32.9)	106	(98.4 – 119)	911
Non-Hispanic Blacks								
1999–2000	38.5 (34.3 – 43.3)	5.23	**	38.1	(33.1 – 44.9)	171	(130 – 382)	690
2001–2002	35.8 (31.0 – 41.3)	5.23	**	36.1	(32.7 – 40.2)	187	(138 – 263)	855
2003–2004	34.1 (30.5 – 38.2)	5.74	(4.17 – 7.50)	33.1	(30.0 – 36.9)	172	(127 – 267)	870
2005–2006	32.7 (30.5 – 35.1)	5.35	(4.67 – 6.15)	34.3	(31.1 – 38.1)	145	(127 – 179)	806
Non-Hispanic Whites								
1999–2000	41.1 (38.4 – 44.0)	9.77	(5.23 – 12.4)	41.0	(35.1 – 47.1)	146	(131 – 181)	838
2001–2002	37.0 (34.2 – 40.1)	6.86	(5.23 – 8.38)	35.5	(32.8 – 38.6)	141	(124 – 188)	1,236
2003–2004	37.7 (35.1 – 40.5)	8.37	(4.79 – 10.0)	38.3	(35.6 – 39.7)	147	(136 – 190)	1,069
2005–2006	37.3 (34.1 – 40.7)	7.57	(6.33 – 8.68)	38.1	(34.4 – 41.1)	135	(113 – 176)	1,020

** The minimum value is reported. The desired percentile does not exist because it is less than the estimated cumulative distribution evaluated at the minimum.

Figure 3.1.b. Serum ferritin: Concentrations by survey cycle

Selected percentiles in ng/mL (95% confidence intervals), National Health and Nutrition Examination Survey, 1999–2006

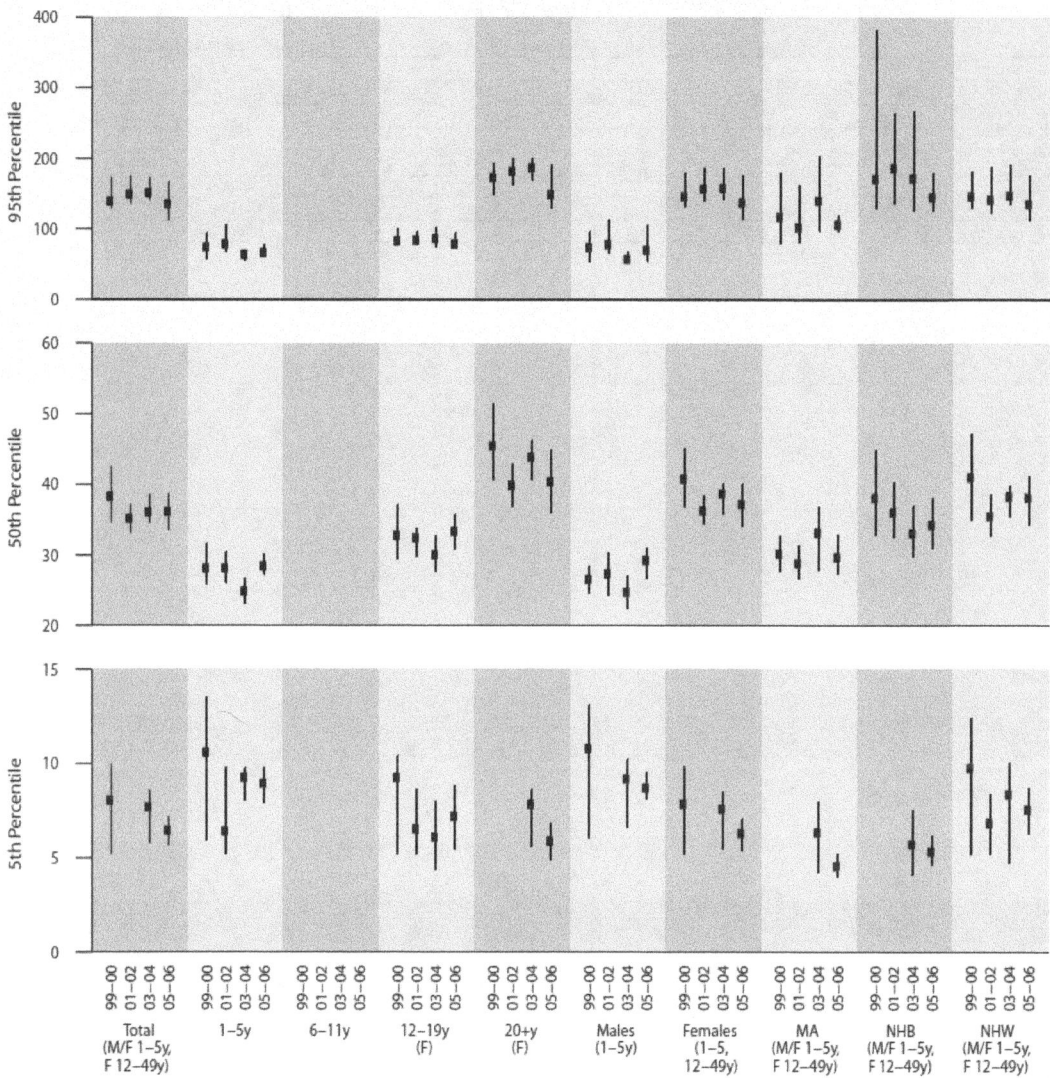

Table 3.1.c.1. Serum ferritin: Prevalence

Prevalence (in percent) of low serum ferritin concentration (< 12 ng/mL) for children in the U.S. population aged 1–5 years, National Health and Nutrition Examination Survey, 2003–2006.

	Sample size	Prevalence (95% conf. interval)	Estimated total number of persons
Children, 1–5 years	1,482	8.9 (7.1 – 11.2)	1,810,000
Gender			
Males	757	9.2 (7.1 – 11.9)	953,000
Females	725	8.6 (6.2 – 11.8)	855,000
Race/ethnicity			
Mexican Americans	468	11.4 (8.6 – 15.1)	348,000
Non-Hispanic Blacks	429	4.9 (3.1 – 7.8)	148,000
Non-Hispanic Whites	416	9.8 (6.9 – 13.7)	1,134,000

Table 3.1.c.2. Serum ferritin: Prevalence

Prevalence (in percent) of low serum ferritin concentration (< 15 ng/mL) for women in the U.S. population aged 12–49 years, National Health and Nutrition Examination Survey, 2003–2006.

	Sample size	Prevalence (95% conf. interval)	Estimated total number of persons
Women, 12–49 years	4,530	13.6 (12.2 – 15.2)	10,748,000
Age group			
12–19 years	1,991	15.2 (12.4 – 18.4)	2,462,000
20–49 years	2,539	13.2 (11.8 – 14.8)	8,299,000
Race/ethnicity			
Mexican Americans	1,236	18.6 (14.9 – 23.0)	1,427,000
Non-Hispanic Blacks	1,247	19.9 (17.9 – 22.1)	2,140,000
Non-Hispanic Whites	1,673	11.3 (9.2 – 13.9)	5,805,000

Table 3.1.c.3. Serum ferritin: Prevalence

Prevalence (in percent) of high serum ferritin concentration (> 150 ng/mL) for women in the U.S. population aged 12–49 years, National Health and Nutrition Examination Survey, 2003–2006.

	Sample size	Prevalence (95% conf. interval)	Estimated total number of persons
Women, 12–49 years	4,530	5.2 (4.2 – 6.4)	4,086,000
Age group			
12–19 years	1,991	0.9‡ (0.5 – 1.8)	149,000‡
20–49 years	2,539	6.2 (5.0 – 7.7)	3,900,000
Race/ethnicity			
Mexican Americans	1,236	4.2 (2.5 – 7.2)	324,000
Non-Hispanic Blacks	1,247	7.1 (5.0 – 9.9)	759,000
Non-Hispanic Whites	1,673	4.9 (3.7 – 6.3)	2,495,000

‡ Estimate flagged: 30% ≤ RSE < 40% for the prevalence estimate.

Table 3.1.d.1. Serum ferritin: Prevalence by survey cycle

Prevalence (in percent) of low serum ferritin concentration (< 12 ng/mL) for children in the U.S. population aged 1–5 years, National Health and Nutrition Examination Survey, 1999–2006.

	Sample size	Prevalence (95% conf. interval)	Estimated total number of persons
Children, 1–5 years			
1999–2000	680	5.7 (3.3 – 9.6)	1,133,000
2001–2002	843	10.0 (7.0 – 13.9)	1,935,000
2003–2004	796	9.0 (6.6 – 12.3)	1,828,000
2005–2006	686	8.8 (6.0 – 12.8)	1,782,000
Gender			
Males			
1999–2000	377	5.9 (3.3 – 10.4)	599,000
2001–2002	428	13.3 (8.6 – 20.1)	1,326,000
2003–2004	415	9.4 (6.6 – 13.3)	970,000
2005–2006	342	9.0 (5.8 – 13.8)	933,000
Females			
1999–2000	303	5.5‡ (2.4 – 12.0)	530,000‡
2001–2002	415	6.5 (4.3 – 9.6)	613,000
2003–2004	381	8.6 (5.6 – 12.8)	854,000
2005–2006	344	8.6 (4.8 – 14.9)	849,000
Race/ethnicity			
Mexican Americans			
1999–2000	269	11.7 (7.7 – 17.4)	305,000
2001–2002	246	10.1 (7.4 – 13.6)	283,000
2003–2004	230	12.5 (7.6 – 19.8)	380,000
2005–2006	238	10.2 (8.1 – 12.8)	329,000
Non-Hispanic Blacks			
1999–2000	168	4.7 (2.6 – 8.4)	142,000
2001–2002	247	§	§
2003–2004	252	6.0 (3.1 – 11.3)	180,000
2005–2006	177	3.4‡ (1.7 – 6.9)	100,000‡
Non-Hispanic Whites			
1999–2000	161	2.9‡ (1.3 – 6.1)	346,000‡
2001–2002	259	11.9 (7.1 – 19.2)	1,357,000
2003–2004	230	9.4 (5.5 – 15.5)	1,088,000
2005–2006	186	10.3 (6.1 – 16.7)	1,157,000

‡ Estimate flagged: 30% ≤ RSE < 40% for the prevalence estimate.
§ Estimate suppressed: RSE ≥ 40% for the prevalence estimate.

Table 3.1.d.2. Serum ferritin: Prevalence by survey cycle

Prevalence (in percent) of low serum ferritin concentration (< 15 ng/mL) for women in the U.S. population aged 12–49 years, National Health and Nutrition Examination Survey, 1999–2006.

	Sample size	Prevalence (95% conf. interval)	Estimated total number of persons
Women, 12–49 years			
1999–2000	2,239	11.4 (9.4 – 13.9)	8,767,000
2001–2002	2,522	13.9 (12.2 – 15.8)	10,821,000
2003–2004	2,185	13.2 (10.7 – 16.3)	10,460,000
2005–2006	2,345	14.0 (12.6 – 15.5)	11,069,000
Age group			
12–19 years			
1999–2000	1,048	11.5 (8.5 – 15.3)	1,781,000
2001–2002	1,120	13.9 (11.2 – 17.1)	2,201,000
2003–2004	998	17.4 (12.8 – 23.3)	2,825,000
2005–2006	993	12.9 (10.0 – 16.5)	2,119,000
20–49 years			
1999–2000	1,191	11.4 (9.2 – 14.2)	6,986,000
2001–2002	1,402	13.9 (12.0 – 16.0)	8,620,000
2003–2004	1,187	12.2 (9.7 – 15.2)	7,670,000
2005–2006	1,352	14.2 (12.8 – 15.7)	8,938,000
Race/ethnicity			
Mexican Americans			
1999–2000	808	18.8 (12.3 – 27.5)	1,140,000
2001–2002	721	21.9 (18.8 – 25.4)	1,541,000
2003–2004	563	16.7 (11.7 – 23.2)	1,276,000
2005–2006	673	20.6 (15.3 – 27.2)	1,632,000
Non-Hispanic Blacks			
1999–2000	522	16.4 (11.2 – 23.4)	1,764,000
2001–2002	608	19.5 (12.3 – 29.6)	2,091,000
2003–2004	618	19.1 (16.4 – 22.0)	2,051,000
2005–2006	629	20.7 (17.5 – 24.4)	2,256,000
Non-Hispanic Whites			
1999–2000	677	9.1 (6.7 – 12.2)	4,741,000
2001–2002	977	11.6 (9.5 – 14.2)	6,025,000
2003–2004	839	11.8 (8.3 – 16.5)	6,032,000
2005–2006	834	10.9 (8.5 – 13.8)	5,500,000

Table 3.1.d.3. Serum ferritin: Prevalence by survey cycle

Prevalence (in percent) of low serum ferritin concentration (< 15 ng/mL) for males in the U.S. population aged 6 years and older, National Health and Nutrition Examination Survey, 1999–2002.

	Sample size	Prevalence (95% conf. interval)	Estimated total number of persons
Males, 6 years and older			
1999–2000	3,488	1.1 (0.6 – 2.0)	1,323,000
2001–2002	3,849	1.3 (0.9 – 1.7)	1,576,000
Age group			
6–11 years			
1999–2000	463	§	§
2001–2002	509	§	§
12–19 years			
1999–2000	1,078	2.1‡ (1.0 – 4.2)	336,000‡
2001–2002	1,094	2.8‡ (1.4 – 5.4)	463,000‡
20–39 years			
1999–2000	632	§	§
2001–2002	724	0.5‡ (0.2 – 1.0)	176,000‡
40–59 years			
1999–2000	570	§	§
2001–2002	770	§	§
60 years and older			
1999–2000	745	§	§
2001–2002	752	2.0 (1.1 – 3.4)	384,000
Race/ethnicity			
Mexican Americans			
1999–2000	1,196	1.0 (0.5 – 1.8)	91,000
2001–2002	958	0.7‡ (0.3 – 1.5)	77,000‡
Non-Hispanic Blacks			
1999–2000	781	§	§
2001–2002	921	1.3‡ (0.7 – 2.7)	187,000‡
Non-Hispanic Whites			
1999–2000	1,223	1.3‡ (0.6 – 2.7)	1,100,000‡
2001–2002	1,678	1.3 (0.9 – 1.9)	1,159,000

‡ Estimate flagged: 30% ≤ RSE < 40% for the prevalence estimate.

§ Estimate suppressed: RSE ≥ 40% for the prevalence estimate.

Table 3.1.d.4. Serum ferritin: Prevalence by survey cycle

Prevalence (in percent) of high serum ferritin concentration (> 150 ng/mL) for women in the U.S. population aged 12–49 years, National Health and Nutrition Examination Survey, 1999–2006.

	Sample size	Prevalence (95% conf. interval)	Estimated total number of persons
Women, 12–49 years			
1999–2000	2,239	5.3 (4.0 – 7.0)	4,069,000
2001–2002	2,522	5.6 (4.5 – 7.0)	4,374,000
2003–2004	2,185	6.0 (4.7 – 7.5)	4,711,000
2005–2006	2,345	4.4 (2.9 – 6.6)	3,470,000
Age group			
12–19 years			
1999–2000	1,048	§	§
2001–2002	1,120	§	§
2003–2004	998	§	§
2005–2006	993	1.4‡ (0.6 – 3.2)	237,000‡
20–49 years			
1999–2000	1,191	6.3 (4.8 – 8.3)	3,878,000
2001–2002	1,402	6.8 (5.3 – 8.5)	4,196,000
2003–2004	1,187	7.3 (5.9 – 9.1)	4,600,000
2005–2006	1,352	5.1 (3.2 – 7.9)	3,202,000
Race/ethnicity			
Mexican Americans			
1999–2000	808	3.7‡ (1.7 – 7.9)	224,000‡
2001–2002	721	3.5 (1.8 – 6.8)	249,000
2003–2004	563	5.6‡ (2.7 – 11.3)	429,000‡
2005–2006	673	2.9‡ (1.4 – 5.7)	226,000‡
Non-Hispanic Blacks			
1999–2000	522	7.8 (5.2 – 11.6)	840,000
2001–2002	608	7.7 (5.0 – 11.8)	828,000
2003–2004	618	8.3 (4.6 – 14.7)	895,000
2005–2006	629	5.7 (4.2 – 7.9)	625,000
Non-Hispanic Whites			
1999–2000	677	5.7 (4.1 – 8.0)	3,000,000
2001–2002	977	5.0 (3.4 – 7.2)	2,579,000
2003–2004	839	5.7 (4.1 – 7.8)	2,926,000
2005–2006	834	4.0 (2.5 – 6.3)	2,026,000

‡ Estimate flagged: 30% ≤ RSE < 40% for the prevalence estimate.
§ Estimate suppressed: RSE ≥ 40% for the prevalence estimate.

Table 3.1.d.5. Serum ferritin: Prevalence by survey cycle

Prevalence (in percent) of high serum ferritin concentration (> 200 ng/mL) for males in the U.S. population aged 12 years and older, National Health and Nutrition Examination Survey, 1999–2002.

	Sample size	Prevalence (95% conf. interval)	Estimated total number of persons
Males, 12 years and older			
1999–2000	3,025	31.8 (27.7 – 36.3)	34,391,000
2001–2002	3,340	32.7 (30.1 – 35.5)	36,644,000
Age group			
12–19 years			
1999–2000	1,078	3.3 (1.8 – 6.0)	538,000
2001–2002	1,094	1.7 (1.0 – 2.9)	283,000
20–39 years			
1999–2000	632	33.1 (26.8 – 40.1)	12,720,000
2001–2002	724	31.0 (27.1 – 35.1)	12,101,000
40–59 years			
1999–2000	570	39.9 (33.0 – 47.1)	13,748,000
2001–2002	770	44.5 (39.0 – 50.2)	16,443,000
60 years and older			
1999–2000	745	39.1 (33.2 – 45.2)	7,336,000
2001–2002	752	37.2 (32.3 – 42.4)	7,219,000
Race/ethnicity			
Mexican Americans			
1999–2000	998	27.4 (23.1 – 32.1)	2,155,000
2001–2002	819	25.8 (21.3 – 31.0)	2,430,000
Non-Hispanic Blacks			
1999–2000	652	37.8 (32.8 – 43.2)	4,574,000
2001–2002	746	33.7 (28.7 – 39.2)	4,079,000
Non-Hispanic Whites			
1999–2000	1,122	32.4 (27.5 – 37.6)	25,539,000
2001–2002	1,518	33.1 (29.9 – 36.5)	26,398,000

Table 3.2.a.1. Serum soluble transferrin receptor: Concentrations

Geometric mean and selected percentiles of serum concentrations (in mg/L) for children aged 1–5 years and women aged 12–49 years in the U.S. population, National Health and Nutrition Examination Survey, 2003–2006.

	Geometric mean (95% conf. interval)	Selected percentiles (95% conf. interval)						Sample size
		2.5th	5th	50th	95th	97.5th		
Total	3.57 (3.51 – 3.63)	1.94 (1.91 – 1.96)	2.11 (1.99 – 2.20)	3.46 (3.37 – 3.55)	6.04 (5.90 – 6.36)	7.06 (6.78 – 7.62)		5,856
(Children 1–5 years, women 12–49 years)								
Age group								
1–5 years (Children)	4.30 (4.24 – 4.37)	2.84 (2.73 – 2.90)	2.98 (2.91 – 3.06)	4.21 (4.11 – 4.29)	6.00 (5.91 – 6.42)	6.67 (6.45 – 7.17)		1,375
12–19 years (Women)	3.50 (3.44 – 3.55)	2.12 (1.96 – 2.21)	2.27 (2.20 – 2.35)	3.38 (3.32 – 3.46)	5.36 (5.22 – 5.82)	6.47 (5.95 – 7.32)		1,968
20–39 years (Women)	3.42 (3.36 – 3.49)	1.91 (1.85 – 1.94)	2.02 (1.95 – 2.13)	3.23 (3.15 – 3.32)	6.00 (5.75 – 6.36)	6.97 (6.50 – 7.88)		1,761
40–49 years (Women)	3.52 (3.38 – 3.65)	1.91 (1.71 – 1.95)	1.97 (1.93 – 2.05)	3.35 (3.17 – 3.56)	6.43 (6.07 – 6.98)	7.96 (7.12 – 9.13)		752
Gender								
Males (1–5 years)	4.38 (4.28 – 4.48)	2.93 (2.75 – 2.98)	3.06 (2.95 – 3.18)	4.26 (4.13 – 4.41)	6.25 (5.94 – 6.63)	6.80 (6.48 – 7.45)		698
Females (1–5, 12–49 years)	3.51 (3.45 – 3.57)	1.93 (1.91 – 1.95)	2.07 (1.97 – 2.18)	3.37 (3.29 – 3.47)	6.02 (5.83 – 6.36)	7.19 (6.79 – 7.67)		5,158
Race/ethnicity								
(Children 1–5 years, women 12–49 years)								
Mexican Americans	3.62 (3.53 – 3.72)	1.97 (1.93 – 2.03)	2.16 (2.06 – 2.24)	3.52 (3.42 – 3.62)	6.38 (5.92 – 7.10)	7.80 (6.96 – 8.77)		1,643
Non-Hispanic Blacks	4.19 (4.10 – 4.29)	2.17 (1.97 – 2.33)	2.47 (2.31 – 2.57)	3.97 (3.91 – 4.04)	8.02 (7.31 – 9.69)	10.3 (9.78 – 12.6)		1,634
Non-Hispanic Whites	3.43 (3.35 – 3.52)	1.92 (1.89 – 1.94)	2.02 (1.94 – 2.17)	3.32 (3.22 – 3.44)	5.59 (5.28 – 6.07)	6.33 (5.96 – 7.33)		2,048

Figure 3.2.a. Serum soluble transferrin receptor: Concentrations by age group

Geometric mean (95% confidence interval), National Health and Nutrition Examination Survey, 2003–2006

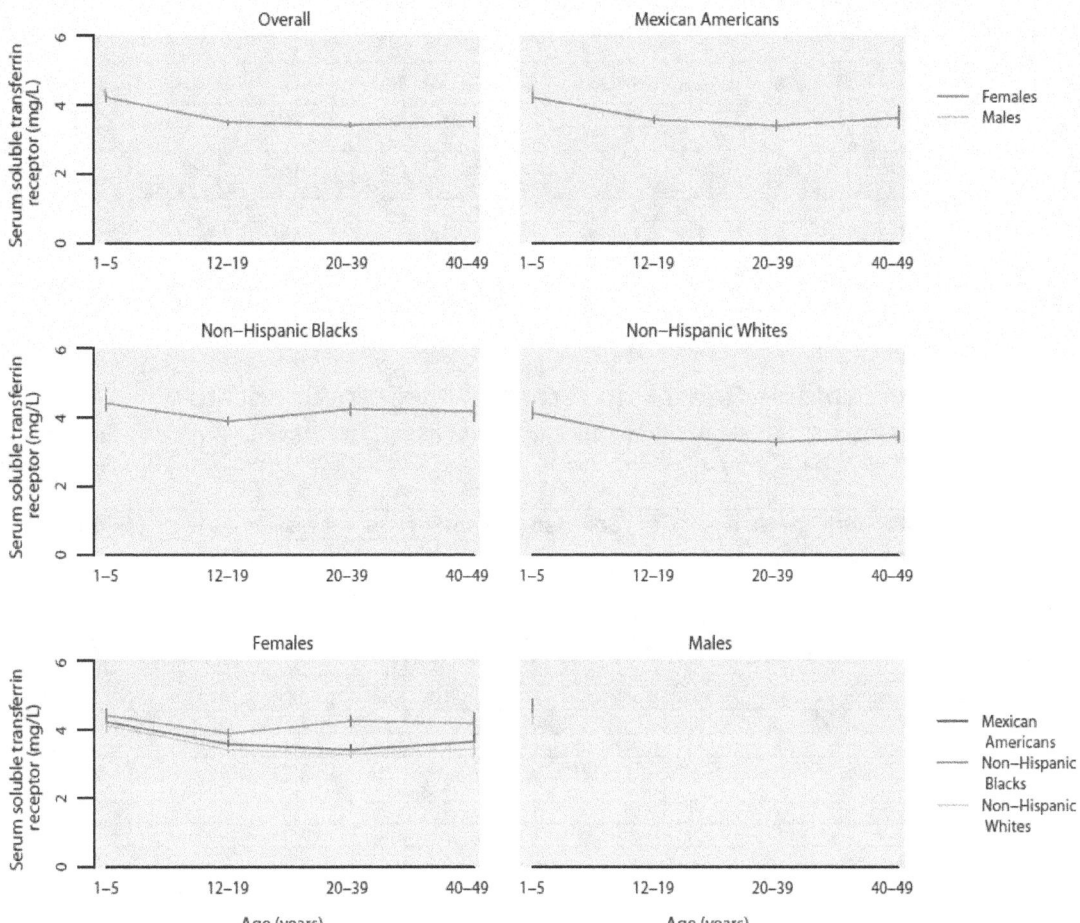

Table 3.2.a.2. Serum soluble transferrin receptor: Total population

Geometric mean and selected percentiles of serum concentrations (in mg/L) for children aged 1–5 years and women aged 12–49 years in the U.S. population, National Health and Nutrition Examination Survey, 2003–2006.

	Geometric mean (95% conf. interval)	Selected percentiles (95% conf. interval)						Sample size
		5th		50th		95th		
Males and Females								
Total, Children 1–5 years, women 12–49 years	3.57	(3.51 – 3.63)	2.11	(1.99 – 2.20)	3.46	(3.37 – 3.55)	6.04 (5.90 – 6.36)	5,856
1–5 years	4.30	(4.24 – 4.37)	2.98	(2.91 – 3.06)	4.21	(4.11 – 4.29)	6.00 (5.91 – 6.42)	1,375
Males								
1–5 years	4.38	(4.28 – 4.48)	3.06	(2.95 – 3.18)	4.26	(4.13 – 4.41)	6.25 (5.94 – 6.63)	698
Females								
Total, 1–5, 12–49 years	3.51	(3.45 – 3.57)	2.07	(1.97 – 2.18)	3.37	(3.29 – 3.47)	6.02 (5.83 – 6.36)	5,158
1–5 years	4.22	(4.12 – 4.31)	2.90	(2.83 – 3.00)	4.10	(3.99 – 4.27)	5.91 (5.68 – 6.16)	677
12–19 years	3.50	(3.44 – 3.55)	2.27	(2.20 – 2.35)	3.38	(3.32 – 3.46)	5.36 (5.22 – 5.82)	1,968
20–39 years	3.42	(3.36 – 3.49)	2.02	(1.95 – 2.13)	3.23	(3.15 – 3.32)	6.00 (5.75 – 6.36)	1,761
40–49 years	3.52	(3.38 – 3.65)	1.97	(1.93 – 2.05)	3.35	(3.17 – 3.56)	6.43 (6.07 – 6.98)	752

Table 3.2.a.3. Serum soluble transferrin receptor: Mexican Americans

Geometric mean and selected percentiles of serum concentrations (in mg/L) for Mexican-American children aged 1–5 years and women aged 12–49 years in the U.S. population, National Health and Nutrition Examination Survey, 2003–2006.

	Geometric mean (95% conf. interval)	Selected percentiles (95% conf. interval)						Sample size
		5th		50th		95th		
Males and Females								
Total, Children 1–5 years, women 12–49 years	3.62	(3.53 – 3.72)	2.16	(2.06 – 2.24)	3.52	(3.42 – 3.62)	6.38 (5.92 – 7.10)	1,643
1–5 years	4.30	(4.17 – 4.43)	2.99	(2.94 – 3.07)	4.15	(3.99 – 4.32)	6.40 (6.06 – 7.18)	422
Males								
1–5 years	4.38	(4.21 – 4.56)	3.09†	(2.90 – 3.21)	4.18	(4.00 – 4.36)	6.89† (6.00 – 8.30)	203
Females								
Total, 1–5, 12–49 years	3.55	(3.45 – 3.65)	2.13	(2.01 – 2.22)	3.41	(3.27 – 3.54)	6.32 (5.85 – 7.25)	1,440
1–5 years	4.21	(4.08 – 4.35)	2.93†	(2.58 – 3.07)	4.10	(3.94 – 4.31)	6.01† (5.66 – 7.53)	219
12–19 years	3.57	(3.46 – 3.68)	2.26	(2.18 – 2.36)	3.44	(3.33 – 3.59)	5.92 (5.27 – 6.92)	637
20–39 years	3.40	(3.27 – 3.54)	2.02	(1.93 – 2.12)	3.19	(3.01 – 3.40)	5.99 (5.62 – 7.63)	430
40–49 years	3.63	(3.32 – 3.96)	2.22†	(1.80 – 2.30)	3.34	(3.02 – 3.71)	7.75† (6.29 – 11.7)	154

† Estimate is subject to greater uncertainty due to small cell size.

Table 3.2.a.4. Serum soluble transferrin receptor: Non-Hispanic blacks

Geometric mean and selected percentiles of serum concentrations (in mg/L) for non-Hispanic black children aged 1–5 years and women aged 12–49 years in the U.S. population, National Health and Nutrition Examination Survey, 2003–2006.

	Geometric mean (95% conf. interval)	Selected percentiles (95% conf. interval)			Sample size
		5th	50th	95th	
Males and Females					
Total, Children 1–5 years, women 12–49 years	4.19 (4.10 – 4.29)	2.47 (2.31 – 2.57)	3.97 (3.91 – 4.04)	8.02 (7.31 – 9.69)	1,634
1–5 years	4.55 (4.43 – 4.67)	3.11 (3.02 – 3.29)	4.37 (4.26 – 4.56)	6.68 (6.31 – 7.16)	401
Males					
1–5 years	4.70 (4.56 – 4.86)	3.24† (3.06 – 3.37)	4.58 (4.30 – 4.89)	6.76† (6.42 – 7.77)	199
Females					
Total, 1–5, 12–49 years	4.15 (4.05 – 4.26)	2.43 (2.27 – 2.55)	3.94 (3.86 – 4.00)	8.49 (7.37 – 9.87)	1,435
1–5 years	4.40 (4.21 – 4.59)	3.05† (2.73 – 3.23)	4.26 (4.00 – 4.47)	6.49† (5.96 – 7.16)	202
12–19 years	3.88 (3.77 – 4.00)	2.42 (2.25 – 2.52)	3.76 (3.66 – 3.87)	6.46 (6.14 – 7.07)	668
20–39 years	4.23 (4.08 – 4.39)	2.41 (2.06 – 2.58)	3.97 (3.85 – 4.15)	9.70 (7.33 – 10.5)	368
40–49 years	4.17 (3.89 – 4.47)	2.34† (1.94 – 2.61)	3.87 (3.51 – 4.08)	9.72† (8.28 – 13.2)	197

† Estimate is subject to greater uncertainty due to small cell size.

Table 3.2.a.5. Serum soluble transferrin receptor: Non-Hispanic whites

Geometric mean and selected percentiles of serum concentrations (in mg/L) for non-Hispanic white children aged 1–5 years and women aged 12–49 years in the U.S. population, National Health and Nutrition Examination Survey, 2003–2006.

	Geometric mean (95% conf. interval)	Selected percentiles (95% conf. interval)			Sample size
		5th	50th	95th	
Males and Females					
Total, Children 1–5 years, women 12–49 years	3.43 (3.35 – 3.52)	2.02 (1.94 – 2.17)	3.32 (3.22 – 3.44)	5.59 (5.28 – 6.07)	2,048
1–5 years	4.22 (4.11 – 4.32)	2.91 (2.78 – 3.04)	4.15 (4.01 – 4.28)	5.90 (5.63 – 6.19)	391
Males					
1–5 years	4.31 (4.16 – 4.46)	2.98† (2.91 – 3.15)	4.22 (3.99 – 4.48)	5.95† (5.67 – 6.83)	215
Females					
Total, 1–5, 12–49 years	3.38 (3.30 – 3.47)	2.00 (1.97 – 2.05)	3.25 (3.14 – 3.37)	5.53 (5.18 – 6.08)	1,833
1–5 years	4.11 (3.96 – 4.27)	2.85† (2.64 – 2.97)	4.05 (3.88 – 4.27)	5.64† (5.36 – 6.64)	176
12–19 years	3.40 (3.33 – 3.46)	2.25 (2.12 – 2.35)	3.29 (3.20 – 3.37)	4.98 (4.78 – 5.49)	514
20–39 years	3.27 (3.18 – 3.36)	1.97 (1.94 – 2.01)	3.10 (3.00 – 3.20)	5.44 (4.96 – 6.01)	806
40–49 years	3.42 (3.26 – 3.59)	1.96 (1.92 – 2.01)	3.31 (3.03 – 3.57)	6.02 (5.41 – 6.76)	337

† Estimate is subject to greater uncertainty due to small cell size.

Table 3.2.b. Serum soluble transferrin receptor: Concentrations by survey cycle

Geometric mean and selected percentiles of serum concentrations (in mg/L) for children aged 1–5 and women aged 12–49 years in the U.S. population, National Health and Nutrition Examination Survey, 2003–2006.

	Geometric mean (95% conf. interval)	Selected percentiles (95% conf. interval)			Sample size
		5th	50th	95th	
Total (Children 1–5 years, women 12–49 years)					
2003–2004	3.63 (3.54 – 3.71)	2.06 (1.94 – 2.36)	3.55 (3.43 – 3.66)	5.96 (5.75 – 6.41)	2,831
2005–2006	3.51 (3.42 – 3.60)	2.13 (2.00 – 2.20)	3.36 (3.28 – 3.47)	6.16 (5.77 – 6.63)	3,025
Age group					
1–5 years (Children)					
2003–2004	4.44 (4.34 – 4.55)	3.28 (3.13 – 3.38)	4.33 (4.21 – 4.45)	5.99 (5.83 – 6.83)	696
2005–2006	4.16 (4.04 – 4.27)	2.86 (2.79 – 2.93)	4.06 (3.89 – 4.21)	6.08 (5.79 – 6.48)	679
12–19 years (Women)					
2003–2004	3.57 (3.48 – 3.66)	2.29 (2.15 – 2.46)	3.49 (3.32 – 3.62)	5.72 (5.26 – 6.39)	975
2005–2006	3.43 (3.36 – 3.49)	2.26 (2.13 – 2.35)	3.33 (3.25 – 3.38)	5.23 (5.01 – 5.81)	993
20–39 years (Women)					
2003–2004	3.49 (3.43 – 3.56)	2.02 (1.93 – 2.27)	3.33 (3.23 – 3.41)	5.96 (5.73 – 6.32)	803
2005–2006	3.35 (3.24 – 3.47)	2.02 (1.90 – 2.13)	3.16 (3.04 – 3.31)	6.07 (5.54 – 6.57)	958
40–49 years (Women)					
2003–2004	3.49 (3.28 – 3.71)	1.96 (1.94 – 1.99)	3.33 (2.98 – 3.63)	6.01 (5.39 – 7.56)	357
2005–2006	3.54 (3.36 – 3.74)	2.05 (1.66 – 2.23)	3.37 (3.19 – 3.65)	6.86 (6.22 – 7.89)	395
Gender					
Males (1–5 years)					
2003–2004	4.54 (4.39 – 4.70)	3.32 (3.20 – 3.41)	4.40 (4.23 – 4.56)	6.38 (5.94 – 7.23)	358
2005–2006	4.21 (4.05 – 4.38)	2.94 (2.74 – 3.02)	4.16 (3.90 – 4.34)	6.04 (5.69 – 6.52)	340
Females (1–5, 12–49 years)					
2003–2004	3.56 (3.47 – 3.65)	2.03 (1.93 – 2.32)	3.45 (3.31 – 3.59)	5.94 (5.64 – 6.37)	2,473
2005–2006	3.46 (3.37 – 3.55)	2.11 (1.96 – 2.19)	3.31 (3.22 – 3.39)	6.17 (5.77 – 6.69)	2,685
Race/ethnicity (Children 1–5 years, women 12–49 years)					
Mexican Americans					
2003–2004	3.63 (3.53 – 3.73)	2.18 (1.99 – 2.37)	3.59 (3.44 – 3.80)	5.88 (5.49 – 6.42)	734
2005–2006	3.62 (3.46 – 3.79)	2.15 (2.02 – 2.24)	3.46 (3.28 – 3.62)	7.32 (6.16 – 8.70)	909
Non-Hispanic Blacks					
2003–2004	4.18 (4.04 – 4.33)	2.54 (2.33 – 2.65)	3.96 (3.89 – 4.06)	7.97 (6.94 – 9.88)	832
2005–2006	4.20 (4.08 – 4.33)	2.36 (2.19 – 2.56)	4.00 (3.86 – 4.13)	8.17 (7.15 – 10.4)	802
Non-Hispanic Whites					
2003–2004	3.51 (3.37 – 3.65)	1.99 (1.98 – 2.03)	3.44 (3.22 – 3.63)	5.68 (5.16 – 6.38)	1,026
2005–2006	3.36 (3.27 – 3.45)	2.09 (1.91 – 2.19)	3.24 (3.15 – 3.33)	5.55 (5.11 – 6.40)	1,022

Figure 3.2.b. Serum soluble transferrin receptor: Concentrations by survey cycle

Selected percentiles in mg/L (95% confidence intervals), National Health and Nutrition Examination Survey, 2003–2006

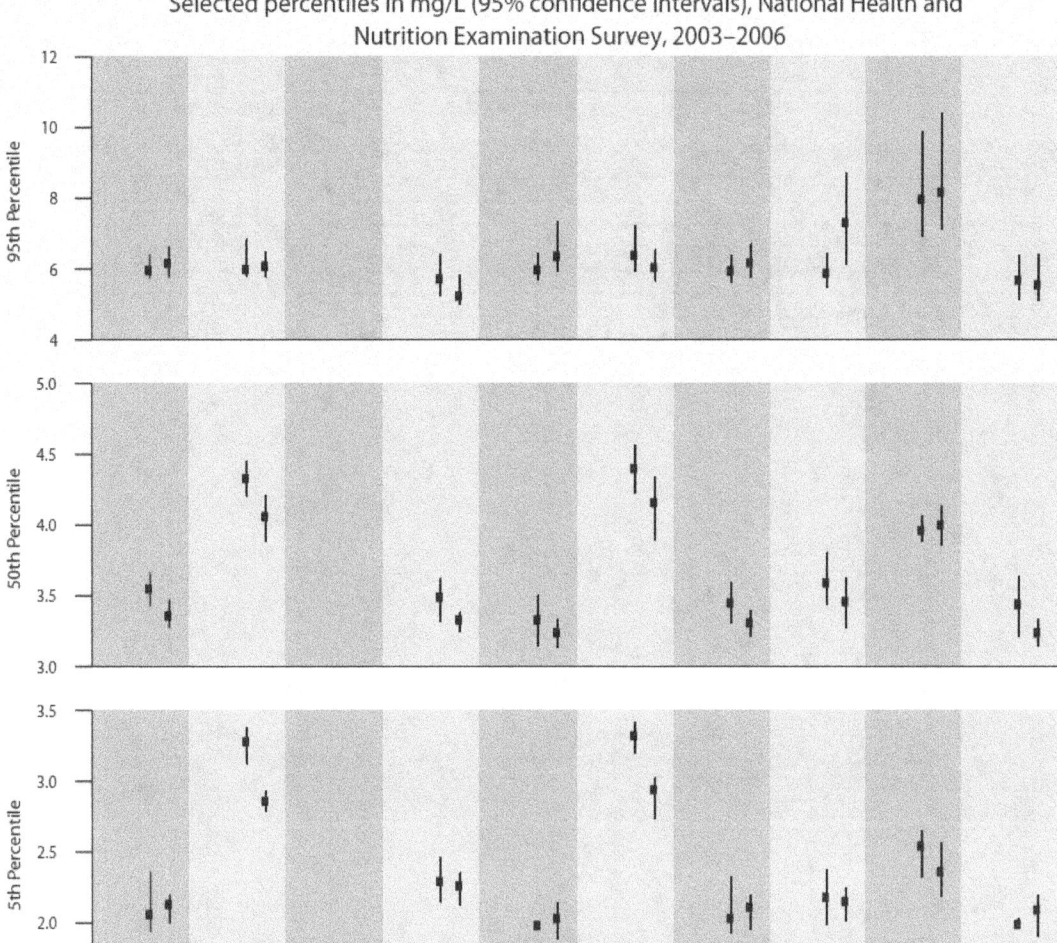

Table 3.2.c. Serum soluble transferrin receptor: Prevalence

Prevalence (in percent) of high serum soluble transferrin receptor concentration (> 4.4 mg/L) for women in the U.S. population aged 12–49 years, National Health and Nutrition Examination Survey, 2003–2006.

	Sample size	Prevalence (95% conf. interval)	Estimated total number of persons
Women, 12–49 years	4,481	18.9 (17.0 – 20.9)	14,918,000
Age group			
12–19 years	1,968	16.9 (14.7 – 19.3)	2,741,000
20–49 years	2,513	19.4 (17.3 – 21.6)	12,159,000
Race/ethnicity			
Mexican Americans	1,221	19.0 (15.5 – 23.0)	1,451,000
Non-Hispanic Blacks	1,233	34.9 (31.6 – 38.4)	3,756,000
Non-Hispanic Whites	1,657	16.0 (13.6 – 18.7)	8,177,000

Table 3.2.d. Serum soluble transferrin receptor: Prevalence by survey cycle

Prevalence (in percent) of high serum soluble transferrin receptor concentration (> 4.4 mg/L) for women in the U.S. population aged 12–49 years, National Health and Nutrition Examination Survey, 2003–2006.

	Sample size	Prevalence (95% conf. interval)	Estimated total number of persons
Women, 12–49 years			
2003–2004	2,135	18.8 (16.3 – 21.6)	14,862,000
2005–2006	2,346	18.9 (16.0 – 22.3)	15,017,000
Age group			
12–19 years			
2003–2004	975	17.4 (14.0 – 21.3)	2,818,000
2005–2006	993	16.4 (13.5 – 19.8)	2,694,000
20–49 years			
2003–2004	1,160	19.2 (16.3 – 22.4)	12,031,000
2005–2006	1,353	19.6 (16.4 – 23.2)	12,296,000
Race/ethnicity			
Mexican Americans			
2003–2004	547	18.7 (13.3 – 25.7)	1,435,000
2005–2006	674	19.2 (14.6 – 24.7)	1,516,000
Non-Hispanic Blacks			
2003–2004	604	33.2 (28.9 – 37.7)	3,568,000
2005–2006	629	36.7 (31.6 – 42.1)	3,988,000
Non-Hispanic Whites			
2003–2004	823	16.1 (12.5 – 20.5)	8,258,000
2005–2006	834	15.8 (12.6 – 19.6)	7,991,000

Table 3.3.a.1. Body iron

Arithmetic mean and selected percentiles of body iron (in mg/kg) for children aged 1–5 years and women aged 12–49 years in the U.S. population, National Health and Nutrition Examination Survey, 2003–2006.

	Arithmetic mean (95% conf. interval)	Selected percentiles (95% conf. interval)					Sample size
		2.5th	5th	50th	95th	97.5th	
Total	5.16 (5.01 – 5.31)	-3.75 (-4.05 – -3.41)	-1.83 (-2.60 – -1.41)	5.43 (5.32 – 5.58)	10.8 (10.6 – 11.2)	12.0 (11.5 – 12.5)	5,845
(Children 1-5 years, women 12-49 years)							
Age group							
1-5 years (Children)	3.47 (3.31 – 3.63)	-2.00 (-3.06 – -1.34)	-.648 (-1.26 – -.159)	3.64 (3.44 – 3.79)	6.89 (6.72 – 7.06)	7.36 (7.17 – 7.87)	1,369
12-19 years (Women)	4.49 (4.26 – 4.72)	-3.37 (-4.28 – -2.61)	-1.59 (-2.69 – -.763)	4.96 (4.71 – 5.16)	8.84 (8.35 – 9.34)	9.61 (9.23 – 10.2)	1,967
20-39 years (Women)	5.51 (5.29 – 5.73)	-3.76 (-4.09 – -3.12)	-1.75 (-2.81 – -1.22)	5.88 (5.69 – 6.17)	10.7 (10.2 – 11.1)	11.6 (11.0 – 12.4)	1,758
40-49 years (Women)	5.88 (5.46 – 6.30)	-4.43 (-5.33 – -3.76)	-2.85 (-3.78 – -1.84)	6.37 (5.86 – 6.82)	12.4 (11.7 – 12.9)	13.1 (12.7 – 14.2)	751
Gender							
Males (1–5 years)	3.38 (3.17 – 3.59)	-1.69 (-3.30 – -1.25)	-.715 (-1.36 – -.262)	3.52 (3.32 – 3.80)	6.91 (6.65 – 7.30)	7.33 (6.93 – 8.12)	695
Females (1–5, 12–49 years)	5.30 (5.13 – 5.46)	-3.78 (-4.06 – -3.50)	-2.01 (-2.70 – -1.43)	5.65 (5.49 – 5.76)	11.0 (10.7 – 11.4)	12.1 (11.6 – 12.6)	5,150
Race/ethnicity							
(Children 1-5 years, women 12-49 years)							
Mexican Americans	4.49 (4.10 – 4.88)	-4.49 (-5.27 – -3.69)	-3.16 (-3.81 – -2.03)	4.75 (4.44 – 5.12)	10.4 (9.73 – 11.2)	11.4 (10.8 – 12.9)	1,641
Non-Hispanic Blacks	4.37 (4.10 – 4.64)	-5.79 (-6.99 – -4.66)	-3.79 (-4.61 – -2.88)	4.66 (4.30 – 5.05)	11.0 (10.3 – 11.6)	12.1 (11.3 – 13.2)	1,633
Non-Hispanic Whites	5.46 (5.24 – 5.69)	-3.17 (-3.99 – -2.25)	-1.21 (-2.34 – -.516)	5.66 (5.49 – 5.81)	10.9 (10.5 – 11.5)	12.0 (11.5 – 12.7)	2,041

Figure 3.3.a. Body iron: by age group

Arithmetic mean (95% confidence interval), National Health and Nutrition Examination Survey, 2003–2006

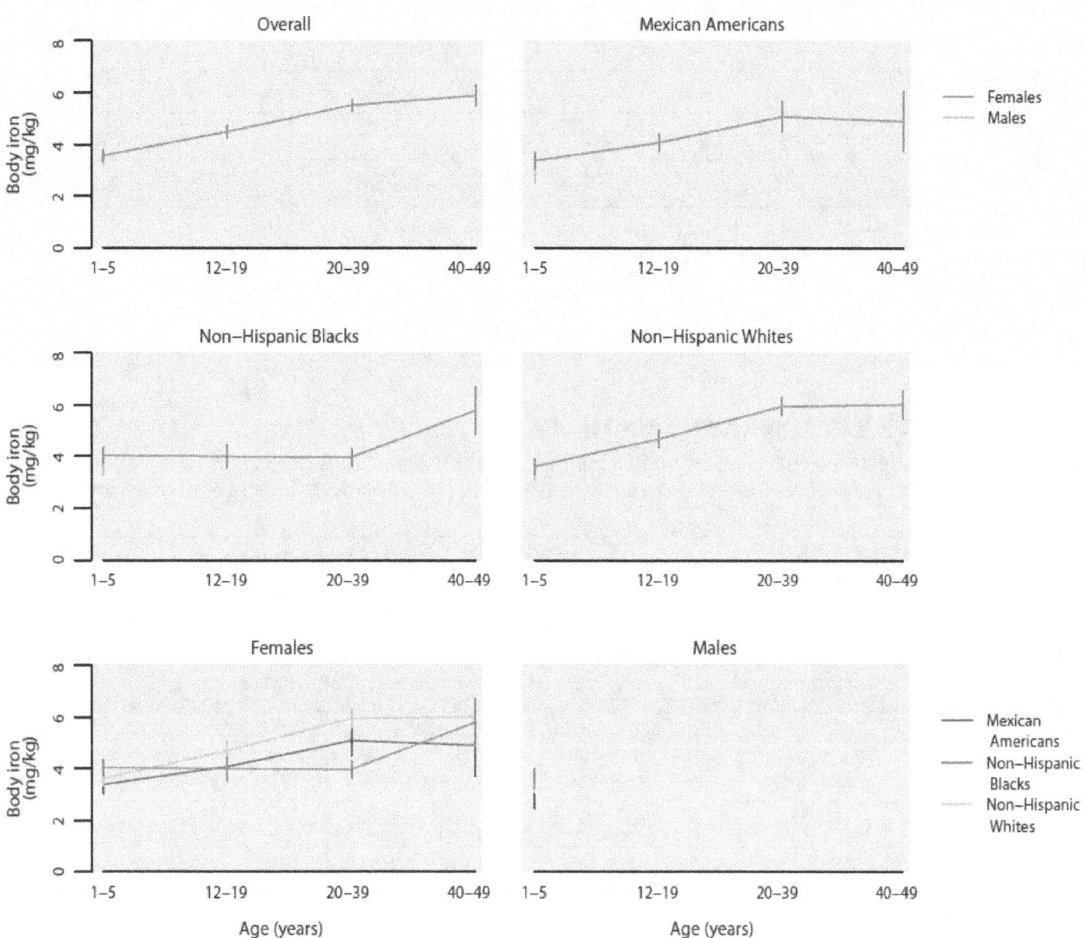

Table 3.3.a.2. Body iron: Total population

Arithmetic mean and selected percentiles of body iron (in mg/kg) for children aged 1–5 years and women aged 12–49 years in the U.S. population, National Health and Nutrition Examination Survey, 2003–2006.

| | Arithmetic mean (95% conf. interval) | Selected percentiles (95% conf. interval) | | | Sample size |
		5th	50th	95th	
Males and Females					
Total, Children 1–5 years, women 12–49 years	5.16 (5.01 – 5.31)	-1.83 (-2.60 – -1.41)	5.43 (5.32 – 5.58)	10.8 (10.6 – 11.2)	5,845
1–5 years	3.47 (3.31 – 3.63)	-.648 (-1.26 – -.159)	3.64 (3.44 – 3.79)	6.89 (6.72 – 7.06)	1,369
Males					
1–5 years	3.38 (3.17 – 3.59)	-.715 (-1.36 – -.262)	3.52 (3.32 – 3.80)	6.91 (6.65 – 7.30)	695
Females					
Total, Children 1–5 years, women 12–49 years	5.30 (5.13 – 5.46)	-2.01 (-2.70 – -1.43)	5.65 (5.49 – 5.76)	11.0 (10.7 – 11.4)	5,150
1–5 years	3.57 (3.36 – 3.78)	-.196 (-2.11 – .411)	3.70 (3.41 – 4.04)	6.89 (6.67 – 7.27)	674
12–19 years	4.49 (4.26 – 4.72)	-1.59 (-2.69 – -.763)	4.96 (4.71 – 5.16)	8.84 (8.35 – 9.34)	1,967
20–39 years	5.51 (5.29 – 5.73)	-1.75 (-2.81 – -1.22)	5.88 (5.69 – 6.17)	10.7 (10.2 – 11.1)	1,758
40–49 years	5.88 (5.46 – 6.30)	-2.85 (-3.78 – -1.84)	6.37 (5.86 – 6.82)	12.4 (11.7 – 12.9)	751

Table 3.3.a.3. Body iron: Mexican Americans

Arithmetic mean and selected percentiles of body iron (in mg/kg) for Mexican American children aged 1–5 years and women aged 12–49 years in the U.S. population, National Health and Nutrition Examination Survey, 2003–2006.

| | Arithmetic mean (95% conf. interval) | Selected percentiles (95% conf. interval) | | | Sample size |
		5th	50th	95th	
Males and Females					
Total, Children 1–5 years, women 12–49 years	4.49 (4.10 – 4.88)	-3.16 (-3.81 – -2.03)	4.75 (4.44 – 5.12)	10.4 (9.73 – 11.2)	1,641
1–5 years	3.16 (2.84 – 3.48)	-2.09 (-3.35 – -1.36)	3.48 (3.13 – 3.78)	6.99 (6.57 – 7.93)	422
Males					
1–5 years	2.95 (2.48 – 3.41)	-2.71† (-4.72 – -1.59)	3.34 (2.99 – 3.77)	6.92† (5.95 – 9.30)	203
Females					
Total, Children 1–5 years, women 12–49 years	4.66 (4.23 – 5.10)	-3.17 (-3.82 – -1.90)	5.02 (4.60 – 5.44)	10.6 (9.79 – 11.4)	1,438
1–5 years	3.38 (3.04 – 3.72)	-1.88† (-2.87 – -.828)	3.55 (3.22 – 4.15)	6.99† (6.78 – 8.13)	219
12–19 years	4.07 (3.76 – 4.39)	-1.76 (-3.29 – -.981)	4.46 (4.26 – 4.68)	8.99 (8.51 – 9.69)	637
20–39 years	5.07 (4.48 – 5.67)	-3.15 (-4.31 – -1.66)	5.72 (4.93 – 6.28)	10.7 (9.89 – 12.0)	429
40–49 years	4.89 (3.74 – 6.04)	-4.89† (-6.96 – -3.40)	5.33 (4.42 – 6.59)	11.1† (10.4 – 15.1)	153

† Estimate is subject to greater uncertainty due to small cell size.

Table 3.3.a.4. Body iron: Non-Hispanic blacks

Arithmetic mean and selected percentiles of body iron (in mg/kg) for non-Hispanic black children aged 1–5 years and women aged 12–49 years in the U.S. population, National Health and Nutrition Examination Survey, 2003–2006.

	Arithmetic mean (95% conf. interval)	Selected percentiles (95% conf. interval) 5th	Selected percentiles (95% conf. interval) 50th	Selected percentiles (95% conf. interval) 95th	Sample size
Males and Females					
Total, Children 1–5 years, women 12–49 years	4.37 (4.10 – 4.64)	-3.79 (-4.61 – -2.88)	4.66 (4.30 – 5.05)	11.0 (10.3 – 11.6)	1,633
1–5 years	3.83 (3.56 – 4.09)	-.115 (-.906 – .776)	3.95 (3.78 – 4.25)	7.51 (6.80 – 8.03)	401
Males					
1–5 years	3.63 (3.25 – 4.00)	-.328† (-2.15 – .070)	3.77 (3.17 – 4.19)	6.90† (6.55 – 8.03)	199
Females					
Total, Children 1–5 years, women 12–49 years	4.43 (4.14 – 4.72)	-3.94 (-4.87 – -3.04)	4.80 (4.35 – 5.16)	11.0 (10.4 – 11.9)	1,434
1–5 years	4.03 (3.73 – 4.34)	.658† (-.541 – .981)	4.17 (3.92 – 4.35)	7.71† (6.93 – 8.09)	202
12–19 years	3.99 (3.56 – 4.42)	-2.53 (-3.91 – -1.71)	4.46 (4.09 – 4.79)	8.91 (8.38 – 9.43)	667
20–39 years	3.96 (3.63 – 4.28)	-4.12 (-5.73 – -3.46)	4.35 (4.08 – 4.86)	9.96 (9.46 – 11.2)	368
40–49 years	5.78 (4.86 – 6.69)	-5.62† (-9.51 – -2.80)	6.68 (5.78 – 7.32)	12.9† (11.9 – 15.4)	197

† Estimate is subject to greater uncertainty due to small cell size.

Table 3.3.a.5. Body iron: Non-Hispanic whites

Arithmetic mean and selected percentiles of body iron (in mg/kg) for non-Hispanic white children aged 1–5 years and women aged 12–49 years in the U.S. population, National Health and Nutrition Examination Survey, 2003–2006.

	Arithmetic mean (95% conf. interval)	Selected percentiles (95% conf. interval) 5th	Selected percentiles (95% conf. interval) 50th	Selected percentiles (95% conf. interval) 95th	Sample size
Males and Females					
Total, Children 1–5 years, women 12–49 years	5.46 (5.24 – 5.69)	-1.21 (-2.34 – -.516)	5.66 (5.49 – 5.81)	10.9 (10.5 – 11.5)	2,041
1–5 years	3.51 (3.27 – 3.74)	-.264 (-1.28 – .300)	3.56 (3.34 – 3.92)	6.89 (6.64 – 7.00)	385
Males					
1–5 years	3.42 (3.09 – 3.75)	-.571† (-1.39 – .140)	3.50 (3.06 – 4.01)	6.91† (6.45 – 7.33)	212
Females					
Total, Children 1–5 years, women 12–49 years	5.60 (5.36 – 5.84)	-1.27 (-2.60 – -.546)	5.81 (5.66 – 6.02)	11.0 (10.7 – 11.5)	1,829
1–5 years	3.61 (3.33 – 3.89)	.062† (-3.13 – .791)	3.67 (3.35 – 4.03)	6.70† (6.45 – 7.27)	173
12–19 years	4.68 (4.35 – 5.02)	-1.48 (-3.15 – -.417)	5.17 (4.86 – 5.50)	8.84 (8.29 – 9.62)	514
20–39 years	5.93 (5.58 – 6.28)	-.640 (-2.73 – .779)	6.16 (5.82 – 6.59)	10.7 (10.2 – 11.4)	805
40–49 years	6.01 (5.45 – 6.57)	-2.26 (-3.78 – -1.01)	6.36 (5.77 – 6.99)	12.4 (11.6 – 13.0)	337

† Estimate is subject to greater uncertainty due to small cell size.

Table 3.3.b. Body iron: By survey cycle

Arithmetic mean and selected percentiles of body iron (in mg/kg) for children aged 1–5 years and women aged 12–49 years in the U.S. population, National Health and Nutrition Examination Survey, 2003–2006.

	Arithmetic mean (95% conf. interval)	Selected percentiles (95% conf. interval)			Sample size
		5th	50th	95th	
Total (Children 1–5 years, women 12–49 years)					
2003–2004	5.21 (5.03 – 5.39)	-1.60 (-2.96 – -.854)	5.43 (5.32 – 5.55)	10.9 (10.7 – 11.3)	2,826
2005–2006	5.11 (4.85 – 5.38)	-2.04 (-2.73 – -1.43)	5.43 (5.08 – 5.71)	10.8 (10.2 – 11.5)	3,019
Age group					
1–5 years (Children)					
2003–2004	3.25 (3.01 – 3.50)	-.651 (-1.73 – .144)	3.34 (2.99 – 3.66)	6.55 (6.39 – 6.73)	694
2005–2006	3.70 (3.47 – 3.94)	-.642 (-1.65 – -.080)	3.91 (3.70 – 4.14)	7.00 (6.92 – 7.33)	675
12–19 years (Women)					
2003–2004	4.27 (3.89 – 4.66)	-2.23 (-3.93 – -.653)	4.71 (4.27 – 5.11)	8.89 (8.29 – 9.73)	974
2005–2006	4.71 (4.45 – 4.96)	-1.45 (-2.64 – -.527)	5.10 (4.85 – 5.33)	8.53 (8.31 – 9.55)	993
20–39 years (Women)					
2003–2004	5.61 (5.33 – 5.89)	-1.21 (-2.14 – -.835)	6.07 (5.69 – 6.25)	10.4 (9.92 – 11.1)	801
2005–2006	5.42 (5.04 – 5.79)	-2.55 (-3.91 – -1.41)	5.83 (5.44 – 6.27)	10.8 (10.2 – 11.9)	957
40–49 years (Women)					
2003–2004	6.22 (5.61 – 6.82)	-3.28 (-3.80 – -1.85)	6.85 (6.21 – 7.33)	12.7 (12.0 – 13.4)	357
2005–2006	5.55 (4.89 – 6.21)	-2.47 (-4.61 – -1.59)	5.96 (5.33 – 6.66)	11.8 (11.1 – 13.1)	394
Gender					
Males (1–5 years)					
2003–2004	3.11 (2.76 – 3.46)	-.719 (-1.89 – -.152)	3.13 (2.70 – 3.65)	6.21 (5.74 – 6.92)	358
2005–2006	3.68 (3.41 – 3.95)	-.746 (-1.32 – -.268)	3.91 (3.48 – 4.41)	7.24 (6.81 – 8.27)	337
Females (1–5, 12–49 years)					
2003–2004	5.38 (5.18 – 5.58)	-1.76 (-3.18 – -.854)	5.66 (5.50 – 5.80)	11.0 (10.7 – 11.5)	2,468
2005–2006	5.22 (4.94 – 5.49)	-2.20 (-2.98 – -1.52)	5.60 (5.32 – 5.84)	10.9 (10.2 – 11.6)	2,682
Race/ethnicity (Children 1–5 years, women 12–49 years)					
Mexican Americans					
2003–2004	4.74 (4.13 – 5.35)	-2.05 (-3.57 – -1.13)	4.94 (4.28 – 5.64)	10.6 (9.69 – 12.5)	734
2005–2006	4.26 (3.78 – 4.73)	-3.70 (-5.21 – -2.73)	4.71 (4.31 – 5.05)	9.91 (9.73 – 10.8)	907
Non-Hispanic Blacks					
2003–2004	4.48 (4.02 – 4.94)	-3.79 (-5.06 – -2.47)	4.68 (4.15 – 5.24)	11.1 (9.95 – 12.7)	831
2005–2006	4.26 (3.94 – 4.58)	-3.96 (-4.99 – -2.62)	4.66 (4.16 – 5.17)	10.6 (9.86 – 11.4)	802
Non-Hispanic Whites					
2003–2004	5.45 (5.14 – 5.75)	-.903 (-3.69 – .285)	5.57 (5.43 – 5.76)	11.0 (10.5 – 11.6)	1,023
2005–2006	5.48 (5.12 – 5.85)	-1.39 (-2.45 – -.593)	5.70 (5.42 – 6.01)	10.9 (10.2 – 12.0)	1,018

Figure 3.3.b. Body iron: By Survey Cycle

Selected percentiles in mg/kg (95% confidence intervals), National Health and Nutrition Examination Survey, 2003–2006

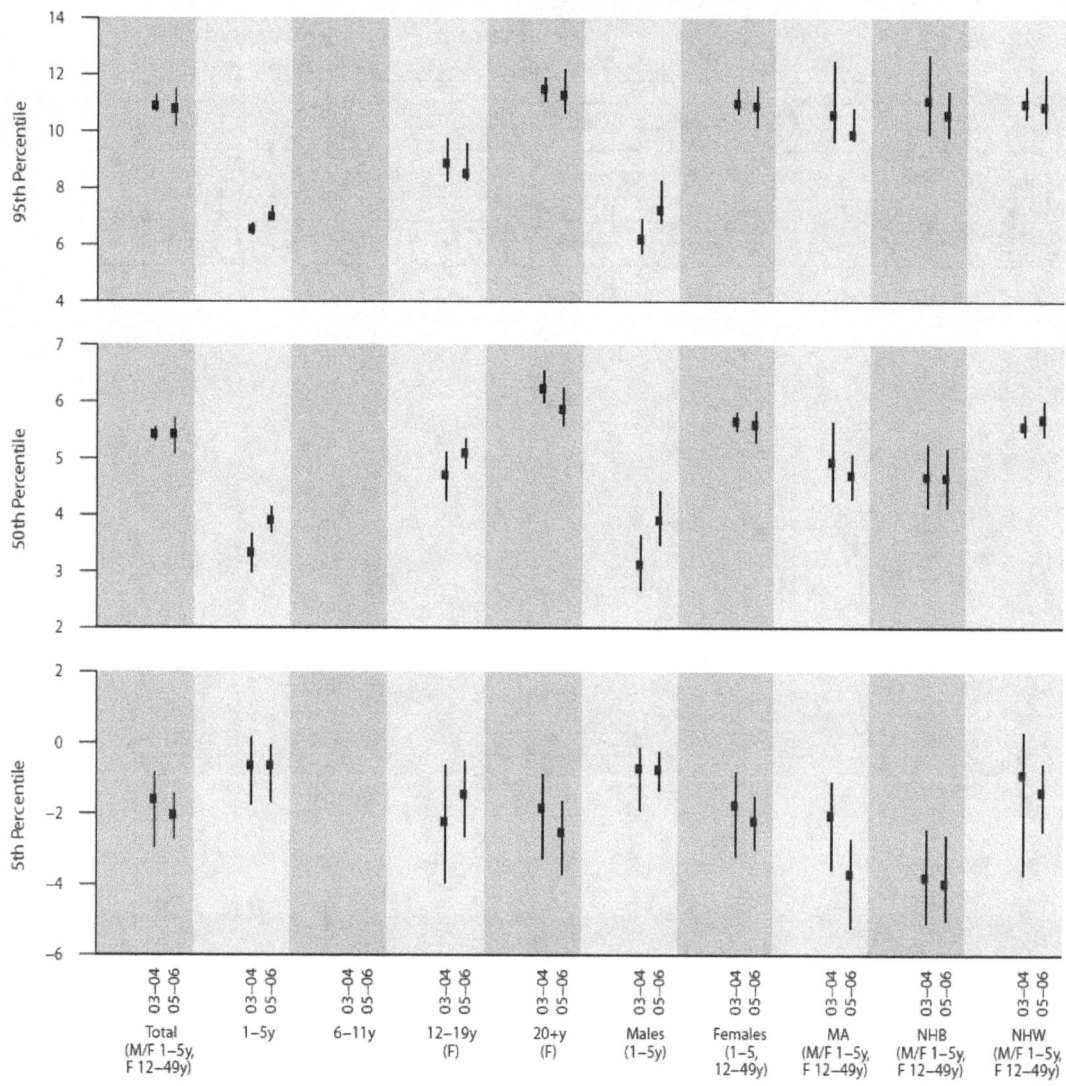

Table 3.3.c.1. Body iron: Prevalence

Prevalence (in percent) of low body iron (< 0 mg/kg) for children in the U.S. population aged 1–5 years, National Health and Nutrition Examination Survey, 2003–2006.

	Sample size	Prevalence (95% conf. interval)	Estimated total number of persons
Children, 1–5 years	1,369	6.7 (5.0 – 8.8)	1,350,000
Gender			
Males	695	7.8 (5.6 – 10.8)	807,000
Females	674	5.4 (3.4 – 8.3)	534,000
Race/ethnicity			
Mexican Americans	422	10.9 (8.1 – 14.6)	333,000
Non-Hispanic Blacks	401	5.1 (3.0 – 8.6)	154,000
Non-Hispanic Whites	385	5.8 (3.6 – 9.1)	670,000

Table 3.3.c.2. Body iron: Prevalence

Prevalence (in percent) of low body iron (< 0 mg/kg) for women in the U.S. population aged 12–49 years, National Health and Nutrition Examination Survey, 2003–2006.

	Sample size	Prevalence (95% conf. interval)	Estimated total number of persons
Women, 12–49 years	4,476	9.5 (8.6 – 10.5)	7,515,000
Age group			
12–19 years	1,967	9.3 (7.4 – 11.6)	1,508,000
20–49 years	2,509	9.6 (8.6 – 10.7)	6,006,000
Race/ethnicity			
Mexican Americans	1,219	13.2 (10.2 – 16.9)	1,007,000
Non-Hispanic Blacks	1,232	16.2 (13.9 – 18.7)	1,739,000
Non-Hispanic Whites	1,656	7.4 (5.8 – 9.4)	3,803,000

Table 3.3.d.1. Body iron: Prevalence by survey cycle

Prevalence (in percent) of low body iron (< 0 mg/kg) for children in the U.S. population aged 1–5 years, National Health and Nutrition Examination Survey, 2003–2006.

	Sample size	Prevalence (95% conf. interval)	Estimated total number of persons
Children, 1–5 years			
2003–2004	694	6.5 (4.3 – 9.8)	1,321,000
2005–2006	675	6.8 (4.5 – 10.2)	1,377,000
Gender			
Males			
2003–2004	358	8.3 (4.9 – 13.7)	854,000
2005–2006	337	7.3 (4.7 – 11.1)	755,000
Females			
2003–2004	336	4.5 (2.7 – 7.4)	449,000
2005–2006	338	6.3‡ (3.1 – 12.4)	620,000‡
Race/ethnicity			
Mexican Americans			
2003–2004	187	13.3 (8.4 – 20.5)	405,000
2005–2006	235	8.6 (6.0 – 12.1)	275,000
Non-Hispanic Blacks			
2003–2004	228	6.1‡ (3.1 – 11.8)	183,000‡
2005–2006	173	§	§
Non-Hispanic Whites			
2003–2004	201	4.6‡ (2.1 – 10.0)	538,000‡
2005–2006	184	7.0 (3.8 – 12.5)	792,000

‡ Estimate flagged: 30% ≤ RSE < 40% for the prevalence estimate.

§ Estimate suppressed: RSE ≥ 40% for the prevalence estimate.

Table 3.3.d.2. Body iron: Prevalence by survey cycle

Prevalence (in percent) of low body iron (< 0 mg/kg) for women in the U.S. population aged 12–49 years, National Health and Nutrition Examination Survey, 2003–2006.

	Sample size	Prevalence (95% conf. interval)		Estimated total number of persons
Women, 12–49 years				
2003–2004	2,132	8.6	(7.0 – 10.4)	6,773,000
2005–2006	2,344	10.4	(9.3 – 11.7)	8,266,000
Age group				
12–19 years				
2003–2004	974	9.0	(6.3 – 12.6)	1,455,000
2005–2006	993	9.6	(6.9 – 13.2)	1,576,000
20–49 years				
2003–2004	1,158	8.5	(6.8 – 10.5)	5,322,000
2005–2006	1,351	10.6	(9.5 – 11.9)	6,681,000
Race/ethnicity				
Mexican Americans				
2003–2004	547	11.2	(7.6 – 16.2)	857,000
2005–2006	672	15.1	(10.5 – 21.2)	1,193,000
Non-Hispanic Blacks				
2003–2004	603	16.0	(12.8 – 19.8)	1,720,000
2005–2006	629	16.3	(13.1 – 20.1)	1,777,000
Non-Hispanic Whites				
2003–2004	822	6.9	(4.4 – 10.6)	3,530,000
2005–2006	834	8.0	(6.0 – 10.5)	4,023,000

References

Beard JL. Iron deficiency and neural development: an update. Arch Latinoam Nutr. 1999;49(3 Suppl 2):34S–39S.

Beard J. Indicators of the iron status of the population: free erythrocyte protoporphyrin and zinc protoporphyrin; serum and plasma iron, total iron binding capacity and transferrin saturation; and serum transferrin receptor. In: WHO/CDC. Assessing the iron status of populations: report of a joint World Health Organization/Centers for Disease Control and Prevention technical consultation on the assessment of iron status at the population level. Geneva: World Health Organization; 2007 [cited 2011]. Available at: http://www.who.int/nutrition/publications/micronutrients/anaemia_iron_deficiency/9789241596107.pdf.

Cogswell ME, Looker AC, Pfeiffer CM, Cook JD, Lacher DA, Beard JL, et al. Assessment of iron deficiency in US preschool children and nonpregnant females of childbearing age: National Health and Nutrition Examination Survey 2003–2006. Am J Clin Nutr. 2009;89:1334–1342.

Cook JD, Flowers CH, Skikne BS. The quantitative assessment of body iron. Blood. 2003;101:3359–3364.

Flowers CH, Skikne BS, Covell AM, Cook JF. The clinical measurement of serum transferrin receptor. J Lab Clin Med. 1989;114:368–377.

Grantham-McGregor S, Ani C. A review of studies on the effect of iron deficiency on cognitive development in children. J Nutr. 2001;131(2S-2):649S–656S.

Haas JD, Brownlie T 4th. Iron deficiency and reduced work capacity: a critical review of the research to determine a causal relationship. J Nutr. 2001;131:691S–696S.

Institute of Medicine, Food and Nutrition Board. Dietary reference intakes: vitamin A, vitamin K, arsenic, boron, chromium, copper, iodine, iron, manganese, molybdenum, nickel, silicon, vanadium and zinc. Washington, D.C.: National Academy Press; 2001.

Kuiper-Kramer EPA, Coenen JLLM, Huisman CMS, Abbes A, van Raan J, van Eijk HG. Relation between soluble transferrin receptors in serum and membrane-bound transferrin receptors. Acta Haematol. 1998;99:8–11.

Looker AC, Gunter EW, Johnson CL. Methods to assess iron status in various NHANES surveys. Nutr Rev. 1995;53:246–254.

Looker AC, Dallman PR, Carroll M, Gunter EW, Johnson CL. Prevalence of iron deficiency in the United States. JAMA. 1997;277:973–975.

Looker AC, Cogswell ME, Gunter EW. Iron deficiency—United States, 1999–2000. Morb Mortal Wkly Rep. 2002;51:897–899.

Miret S, Simpson RJ, McKie AT. Physiology and molecular biology of dietary iron absorption. Annu Rev Nutr. 2003;23:283–301.

Pfeiffer CM, Cook JD, Mei Z, Cogswell ME, Looker AC, Lacher DA. Evaluation of an automated soluble transferrin receptor (sTfR) assay on the Roche Hitachi analyzer and its comparison to two ELISA assays. Clin Chim Acta 2007;382:112–116.

Pietrangelo A. Hereditary hemochromatosis—a new look at an old disease. N Engl J Med. 2004;350:2382–2397.

Pilch SM, Senti FR, editors. Assessment of iron nutritional status of the U.S. population based on data collected in the Second National Health and Nutrition Examination Survey, 1976–1980. Bethesda (MD): Federation of American Societies for Experimental Biology; 1984.

Schorr TO, Hediger ML. Anemia and iron-deficiency anemia: compilation of data on pregnancy outcome. Am J Clin Nutr. 1994;59(Suppl):492S–501S.

Skikne BS, Flowers CH, Cook JD. Serum transferrin receptor: a quantitative measure of tissue iron deficiency. Blood. 1990;75:1870–1876.

Thorpe SJ. The development and role of international biological reference materials in the diagnosis of anaemia. Biologicals 2010;38:449–458.

U.S. Department of Agriculture and U.S. Department of Health and Human Services. Dietary Guidelines for Americans, 2010. 7th Edition, Washington, DC: U.S. Government Printing Office, December 2010 [cited 2011]. Available at: http://www.cnpp.usda.gov/DGAs2010-PolicyDocument.htm.

World Health Organization (WHO)/UNICEF/UNU. Iron deficiency anaemia: assessment, prevention, and control. A guide for programme managers. Geneva: World Health Organization; 2001 (WHO/NHD/01.3) [cited 2011]. Available at:

http://www.who.int/nutrition/publications/micronutrients/anaemia_iron_deficiency/WHO_NHD_01.3/en/index.html.

World Health Organization (WHO)/CDC. Assessing the iron status of populations: report of a joint World Health Organization/Centers for Disease Control and Prevention technical consultation on the assessment of iron status at the population level. Geneva: World Health Organization; 2005 [cited 2011]. Available at: http://whqlibdoc.who.int/publications/2004/9241593156_eng.pdf.

WHO. Serum ferritin concentrations for the assessment of iron status and iron deficiency in populations. Vitamin and Mineral Nutrition Information System. Geneva, World Health Organization; 2011 (WHO/NMH/NHD/MNM/11.2). (http://www.who.int/vmnis/indicators/serum_ferritin.pdf, accessed February 14, 2012).

Worwood M. The measurement of ferritin. In: Rowan, van Assendelft, Preston, editors. Advanced Laboratory Methods in Haematology. Hodder Arnold; 2002a. pp. 241–263.

Worwood M. Serum transferrin receptor assays and their application. Ann Clin Biochem. 2002b;39:221–230.

Worwood M. Indicators of the iron status of populations: ferritin. In: WHO/CDC. Assessing the iron status of populations: report of a joint World Health Organization/Centers for Disease Control and Prevention technical consultation on the assessment of iron status at the population level. Geneva: World Health Organization; 2007 [cited 2011]. Available at: http://www.who.int/nutrition/publications/micronutrients/anaemia_iron_deficiency/9789241596107.pdf.

Iodine

Background Information

Sources and Physiological Functions. Iodine, a trace element found in soil, is an essential component of the thyroid hormones involved in regulating the body's metabolic processes related to normal growth and development. Across the world, iodized salt and seafood are the major dietary sources of iodine. In the United States, where the addition of iodine to salt is not mandatory, most people get their iodine from dairy products and grains (bread) (Murray 2008). In the United States, salt is iodized with potassium iodide at 100 parts per million (76 milligram [mg] of iodine per kilogram [kg] of salt). Iodized salt is chosen by about 50–60% of the U.S. population (Institute of Medicine 2001). Still, most ingested salt comes from processed food (approximately 70%), which is typically not iodized in either the United States or in Canada (The Public Health Committee of the American Thyroid Association 2006). Dairy products have been identified as another important contributor to iodine status among reproductive-age women in the United States (Perrine 2010).

Health Effects. Iodine deficiency disorders include mental retardation, hypothyroidism, goiter, cretinism, and varying degrees of other growth and developmental abnormalities. Iodine deficiency is the most preventable cause of mental retardation in the world (World Health Organization 2007). Thyroid enlargement (goiter) is usually the earliest clinical feature of iodine deficiency. Thyroid hormone is particularly important in the development of the central nervous system during the fetal and early postnatal periods. In areas where iodized salt is common, iodine deficiency is rare. The most critical period for iodine sufficiency is in utero through the first two years of life, when thyroid hormones are required for normal brain development (World Health Organization 2007).

Excess iodine intake may also result in goiter, as well as in hyper- or hypothyroidism. High iodine intake has also been associated with increased risk for thyroid papillary cancer (Institute of Medicine 2001). For most people, iodine intake from usual foods and supplements is unlikely to exceed the tolerable upper intake level (1100 μg/day) (Institute of Medicine 2001).

Intake Recommendations. The Institute of Medicine recommends the following daily intake of iodine: 90 μg for children 1 to 8 years, 120 μg for children 9 to 13 years, 150 μg for adolescents (14 to 18 years) and for nonpregnant adults, 220 μg per day for pregnant women, and 290 μg per day during lactation (Institute of Medicine 2001). Dietary iodine requirements are higher in pregnancy because of increased thyroid hormone production, increased renal iodine excretion, and fetal iodine requirements (Glinoer 2007).

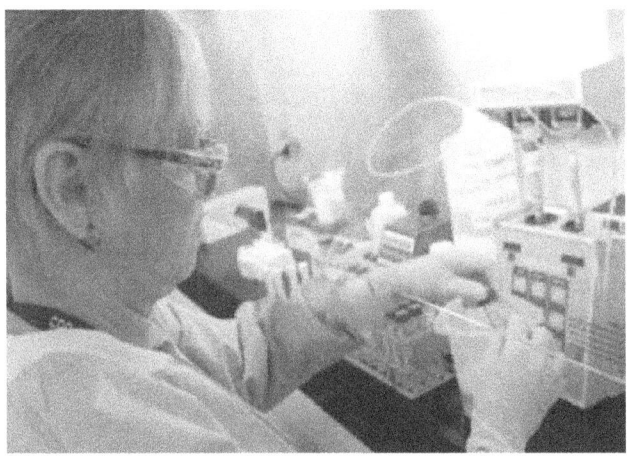

The World Health Organization (WHO) recommends the following daily intake of iodine: 90 μg for preschool children (0 to 59 months); 120 μg for schoolchildren (6 to 12 years); 150 μg for adolescents (above 12 years) and adults; and 250 μg for pregnant and lactating women (World Health Organization 2007). The American Thyroid Association recommends that North American women receive dietary supplements containing 150 μg iodine daily during pregnancy and lactation and that all prenatal vitamins contain 150 μg of iodine (Becker 2006). An Endocrine Society Clinical Practice Guideline on the management of thyroid dysfunction during pregnancy and postpartum recommends an average daily intake of 250 µg iodine for pregnant women (Abalovich 2007). These recommendations have not yet been widely adopted. A current survey of prenatal multivitamins marketed in the United States showed that 49% did not contain iodine (Leung 2009). Furthermore, the majority of women of childbearing age (> 80%) are not consuming supplements containing iodine (Gregory 2009).

Biochemical Indicators. Iodine deficiency develops when iodide intake is less than 20 µg/day (Beers 2006). Most dietary iodine absorbed in the body eventually appears in the urine; thus, urinary iodine excretion is recommended for assessing recent dietary iodine intake worldwide (World Health Organization 2007).

WHO categories for median urinary iodine concentrations in school-age children and adults (excluding pregnant and lactating women) are widely used to define iodine intake and nutrition status for populations (World Health Organization 2007). An additional adequacy criterion is that not more than 20% of samples from children and non-pregnant women be below 50 nanograms per milliliter (ng/mL) of iodine. These categories are useful for classifying population risk, but they are not categories to define individual risk for adverse health outcomes. The large day-to-day variations in urine iodine excretion, even among individuals with stable iodine intake, tend to offset one another when the sample includes an adequately large number (100–500 spot urine samples per group or subgroup) of representative individuals (Andersen 2008).

Epidemiological criteria for assessing iodine nutrition based on median urinary iodine concentrations of school-age children ($\geq$ 6 years)* (World Health Organization 2007)

Median Urinary Iodine (ng/mL)	Iodine Intake	Iodine Status
< 20	Insufficient	Severe iodine deficiency
20–49	Insufficient	Moderate iodine deficiency
50–99	Insufficient	Mild iodine deficiency
100–199	Adequate	Adequate iodine nutrition
200–299	Above requirements	Likely to provide adequate intake for pregnant/lactating women but may pose a slight risk of more than adequate intake in the overall population
$\geq$ 300	Excessive	Risk for adverse health consequences (e.g., iodine-induced hyperthyroidism, autoimmune thyroid diseases)

* Applies to adults but not to pregnant and lactating women.

For pregnant women, median urinary iodine concentrations of 150–249 ng/mL represent adequate iodine intake (World Health Organization 2007; Andersson 2007). Median urinary iodine concentrations of < 150 ng/mL represent insufficient intake; 250–499 ng/mL represent an intake above requirements, and $\geq$ 500 ng/mL represent an excessive intake. For lactating women and children less than 2 years of age, median urinary iodine concentrations of 100 ng/mL represent adequate iodine intake, but no other categories of iodine intake are defined (World Health Organization 2007; Andersson 2007).

Data in NHANES. NHANES has measured urinary iodine since 1971. The NHANES III survey (1988–1994) showed a sizable decrease in urinary iodine concentrations compared to concentrations measured during NHANES I (1971–1974) (Hollowell 1998). This decline may have been due to the dairy industry's effort in the mid-1980s to reduce the iodine residue in milk from feed supplements and iodophor sanitizing agents (Pennington 1996). Decreased concentrations of iodine in fruit-flavored breakfast cereals resulted from a ban on erythrosine (an iodine-containing food dye) and could also have contributed to the decline in urinary iodine concentrations (Pennington 1996). Since 2000, urinary iodine has been measured in the continuous NHANES survey. Starting with NHANES 2000, CDC used a new method, inductively coupled plasma mass spectrometry (ICP-MS), to make these measurements (Caldwell 2003). This method produced comparable data to the established Sandell-Kolthoff spectrophotometric method used in NHANES III (Pino 1998). When CDC laboratory scientists measured urinary iodine concentrations in NHANES 2001–2002 Caldwell 2005 , 2003–2004 (Caldwell 2008 , and 2005–2006 and 2007–2008 (Caldwell 2011), they found that the U.S. median urinary iodine concentration had stabilized since the initial drop that had occurred from NHANES I to NHANES III and that it represented adequate iodine intake for the overall population 6 years and older. The median (95% confidence interval) urinary iodine concentration for pregnant women [125 (86–198) ng/mL] was below the cutoff value of 150 ng/mL indicating iodine deficiency, however the sample was small (n = 184) (Caldwell 2011). Continued monitoring of the population for iodine sufficiency is warranted because of groups at risk for iodine deficiency disorders.

For more information about iodine, see the Institute of Medicine's Dietary Reference Intake report (Institute of Medicine 2001 .

Highlights

Urinary iodine concentrations in the U.S. population showed the following demographic patterns and characteristics:

- The lowest concentrations were observed in young women, while the highest concentrations were observed in children.
- No consistent pattern was observed with regard to race/ethnicity.
- Concentrations have been relatively stable since the late 1980's.

The iodine intake of the U.S. population appeared to be adequate on the basis of median urinary iodine concentrations. However, women aged 20–39 years had the lowest iodine intake, just slightly above insufficient intake (Figure H.3.e). Young women merit special attention to ensure the best possible brain development of the fetus during pregnancy. While no age group had a median urinary iodine concentration that represented excessive iodine intake, boys 6–11 years of age had the highest intake, and the upper confidence limit of the median was just slightly within the range of excessive intake (Figure H.3.e .

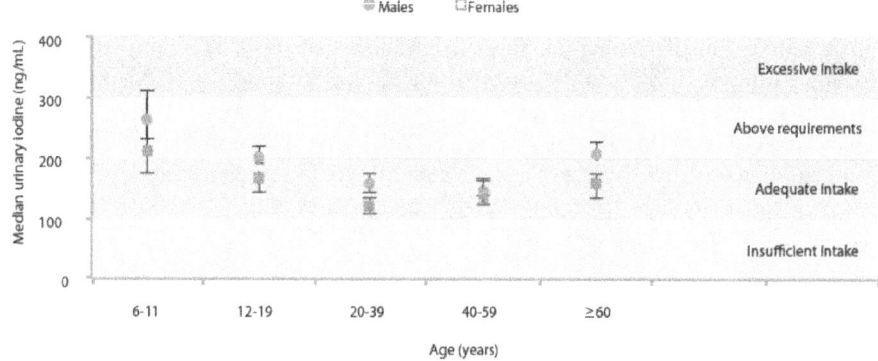

Figure H.3.e. Median concentrations of urinary iodine in the U.S. population aged 6 years and older by age group and gender associated with estimated iodine intake, National Health and Nutrition Examination Survey, 2001–2006.

Error bars represent 95% confidence intervals.

Urinary iodine concentrations have been relatively stable over almost two decades between 1988–2006 (Figure H.3.f). They increased slightly (< 20%) between 1988–1994 and 2001–2002 in the total population, in males, in females, and in non-Hispanic whites. However, they remained unchanged in non-Hispanic blacks and Mexican Americans.

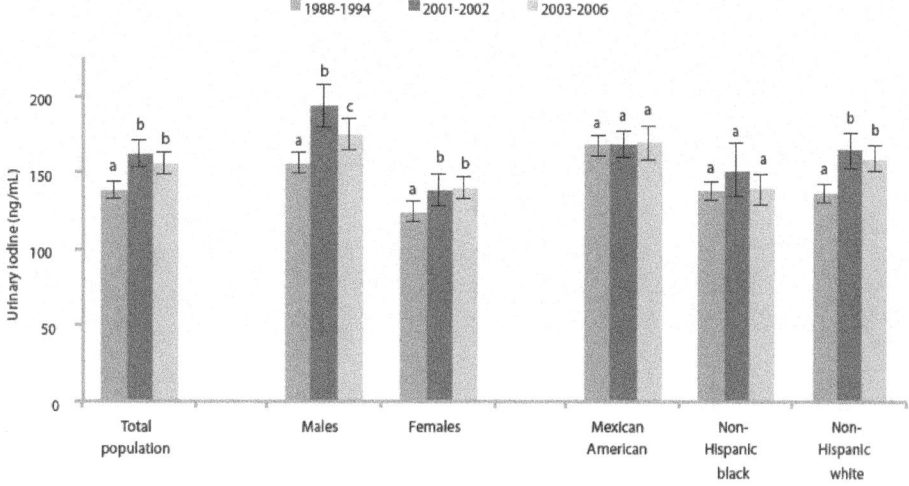

Figure H.3.f. *Age-adjusted geometric mean concentrations of urinary iodine in the U.S. population aged 6 years and older by gender or race/ethnicity, National Health and Nutrition Examination Survey, 1988–2006.*

Error bars represent 95% confidence intervals. Within a demographic group, bars not sharing a common letter differ (p < 0.05).

Detailed Observations

The selected observations mentioned below are derived from the uncorrected tables and figures presented next. The NHANES population is of sufficient size to allow group comparisons based on uncorrected data. Statements about categorical differences between demographic groups noted below are based on non-overlapping confidence limits from univariate analysis without adjusting for demographic variables (i.e., age, sex, race/ethnicity) or other determinants of these urine concentrations (i.e., dietary intake, supplement usage, smoking, BMI). A multivariate analysis may alter the size and statistical significance of these categorical differences. Furthermore, additional significant differences of smaller magnitude may be present despite their lack of mention here (e.g., if confidence limits slightly overlap or if differences are not statistically significant before covariate adjustment has occurred). For a selection of citations of descriptive NHANES papers related to these biochemical indicators of diet and nutrition, see **Appendix G**.

Geometric mean concentrations (NHANES 2003–2006):

- Urinary iodine concentrations followed a U-shaped age pattern, with the lowest concentrations seen in young and middle-aged adults (Table 3.4.a.1 and Figure 3.4.a).
- Females had lower urinary iodine concentrations than males (Table 3.4.a.1 and Figure 3.4.a).
- Non-Hispanic blacks had lower urinary iodine concentrations than either non-Hispanic whites or Mexican Americans (Table 3.4.a.1 and Figure 3.4.a).

Changes in geometric mean concentrations across survey cycles:

- We observed no change in urinary iodine concentrations between 2001 and 2006 (Table 3.4.b).

Table 3.4.a.1. Urinary iodine: Concentrations

Geometric mean and selected percentiles of urine concentrations (in ng/mL) for the total U.S. population aged 6 years and older, National Health and Nutrition Examination Survey, 2003–2006.

	Geometric mean (95% conf. interval)	Selected percentiles (95% conf. interval)						Sample size
		2.5th	5th	50th	95th	97.5th	
Total	156 (148 – 163)	23.3 (19.4 – 26.0)	33.0 (29.0 – 36.5)	162 (154 – 170)	603 (565 – 676)	816 (719 – 1,040)	5,175
(Children 1–5 years, women 12–49 years)							
Age group							
6–11 years	222 (201 – 245)	36.4 (25.8 – 43.0)	51.6 (37.5 – 55.9)	232 (208 – 270)	764 (631 – 1,080)	1,040 (756 – 6,960)	666
12–19 years	179 (161 – 199)	24.9 (18.0 – 30.8)	36.7 (25.0 – 45.7)	186 (171 – 203)	741 (644 – 903)	936 (808 – 1,240)	1,443
20–39 years	135 (126 – 144)	20.0 (17.6 – 23.8)	29.4 (22.5 – 33.6)	140 (129 – 149)	515 (453 – 614)	679 (599 – 872)	1,134
40–59 years	137 (128 – 147)	20.0 (13.2 – 26.0)	28.4 (21.5 – 35.2)	145 (136 – 156)	489 (457 – 574)	674 (556 – 906)	919
60 years and older	187 (170 – 205)	30.3 (25.9 – 37.7)	41.9 (36.9 – 49.0)	181 (168 – 202)	707 (616 – 1,080)	1,530 (1,050 – 4,320)	1,013
Gender							
Males	174 (164 – 185)	28.0 (22.4 – 32.9)	38.1 (34.9 – 42.5)	180 (172 – 189)	673 (581 – 760)	935 (743 – 1,260)	2,477
Females	140 (133 – 147)	20.0 (17.5 – 24.0)	28.5 (24.0 – 32.0)	144 (137 – 153)	571 (541 – 606)	762 (664 – 953)	2,698
Race/ethnicity							
(Children 1–5 years, women 12–49 years)							
Mexican Americans	173 (161 – 185)	30.7 (19.0 – 38.6)	40.2 (34.0 – 49.4)	186 (173 – 195)	591 (539 – 730)	768 (687 – 1,130)	1,320
Non-Hispanic Blacks	141 (131 – 151)	28.7 (25.7 – 30.8)	38.2 (31.1 – 44.0)	141 (128 – 152)	482 (442 – 554)	606 (535 – 770)	1,363
Non-Hispanic Whites	159 (151 – 168)	22.5 (18.9 – 25.8)	32.0 (27.9 – 36.6)	166 (156 – 176)	634 (570 – 714)	835 (731 – 1,170)	2,085

Figure 3.4.a. Urinary iodine: Concentrations by age group

Geometric mean (95% confidence interval), National Health and Nutrition Examination Survey, 2003–2006

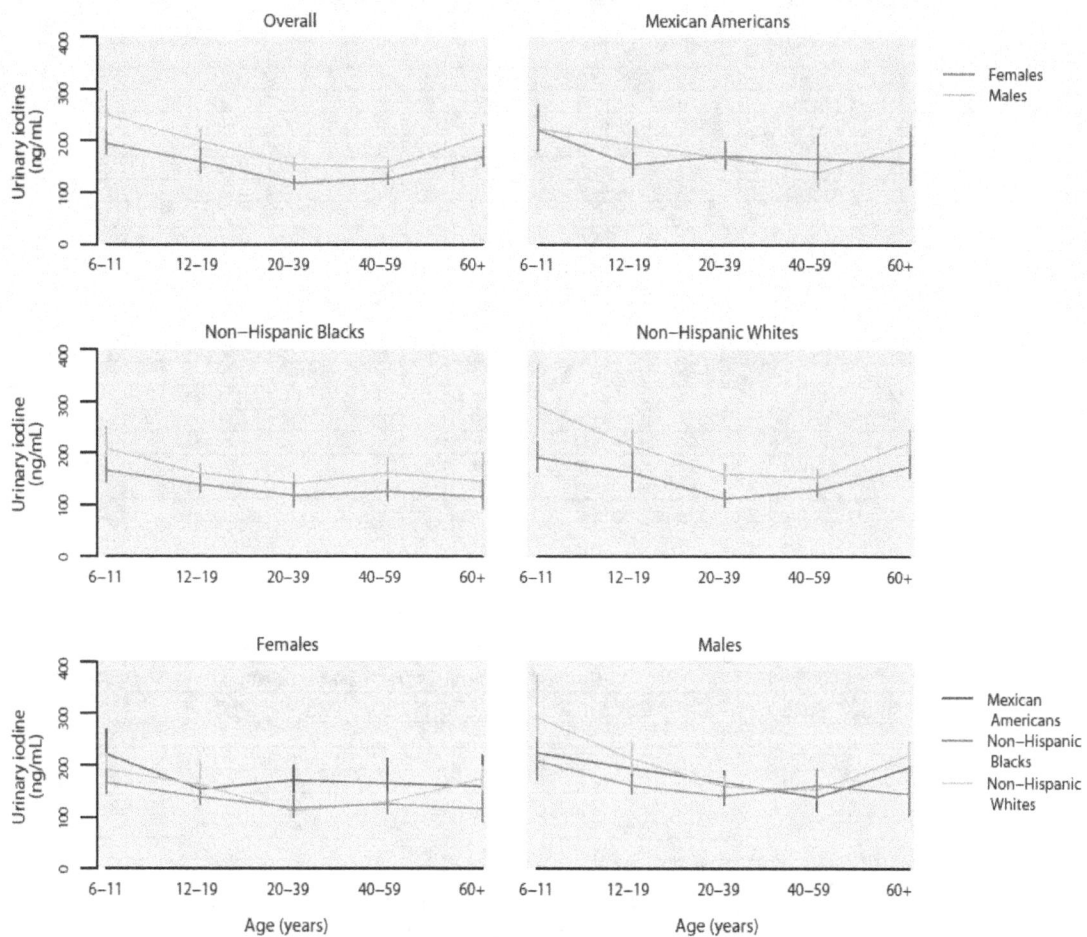

Table 3.4.a.2. Urinary iodine: Total population

Geometric mean and selected percentiles of urine concentrations (in ng/mL) for the total U.S. population aged 6 years and older, National Health and Nutrition Examination Survey, 2003–2006.

	Geometric mean (95% conf. interval)		Selected percentiles (95% conf. interval)						Sample size
			10th		50th		90th		
Males and Females									
Total, 6 years and older	156	(148 – 163)	47.9	(42.9 – 53.9)	162	(154 – 170)	444	(422 – 467)	5,175
6–11 years	222	(201 – 245)	77.6	(55.8 – 94.7)	232	(208 – 270)	581	(515 – 754)	666
12–19 years	179	(161 – 199)	55.5	(44.3 – 68.0)	186	(171 – 203)	518	(465 – 658)	1,443
20–39 years	135	(126 – 144)	42.0	(33.9 – 52.9)	140	(129 – 149)	368	(323 – 416)	1,134
40–59 years	137	(128 – 147)	40.4	(36.9 – 45.7)	145	(136 – 156)	388	(359 – 423)	919
60 years and older	187	(170 – 205)	61.3	(52.0 – 68.5)	181	(168 – 202)	523	(463 – 580)	1,013
Males									
Total, 6 years and older	174	(164 – 185)	56.4	(48.0 – 65.2)	180	(172 – 189)	465	(441 – 500)	2,477
6–11 years	250	(212 – 295)	94.3	(55.4 – 115)	264	(212 – 313)	653	(498 – 1,080)	307
12–19 years	200	(181 – 222)	73.1	(54.8 – 87.7)	198	(184 – 220)	525	(479 – 707)	693
20–39 years	154	(142 – 167)	53.6	(38.8 – 65.1)	160	(143 – 174)	408	(327 – 478)	512
40–59 years	149	(137 – 163)	48.3	(38.6 – 59.5)	148	(138 – 166)	395	(363 – 458)	454
60 years and older	211	(191 – 233)	65.1	(46.9 – 88.2)	205	(193 – 228)	538	(469 – 652)	511
Females									
Total, 6 years and older	140	(133 – 147)	41.4	(37.7 – 46.8)	144	(137 – 153)	412	(389 – 453)	2,698
6–11 years	195	(176 – 215)	61.8	(45.8 – 81.5)	210	(174 – 232)	549	(423 – 718)	359
12–19 years	160	(137 – 186)	46.1	(29.2 – 59.0)	166	(143 – 191)	487	(421 – 633)	750
20–39 years	118	(107 – 131)	35.4	(30.4 – 43.8)	119	(108 – 136)	333	(300 – 406)	622
40–59 years	127	(116 – 139)	36.4	(28.2 – 40.1)	140	(123 – 161)	368	(333 – 418)	465
60 years and older	169	(151 – 189)	60.2	(48.9 – 67.7)	157	(134 – 176)	483	(413 – 590)	502

Table 3.4.a.3. Urinary iodine: Mexican Americans

Geometric mean and selected percentiles of urine concentrations (in ng/mL) for Mexican Americans in the U.S. population aged 6 years and older, National Health and Nutrition Examination Survey, 2003–2006.

	Geometric mean (95% conf. interval)		Selected percentiles (95% conf. interval)						Sample size
			10th		50th		90th		
Males and Females									
Total, 6 years and older	173	(161 – 185)	59.9	(52.3 – 68.3)	186	(173 – 195)	450	(404 – 518)	1,320
6–11 years	223	(196 – 253)	80.8	(54.8 – 98.9)	235	(208 – 265)	544	(469 – 713)	217
12–19 years	174	(155 – 194)	56.6	(44.9 – 62.7)	176	(163 – 203)	488	(414 – 596)	466
20–39 years	169	(153 – 186)	65.7	(55.6 – 78.5)	187	(165 – 198)	401	(352 – 547)	283
40–59 years	151	(124 – 184)	45.4	(33.9 – 59.5)	158	(123 – 196)	382	(305 – 699)	165
60 years and older	175	(148 – 207)	57.2	(43.7 – 69.2)	159	(128 – 193)	444	(377 – 690)	189
Males									
Total, 6 years and older	173	(162 – 185)	61.8	(56.1 – 71.9)	184	(165 – 199)	454	(404 – 510)	623
6–11 years	224	(187 – 269)	85.2†	(41.0 – 133)	236	(209 – 271)	519†	(422 – 836)	96
12–19 years	194	(164 – 230)	60.8	(46.1 – 78.1)	199	(169 – 234)	549	(432 – 747)	221
20–39 years	167	(148 – 189)	62.3	(58.5 – 78.1)	184	(146 – 202)	386	(334 – 591)	134
40–59 years	139	(112 – 171)	45.1†	(31.2 – 61.1)	122	(107 – 168)	369†	(298 – 1,260)	77
60 years and older	196	(166 – 232)	70.5†	(30.1 – 92.3)	196	(155 – 243)	495†	(365 – 6,920)	95
Females									
Total, 6 years and older	172	(159 – 187)	57.0	(45.9 – 67.4)	190	(164 – 205)	444	(373 – 566)	697
6–11 years	221	(182 – 269)	75.9	(47.0 – 94.8)	226	(180 – 270)	584	(456 – 1,110)	121
12–19 years	154	(134 – 178)	49.4	(34.7 – 61.1)	163	(142 – 188)	428	(338 – 695)	245
20–39 years	171	(148 – 198)	68.9	(39.1 – 81.4)	187	(145 – 219)	402	(348 – 569)	149
40–59 years	165	(128 – 212)	45.9†	(20.2 – 64.8)	199	(145 – 218)	385†	(295 – 1,150)	88
60 years and older	159	(117 – 218)	52.5†	(34.2 – 61.4)	128	(107 – 163)	425†	(283 – 1,010,900)	94

† Estimate is subject to greater uncertainty due to small cell size.

Table 3.4.a.4. Urinary iodine: Non-Hispanic blacks

Geometric mean and selected percentiles of urine concentrations (in ng/mL) for non-Hispanic blacks in the U.S. population aged 6 years and older, National Health and Nutrition Examination Survey, 2003–2006.

	Geometric mean (95% conf. interval)		Selected percentiles (95% conf. interval)						Sample size
			10th		50th		90th		
Males and Females									
Total, 6 years and older	141	(131 – 151)	51.7	(47.6 – 57.0)	141	(128 – 152)	374	(322 – 423)	1,363
6–11 years	186	(163 – 213)	62.4	(45.7 – 76.1)	190	(168 – 217)	459	(387 – 682)	221
12–19 years	149	(137 – 163)	55.0	(47.9 – 61.0)	148	(138 – 168)	394	(351 – 475)	515
20–39 years	128	(113 – 145)	57.3	(47.2 – 66.3)	125	(116 – 160)	283	(242 – 310)	238
40–59 years	140	(124 – 160)	48.3	(35.7 – 59.1)	134	(122 – 144)	428	(337 – 485)	219
60 years and older	128	(108 – 151)	42.1	(35.0 – 50.6)	128	(102 – 146)	326	(259 – 529)	170
Males									
Total, 6 years and older	158	(145 – 172)	58.1	(51.7 – 69.8)	159	(142 – 176)	408	(335 – 456)	663
6–11 years	208	(172 – 251)	75.9†	(48.1 – 102)	205	(172 – 284)	500†	(393 – 952)	106
12–19 years	161	(145 – 178)	61.4	(47.3 – 76.3)	155	(141 – 177)	409	(342 – 588)	260
20–39 years	141	(125 – 160)	61.0†	(46.8 – 72.0)	154	(117 – 185)	292†	(259 – 398)	108
40–59 years	161	(134 – 192)	55.5†	(34.1 – 77.7)	145	(125 – 198)	429†	(329 – 518)	104
60 years and older	145	(105 – 200)	42.6†	(31.1 – 55.9)	141	(93.6 – 204)	414†	(249 – 8,300)	85
Females									
Total, 6 years and older	127	(117 – 138)	49.0	(41.9 – 53.8)	128	(121 – 136)	329	(307 – 380)	700
6–11 years	166	(145 – 190)	44.7	(39.2 – 67.1)	168	(151 – 211)	409	(381 – 581)	115
12–19 years	139	(124 – 156)	50.9	(36.2 – 59.2)	139	(125 – 164)	387	(312 – 475)	255
20–39 years	118	(98.4 – 142)	54.2	(27.1 – 66.6)	123	(105 – 148)	237	(212 – 342)	130
40–59 years	125	(107 – 147)	44.8	(30.9 – 53.4)	122	(103 – 137)	390	(290 – 516)	115
60 years and older	116	(91.7 – 148)	42.0†	(12.9 – 50.6)	115	(83.6 – 146)	271†	(244 – 466)	85

† Estimate is subject to greater uncertainty due to small cell size.

Table 3.4.a.5. Urinary iodine: Non-Hispanic whites

Geometric mean and selected percentiles of urine concentrations (in ng/mL) for non-Hispanic whites in the U.S. population aged 6 years and older, National Health and Nutrition Examination Survey, 2003–2006.

	Geometric mean (95% conf. interval)		Selected percentiles (95% conf. interval)						Sample size
			10th		50th		90th		
Males and Females									
Total, 6 years and older	159	(151 – 168)	47.0	(41.1 – 54.3)	166	(156 – 176)	461	(427 – 489)	2,085
6–11 years	237	(208 – 271)	81.0	(55.0 – 103)	267	(202 – 315)	620	(536 – 978)	169
12–19 years	187	(160 – 218)	48.9	(36.7 – 73.4)	194	(172 – 224)	561	(481 – 744)	365
20–39 years	133	(122 – 145)	39.9	(32.0 – 49.0)	139	(125 – 150)	378	(318 – 461)	494
40–59 years	140	(131 – 151)	40.3	(35.6 – 48.7)	153	(139 – 167)	389	(361 – 424)	453
60 years and older	193	(175 – 214)	65.3	(55.5 – 74.1)	193	(172 – 211)	538	(460 – 598)	604
Males									
Total, 6 years and older	182	(170 – 195)	58.0	(47.5 – 69.5)	187	(176 – 199)	481	(450 – 548)	996
6–11 years	292	(230 – 371)	112†	(46.9 – 132)	315	(229 – 381)	741†	(503 – 1,600)	76
12–19 years	213	(185 – 246)	77.2	(38.8 – 102)	208	(187 – 242)	564	(483 – 770)	174
20–39 years	159	(141 – 179)	51.0	(36.9 – 71.6)	163	(139 – 186)	413	(322 – 516)	211
40–59 years	153	(140 – 168)	49.7	(38.4 – 65.5)	153	(137 – 173)	396	(355 – 464)	229
60 years and older	220	(198 – 245)	66.6	(45.4 – 93.4)	218	(197 – 249)	548	(483 – 666)	306
Females									
Total, 6 years and older	141	(132 – 149)	39.6	(33.9 – 44.0)	148	(137 – 157)	423	(390 – 471)	1,089
6–11 years	191	(166 – 221)	58.9†	(38.5 – 81.6)	194	(150 – 251)	554†	(423 – 855)	93
12–19 years	162	(127 – 206)	36.9	(18.6 – 58.0)	171	(138 – 227)	538	(431 – 793)	191
20–39 years	112	(98.2 – 129)	32.3	(22.5 – 41.6)	115	(102 – 130)	327	(278 – 461)	283
40–59 years	129	(117 – 143)	33.6	(24.7 – 40.7)	150	(123 – 178)	368	(334 – 425)	224
60 years and older	174	(153 – 197)	63.3	(50.0 – 72.8)	166	(137 – 191)	482	(401 – 613)	298

† Estimate is subject to greater uncertainty due to small cell size.

Table 3.4.b. Urinary iodine: Concentrations by survey cycle

Geometric mean and selected percentiles of urine concentrations (in ng/mL) for the U.S. population, National Health and Nutrition Examination Survey, 2001–2006.

	Geometric mean (95% conf. interval)	Selected percentiles (95% conf. interval) 5th	50th	95th	Sample size
Total, 6 years and older					
2001–2002	162 (152 – 172)	30.1 (24.9 – 35.5)	168 (158 – 177)	713 (627 – 809)	2,837
2003–2004	150 (141 – 160)	28.9 (24.9 – 33.7)	160 (146 – 172)	569 (493 – 660)	2,526
2005–2006	161 (150 – 174)	36.0 (29.0 – 39.1)	164 (154 – 174)	665 (580 – 762)	2,649
Age group					
6–11 years					
2001–2002	235 (208 – 266)	51.8 (25.5 – 65.9)	249 (220 – 288)	771 (700 – 918)	374
2003–2004	209 (183 – 239)	45.7 (37.4 – 54.0)	229 (187 – 279)	613 (553 – 1,180)	315
2005–2006	235 (201 – 276)	60.2 (28.0 – 80.9)	238 (197 – 279)	967 (673 – 2,950)	351
12–19 years					
2001–2002	192 (178 – 207)	38.3 (23.5 – 47.2)	205 (189 – 214)	803 (710 – 968)	831
2003–2004	166 (141 – 195)	33.5 (17.9 – 46.4)	178 (144 – 203)	645 (503 – 924)	721
2005–2006	193 (167 – 224)	38.2 (25.1 – 51.8)	194 (177 – 224)	797 (713 – 1,160)	722
20–39 years					
2001–2002	148 (132 – 166)	27.8 (22.0 – 40.6)	153 (136 – 173)	536 (473 – 762)	627
2003–2004	138 (125 – 151)	23.8 (18.5 – 32.3)	146 (123 – 165)	564 (446 – 746)	517
2005–2006	132 (120 – 145)	31.9 (22.3 – 40.0)	134 (124 – 143)	483 (412 – 601)	617
40–59 years					
2001–2002	140 (121 – 162)	24.5 (21.1 – 30.0)	141 (119 – 169)	689 (525 – 1,330)	496
2003–2004	132 (119 – 147)	24.9 (13.1 – 35.0)	142 (128 – 161)	478 (422 – 690)	434
2005–2006	143 (129 – 158)	34.6 (20.1 – 38.3)	148 (131 – 173)	519 (431 – 640)	485
60 years and older					
2001–2002	177 (156 – 200)	40.7 (30.1 – 48.7)	171 (152 – 198)	744 (617 – 1,250)	509
2003–2004	169 (152 – 189)	39.7 (29.9 – 45.9)	170 (148 – 196)	635 (518 – 776)	539
2005–2006	205 (175 – 240)	47.9 (35.6 – 59.7)	195 (172 – 223)	826 (620 – 4,220)	474
Gender					
Males					
2001–2002	192 (178 – 208)	41.7 (35.0 – 48.0)	196 (179 – 209)	769 (630 – 981)	1,333
2003–2004	169 (156 – 183)	38.8 (25.9 – 44.3)	178 (164 – 193)	584 (475 – 786)	1,229
2005–2006	179 (163 – 197)	38.0 (32.9 – 44.8)	182 (172 – 195)	702 (595 – 960)	1,248
Females					
2001–2002	137 (127 – 148)	24.6 (21.3 – 29.2)	140 (126 – 156)	653 (576 – 736)	1,504
2003–2004	134 (125 – 145)	25.0 (23.0 – 29.0)	141 (127 – 155)	559 (493 – 584)	1,297
2005–2006	146 (136 – 158)	31.2 (20.6 – 39.0)	147 (137 – 155)	592 (544 – 693)	1,401
Race/ethnicity					
Mexican Americans					
2001–2002	176 (163 – 189)	33.7 (29.0 – 42.3)	187 (168 – 206)	673 (527 – 883)	720
2003–2004	168 (152 – 187)	38.7 (19.9 – 52.0)	186 (166 – 194)	568 (444 – 1,020)	617
2005–2006	177 (161 – 195)	44.6 (34.7 – 54.0)	184 (165 – 210)	640 (531 – 1,030)	703
Non-Hispanic Blacks					
2001–2002	156 (137 – 178)	38.6 (30.6 – 45.7)	143 (124 – 172)	716 (608 – 918)	670
2003–2004	134 (120 – 149)	42.3 (33.6 – 44.9)	131 (121 – 146)	456 (386 – 599)	634
2005–2006	147 (133 – 163)	34.3 (27.8 – 42.0)	149 (137 – 164)	510 (440 – 678)	729
Non-Hispanic Whites					
2001–2002	163 (150 – 176)	29.2 (22.7 – 35.6)	169 (160 – 181)	734 (604 – 875)	1,222
2003–2004	154 (144 – 164)	28.8 (23.9 – 33.8)	166 (151 – 181)	572 (486 – 684)	1,080
2005–2006	165 (151 – 180)	35.3 (26.3 – 39.1)	166 (154 – 179)	678 (583 – 831)	1,005

Figure 3.4.b. Urinary iodine: Concentrations by survey cycle

Selected percentiles in ng/mL (95% confidence intervals), National Health and Nutrition Examination Survey, 2001–2006

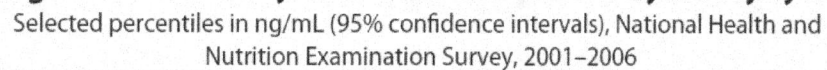

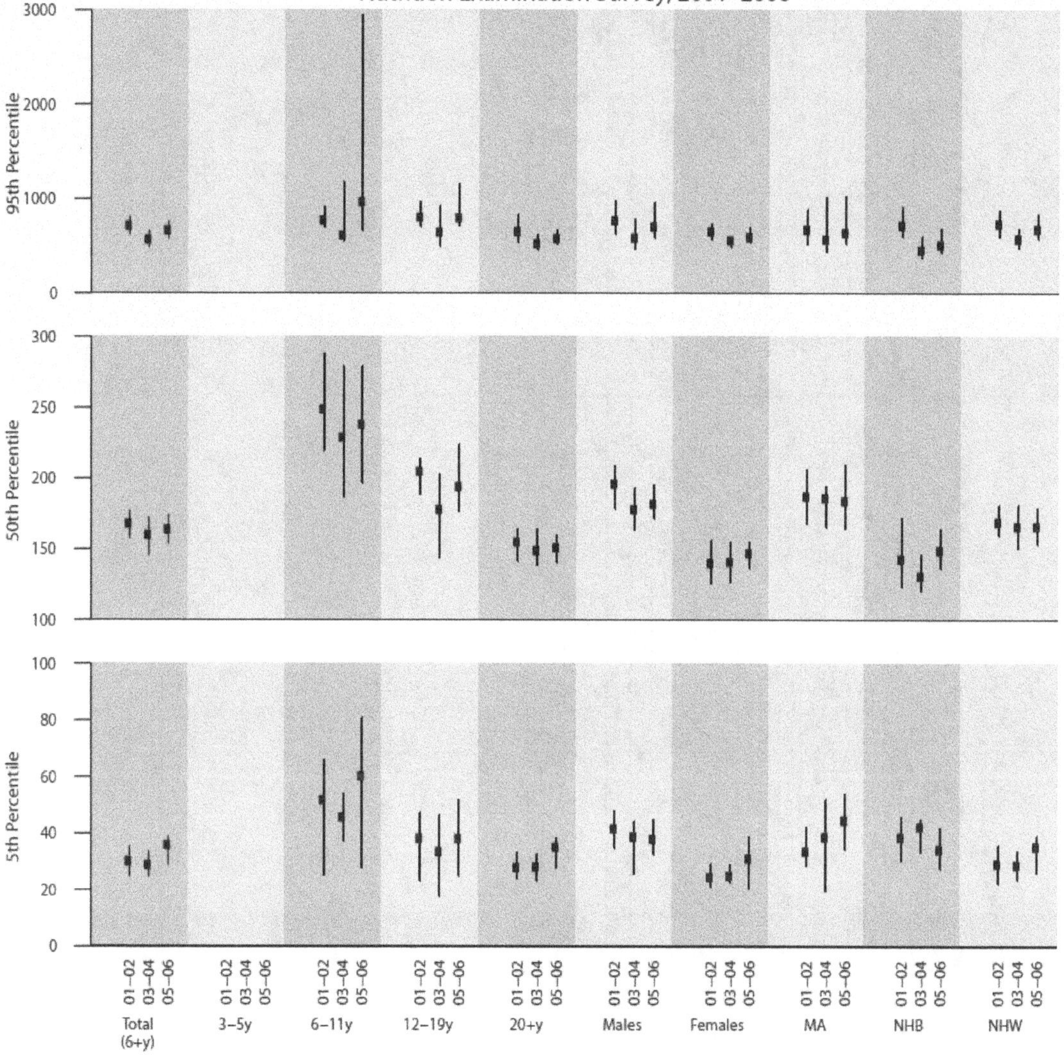

Table 3.5.a.1. Urinary iodine (creatinine corrected): Concentrations

Geometric mean and selected percentiles of urine concentrations (in µg/g creatinine) for the total U.S. population aged 6 years and older, National Health and Nutrition Examination Survey, 2003–2006.

	Geometric mean (95% conf. interval)	Selected percentiles (95% conf. interval)					Sample size
		2.5th	5th	50th	95th	97.5th	
Total, 6 years and older	155 (147 – 163)	39.3 (37.1 – 41.7)	46.7 (44.7 – 50.0)	149 (140 – 156)	572 (525 – 628)	763 (663 – 932)	5,174
Age group							
6–11 years	269 (244 – 297)	73.3 (56.4 – 81.6)	84.3 (77.6 – 92.2)	266 (240 – 293)	840 (653 – 1,190)	1,150 (827 – 7,820)	666
12–19 years	134 (124 – 145)	38.4 (35.1 – 42.1)	45.4 (41.0 – 49.7)	125 (115 – 137)	473 (406 – 555)	616 (528 – 835)	1,442
20–39 years	119 (111 – 127)	35.2 (32.5 – 38.8)	40.4 (37.5 – 44.9)	111 (103 – 119)	392 (347 – 485)	557 (450 – 903)	1,134
40–59 years	145 (136 – 156)	39.9 (34.1 – 42.0)	45.7 (41.2 – 50.6)	146 (132 – 158)	482 (421 – 526)	600 (519 – 738)	919
60 years and older	224 (209 – 241)	60.9 (53.6 – 65.5)	67.9 (65.6 – 71.0)	214 (191 – 237)	727 (660 – 891)	1,320 (863 – 5,710)	1,013
Gender							
Males	145 (137 – 153)	37.5 (35.0 – 39.6)	44.9 (41.2 – 47.7)	138 (129 – 149)	523 (479 – 591)	642 (584 – 1,140)	2,477
Females	165 (156 – 174)	42.1 (37.8 – 45.4)	49.7 (45.4 – 55.6)	157 (148 – 169)	617 (558 – 693)	807 (716 – 944)	2,697
Race/ethnicity							
Mexican Americans	160 (151 – 170)	46.2 (42.1 – 49.9)	54.1 (50.2 – 58.7)	156 (146 – 163)	494 (470 – 617)	695 (588 – 1,060)	1,319
Non-Hispanic Blacks	98.6 (91.2 – 106)	29.1 (25.8 – 30.7)	33.1 (30.4 – 34.6)	90.4 (83.4 – 99.1)	360 (325 – 395)	493 (437 – 588)	1,363
Non-Hispanic Whites	167 (161 – 174)	45.0 (41.4 – 46.9)	53.2 (48.7 – 57.4)	158 (151 – 169)	602 (539 – 669)	819 (697 – 1,060)	2,085

Figure 3.5.a. Urinary iodine (creatinine corrected): Concentrations by age group

Geometric mean (95% confidence interval), National Health and Nutrition Examination Survey, 2003–2006

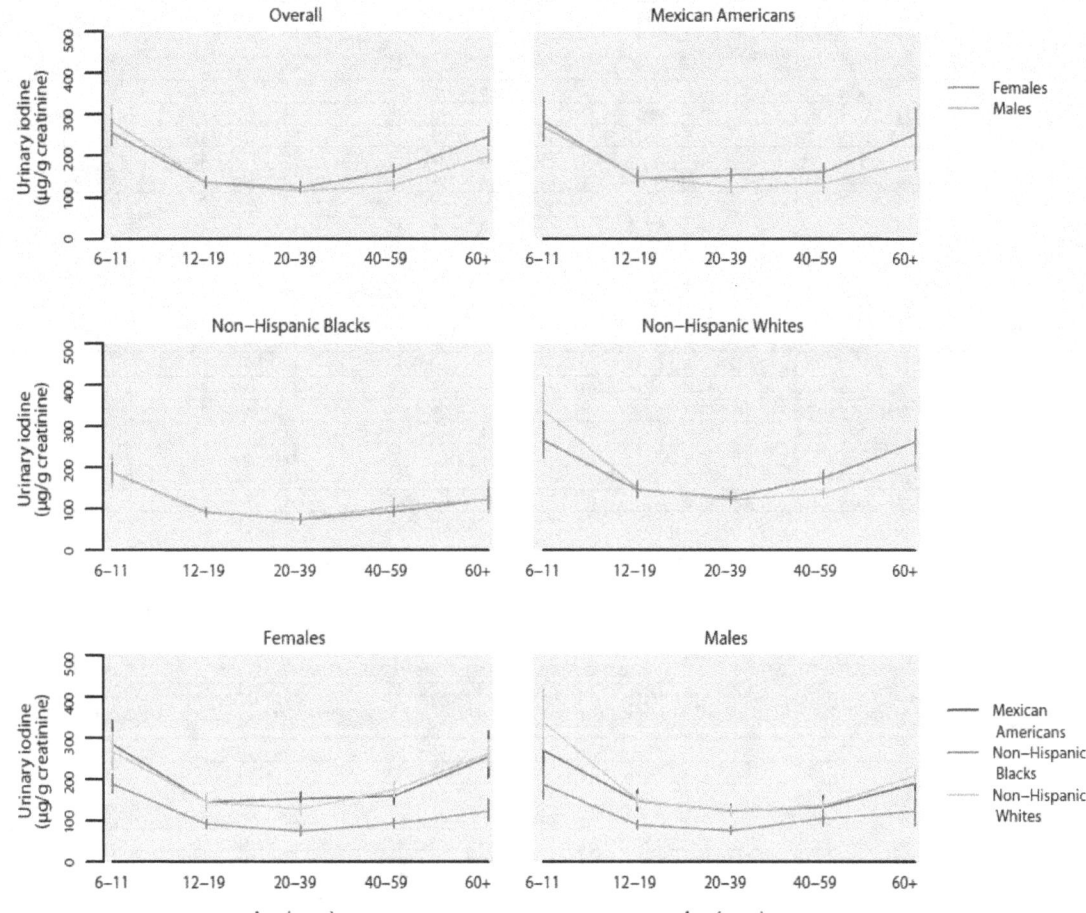

Table 3.5.a.2. Urinary iodine (creatinine corrected): Total population

Geometric mean and selected percentiles of urine concentrations (in µg/g creatinine) for the total U.S. population aged 6 years and older, National Health and Nutrition Examination Survey, 2003–2006.

| | Geometric mean (95% conf. interval) | Selected percentiles (95% conf. interval) | | | Sample size |
		10th	50th	90th	
Males and Females					
Total, 6 years and older	155 (147 – 163)	59.8 (56.4 – 64.0)	149 (140 – 156)	410 (391 – 438)	5,174
6–11 years	269 (244 – 297)	105 (92.1 – 115)	266 (240 – 293)	631 (590 – 820)	666
12–19 years	134 (124 – 145)	55.9 (49.7 – 61.9)	125 (115 – 137)	346 (301 – 386)	1,442
20–39 years	119 (111 – 127)	50.5 (46.7 – 55.0)	111 (103 – 119)	289 (271 – 324)	1,134
40–59 years	145 (136 – 156)	58.4 (50.9 – 63.7)	146 (132 – 158)	357 (322 – 408)	919
60 years and older	224 (209 – 241)	83.6 (75.9 – 92.3)	214 (191 – 237)	552 (481 – 635)	1,013
Males					
Total, 6 years and older	145 (137 – 153)	56.5 (52.3 – 60.2)	138 (129 – 149)	382 (357 – 414)	2,477
6–11 years	283 (248 – 323)	108 (83.8 – 131)	280 (245 – 322)	631 (589 – 1,060)	307
12–19 years	134 (122 – 148)	52.4 (46.2 – 58.2)	132 (117 – 149)	347 (300 – 413)	693
20–39 years	114 (106 – 123)	50.3 (44.9 – 54.6)	103 (93.8 – 114)	276 (264 – 335)	512
40–59 years	129 (119 – 140)	52.1 (45.8 – 60.0)	126 (113 – 136)	311 (274 – 392)	454
60 years and older	198 (183 – 215)	73.1 (67.3 – 83.9)	180 (168 – 205)	440 (407 – 481)	511
Females					
Total, 6 years and older	165 (156 – 174)	63.9 (57.9 – 69.6)	157 (148 – 169)	439 (403 – 481)	2,697
6–11 years	256 (228 – 286)	99.9 (87.8 – 114)	247 (227 – 293)	630 (529 – 821)	359
12–19 years	134 (121 – 148)	59.3 (51.3 – 64.9)	121 (111 – 131)	332 (292 – 403)	749
20–39 years	123 (112 – 136)	51.0 (45.8 – 57.9)	118 (107 – 130)	292 (254 – 359)	622
40–59 years	162 (148 – 178)	63.8 (55.7 – 70.9)	166 (145 – 188)	408 (344 – 482)	465
60 years and older	247 (224 – 272)	92.2 (79.1 – 104)	243 (221 – 262)	617 (554 – 696)	502

Table 3.5.a.3. Urinary iodine (creatinine corrected): Mexican Americans

Geometric mean and selected percentiles of urine concentrations (in µg/g creatinine) for Mexican Americans in the U.S. population aged 6 years and older, National Health and Nutrition Examination Survey, 2003–2006.

| | Geometric mean (95% conf. interval) | Selected percentiles (95% conf. interval) | | | Sample size |
		10th	50th	90th	
Males and Females					
Total, 6 years and older	160 (151 – 170)	67.5 (60.4 – 70.6)	156 (146 – 163)	383 (343 – 470)	1,319
6–11 years	276 (246 – 311)	123 (103 – 138)	267 (242 – 293)	619 (468 – 925)	217
12–19 years	146 (131 – 163)	61.9 (53.6 – 72.7)	143 (128 – 157)	344 (285 – 468)	465
20–39 years	137 (125 – 149)	59.7 (53.7 – 71.1)	137 (120 – 147)	293 (261 – 384)	283
40–59 years	146 (129 – 164)	66.0 (55.3 – 69.3)	148 (124 – 161)	317 (292 – 382)	165
60 years and older	222 (193 – 255)	85.2 (67.8 – 101)	210 (167 – 247)	459 (385 – 725)	189
Males					
Total, 6 years and older	148 (137 – 159)	60.0 (56.3 – 65.7)	147 (131 – 163)	361 (319 – 428)	623
6–11 years	269 (236 – 307)	126† (81.6 – 166)	278 (226 – 318)	541† (454 – 725)	96
12–19 years	147 (125 – 173)	58.5 (46.3 – 72.5)	141 (121 – 168)	346 (282 – 519)	221
20–39 years	124 (111 – 139)	55.7 (46.1 – 64.8)	121 (109 – 146)	244 (220 – 435)	134
40–59 years	133 (111 – 160)	58.9† (40.2 – 67.6)	136 (101 – 161)	318† (285 – 383)	77
60 years and older	189 (167 – 213)	81.1† (67.3 – 99.9)	168 (144 – 204)	410† (319 – 1,020)	95
Females					
Total, 6 years and older	174 (164 – 186)	73.4 (67.6 – 78.3)	162 (156 – 177)	416 (352 – 488)	696
6–11 years	284 (237 – 340)	116 (101 – 134)	250 (224 – 299)	656 (468 – 2,530)	121
12–19 years	145 (129 – 162)	67.1 (55.5 – 74.4)	144 (123 – 157)	333 (267 – 492)	244
20–39 years	153 (139 – 168)	73.4 (51.7 – 84.7)	143 (125 – 162)	344 (293 – 446)	149
40–59 years	160 (141 – 182)	68.0† (59.1 – 82.3)	160 (141 – 181)	308† (264 – 434)	88
60 years and older	253 (204 – 315)	86.1† (23.2 – 124)	232 (196 – 265)	502† (415 – 2,790)	94

† Estimate is subject to greater uncertainty due to small cell size.

Table 3.5.a.4. Urinary iodine (creatinine corrected): Non-Hispanic blacks

Geometric mean and selected percentiles of urine concentrations (in µg/g creatinine) for non-Hispanic blacks in the U.S. population aged 6 years and older, National Health and Nutrition Examination Survey, 2003–2006.

| | Geometric mean (95% conf. interval) | | Selected percentiles (95% conf. interval) | | | | | | Sample size |
			10th		50th		90th		
Males and Females									
Total, 6 years and older	98.6	(91.2 – 106)	39.0	(35.8 – 41.7)	90.4	(83.4 – 99.1)	264	(248 – 293)	1,363
6–11 years	188	(164 – 214)	80.2	(67.6 – 87.6)	180	(152 – 221)	448	(376 – 558)	221
12–19 years	90.8	(83.6 – 98.6)	40.5	(36.5 – 42.5)	87.0	(78.8 – 95.5)	223	(191 – 258)	515
20–39 years	75.5	(67.9 – 83.9)	35.6	(31.1 – 38.6)	72.6	(63.6 – 80.4)	209	(137 – 254)	238
40–59 years	98.3	(88.0 – 110)	38.1	(32.9 – 45.4)	90.5	(78.2 – 103)	257	(217 – 296)	219
60 years and older	123	(106 – 143)	46.0	(40.3 – 50.9)	108	(98.4 – 129)	337	(251 – 498)	170
Males									
Total, 6 years and older	101	(90.7 – 112)	37.6	(33.7 – 41.2)	92.1	(80.8 – 103)	294	(254 – 360)	663
6–11 years	187	(152 – 231)	73.7†	(52.4 – 87.7)	178	(142 – 244)	447†	(360 – 898)	106
12–19 years	90.1	(81.4 – 99.7)	37.4	(31.5 – 41.8)	84.8	(75.5 – 97.0)	224	(196 – 264)	260
20–39 years	76.2	(67.5 – 85.9)	35.3†	(27.7 – 38.4)	71.7	(62.5 – 78.5)	215†	(127 – 285)	108
40–59 years	105	(87.6 – 126)	34.3†	(29.7 – 47.5)	93.8	(73.4 – 130)	286†	(239 – 559)	104
60 years and older	123	(89.2 – 170)	41.0†	(34.7 – 49.6)	103	(78.5 – 159)	365†	(242 – 4,440)	85
Females									
Total, 6 years and older	96.5	(89.3 – 104)	39.3	(35.7 – 44.7)	89.3	(84.3 – 97.6)	247	(218 – 285)	700
6–11 years	188	(167 – 211)	83.8	(68.1 – 98.7)	185	(152 – 220)	442	(375 – 548)	115
12–19 years	91.5	(82.1 – 102)	42.8	(36.5 – 46.2)	88.5	(76.0 – 99.7)	205	(164 – 311)	255
20–39 years	74.9	(64.2 – 87.5)	36.1	(30.0 – 39.1)	72.7	(60.5 – 84.3)	196	(130 – 248)	130
40–59 years	92.9	(83.6 – 103)	39.5	(29.3 – 47.1)	88.5	(73.7 – 99.0)	217	(196 – 284)	115
60 years and older	123	(99.9 – 152)	50.2†	(30.9 – 61.9)	111	(97.1 – 134)	255†	(229 – 540)	85

† Estimate is subject to greater uncertainty due to small cell size.

Table 3.5.a.5. Urinary iodine (creatinine corrected): Non-Hispanic whites

Geometric mean and selected percentiles of urine concentrations (in µg/g creatinine) for non-Hispanic whites in the U.S. population aged 6 years and older, National Health and Nutrition Examination Survey, 2003–2006.

| | Geometric mean (95% conf. interval) | | Selected percentiles (95% conf. interval) | | | | | | Sample size |
			10th		50th		90th		
Males and Females									
Total, 6 years and older	167	(161 – 174)	67.2	(63.6 – 69.2)	158	(151 – 169)	430	(404 – 472)	2,085
6–11 years	299	(261 – 342)	114	(92.8 – 132)	289	(259 – 348)	663	(616 – 1,050)	169
12–19 years	147	(134 – 161)	63.3	(54.3 – 69.8)	135	(122 – 155)	374	(311 – 447)	365
20–39 years	125	(118 – 133)	55.5	(47.8 – 62.1)	115	(107 – 124)	298	(274 – 345)	494
40–59 years	155	(145 – 166)	62.7	(56.4 – 69.7)	155	(140 – 174)	364	(327 – 419)	453
60 years and older	236	(218 – 256)	94.3	(82.5 – 102)	233	(196 – 248)	559	(481 – 657)	604
Males									
Total, 6 years and older	157	(149 – 165)	64.0	(61.1 – 67.2)	150	(140 – 156)	396	(368 – 428)	996
6–11 years	337	(272 – 417)	131†	(63.9 – 170)	326	(268 – 429)	811†	(610 – 2,040)	76
12–19 years	149	(135 – 163)	59.4	(49.6 – 67.3)	143	(129 – 170)	378	(301 – 455)	174
20–39 years	122	(111 – 135)	57.5	(46.5 – 65.4)	104	(93.8 – 122)	292	(265 – 349)	211
40–59 years	137	(126 – 149)	59.3	(48.9 – 64.1)	136	(120 – 152)	313	(274 – 414)	229
60 years and older	208	(192 – 226)	82.9	(70.7 – 95.2)	189	(173 – 215)	440	(402 – 522)	306
Females									
Total, 6 years and older	178	(169 – 188)	70.6	(64.9 – 74.3)	169	(156 – 183)	464	(431 – 514)	1,089
6–11 years	265	(225 – 311)	99.1†	(84.0 – 118)	262	(227 – 315)	640†	(474 – 1,020)	93
12–19 years	145	(127 – 167)	65.0	(56.0 – 74.0)	127	(112 – 152)	368	(292 – 499)	191
20–39 years	128	(116 – 142)	51.3	(45.4 – 62.5)	123	(110 – 141)	295	(242 – 391)	283
40–59 years	175	(159 – 193)	70.6	(58.0 – 79.3)	179	(152 – 202)	433	(362 – 496)	224
60 years and older	261	(232 – 294)	104	(81.2 – 119)	255	(236 – 280)	630	(556 – 697)	298

† Estimate is subject to greater uncertainty due to small cell size.

Table 3.5.b. Urinary iodine (creatinine corrected): Concentrations by survey cycle

Geometric mean and selected percentiles of urine concentrations (in µg/g creatinine) for the U.S. population, National Health and Nutrition Examination Survey, 2001–2006.

	Geometric mean (95% conf. interval)	Selected percentiles (95% conf. interval) 5th		Selected percentiles 50th		Selected percentiles 95th		Sample size
Total, 6 years and older								
2001–2002	163 (153 – 173)	50.0	(46.8 – 54.0)	151	(141 – 165)	620	(567 – 687)	2,835
2003–2004	146 (135 – 158)	45.4	(39.4 – 49.3)	142	(130 – 154)	492	(449 – 585)	2,525
2005–2006	163 (153 – 175)	50.0	(45.0 – 54.7)	155	(143 – 169)	620	(549 – 733)	2,649
Age group								
6–11 years								
2001–2002	273 (246 – 304)	94.5	(75.7 – 106)	257	(220 – 319)	923	(772 – 1,140)	374
2003–2004	254 (228 – 283)	84.4	(71.9 – 98.7)	246	(233 – 269)	718	(615 – 1,210)	315
2005–2006	286 (242 – 339)	82.5	(64.3 – 98.9)	288	(236 – 362)	947	(654 – 2,300)	351
12–19 years								
2001–2002	149 (137 – 161)	52.5	(47.8 – 58.9)	138	(129 – 146)	601	(450 – 721)	830
2003–2004	124 (109 – 141)	45.4	(36.3 – 49.9)	117	(104 – 132)	381	(314 – 532)	720
2005–2006	145 (130 – 162)	45.4	(39.8 – 51.9)	138	(117 – 163)	477	(434 – 829)	722
20–39 years								
2001–2002	135 (127 – 143)	46.7	(42.2 – 49.5)	128	(118 – 136)	470	(443 – 577)	627
2003–2004	115 (104 – 127)	39.2	(33.9 – 44.9)	108	(99.3 – 119)	407	(319 – 559)	517
2005–2006	123 (112 – 135)	43.9	(39.1 – 49.0)	114	(97.7 – 131)	378	(339 – 592)	617
40–59 years								
2001–2002	151 (130 – 175)	44.7	(37.9 – 54.5)	142	(120 – 176)	522	(427 – 712)	496
2003–2004	138 (126 – 152)	42.0	(34.9 – 49.9)	136	(126 – 150)	436	(392 – 561)	434
2005–2006	152 (137 – 170)	47.0	(40.9 – 56.5)	153	(126 – 179)	492	(429 – 544)	485
60 years and older								
2001–2002	216 (192 – 244)	67.1	(51.2 – 75.5)	199	(179 – 230)	751	(632 – 1,000)	508
2003–2004	204 (188 – 222)	67.2	(60.3 – 74.0)	197	(178 – 233)	595	(521 – 726)	539
2005–2006	246 (218 – 277)	68.4	(65.8 – 72.8)	235	(193 – 256)	858	(697 – 5,190)	474
Gender								
Males								
2001–2002	156 (143 – 171)	47.0	(43.7 – 51.1)	145	(137 – 160)	578	(514 – 674)	1,333
2003–2004	137 (127 – 148)	41.7	(36.3 – 46.4)	132	(121 – 146)	481	(417 – 590)	1,229
2005–2006	152 (140 – 165)	47.8	(42.6 – 50.4)	147	(132 – 158)	540	(480 – 795)	1,248
Females								
2001–2002	170 (161 – 179)	55.2	(48.0 – 57.1)	158	(146 – 168)	670	(585 – 748)	1,502
2003–2004	155 (142 – 169)	46.9	(41.8 – 52.7)	151	(133 – 167)	532	(452 – 630)	1,296
2005–2006	176 (163 – 189)	54.4	(44.6 – 60.3)	164	(150 – 179)	687	(598 – 829)	1,401
Race/ethnicity								
Mexican Americans								
2001–2002	164 (152 – 176)	56.0	(49.4 – 61.0)	154	(140 – 177)	589	(469 – 754)	720
2003–2004	152 (138 – 169)	51.3	(42.1 – 58.9)	147	(133 – 164)	481	(389 – 1,100)	616
2005–2006	167 (154 – 181)	56.2	(51.7 – 60.0)	163	(153 – 179)	544	(454 – 728)	703
Non-Hispanic Blacks								
2001–2002	113 (103 – 124)	36.8	(27.9 – 42.8)	103	(93.5 – 115)	440	(361 – 645)	669
2003–2004	92.1 (81.2 – 104)	33.1	(29.7 – 33.8)	84.6	(73.1 – 97.6)	336	(296 – 375)	634
2005–2006	105 (96.7 – 115)	33.7	(29.8 – 37.7)	96.6	(87.0 – 111)	397	(315 – 513)	729
Non-Hispanic Whites								
2001–2002	175 (163 – 188)	55.1	(48.3 – 58.2)	164	(151 – 176)	652	(576 – 749)	1,221
2003–2004	159 (150 – 168)	50.9	(46.3 – 58.2)	153	(147 – 161)	526	(442 – 621)	1,080
2005–2006	177 (166 – 188)	55.0	(45.8 – 59.4)	168	(152 – 179)	656	(561 – 868)	1,005

Figure 3.5.b. Urinary iodine (creatinine corrected): Concentrations by survey cycle
Selected percentiles in µg/g creatinine (95% confidence intervals),
National Health and Nutrition Examination Survey, 2001–2006

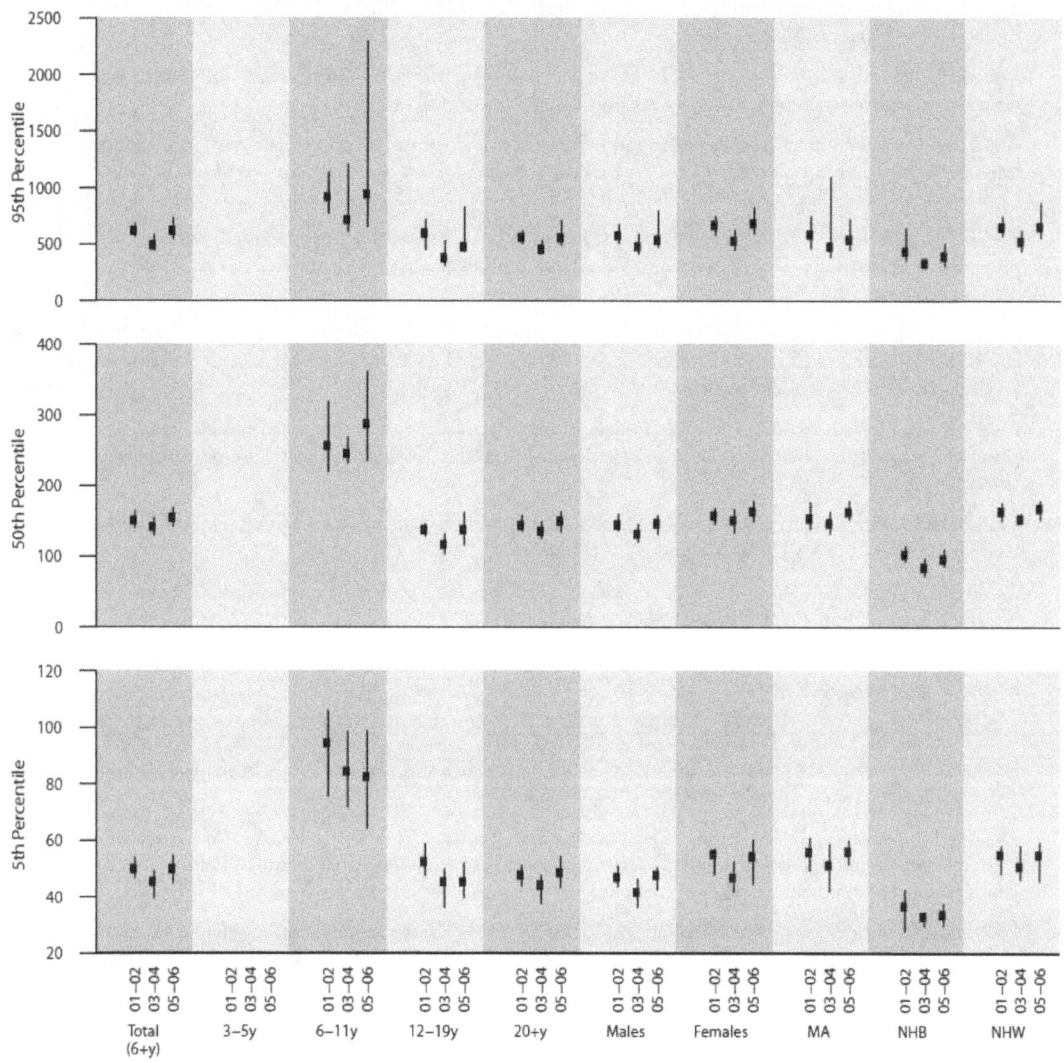

References

Abalovich M, Amino N, Barbour LA, Cobin RH, De Groot LJ, Glinoer D, et al. Management of thyroid dysfunction during pregnancy and postpartum: an Endocrine Society Clinical Practice Guideline. J Clin Endocrinol & Metabol. 2007;92:s1–s47.

Andersen S, Karmisholt J, Pdersen KM, Laurberg P. Reliability of studies of iodine intake and recommendations for number of samples in groups and in individuals. Br J Nutr. 2008;99:813–818.

Andersson M, de Benoist B, Delange F, Zupan J. Prevention and control of iodine deficiency in pregnant and lactating women and in children less than 2-years-old: conclusions and recommendations of the Technical Consultation. Public Health Nutrition 2007;10(12A):1606–1611.

Becker DV, Braverman LE, Delange F, Dunn JT, Franklyn JA, Hollowell JG, et al. Iodine supplementation for pregnancy and lactation—United States and Canada: recommendations of the American Thyroid Association. Thyroid. 2006;16:949–951.

Beers MH, editor. Vitamin deficiency, dependency, and toxicity. In: Merck Manual of Diagnosis and Therapy. 18th ed. Whitehouse Station (NJ): Merck & Co., Inc.; 2006 [cited 2011]. Available at: http://www.merckmanuals.com/professional/sec01/ch005/ch005e.html.

Caldwell KL, Maxwell B, Makhmudov A, Pino S, Braverman LE, Jones RL, et al. Use of inductively coupled plasma mass spectrometry to measure urinary iodine in NHANES 2000: comparison with previous method. Clin Chem. 2003;49:1019–1021.

Caldwell KL, Jones R, Hollowell JG. Urinary iodine concentration: United States National Health and Nutrition Examination Survey 2001–2002. Thyroid. 2005;15:692–699.

Caldwell KL, Miller GA, Wang RY, Jain RB, Jones RL. Iodine status of the U.S. population, National Health and Nutrition Examination Survey 2003–2004. Thyroid. 2008;18:1207–1214.

Caldwell KL, Makhmudov A, Ely E, Jones RL, Wang R. Iodine status of the U.S. population, National Health and Nutrition Examination Survey, 2005–2006 and 2007–2008. Thyroid. 2011;21:419–427.

Glinoer D. The importance of iodine nutrition during pregnancy. Publ Health Nutr. 2007;10:1542–1546.

Gregory CO, Serdula MK, Sullivan KM. Use of supplements with and without iodine in women of childbearing age in the United States. Thyroid. 2009;19:1019–1020.

Hollowell JG, Staehling NW, Hannon WH, Flanders DW, Gunter EW, Maberly GF, et al. Iodine nutrition in the United States. Trends and public health implications: iodine excretion data from National Health and Nutrition Examination Surveys I and III (1971–1974 and 1988–1994). J Clin Endocrinol Metab. 1998;83:3401–3408.

Institute of Medicine, Food and Nutrition Board. Dietary Reference Intakes: vitamin A, vitamin K, arsenic, boron, chromium, copper, iodine, iron, manganese, molybdenum, nickel, silicon, vanadium, and zinc. Washington, D.C.: National Academy Press; 2001.

Murray CW, Egan SK, Kim H, Beru N, Bolger PM. US Food and Drug Administration's Total Diet Study: Dietary intake of perchlorate and iodine. J Exposure Sci Environ Epidem. 2008;18:571–580.

Pennington JAT, Schoen SA. Total Diet Study: estimated dietary intakes of nutritional elements, 1982–1991. Int J Vit Nutr Res. 1996;66:350–362.

Perrine CG, Herrick K, Serdula MK, Sullivan KM. Some subgroups of reproductive age women in the United States may be at risk for iodine deficiency. J Nutr. 2010;140:1489–1494.

Pino S, Fang SL, Braverman LE. Ammonium persulfate: a new and safe method for measuring urinary iodine by ammonium persulfate oxidation. Exp Clin Endocrinol Diabetes. 1998;106 Suppl 3:S22–S27.

World Health Organization. Assessment of iodine deficiency disorders and monitoring their elimination: a guide for programme managers. 3rd ed. Geneva (Switzerland): World Health Organization, 2007 (WHO/NHD/01.1) [cited 2011]. Available at: http://whqlibdoc.who.int/publications/2007/9789241595827_eng.pdf.

4. Isoflavones and Lignans

Isoflavones
- Genistein
- Daidzein
- Equol
- O-Desmethylangolensin

Lignans
- Enterodiol
- Enterolactone

Isoflavones and Lignans

Background Information

Sources and Physiological Functions. Isoflavones and lignans are secondary plant metabolites frequently encountered in the diet. When ingested and metabolized, these compounds have the potential to act as phytoestrogens, a class of compounds that have weak estrogenic effects. This report considers urinary concentrations of four isoflavones (daidzein, genistein, O-desmethylangolensin [ODMA], and equol) and two lignans (enterodiol and enterolactone).

Diet is the primary source of human exposure to phytoestrogens. Plant sources of isoflavones include legumes, with the largest contribution coming from soy-based foods. Since soy flour and soy protein isolates may be added to processed meats, meat substitutes, breads, and protein-food bars, these items can be a major source of isoflavones (Lampe 1999; Grace 2004). However, the isoflavone content of soy protein preparations can vary widely, and it is affected by production techniques (Erdman 2004). Daidzein and genistein are the main soy isoflavones. Kudzu root, used in some dietary supplements, also contains appreciable amounts of daidzein. Naringenin, a precursor to genistein, is found in some citrus fruits. Formononetin and biochanin A are methylated isoflavones found in clover, which may be used in red clover dietary supplements, and they are metabolized in the body to daidzein and genistein, respectively. Lignans are found in flax seeds, whole wheat flour, tea, some fruits, and other cereal grains. Lignans include matairesinol and secoisolariciresinol, which are transformed by intestinal bacteria into the estrogenic coumpounds enterolactone and enterodiol, respectively (Rowland 2003; Cornwell 2004). Enterodiol may also convert into enterolactone and vice versa. Isoflavone intake is typically higher in Asian populations than in Western populations, primarily due to the higher soy consumption and the significant role that such fermented food products as tempeh, miso, or natto play in Asian diets (Mortensen 2009). Lignan intake varies greatly from country to country because of different dietary sources; however, completeness of food composition data is also a confounding factor in interpreting these data (Peterson 2010).

The absorption and metabolism of phytoestrogens varies considerably among individuals. The variation may relate to differences in absorption, enterohepatic circulation, and metabolism by intestinal bacteria. Isoflavones and lignans occur primarily as glycosides in unfermented foods with a small percentage of aglycones present. Aglycones represent a larger portion of the phytoestrogens present in fermented foods due to bacterial hydrolysis of the glycosides. Glycosidic forms are hydrolyzed to their aglycones in the intestine, absorbed, and then linked in the intestinal wall and liver with glucuronic acid to make them more water-soluble, a process known as glucuronidation. The glucuronidated metabolites of isoflavones predominate in blood and urine (Doerge 2000; Rowland 2003; Clavel 2006; Nielsen 2007). Ingested daidzein is further metabolized to ODMA and to equol by intestinal bacteria. Equol, but not ODMA, has estrogenic activity. About 30 percent of adults produce equol and have higher serum equol concentrations after they consume daidzein (Setchell 2003a; Cassidy 2006). This ability to produce equol may be related to an individual's intestinal microflora and influenced by dietary habits and genetic factors (Rowland 2000; Setchell 2002; Setchell 2006). It is unclear whether the ability to produce equol results in any health-related effects (Vafeiadou 2006).

Generally, phytoestrogens are much less potent than endogenously produced estrogens, but phytoestrogens can be present in much greater quantities (100 to 1000 times the concentration of endogenous estrogens). Additionally, phytoestrogens bind less tightly to steroid-hormone serum-transport proteins than do endogenous estrogens (Nagel 1998). Equol has more potent estrogen activity than its precursor daidzein and has been proposed to be most important in explaining the possible mechanism of action of isoflavones in disease prevention (Setchell 2002).

Health Effects. The dietary consumption of phytoestrogens is believed to be associated with a reduced risk of hormone-dependent cancers, such as breast (Dong 2010; Buck 2010) and prostate cancer (Yan 2009; Hamilton-Reeves 2010), due to antagonistic mechanisms related to hormone receptor binding. Other health benefits related to the consumption of phytoestrogen-rich diets have also been proposed: reduced

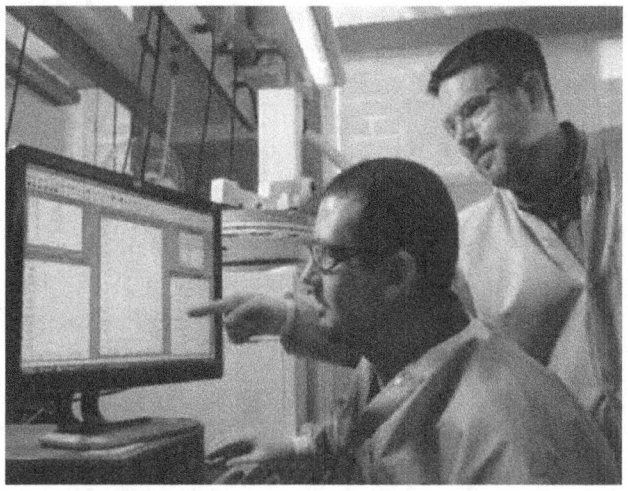

severity of menopause-related symptoms (Howes 2006; Jacobs 2009); cardiovascular health (Pan 2009; Peterson 2010); and modulation of osteoporosis (Liu 2010). A report from the Agency for Healthcare Research and Quality (Balk 2005) about the effects of soy on health outcomes reported that there is no conclusive evidence of a dose-response effect of either soy protein or isoflavone on cardiovascular diseases, menopausal symptoms, endocrine function, cancer, bone health, reproductive health, kidney diseases, cognitive function, or glucose metabolism. For reducing low-density lipoprotein concentrations, however, soy protein could possibly have a dose-response effect. As for lignan intake, flaxseed has been shown to significantly reduce LDL- and total cholesterol depending on the type of intervention, sex, and lipid profiles of the subjects (Pan 2009).

Adverse effects on fertility have been observed in animals that graze on red clover. Results of chronic feeding studies in pregnant animals suggest that high doses of phytoestrogens alter the fetal hormonal environment (Cornwell 2004). Infants who consume soy-based formula can have plasma concentrations of isoflavones that are 13,000–22,000 times higher than concentrations of endogenous estrogen in infants (Setchell 1997). Yet, studies of children who had been fed soy-based formula as infants and who were followed through adolescence (Klein 1998) and young adulthood (Strom 2001) found no adverse reproductive or endocrine effects. A meta-analysis of 32 studies in which adult men consumed soy foods, isolated soy protein, or isoflavone extracts (from soy or red clover) found that neither soy foods nor isoflavone supplements alter measures of bioavailable testosterone concentrations in men (Hamilton-Reeves 2010). In vitro and animal studies also suggest that soy isoflavones may have immunologic and thyroid effects (Doerge 2002). The Center for the Evaluation of Risks to Human Reproduction (CERHR) of the National Toxicology Program reviewed the developmental and reproductive toxicity of both soy formula and genistein and concluded that available data were inadequate to determine the effects of soy formula on developmental or reproductive toxicity (Rozman 2006a). The expert review panel expressed negligible concern for adverse effects in the general population of consuming dietary sources of genistein: under current exposure conditions, adults would be unlikely to consume sufficient daily levels of genistein to cause adverse reproductive and/or developmental effects (Rozman 2006b). A subsequent review by CERHR that included new study data from 2006–2009 and focused specifically on the developmental toxicity of soy infant formula and its major isoflavone components found minimal concern for adverse effects on development in infants who consume soy infant formula (McCarver 2011).

Biochemical Indicators and Methods. A systematic review of intervention studies has shown that urinary concentrations of daidzein, genistein, and enterolactone are good biomarkers of dietary intake (Pearson r = 0.78–0.87) as compared to equol, ODMA (0.38–0.40) and enterodiol (-0.14) (Pérez-Jiménez 2010). Linear dose-response relations are typically observed for the lignans (Nesbitt 1999; Hutchins 2000). Saturation in urine recovery has been observed with the isoflavones (Setchell 2003a). Isoflavones and lignans have been measured in biologic matrices such as plasma, serum, and urine by use of high performance liquid chromatography (HPLC) or gas chromatography (GC) with various modes of detection (Hoikkala 2003; Prasain 2004). Liquid chromatography coupled to tandem mass spectrometry (LC-MS/MS) methods that measure isoflavones and lignans concentrations after deconjugation of glucuronides and sulfates are most commonly used at present.

Data in NHANES. Phytoestrogens have been measured in NHANES since 1999. In NHANES 1999–2000, CDC scientists detected enterolactone in the highest concentration, and daidzein was detected with the highest frequency among the six measured phytoestrogens (Valentin-Blasini 2005). CDC's Fourth National Report on Human Exposure to Environmental Chemicals presented geometric means and selected percentiles (50th, 75th, 90th, and 95th) for concentrations of phytoestrogens by age, sex, or race/ethnicity for participants in NHANES 1999–2000, 2001–2002, and 2003–2004 (U.S. Centers for Disease Control and Prevention 2009).

Urinary daidzein, genistein, equol, ODMA, enterolactone, and enterodiol data presented in this report were generated by use of LC-MS/MS using electrospray ionization (ESI) for NHANES 2003–2004 (Rybak 2008) and LC-MS/MS using atmospheric pressure photoionization (APPI) for NHANES 2005–2006 (Parker 2011). Crossover studies comparing samples analyzed by LC-ESI-MS/MS and LC-APPI-MS/MS demonstrated high correlation coefficients (r >0.99) and regression slopes approximately equal to 1 and intercepts close to 0 (U.S. Centers for Disease Control and Prevention 2011).

For more information about soy isoflavones, see the fact sheet from the National Institutes of Health, Office of Dietary Supplements (http://ods.od.nih.gov/Health_Information/Information_About_Individual_Dietary_Supplements.aspx).

Highlights

Urinary isoflavone and lignan concentrations in the U.S. population showed the following demographic patterns and characteristics:

- No consistent patterns were observed with regard to age, gender, or race/ethnicity.
- Concentrations have been relatively similar from 1999–2006.

Urinary isoflavone and lignan concentrations showed only small variations by demographic variables, such as age, gender, or race/ethnicity, or by survey cycle. However, as reported previously (Valentin-Blasini 2005), we observed large differences in the concentration of different urinary phytoestrogens. The enterolactone concentration was approximately one order of magnitude higher than the concentrations of genistein, daidzein, and enterodiol, which in turn were approximately one order of magnitude higher than the concentrations of equol and ODMA (Figure H.4.a). These phytoestrogens were detected in >99% of all samples, with the exception of ODMA, which was detected in only 93% of all samples.

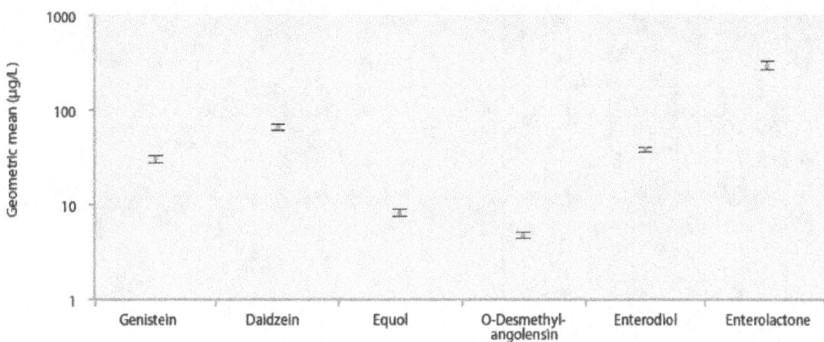

Figure H.4.a. *Geometric mean concentrations of urinary isoflavones and lignans in the U.S. population aged 6 years and older, National Health and Nutrition Examination Survey, 2003–2006.*

Error bars represent 95 percent confidence intervals. The y-axis is displayed on the logarithmic scale.

Detailed Observations

The selected observations mentioned below are derived from the uncorrected tables and figures presented next. The NHANES population is of sufficient size to allow group comparisons based on uncorrected data. Statements about categorical differences between demographic groups noted below are based on non-overlapping confidence limits from univariate analysis without adjusting for demographic variables (i.e., age, sex, race/ethnicity) or other determinants of these urine concentrations (i.e., dietary intake, supplement usage, smoking, BMI). A multivariate analysis may alter the size and statistical significance of these categorical differences. Furthermore, additional significant differences of smaller magnitude may be present despite their lack of mention here (e.g., if confidence limits slightly overlap or if differences are not statistically significant before covariate adjustment has occurred). For a selection of citations of descriptive NHANES papers related to these biochemical indicators of diet and nutrition, see **Appendix G.**

Geometric mean concentrations (NHANES 2003–2006):

- Urinary concentrations of daidzein (Table 4.3.a.1 and Figure 4.3.a), equol (Table 4.5.a.1 and Figure 4.5.a), and ODMA (Table 5.7.a.1 and Figure 5.7.1) were highest in children and adolescents than for other age groups, while urinary concentrations of genistein and the two lignans were similar across age groups (Tables 4.1.a.1, 4.9.a.1, 5.11.a.1 and Figures 4.1.a, 4.9.a, 4.11.a).

- Males and females had similar phytoestrogen concentrations with the exception of daidzein and genistein concentrations which were lower in females.

- Urinary concentrations of phytoestrogens were similar across the three race/ethnic groups, with the exception of ODMA concentrations, which were lowest in Mexican Americans.

Changes in geometric mean concentrations across survey cycles:

- Urinary genistein, equol, ODMA, and enterolactone concentrations were similar across the four survey cycles (Tables 4.1.b, 4.5.b, 4.7.b, and 4.11.b).

- Urinary daidzein concentrations were lower in 2001–2002 than in the other three survey cycles (Table 4.3.b).

- Urinary enterodiol concentrations were lower in 1999-2000 than in the other three survey cycles (Table 4.9.b).

Table 4.1.a.1. Urinary genistein: Concentrations

Geometric mean and selected percentiles of urine concentrations (in μg/L) for the total U.S. population aged 6 years and older, National Health and Nutrition Examination Survey, 2003–2006.

	Geometric mean (95% conf. interval)	Selected percentiles (95% conf. interval)					Sample size
		2.5th	5th	50th	95th	97.5th	
Total, 6 years and older	29.9 (28.0 – 31.8)	1.51 (1.24 – 1.78)	2.45 (2.14 – 2.78)	26.1 (23.8 – 28.5)	523 (459 – 578)	852 (706 – 1,060)	5,122
Age group							
6–11 years	36.0 (30.9 – 41.9)	3.05 (1.06 – 3.78)	4.20 (2.59 – 5.15)	31.7 (26.6 – 35.8)	414 (357 – 819)	846 (579 – 2,730)	692
12–19 years	34.4 (30.7 – 38.6)	2.39 (1.92 – 2.78)	3.33 (2.72 – 3.84)	27.6 (23.6 – 33.2)	514 (409 – 651)	946 (659 – 1,510)	1,422
20–39 years	28.5 (25.0 – 32.5)	1.54 (1.04 – 1.95)	2.27 (1.68 – 3.27)	23.7 (20.4 – 27.5)	516 (412 – 596)	810 (639 – 1,280)	1,137
40–59 years	28.1 (25.1 – 31.5)	1.33 (1.04 – 1.73)	2.17 (1.68 – 2.72)	26.2 (20.7 – 30.2)	589 (423 – 703)	767 (631 – 1,500)	901
60 years and older	29.5 (26.1 – 33.3)	1.15 (< LOD – 1.48)	2.16 (1.41 – 2.69)	27.5 (22.4 – 31.7)	435 (341 – 559)	794 (558 – 2,580)	970
Gender							
Males	32.9 (30.2 – 35.7)	1.96 (1.41 – 2.35)	3.22 (2.55 – 3.62)	28.5 (25.7 – 32.0)	544 (461 – 591)	805 (701 – 1,120)	2,496
Females	27.2 (24.9 – 29.9)	1.25 (1.05 – 1.53)	2.01 (1.76 – 2.31)	23.8 (20.8 – 27.0)	514 (398 – 618)	867 (654 – 1,150)	2,626
Race/ethnicity							
Mexican Americans	29.3 (26.8 – 32.0)	1.67 (1.10 – 2.05)	2.47 (1.90 – 3.28)	25.8 (22.2 – 29.0)	570 (434 – 695)	929 (763 – 1,290)	1,287
Non-Hispanic Blacks	31.8 (27.1 – 37.3)	1.88 (1.21 – 2.30)	3.03 (2.34 – 3.53)	27.8 (23.0 – 34.7)	466 (387 – 743)	899 (642 – 1,260)	1,343
Non-Hispanic Whites	28.8 (26.7 – 31.1)	1.38 (1.13 – 1.65)	2.18 (1.84 – 2.71)	25.3 (22.3 – 28.3)	502 (417 – 589)	761 (682 – 1,100)	2,108

< LOD means less than the limit of detection, which may vary for some compounds by year. See Appendix D for LOD.

Figure 4.1.a. Urinary genistein: Concentrations by age group

Geometric mean (95% confidence interval), National Health and Nutrition Examination Survey, 2003–2006

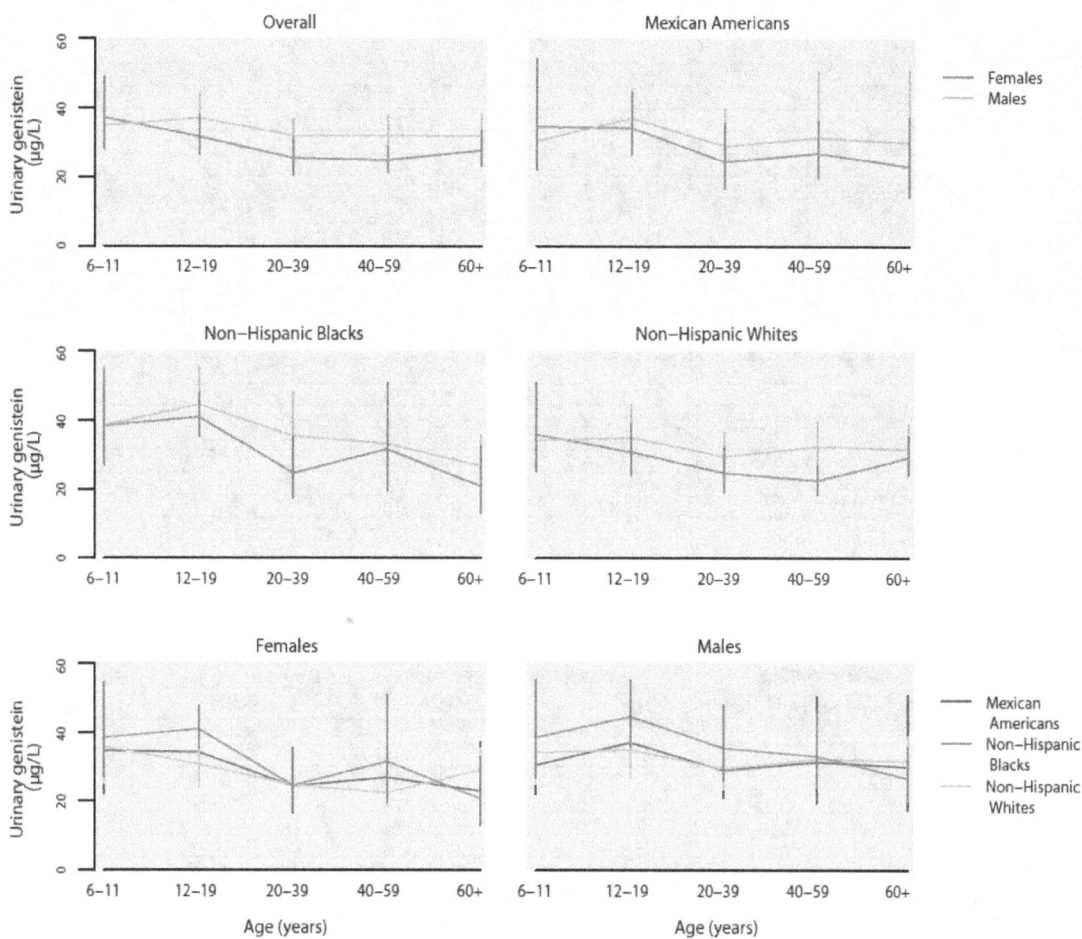

Table 4.1.a.2. Urinary genistein: Total population

Geometric mean and selected percentiles of urine concentrations (in μg/L) for the total U.S. population aged 6 years and older, National Health and Nutrition Examination Survey, 2003–2006.

	Geometric mean (95% conf. interval)		Selected percentiles (95% conf. interval)						Sample size
			10th		50th		90th		
Males and Females									
Total, 6 years and older	29.9	(28.0 – 31.8)	4.18	(3.88 – 4.51)	26.1	(23.8 – 28.5)	274	(246 – 304)	5,122
6–11 years	36.0	(30.9 – 41.9)	6.11	(4.50 – 7.43)	31.7	(26.6 – 35.8)	276	(215 – 355)	692
12–19 years	34.4	(30.7 – 38.6)	4.87	(4.11 – 5.91)	27.6	(23.6 – 33.2)	303	(237 – 367)	1,422
20–39 years	28.5	(25.0 – 32.5)	4.25	(3.30 – 5.01)	23.7	(20.4 – 27.5)	237	(185 – 322)	1,137
40–59 years	28.1	(25.1 – 31.5)	3.76	(3.33 – 3.96)	26.2	(20.7 – 30.2)	307	(242 – 374)	901
60 years and older	29.5	(26.1 – 33.3)	4.09	(3.31 – 4.77)	27.5	(22.4 – 31.7)	244	(212 – 311)	970
Males									
Total, 6 years and older	32.9	(30.2 – 35.7)	4.91	(4.35 – 5.39)	28.5	(25.7 – 32.0)	301	(247 – 337)	2,496
6–11 years	34.9	(28.9 – 42.1)	6.44	(4.51 – 8.48)	29.8	(22.4 – 35.8)	215	(177 – 369)	340
12–19 years	37.1	(31.3 – 44.0)	5.45	(4.48 – 6.96)	31.9	(24.2 – 42.5)	261	(209 – 402)	728
20–39 years	32.0	(27.8 – 36.7)	4.95	(3.48 – 5.71)	25.9	(21.5 – 32.0)	300	(197 – 397)	499
40–59 years	32.0	(26.9 – 38.0)	4.14	(3.42 – 5.17)	29.1	(21.7 – 34.2)	324	(227 – 510)	451
60 years and older	31.9	(26.6 – 38.3)	4.73	(3.78 – 5.83)	28.9	(20.6 – 36.6)	230	(183 – 337)	478
Females									
Total, 6 years and older	27.2	(24.9 – 29.9)	3.73	(3.23 – 4.07)	23.8	(20.8 – 27.0)	253	(222 – 302)	2,626
6–11 years	37.2	(28.2 – 49.0)	5.55	(3.39 – 7.52)	34.9	(25.3 – 44.7)	278	(239 – 407)	352
12–19 years	31.7	(26.6 – 37.9)	3.85	(3.34 – 5.15)	24.3	(20.0 – 31.7)	321	(220 – 413)	694
20–39 years	25.5	(20.7 – 31.3)	3.81	(2.25 – 4.32)	22.1	(18.9 – 26.9)	208	(154 – 318)	638
40–59 years	24.9	(21.3 – 29.0)	3.14	(2.70 – 3.91)	20.4	(16.6 – 27.0)	256	(175 – 408)	450
60 years and older	27.7	(23.1 – 33.2)	3.34	(2.11 – 4.74)	26.6	(19.2 – 32.0)	243	(208 – 322)	492

Table 4.1.a.3. Urinary genistein: Mexican Americans

Geometric mean and selected percentiles of urine concentrations (in μg/L) for Mexican Americans in the U.S. population aged 6 years and older, National Health and Nutrition Examination Survey, 2003–2006.

	Geometric mean (95% conf. interval)		Selected percentiles (95% conf. interval)						Sample size
			10th		50th		90th		
Males and Females									
Total, 6 years and older	29.3	(26.8 – 32.0)	4.38	(3.48 – 5.15)	25.8	(22.2 – 29.0)	301	(242 – 341)	1,287
6–11 years	32.4	(24.4 – 43.1)	5.65	(4.27 – 6.93)	27.5	(19.2 – 35.8)	293	(127 – 645)	231
12–19 years	35.6	(29.8 – 42.6)	5.60	(4.70 – 6.58)	30.7	(26.9 – 36.0)	315	(171 – 493)	445
20–39 years	26.8	(23.1 – 31.0)	4.03	(2.23 – 5.44)	21.3	(16.7 – 26.1)	325	(229 – 461)	282
40–59 years	29.1	(21.9 – 38.8)	4.18	(2.24 – 5.48)	27.5	(17.8 – 38.2)	253	(132 – 506)	157
60 years and older	25.9	(20.6 – 32.6)	3.09	(2.42 – 3.67)	29.8	(17.7 – 35.2)	228	(138 – 335)	172
Males									
Total, 6 years and older	30.9	(26.4 – 36.3)	4.76	(3.89 – 5.84)	25.9	(21.4 – 31.5)	304	(200 – 457)	625
6–11 years	30.5	(22.1 – 42.0)	6.04	(3.33 – 7.64)	23.1	(17.9 – 34.9)	212	(101 – 566)	112
12–19 years	37.0	(30.3 – 45.3)	6.17	(4.86 – 7.61)	31.6	(26.1 – 40.7)	243	(160 – 424)	228
20–39 years	29.0	(21.3 – 39.5)	4.54	(2.37 – 5.97)	21.0	(15.5 – 36.1)	331	(185 – 646)	117
40–59 years	31.4	(19.5 – 50.6)	3.89†	(1.51 – 6.76)	27.8	(13.3 – 43.9)	259†	(86.0 – 4,840)	85
60 years and older	30.0	(17.7 – 50.9)	3.47†	(1.78 – 5.40)	34.5	(16.9 – 56.7)	178†	(97.8 – 2,730)	83
Females									
Total, 6 years and older	27.5	(23.3 – 32.5)	3.76	(2.76 – 4.71)	25.2	(19.3 – 31.2)	286	(206 – 371)	662
6–11 years	34.6	(22.2 – 54.1)	5.17	(2.04 – 6.90)	34.0	(21.2 – 44.3)	303	(118 – 2,670)	119
12–19 years	34.2	(26.4 – 44.3)	5.03	(3.49 – 6.31)	29.4	(19.4 – 38.1)	407	(192 – 554)	217
20–39 years	24.4	(16.8 – 35.4)	3.41	(1.71 – 4.29)	20.3	(15.3 – 34.0)	251	(97.7 – 827)	165
40–59 years	26.9	(19.9 – 36.3)	4.15†	(1.15 – 5.49)	26.5	(18.5 – 43.2)	199†	(79.1 – 832)	72
60 years and older	23.0	(14.2 – 37.1)	2.53†	(< LOD – 4.40)	17.8	(12.5 – 36.4)	258†	(108 – 681)	89

< LOD means less than the limit of detection, which may vary for some compounds by year. See Appendix D for LOD.

† Estimate is subject to greater uncertainty due to small cell size.

Table 4.1.a.4. Urinary genistein: Non-Hispanic blacks

Geometric mean and selected percentiles of urine concentrations (in µg/L) for non-Hispanic blacks in the U.S. population aged 6 years and older, National Health and Nutrition Examination Survey, 2003–2006.

	Geometric mean (95% conf. interval)	Selected percentiles (95% conf. interval)			Sample size
		10th	50th	90th	
Males and Females					
Total, 6 years and older	31.8 (27.1 – 37.3)	5.01 (4.16 – 5.69)	27.8 (23.0 – 34.7)	269 (206 – 331)	1,343
6–11 years	38.4 (29.9 – 49.4)	5.60 (3.37 – 7.09)	34.7 (25.1 – 46.0)	311 (215 – 640)	207
12–19 years	42.7 (37.0 – 49.2)	6.66 (5.91 – 7.91)	35.3 (29.1 – 44.4)	286 (227 – 400)	496
20–39 years	29.0 (22.5 – 37.4)	5.04 (3.86 – 6.11)	24.7 (17.2 – 33.2)	198 (152 – 390)	249
40–59 years	32.2 (24.2 – 43.0)	4.30 (2.56 – 6.18)	29.9 (20.7 – 45.8)	318 (167 – 547)	231
60 years and older	22.9 (17.5 – 30.0)	3.42 (3.12 – 4.54)	20.6 (14.9 – 32.7)	171 (99.8 – 326)	160
Males					
Total, 6 years and older	35.4 (30.1 – 41.7)	5.67 (4.64 – 6.71)	30.4 (26.5 – 36.3)	293 (214 – 401)	661
6–11 years	38.5 (26.8 – 55.3)	4.06† (1.87 – 7.03)	36.7 (18.6 – 54.7)	360† (205 – 747)	99
12–19 years	44.5 (36.0 – 55.0)	6.90 (4.87 – 8.70)	35.4 (27.4 – 48.1)	282 (193 – 844)	258
20–39 years	35.4 (26.1 – 48.0)	6.47 (4.28 – 9.07)	27.4 (18.8 – 43.5)	310 (158 – 413)	116
40–59 years	33.1 (24.0 – 45.8)	4.50 (2.29 – 7.00)	30.7 (20.4 – 47.7)	265 (153 – 434)	114
60 years and older	26.7 (20.0 – 35.6)	4.67† (3.31 – 6.20)	24.1 (17.1 – 35.7)	145† (110 – 525)	74
Females					
Total, 6 years and older	29.1 (23.5 – 35.9)	4.46 (3.51 – 5.35)	24.9 (19.1 – 35.1)	249 (172 – 336)	682
6–11 years	38.4 (27.0 – 54.5)	6.52† (4.22 – 7.95)	31.4 (19.2 – 45.9)	272† (170 – 1,510)	108
12–19 years	40.9 (35.2 – 47.6)	6.54 (4.59 – 8.23)	35.2 (26.4 – 47.9)	286 (223 – 376)	238
20–39 years	24.6 (17.4 – 35.0)	4.47 (1.60 – 5.45)	20.2 (13.7 – 31.3)	165 (103 – 387)	133
40–59 years	31.5 (19.5 – 51.0)	3.75 (2.08 – 6.18)	27.6 (15.3 – 58.7)	349 (148 – 870)	117
60 years and older	20.8 (13.2 – 32.7)	3.22† (2.12 – 4.03)	18.2 (9.40 – 33.0)	170† (50.8 – 19,800)	86

† Estimate is subject to greater uncertainty due to small cell size.

Table 4.1.a.5. Urinary genistein: Non-Hispanic whites

Geometric mean and selected percentiles of urine concentrations (in µg/L) for non-Hispanic whites in the U.S. population aged 6 years and older, National Health and Nutrition Examination Survey, 2003–2006.

	Geometric mean (95% conf. interval)	Selected percentiles (95% conf. interval)			Sample size
		10th	50th	90th	
Males and Females					
Total, 6 years and older	28.8 (26.7 – 31.1)	4.00 (3.69 – 4.23)	25.3 (22.3 – 28.3)	257 (229 – 302)	2,108
6–11 years	34.9 (28.4 – 42.9)	5.95 (4.33 – 7.79)	29.1 (22.3 – 41.7)	247 (179 – 378)	193
12–19 years	32.8 (28.4 – 37.9)	4.48 (3.60 – 5.63)	24.7 (20.4 – 32.0)	298 (223 – 368)	378
20–39 years	26.9 (22.6 – 32.2)	3.82 (2.28 – 4.71)	22.8 (19.1 – 27.9)	218 (163 – 319)	494
40–59 years	27.0 (23.4 – 31.1)	3.44 (2.90 – 3.98)	26.0 (18.7 – 30.3)	307 (225 – 421)	448
60 years and older	30.2 (26.6 – 34.2)	4.23 (3.01 – 5.32)	28.0 (22.3 – 32.2)	242 (211 – 308)	595
Males					
Total, 6 years and older	31.8 (28.5 – 35.5)	4.75 (4.15 – 5.31)	27.0 (22.4 – 31.9)	274 (227 – 340)	1,035
6–11 years	34.1 (25.0 – 46.4)	6.75† (4.40 – 9.87)	26.6 (18.1 – 42.0)	209† (154 – 400)	99
12–19 years	34.9 (27.3 – 44.7)	5.07 (4.12 – 7.35)	25.4 (19.0 – 41.1)	262 (205 – 392)	191
20–39 years	29.4 (23.6 – 36.6)	4.32 (2.26 – 5.49)	23.6 (18.7 – 32.9)	233 (155 – 418)	217
40–59 years	32.3 (26.3 – 39.7)	4.15 (3.03 – 5.45)	29.0 (21.1 – 37.1)	336 (225 – 590)	229
60 years and older	31.6 (25.7 – 38.8)	4.77 (3.79 – 6.83)	28.5 (19.5 – 39.4)	220 (172 – 341)	299
Females					
Total, 6 years and older	26.2 (23.4 – 29.2)	3.30 (2.72 – 3.94)	23.6 (19.4 – 27.3)	243 (207 – 306)	1,073
6–11 years	35.8 (25.2 – 50.9)	4.98† (1.29 – 7.17)	39.3 (20.8 – 54.2)	271† (153 – 919)	94
12–19 years	30.7 (24.1 – 39.0)	3.62 (2.73 – 5.14)	22.4 (17.2 – 33.7)	311 (207 – 416)	187
20–39 years	24.7 (19.0 – 32.1)	3.18 (1.91 – 4.28)	22.2 (16.3 – 29.1)	210 (149 – 353)	277
40–59 years	22.5 (18.4 – 27.4)	2.93 (1.90 – 3.80)	18.3 (14.9 – 26.8)	232 (154 – 472)	219
60 years and older	29.1 (24.0 – 35.3)	3.67 (1.76 – 5.32)	27.5 (21.6 – 32.3)	244 (197 – 336)	296

† Estimate is subject to greater uncertainty due to small cell size.

Table 4.1.b. Urinary genistein: Concentrations by survey cycle

Geometric mean and selected percentiles of urine concentrations (in µg/L) for the U.S. population, National Health and Nutrition Examination Survey, 1999–2006.

	Geometric mean (95% conf. interval)	Selected percentiles (95% conf. interval) 5th		Selected percentiles 50th		Selected percentiles 95th		Sample size
Total, 6 years and older								
1999–2000	24.4	(19.7 – 30.3)	< LOD		27.0	(22.5 – 32.4)	563 (437 – 727)	2,557
2001–2002	33.0	(30.1 – 36.2)	2.64	(2.24 – 2.89)	28.9	(26.8 – 31.7)	619 (536 – 720)	2,794
2003–2004	31.1	(29.0 – 33.3)	2.63	(1.99 – 3.28)	26.2	(23.8 – 29.6)	525 (411 – 619)	2,594
2005–2006	28.7	(25.8 – 32.0)	2.33	(1.93 – 2.74)	25.9	(20.9 – 29.6)	522 (438 – 590)	2,528
Age group								
6–11 years								
1999–2000	27.6	(21.1 – 36.1)	.922	(< LOD – 3.07)	31.7	(18.4 – 42.6)	376 (287 – 712)	331
2001–2002	39.2	(33.4 – 46.0)	5.09	(3.88 – 6.13)	31.5	(25.8 – 39.2)	501 (329 – 1,150)	396
2003–2004	33.6	(27.8 – 40.6)	4.40	(3.23 – 5.98)	29.2	(22.9 – 37.8)	351 (220 – 433)	341
2005–2006	38.6	(29.8 – 49.9)	3.84	(< LOD – 5.12)	34.3	(25.3 – 42.4)	625 (402 – 2,960)	351
12–19 years								
1999–2000	43.7	(34.2 – 55.7)	2.85	(1.97 – 4.17)	44.9	(34.5 – 59.5)	543 (363 – 842)	754
2001–2002	34.1	(27.2 – 42.8)	3.70	(2.00 – 5.17)	29.0	(26.0 – 32.8)	469 (380 – 708)	744
2003–2004	34.7	(29.3 – 41.0)	3.24	(2.06 – 4.10)	29.0	(23.3 – 37.4)	522 (367 – 675)	729
2005–2006	34.1	(28.8 – 40.5)	3.35	(2.39 – 4.19)	26.7	(20.5 – 35.4)	481 (404 – 1,070)	693
20–39 years								
1999–2000	28.7	(21.7 – 37.8)	< LOD		28.5	(23.2 – 35.8)	704 (453 – 1,540)	536
2001–2002	34.4	(28.2 – 41.9)	2.42	(1.37 – 3.16)	30.4	(25.3 – 38.5)	611 (489 – 797)	604
2003–2004	29.1	(24.5 – 34.6)	2.41	(1.40 – 3.83)	24.9	(21.0 – 29.6)	436 (396 – 567)	554
2005–2006	27.9	(22.7 – 34.4)	2.16	(1.42 – 3.27)	22.3	(18.6 – 29.0)	556 (412 – 938)	583
40–59 years								
1999–2000	15.5	(10.1 – 23.7)	< LOD		21.3	(13.0 – 28.2)	464 (313 – 1,320)	420
2001–2002	32.9	(27.6 – 39.4)	2.74	(.916 – 3.38)	29.3	(24.3 – 34.7)	719 (541 – 1,210)	531
2003–2004	32.4	(27.6 – 38.1)	2.44	(1.75 – 3.38)	27.3	(20.8 – 33.1)	664 (535 – 1,110)	452
2005–2006	24.5	(20.8 – 29.0)	2.06	(1.14 – 2.70)	24.9	(17.5 – 30.1)	466 (348 – 637)	449
60 years and older								
1999–2000	21.7	(16.9 – 27.9)	< LOD		22.5	(17.7 – 30.3)	352 (279 – 904)	516
2001–2002	26.7	(21.8 – 32.7)	1.94	(1.26 – 2.56)	25.0	(20.0 – 32.2)	496 (280 – 1,240)	519
2003–2004	28.6	(24.2 – 33.9)	2.13	(1.26 – 2.66)	25.9	(20.1 – 34.2)	386 (314 – 575)	518
2005–2006	30.3	(25.2 – 36.5)	2.18	(1.17 – 3.21)	28.8	(22.1 – 33.0)	469 (318 – 867)	452
Gender								
Males								
1999–2000	29.8	(22.2 – 40.0)	< LOD		31.8	(26.4 – 37.0)	684 (441 – 1,440)	1,222
2001–2002	32.2	(27.9 – 37.2)	2.61	(1.94 – 3.33)	29.3	(25.6 – 33.7)	474 (348 – 727)	1,375
2003–2004	33.7	(29.6 – 38.4)	3.33	(2.46 – 4.18)	27.3	(23.8 – 33.0)	561 (444 – 655)	1,244
2005–2006	32.0	(28.6 – 36.0)	2.83	(2.34 – 3.45)	29.1	(23.0 – 33.8)	488 (411 – 622)	1,252
Females								
1999–2000	20.3	(17.0 – 24.2)	< LOD		23.1	(20.2 – 26.2)	442 (345 – 674)	1,335
2001–2002	33.7	(30.9 – 36.8)	2.62	(2.25 – 2.87)	28.6	(26.3 – 31.9)	663 (602 – 811)	1,419
2003–2004	28.7	(25.5 – 32.4)	2.05	(1.71 – 2.65)	25.0	(22.5 – 28.4)	466 (362 – 621)	1,350
2005–2006	25.9	(22.3 – 29.9)	1.93	(1.58 – 2.34)	22.3	(17.8 – 27.4)	524 (413 – 694)	1,276
Race/ethnicity								
Mexican Americans								
1999–2000	31.1	(25.1 – 38.5)	.628	(< LOD – 2.04)	30.0	(25.2 – 37.4)	572 (471 – 1,550)	819
2001–2002	28.3	(22.0 – 36.4)	2.80	(1.56 – 3.90)	25.4	(19.9 – 32.4)	423 (340 – 543)	679
2003–2004	31.1	(27.5 – 35.2)	3.38	(2.23 – 4.24)	25.2	(19.2 – 32.2)	643 (566 – 865)	653
2005–2006	27.6	(24.4 – 31.2)	2.11	(1.23 – 2.93)	26.3	(21.7 – 29.8)	412 (333 – 626)	634
Non-Hispanic Blacks								
1999–2000	26.5	(19.0 – 36.9)	< LOD		32.8	(24.6 – 41.4)	456 (363 – 766)	597
2001–2002	37.9	(27.3 – 52.6)	2.49	(1.53 – 4.06)	35.9	(23.9 – 51.2)	598 (446 – 1,300)	692
2003–2004	32.6	(24.2 – 44.0)	3.00	(2.00 – 4.16)	27.7	(19.4 – 44.9)	506 (334 – 875)	681
2005–2006	31.0	(26.7 – 36.1)	3.00	(2.16 – 3.55)	27.8	(23.1 – 34.9)	452 (372 – 883)	662
Non-Hispanic Whites								
1999–2000	23.7	(19.1 – 29.4)	< LOD		25.6	(22.0 – 32.0)	564 (413 – 742)	901
2001–2002	30.9	(27.7 – 34.3)	2.43	(2.03 – 2.75)	27.3	(24.5 – 30.7)	623 (521 – 746)	1,211
2003–2004	30.9	(28.4 – 33.6)	2.34	(1.71 – 3.29)	26.2	(22.8 – 30.9)	501 (384 – 619)	1,069
2005–2006	26.9	(23.6 – 30.6)	2.10	(1.58 – 2.57)	23.7	(19.0 – 29.0)	500 (397 – 623)	1,039

< LOD means less than the limit of detection, which may vary for some compounds by year. See Appendix D for LOD.

Figure 4.1.b. Urinary genistein: Concentrations by survey cycle

Selected percentiles in µg/L (95% confidence intervals), National Health and Nutrition Examination Survey, 1999–2006

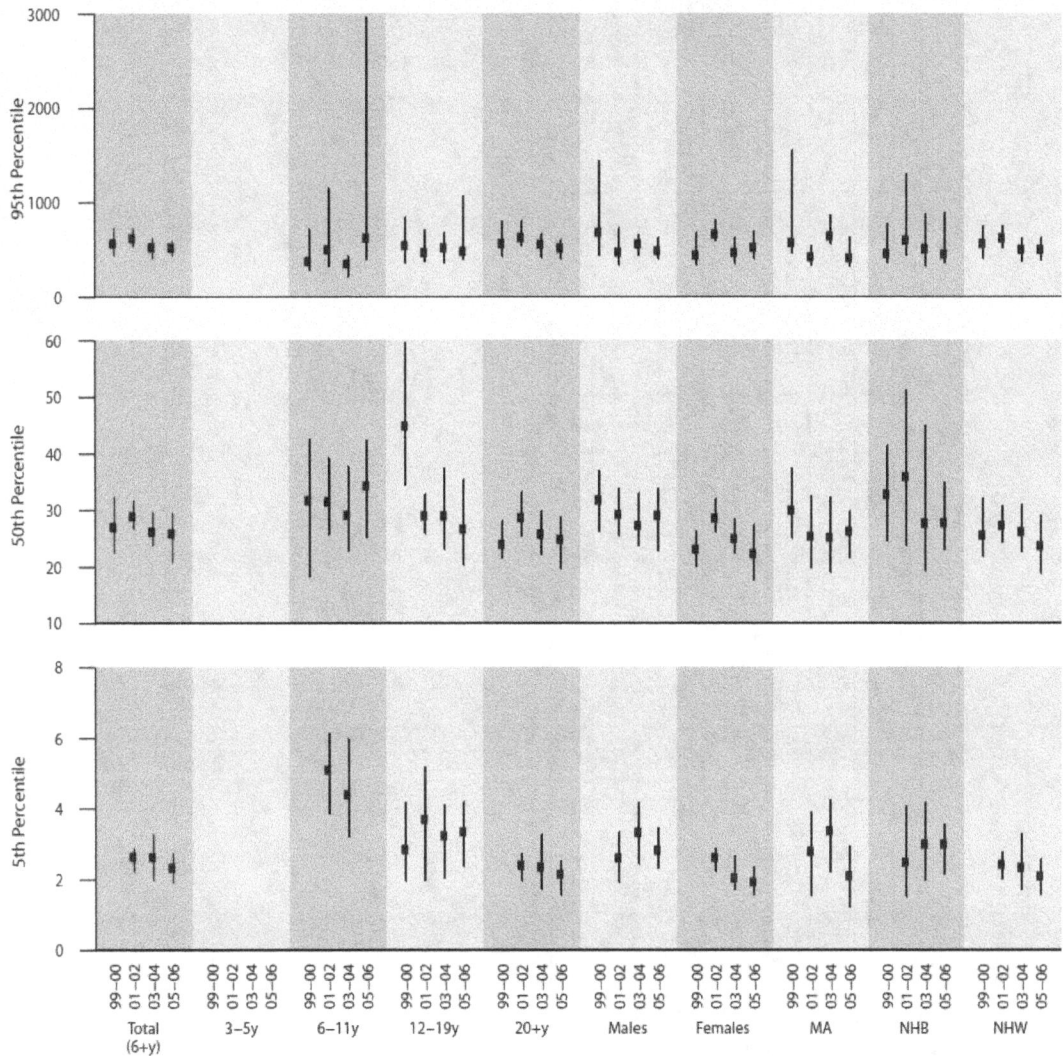

Values in the graph are suppressed if either the point estimate or the lower 95% confidence limit is noted as "< LOD" in the accompanying table.

Table 4.2.a.1. Urinary genistein (creatinine corrected): Concentrations

Geometric mean and selected percentiles of urine concentrations (in µg/g creatinine) for the total U.S. population aged 6 years and older, National Health and Nutrition Examination Survey, 2003–2006.

	Geometric mean (95% conf. interval)	Selected percentiles (95% conf. interval)					Sample size
		2.5th	5th	50th	95th	97.5th	
Total, 6 years and older	28.5 (26.9 – 30.2)	2.22 (1.97 – 2.46)	3.14 (2.83 – 3.45)	23.8 (21.6 – 26.1)	534 (438 – 627)	910 (796 – 1,210)	5,122
Age group							
6–11 years	39.0 (33.7 – 45.1)	3.68 (1.15 – 4.62)	5.09 (3.51 – 6.16)	34.5 (27.4 – 38.3)	626 (412 – 1,060)	1,240 (740 – 2,140)	692
12–19 years	25.6 (23.0 – 28.5)	2.25 (1.60 – 2.74)	3.36 (2.73 – 3.66)	20.4 (17.8 – 24.8)	367 (293 – 440)	730 (439 – 1,120)	1,422
20–39 years	24.3 (21.8 – 27.1)	2.14 (1.81 – 2.43)	2.81 (2.37 – 3.50)	20.7 (17.8 – 23.6)	355 (291 – 530)	749 (563 – 1,220)	1,137
40–59 years	28.4 (25.2 – 32.1)	1.89 (1.35 – 2.35)	2.66 (2.10 – 3.14)	23.6 (19.1 – 27.8)	645 (445 – 1,020)	1,210 (779 – 1,970)	901
60 years and older	34.5 (31.4 – 38.0)	2.97 (< LOD – 3.38)	3.82 (3.36 – 4.47)	28.6 (24.5 – 32.6)	576 (464 – 668)	913 (661 – 1,470)	970
Gender							
Males	26.1 (24.0 – 28.3)	2.12 (1.80 – 2.48)	3.03 (2.60 – 3.42)	22.1 (19.5 – 24.9)	422 (348 – 557)	811 (629 – 1,140)	2,496
Females	31.1 (28.3 – 34.1)	2.35 (1.97 – 2.77)	3.20 (2.80 – 3.76)	25.8 (22.9 – 28.1)	617 (448 – 778)	1,000 (853 – 1,610)	2,626
Race/ethnicity							
Mexican Americans	26.4 (24.2 – 28.8)	1.87 (1.19 – 2.49)	2.97 (2.24 – 3.47)	22.4 (19.5 – 24.6)	441 (355 – 656)	955 (723 – 1,330)	1,287
Non-Hispanic Blacks	22.3 (19.6 – 25.5)	2.02 (1.38 – 2.51)	2.76 (2.31 – 3.16)	19.1 (15.7 – 22.2)	319 (261 – 488)	561 (489 – 793)	1,343
Non-Hispanic Whites	29.3 (27.3 – 31.4)	2.21 (1.84 – 2.54)	3.08 (2.67 – 3.58)	24.9 (22.1 – 27.7)	594 (437 – 687)	915 (834 – 1,250)	2,108

< LOD means less than the limit of detection for the uncorrected urine values, which may vary for some compounds by year. See Appendix D for LOD.

Figure 4.2.a. Urinary genistein (creatinine corrected): Concentrations by age group

Geometric mean (95% confidence interval), National Health and Nutrition Examination Survey, 2003–2006

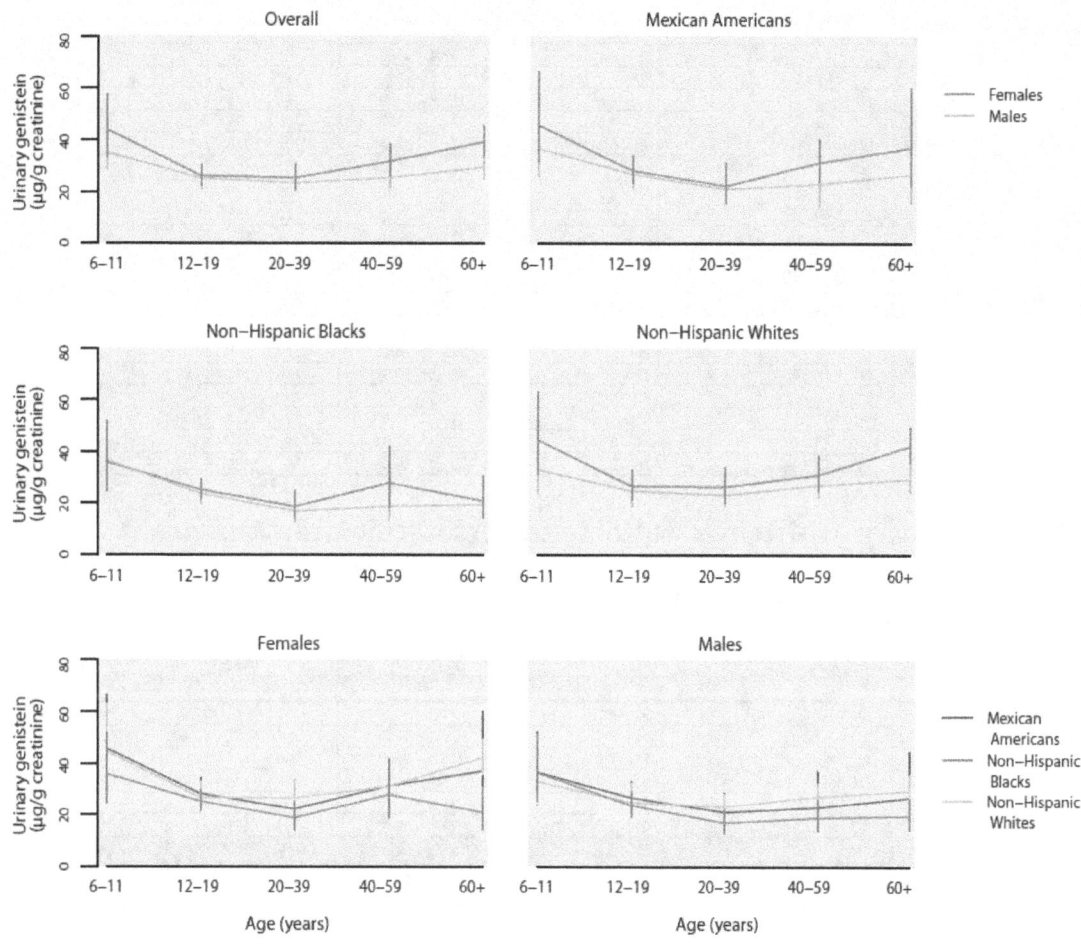

Table 4.2.a.2. Urinary genistein (creatinine corrected): Total population

Geometric mean and selected percentiles of urine concentrations (in µg/g creatinine) for the total U.S. population aged 6 years and older, National Health and Nutrition Examination Survey, 2003–2006.

	Geometric mean (95% conf. interval)	Selected percentiles (95% conf. interval)						Sample size
		10th		50th		90th		
Males and Females								
Total, 6 years and older	28.5	(26.9 – 30.2)	4.53	(4.29 – 4.79)	23.8	(21.6 – 26.1)	236	(210 – 270)	5,122
6–11 years	39.0	(33.7 – 45.1)	6.68	(5.55 – 8.43)	34.5	(27.4 – 38.3)	271	(216 – 388)	692
12–19 years	25.6	(23.0 – 28.5)	4.36	(3.90 – 4.67)	20.4	(17.8 – 24.8)	189	(151 – 236)	1,422
20–39 years	24.3	(21.8 – 27.1)	4.15	(3.81 – 4.55)	20.7	(17.8 – 23.6)	184	(144 – 236)	1,137
40–59 years	28.4	(25.2 – 32.1)	4.04	(3.52 – 4.65)	23.6	(19.1 – 27.8)	270	(207 – 415)	901
60 years and older	34.5	(31.4 – 38.0)	5.51	(4.85 – 6.21)	28.6	(24.5 – 32.6)	287	(226 – 398)	970
Males								
Total, 6 years and older	26.1	(24.0 – 28.3)	4.29	(4.03 – 4.56)	22.1	(19.5 – 24.9)	205	(179 – 237)	2,496
6–11 years	35.0	(28.8 – 42.4)	6.30	(5.10 – 7.99)	29.8	(21.2 – 38.2)	272	(158 – 503)	340
12–19 years	25.2	(21.1 – 30.0)	4.38	(3.66 – 4.66)	20.3	(17.0 – 29.0)	154	(128 – 256)	728
20–39 years	23.3	(20.8 – 26.1)	3.96	(3.39 – 4.38)	20.0	(16.0 – 24.4)	204	(149 – 244)	499
40–59 years	25.4	(21.6 – 29.8)	3.68	(3.27 – 4.51)	20.2	(16.8 – 25.5)	228	(155 – 386)	451
60 years and older	29.4	(24.8 – 34.7)	5.20	(4.11 – 6.32)	25.0	(20.0 – 30.4)	200	(151 – 259)	478
Females								
Total, 6 years and older	31.1	(28.3 – 34.1)	4.80	(4.35 – 5.45)	25.8	(22.9 – 28.1)	274	(230 – 320)	2,626
6–11 years	43.8	(33.4 – 57.4)	8.16	(4.38 – 10.4)	37.7	(26.4 – 50.0)	270	(212 – 798)	352
12–19 years	26.1	(22.5 – 30.3)	4.35	(3.72 – 5.23)	20.6	(16.5 – 24.8)	208	(164 – 269)	694
20–39 years	25.3	(20.9 – 30.7)	4.50	(3.83 – 5.53)	21.0	(17.6 – 26.9)	170	(124 – 289)	638
40–59 years	31.7	(26.2 – 38.3)	4.34	(2.99 – 5.61)	26.6	(21.3 – 32.6)	340	(210 – 631)	450
60 years and older	39.2	(33.9 – 45.4)	5.70	(4.76 – 6.64)	31.6	(25.8 – 39.0)	361	(289 – 530)	492

Table 4.2.a.3. Urinary genistein (creatinine corrected): Mexican Americans

Geometric mean and selected percentiles of urine concentrations (in µg/g creatinine) for Mexican Americans in the U.S. population aged 6 years and older, National Health and Nutrition Examination Survey, 2003–2006.

	Geometric mean (95% conf. interval)	Selected percentiles (95% conf. interval)						Sample size
		10th		50th		90th		
Males and Females								
Total, 6 years and older	26.4	(24.2 – 28.8)	4.25	(3.81 – 4.70)	22.4	(19.5 – 24.6)	212	(186 – 275)	1,287
6–11 years	40.7	(31.0 – 53.5)	7.48	(5.51 – 9.00)	31.6	(22.8 – 44.7)	304	(161 – 1,100)	231
12–19 years	27.5	(23.7 – 32.0)	5.58	(4.31 – 6.56)	22.4	(18.9 – 26.4)	208	(139 – 366)	445
20–39 years	21.6	(18.6 – 25.2)	3.65	(2.96 – 4.28)	16.2	(13.1 – 20.9)	204	(138 – 255)	282
40–59 years	26.7	(20.1 – 35.4)	3.71	(2.37 – 4.69)	25.4	(16.8 – 33.8)	229	(131 – 629)	157
60 years and older	32.0	(23.9 – 42.9)	5.10	(2.91 – 6.94)	31.2	(22.8 – 40.4)	233	(141 – 535)	172
Males								
Total, 6 years and older	24.4	(20.6 – 28.9)	4.10	(3.50 – 4.54)	22.2	(17.2 – 26.4)	203	(136 – 275)	625
6–11 years	36.6	(25.7 – 52.1)	7.40	(5.50 – 9.04)	30.2	(19.7 – 43.0)	251	(129 – 659)	112
12–19 years	26.8	(21.9 – 32.8)	5.68	(4.54 – 6.56)	23.0	(16.8 – 30.7)	151	(116 – 347)	228
20–39 years	21.1	(15.6 – 28.5)	3.54	(2.60 – 4.32)	17.2	(12.4 – 23.3)	199	(112 – 328)	117
40–59 years	23.0	(14.4 – 36.9)	3.31†	(1.22 – 4.36)	20.9	(8.19 – 31.2)	192†	(92.0 – 2,070)	85
60 years and older	26.7	(16.1 – 44.4)	4.18†	(1.75 – 7.13)	29.0	(10.9 – 49.6)	159†	(59.4 – 4,830)	83
Females								
Total, 6 years and older	28.7	(25.0 – 32.9)	4.59	(3.67 – 5.88)	22.9	(18.5 – 27.1)	262	(189 – 391)	662
6–11 years	45.6	(31.5 – 66.2)	7.46	(4.51 – 9.99)	37.3	(20.3 – 68.7)	311	(166 – 1,460)	119
12–19 years	28.2	(23.4 – 34.1)	5.47	(2.84 – 7.19)	21.7	(17.8 – 28.9)	269	(155 – 425)	217
20–39 years	22.3	(15.8 – 31.3)	3.60	(2.14 – 6.28)	15.8	(12.0 – 23.4)	199	(116 – 728)	165
40–59 years	31.3	(24.2 – 40.4)	4.10†	(.565 – 6.37)	32.5	(18.1 – 44.1)	296†	(151 – 594)	72
60 years and older	37.0	(22.8 – 60.0)	5.54†	(< LOD – 8.83)	31.6	(13.4 – 82.7)	261†	(142 – 745)	89

< LOD means less than the limit of detection for the uncorrected urine values, which may vary for some compounds by year. See Appendix D for LOD.

† Estimate is subject to greater uncertainty due to small cell size.

Table 4.2.a.4. Urinary genistein (creatinine corrected): Non-Hispanic blacks

Geometric mean and selected percentiles of urine concentrations (in µg/g creatinine) for non-Hispanic blacks in the U.S. population aged 6 years and older, National Health and Nutrition Examination Survey, 2003–2006.

	Geometric mean (95% conf. interval)	Selected percentiles (95% conf. interval) 10th		Selected percentiles (95% conf. interval) 50th		Selected percentiles (95% conf. interval) 90th		Sample size
Males and Females								
Total, 6 years and older	22.3 (19.6 – 25.5)	3.95	(3.34 – 4.63)	19.1	(15.7 – 22.2)	159	(137 – 211)	1,343
6–11 years	36.1 (28.1 – 46.3)	6.36	(4.62 – 7.24)	25.2	(22.0 – 37.0)	325	(198 – 811)	207
12–19 years	24.5 (21.6 – 27.9)	4.32	(3.87 – 5.01)	22.0	(16.7 – 25.6)	150	(125 – 214)	496
20–39 years	17.9 (14.7 – 21.9)	3.49	(2.75 – 4.31)	14.0	(11.3 – 19.5)	123	(82.7 – 209)	249
40–59 years	23.4 (18.7 – 29.3)	3.30	(2.54 – 4.71)	21.4	(17.4 – 26.3)	173	(128 – 458)	231
60 years and older	20.4 (16.4 – 25.5)	4.39	(3.33 – 4.93)	17.5	(11.4 – 22.8)	130	(84.1 – 218)	160
Males								
Total, 6 years and older	20.7 (17.9 – 23.8)	3.40	(2.80 – 4.38)	17.6	(13.9 – 21.4)	173	(137 – 213)	661
6–11 years	36.4 (25.8 – 51.2)	4.60†	(3.12 – 7.24)	24.9	(19.2 – 47.2)	396†	(214 – 869)	99
12–19 years	23.8 (19.6 – 28.8)	3.95	(3.32 – 4.73)	21.2	(14.5 – 25.8)	159	(122 – 246)	258
20–39 years	17.0 (13.0 – 22.1)	3.20	(2.32 – 3.87)	12.6	(9.92 – 20.3)	150	(86.4 – 209)	116
40–59 years	18.9 (13.8 – 26.0)	2.97	(1.59 – 4.57)	17.4	(9.55 – 25.7)	140	(86.9 – 359)	114
60 years and older	19.6 (14.6 – 26.3)	3.86†	(2.60 – 5.06)	18.3	(11.1 – 25.0)	112†	(65.3 – 220)	74
Females								
Total, 6 years and older	23.8 (19.8 – 28.6)	4.65	(3.49 – 5.61)	20.4	(16.4 – 25.3)	156	(123 – 244)	682
6–11 years	35.8 (24.8 – 51.6)	6.98†	(5.89 – 8.65)	25.0	(20.5 – 37.1)	261†	(113 – 1,290)	108
12–19 years	25.3 (21.7 – 29.4)	4.87	(3.83 – 5.77)	22.7	(15.5 – 28.5)	143	(105 – 292)	238
20–39 years	18.8 (14.2 – 24.8)	3.79	(2.53 – 5.95)	14.3	(10.5 – 21.9)	119	(77.3 – 252)	133
40–59 years	27.9 (18.7 – 41.8)	3.62	(2.57 – 5.58)	24.7	(17.9 – 34.9)	221	(114 – 570)	117
60 years and older	21.0 (14.5 – 30.3)	4.51†	(2.75 – 6.49)	16.5	(9.90 – 29.0)	134†	(83.9 – 254)	86

† Estimate is subject to greater uncertainty due to small cell size.

Table 4.2.a.5. Urinary genistein (creatinine corrected): Non-Hispanic whites

Geometric mean and selected percentiles of urine concentrations (in µg/g creatinine) for non-Hispanic whites in the U.S. population aged 6 years and older, National Health and Nutrition Examination Survey, 2003–2006.

	Geometric mean (95% conf. interval)	Selected percentiles (95% conf. interval) 10th		Selected percentiles (95% conf. interval) 50th		Selected percentiles (95% conf. interval) 90th		Sample size
Males and Females								
Total, 6 years and older	29.3 (27.3 – 31.4)	4.55	(4.17 – 4.93)	24.9	(22.1 – 27.7)	241	(209 – 291)	2,108
6–11 years	37.8 (31.2 – 45.8)	6.34	(5.11 – 8.41)	34.8	(24.5 – 43.0)	255	(175 – 577)	193
12–19 years	25.8 (22.3 – 29.7)	4.33	(3.67 – 4.93)	19.5	(16.7 – 26.0)	181	(143 – 247)	378
20–39 years	24.8 (21.4 – 28.9)	4.16	(3.52 – 4.76)	21.7	(18.1 – 28.3)	181	(134 – 289)	494
40–59 years	29.0 (25.3 – 33.2)	4.00	(3.18 – 4.90)	23.6	(17.7 – 30.3)	273	(202 – 477)	448
60 years and older	36.0 (32.8 – 39.6)	5.83	(4.85 – 6.54)	30.0	(26.4 – 34.1)	292	(224 – 431)	595
Males								
Total, 6 years and older	26.6 (23.9 – 29.5)	4.40	(3.87 – 4.86)	22.7	(19.4 – 26.2)	204	(169 – 261)	1,035
6–11 years	33.0 (23.9 – 45.6)	5.93†	(4.89 – 8.18)	24.8	(17.3 – 40.0)	195†	(126 – 945)	99
12–19 years	24.9 (19.3 – 32.3)	4.34	(3.13 – 5.24)	18.9	(14.5 – 31.4)	144	(121 – 311)	191
20–39 years	23.3 (19.3 – 28.2)	3.96	(2.52 – 4.69)	20.7	(15.9 – 28.7)	189	(105 – 339)	217
40–59 years	27.1 (22.5 – 32.5)	3.85	(3.22 – 4.95)	21.3	(16.4 – 27.9)	244	(155 – 623)	229
60 years and older	29.4 (24.5 – 35.4)	5.47	(3.88 – 6.92)	26.2	(20.0 – 33.5)	190	(147 – 263)	299
Females								
Total, 6 years and older	32.3 (29.0 – 35.9)	4.69	(4.14 – 5.40)	27.4	(23.5 – 32.6)	289	(227 – 361)	1,073
6–11 years	44.4 (31.3 – 62.8)	8.19†	(2.79 – 11.4)	43.0	(26.0 – 58.2)	266†	(164 – 1,300)	94
12–19 years	26.7 (21.7 – 32.8)	4.15	(3.63 – 5.22)	20.5	(15.8 – 26.1)	203	(156 – 342)	187
20–39 years	26.5 (20.8 – 33.7)	4.51	(3.50 – 5.62)	22.3	(18.1 – 33.0)	172	(126 – 300)	277
40–59 years	31.1 (25.1 – 38.6)	3.92	(2.63 – 5.82)	25.6	(17.7 – 34.1)	317	(180 – 675)	219
60 years and older	42.2 (36.1 – 49.3)	6.05	(4.82 – 7.49)	33.7	(27.6 – 42.2)	404	(291 – 567)	296

† Estimate is subject to greater uncertainty due to small cell size.

Table 4.2.b. Urinary genistein (creatinine corrected): Concentrations by survey cycle

Geometric mean and selected percentiles of urine concentrations (in µg/g creatinine) for the U.S. population, National Health and Nutrition Examination Survey, 1999–2006.

	Geometric mean (95% conf. interval)	Selected percentiles (95% conf. interval) 5th		Selected percentiles 50th		Selected percentiles 95th		Sample size
Total, 6 years and older								
1999–2000	22.3 (17.7 – 28.1)	<LOD		23.8	(18.9 – 28.7)	380	(341 – 523)	2,557
2001–2002	30.9 (28.5 – 33.6)	3.52	(3.07 – 3.80)	25.8	(23.5 – 29.2)	426	(375 – 491)	2,794
2003–2004	29.1 (27.3 – 31.0)	3.39	(2.80 – 3.69)	24.5	(21.4 – 27.4)	507	(399 – 619)	2,594
2005–2006	28.0 (25.3 – 31.0)	2.98	(2.42 – 3.44)	23.2	(20.4 – 26.4)	576	(423 – 759)	2,528
Age group								
6–11 years								
1999–2000	28.3 (21.1 – 37.9)	1.84	(<LOD – 3.04)	27.8	(15.8 – 41.1)	489	(282 – 794)	331
2001–2002	44.5 (37.0 – 53.5)	6.82	(4.89 – 8.11)	37.7	(30.0 – 48.3)	489	(276 – 934)	396
2003–2004	35.8 (29.7 – 43.0)	5.15	(3.19 – 6.46)	34.7	(25.3 – 43.1)	293	(175 – 1,130)	341
2005–2006	42.5 (33.1 – 54.6)	4.86	(< LOD – 6.37)	34.0	(24.2 – 40.9)	985	(580 – 1,850)	351
12–19 years								
1999–2000	29.4 (22.3 – 38.8)	2.12	(.684 – 3.24)	31.9	(24.3 – 41.6)	331	(199 – 1,360)	754
2001–2002	26.3 (21.3 – 32.5)	3.43	(2.34 – 4.13)	21.0	(18.1 – 26.5)	321	(294 – 487)	744
2003–2004	25.9 (21.8 – 30.9)	3.45	(2.56 – 4.00)	21.8	(17.0 – 28.6)	366	(322 – 464)	729
2005–2006	25.3 (22.1 – 29.0)	3.32	(2.25 – 3.67)	19.5	(16.3 – 23.8)	367	(238 – 617)	693
20–39 years								
1999–2000	22.7 (17.3 – 29.9)	<LOD		22.8	(17.0 – 27.2)	417	(355 – 738)	536
2001–2002	27.8 (23.8 – 32.4)	3.29	(2.22 – 3.92)	22.9	(18.7 – 29.8)	379	(329 – 476)	604
2003–2004	24.5 (21.9 – 27.4)	2.97	(2.55 – 3.69)	19.7	(17.3 – 23.4)	320	(271 – 557)	554
2005–2006	24.1 (19.8 – 29.3)	2.55	(1.85 – 3.76)	21.3	(16.5 – 27.5)	447	(288 – 734)	583
40–59 years								
1999–2000	15.7 (10.3 – 24.1)	<LOD		16.3	(12.5 – 26.8)	374	(246 – 894)	420
2001–2002	32.7 (27.8 – 38.6)	3.54	(2.26 – 4.12)	28.7	(24.2 – 32.1)	461	(377 – 1,260)	531
2003–2004	31.1 (26.4 – 36.6)	3.18	(1.96 – 3.75)	24.9	(19.7 – 29.8)	676	(496 – 1,670)	452
2005–2006	26.1 (21.5 – 31.7)	2.46	(1.82 – 2.97)	21.5	(16.8 – 29.2)	578	(326 – 1,220)	449
60 years and older								
1999–2000	26.1 (21.7 – 31.3)	<LOD		27.3	(20.4 – 35.9)	371	(252 – 691)	516
2001–2002	31.6 (25.8 – 38.8)	3.00	(2.36 – 3.76)	25.5	(20.7 – 33.3)	491	(323 – 1,310)	519
2003–2004	33.9 (29.7 – 38.7)	3.39	(2.78 – 4.33)	29.5	(23.8 – 34.6)	539	(444 – 754)	518
2005–2006	35.2 (30.3 – 40.8)	4.13	(3.34 – 5.27)	27.9	(23.0 – 35.0)	589	(402 – 776)	452
Gender								
Males								
1999–2000	23.3 (16.8 – 32.3)	<LOD		23.8	(17.7 – 31.9)	510	(329 – 893)	1,222
2001–2002	26.2 (23.1 – 29.8)	3.62	(2.52 – 4.01)	22.0	(19.4 – 26.2)	341	(282 – 427)	1,375
2003–2004	26.4 (22.8 – 30.5)	3.40	(2.66 – 3.63)	21.5	(17.6 – 26.3)	414	(346 – 574)	1,244
2005–2006	25.8 (23.4 – 28.4)	2.68	(1.98 – 3.40)	22.7	(19.3 – 26.2)	430	(319 – 629)	1,252
Females								
1999–2000	21.3 (17.5 – 26.0)	<LOD		23.1	(17.5 – 29.2)	357	(309 – 432)	1,335
2001–2002	36.2 (32.8 – 39.9)	3.50	(3.02 – 3.85)	29.5	(25.4 – 34.1)	540	(430 – 756)	1,419
2003–2004	31.9 (28.7 – 35.5)	3.29	(2.60 – 4.33)	27.1	(23.6 – 31.6)	545	(410 – 775)	1,350
2005–2006	30.3 (25.8 – 35.5)	3.07	(2.34 – 3.76)	23.5	(20.1 – 29.4)	658	(446 – 912)	1,276
Race/ethnicity								
Mexican Americans								
1999–2000	28.4 (23.3 – 34.7)	1.40	(<LOD – 2.74)	27.9	(22.5 – 35.0)	557	(322 – 1,290)	819
2001–2002	26.6 (21.6 – 32.9)	3.75	(2.96 – 4.09)	20.9	(16.1 – 28.7)	371	(280 – 484)	679
2003–2004	28.0 (24.8 – 31.8)	3.35	(2.29 – 3.99)	23.4	(18.8 – 28.1)	594	(426 – 884)	653
2005–2006	24.9 (22.1 – 28.0)	2.66	(1.46 – 3.47)	21.7	(18.1 – 23.7)	334	(277 – 520)	634
Non-Hispanic Blacks								
1999–2000	17.0 (12.2 – 23.6)	<LOD		19.4	(15.7 – 26.1)	284	(229 – 449)	597
2001–2002	26.4 (19.2 – 36.4)	2.91	(2.56 – 3.44)	22.7	(16.4 – 33.4)	369	(237 – 788)	692
2003–2004	23.0 (18.1 – 29.1)	3.11	(2.73 – 3.33)	20.4	(14.3 – 27.3)	304	(210 – 547)	681
2005–2006	21.7 (18.8 – 25.1)	2.58	(1.59 – 3.17)	18.5	(14.9 – 21.5)	350	(247 – 548)	662
Non-Hispanic Whites								
1999–2000	23.3 (18.5 – 29.3)	<LOD		25.6	(19.4 – 31.7)	380	(346 – 574)	901
2001–2002	30.5 (28.1 – 33.0)	3.54	(2.96 – 3.81)	25.2	(23.3 – 28.7)	424	(376 – 494)	1,211
2003–2004	30.5 (28.1 – 33.1)	3.37	(2.66 – 3.83)	26.3	(21.7 – 31.4)	544	(362 – 747)	1,069
2005–2006	28.2 (25.1 – 31.8)	2.98	(2.18 – 3.59)	23.5	(20.0 – 29.0)	615	(427 – 810)	1,039

< LOD means less than the limit of detection for the uncorrected urine values, which may vary for some compounds by year. See Appendix D for LOD.

Figure 4.2.b. Urinary genistein (creatinine corrected): Concentrations by survey cycle

Selected percentiles in μg/g creatinine (95% confidence intervals), National Health and Nutrition Examination Survey, 1999–2006

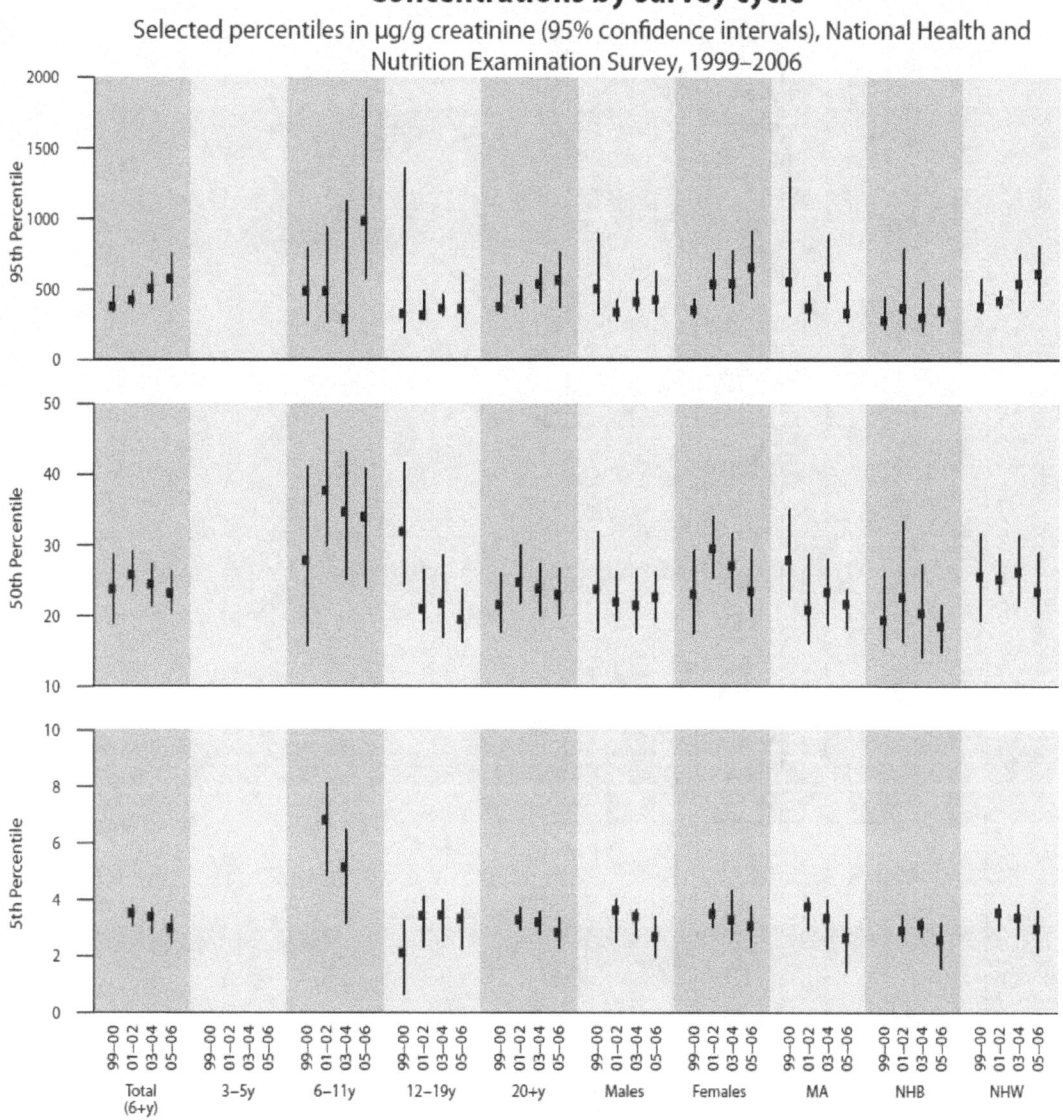

Values in the graph are suppressed if either the point estimate or the lower 95% confidence limit is noted as "< LOD" in the accompanying table.

Table 4.3.a.1. Urinary daidzein: Concentrations

Geometric mean and selected percentiles of urine concentrations (in μg/L) for the total U.S. population aged 6 years and older, National Health and Nutrition Examination Survey, 2003–2006.

	Geometric mean (95% conf. interval)	Selected percentiles (95% conf. interval)						Sample size
		2.5th	5th	50th	95th	97.5th		
Total, 6 years and older	66.6 (62.1 – 71.5)	3.31 (2.74 – 3.72)	5.35 (4.25 – 6.22)	60.4 (54.7 – 65.9)	1,170 (1,000 – 1,290)	1,850 (1,590 – 2,200)		5,122
Age group								
6–11 years	89.4 (77.7 – 103)	7.38 (5.07 – 8.35)	10.2 (7.62 – 13.1)	68.4 (59.2 – 86.6)	1,180 (996 – 1,870)	2,250 (1,550 – 6,320)		692
12–19 years	91.6 (80.5 – 104)	5.85 (3.92 – 6.63)	9.07 (6.69 – 9.60)	77.3 (65.0 – 94.5)	1,310 (989 – 1,760)	2,180 (1,710 – 3,350)		1,422
20–39 years	61.6 (53.3 – 71.3)	3.32 (1.80 – 3.99)	4.82 (3.43 – 6.14)	54.3 (47.2 – 65.9)	1,210 (835 – 1,560)	1,860 (1,490 – 2,430)		1,137
40–59 years	60.9 (54.9 – 67.6)	3.04 (1.89 – 3.48)	4.56 (3.42 – 5.90)	56.5 (47.0 – 65.5)	1,120 (893 – 1,340)	1,510 (1,270 – 3,510)		901
60 years and older	60.9 (52.7 – 70.5)	2.24 (1.47 – 3.58)	4.31 (2.73 – 6.34)	60.5 (48.9 – 73.4)	839 (709 – 1,310)	1,600 (1,210 – 2,660)		970
Gender								
Males	73.8 (67.2 – 81.1)	3.63 (2.74 – 4.56)	6.35 (4.53 – 7.62)	66.0 (58.0 – 73.7)	1,200 (1,060 – 1,350)	1,750 (1,520 – 2,220)		2,496
Females	60.4 (55.3 – 66.0)	3.04 (2.39 – 3.41)	4.47 (3.72 – 5.61)	55.5 (49.5 – 61.5)	1,000 (836 – 1,270)	1,910 (1,490 – 2,630)		2,626
Race/ethnicity								
Mexican Americans	59.0 (54.1 – 64.4)	3.07 (2.14 – 3.68)	4.71 (3.62 – 5.66)	48.6 (44.8 – 56.8)	1,350 (1,130 – 1,500)	1,800 (1,560 – 2,450)		1,287
Non-Hispanic Blacks	78.4 (67.6 – 90.9)	4.48 (3.48 – 5.77)	7.05 (5.74 – 7.82)	72.3 (61.3 – 85.2)	1,180 (886 – 1,610)	2,220 (1,500 – 3,390)		1,343
Non-Hispanic Whites	63.9 (58.7 – 69.6)	3.03 (2.26 – 3.41)	4.66 (3.69 – 6.11)	58.5 (52.0 – 65.3)	1,040 (930 – 1,250)	1,600 (1,420 – 2,150)		2,108

Figure 4.3.a. Urinary daidzein: Concentrations by age group

Geometric mean (95% confidence interval), National Health and Nutrition Examination Survey, 2003–2006

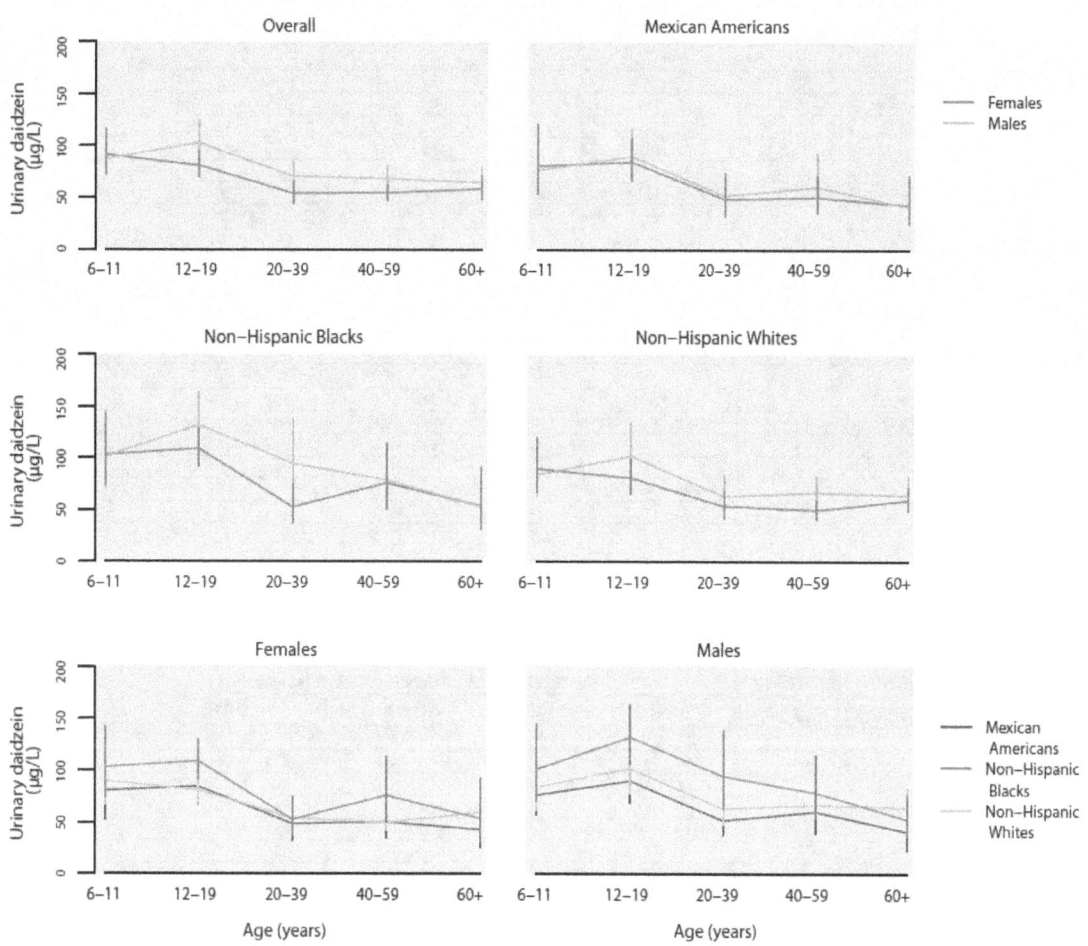

Table 4.3.a.2. Urinary daidzein: Total population

Geometric mean and selected percentiles of urine concentrations (in µg/L) for the total U.S. population aged 6 years and older, National Health and Nutrition Examination Survey, 2003–2006.

	Geometric mean (95% conf. interval)	Selected percentiles (95% conf. interval)						Sample size
		10th		50th		90th		
Males and Females								
Total, 6 years and older	66.6 (62.1 – 71.5)	8.65	(7.74 – 9.48)	60.4	(54.7 – 65.9)	613	(525 – 684)	5,122
6–11 years	89.4 (77.7 – 103)	15.7	(12.2 – 18.1)	68.4	(59.2 – 86.6)	653	(619 – 916)	692
12–19 years	91.6 (80.5 – 104)	14.5	(11.8 – 15.8)	77.3	(65.0 – 94.5)	834	(659 – 969)	1,422
20–39 years	61.6 (53.3 – 71.3)	8.20	(6.00 – 10.4)	54.3	(47.2 – 65.9)	571	(422 – 752)	1,137
40–59 years	60.9 (54.9 – 67.6)	7.71	(6.35 – 8.67)	56.5	(47.0 – 65.5)	572	(410 – 807)	901
60 years and older	60.9 (52.7 – 70.5)	7.92	(6.54 – 9.19)	60.5	(48.9 – 73.4)	471	(399 – 618)	970
Males								
Total, 6 years and older	73.8 (67.2 – 81.1)	9.92	(8.68 – 11.9)	66.0	(58.0 – 73.7)	695	(589 – 786)	2,496
6–11 years	87.3 (72.9 – 105)	17.5	(12.2 – 21.0)	64.0	(51.5 – 91.4)	874	(497 – 1,150)	340
12–19 years	103 (85.2 – 124)	17.3	(13.9 – 19.4)	86.6	(64.8 – 107)	863	(526 – 1,320)	728
20–39 years	70.4 (58.8 – 84.2)	9.80	(5.43 – 12.8)	65.3	(51.7 – 75.0)	729	(544 – 968)	499
40–59 years	68.4 (57.9 – 80.8)	8.55	(7.15 – 9.37)	66.2	(47.7 – 84.7)	671	(409 – 930)	451
60 years and older	64.4 (52.0 – 79.9)	9.16	(7.75 – 11.8)	57.7	(43.8 – 78.5)	561	(417 – 749)	478
Females								
Total, 6 years and older	60.4 (55.3 – 66.0)	7.79	(6.41 – 8.76)	55.5	(49.5 – 61.5)	507	(431 – 619)	2,626
6–11 years	91.6 (72.4 – 116)	14.3	(9.67 – 17.9)	78.1	(57.3 – 99.4)	643	(455 – 882)	352
12–19 years	81.0 (69.6 – 94.3)	11.1	(9.30 – 14.5)	71.1	(59.6 – 93.6)	812	(604 – 936)	694
20–39 years	54.0 (44.1 – 66.2)	7.31	(5.72 – 9.03)	47.9	(38.1 – 63.6)	383	(309 – 585)	638
40–59 years	54.6 (47.9 – 62.3)	6.98	(4.64 – 8.60)	48.2	(40.6 – 58.2)	511	(395 – 736)	450
60 years and older	58.3 (48.5 – 70.2)	7.04	(4.21 – 8.11)	60.9	(46.8 – 80.2)	403	(362 – 562)	492

Table 4.3.a.3. Urinary daidzein: Mexican Americans

Geometric mean and selected percentiles of urine concentrations (in µg/L) for Mexican Americans in the U.S. population aged 6 years and older, National Health and Nutrition Examination Survey, 2003–2006.

	Geometric mean (95% conf. interval)	Selected percentiles (95% conf. interval)						Sample size
		10th		50th		90th		
Males and Females								
Total, 6 years and older	59.0 (54.1 – 64.4)	7.94	(6.47 – 8.95)	48.6	(44.8 – 56.8)	671	(496 – 848)	1,287
6–11 years	78.3 (61.0 – 100)	16.6	(11.6 – 18.1)	64.5	(51.3 – 83.2)	588	(321 – 2,270)	231
12–19 years	87.3 (72.5 – 105)	12.3	(8.90 – 16.5)	74.6	(62.2 – 96.1)	812	(558 – 1,000)	445
20–39 years	50.5 (42.9 – 59.3)	6.19	(4.34 – 8.14)	35.3	(28.1 – 47.1)	821	(468 – 1,160)	282
40–59 years	55.4 (43.6 – 70.3)	7.50	(4.68 – 10.4)	48.2	(38.0 – 62.6)	475	(347 – 1,260)	157
60 years and older	42.1 (31.0 – 57.3)	5.61	(2.89 – 7.89)	40.7	(22.8 – 61.7)	366	(222 – 1,200)	172
Males								
Total, 6 years and older	60.8 (52.2 – 70.9)	8.82	(7.42 – 9.78)	48.2	(40.1 – 56.8)	742	(484 – 1,050)	625
6–11 years	76.3 (57.3 – 102)	17.3	(7.01 – 20.6)	60.0	(41.0 – 109)	481	(312 – 1,370)	112
12–19 years	90.0 (69.7 – 116)	16.0	(9.79 – 17.8)	84.7	(53.8 – 129)	590	(408 – 1,270)	228
20–39 years	52.0 (37.9 – 71.3)	7.67	(3.36 – 10.2)	36.0	(27.9 – 48.7)	846	(468 – 1,330)	117
40–59 years	60.4 (39.7 – 92.0)	8.25†	(4.94 – 10.0)	47.8	(21.4 – 81.5)	790†	(356 – 4,980)	85
60 years and older	41.1 (23.7 – 71.4)	7.55†	(1.89 – 9.13)	40.0	(15.3 – 84.1)	329†	(154 – 2,020)	83
Females								
Total, 6 years and older	57.1 (48.9 – 66.7)	6.73	(5.24 – 8.15)	49.8	(42.3 – 64.2)	556	(418 – 871)	662
6–11 years	80.5 (53.3 – 121)	14.4	(5.79 – 22.1)	65.4	(49.0 – 98.4)	735	(283 – 3,410)	119
12–19 years	84.6 (67.0 – 107)	10.4	(8.24 – 13.6)	71.1	(56.2 – 97.1)	867	(623 – 1,380)	217
20–39 years	48.7 (32.2 – 73.6)	5.71	(3.33 – 8.01)	32.3	(23.7 – 67.2)	594	(295 – 1,790)	165
40–59 years	50.4 (35.6 – 71.2)	5.24†	(3.72 – 11.2)	48.4	(35.4 – 84.6)	346†	(267 – 484)	72
60 years and older	42.9 (25.7 – 71.5)	5.28†	(1.79 – 7.45)	40.1	(18.6 – 73.7)	381†	(226 – 2,270)	89

† Estimate is subject to greater uncertainty due to small cell size.

Table 4.3.a.4. Urinary daidzein: Non-Hispanic blacks

Geometric mean and selected percentiles of urine concentrations (in µg/L) for non-Hispanic blacks in the U.S. population aged 6 years and older, National Health and Nutrition Examination Survey, 2003–2006.

	Geometric mean (95% conf. interval)		Selected percentiles (95% conf. interval)						Sample size
			10th		50th		90th		
Males and Females									
Total, 6 years and older	78.4	(67.6 – 90.9)	9.87	(8.52 – 11.6)	72.3	(61.3 – 85.2)	639	(474 – 766)	1,343
6–11 years	102	(80.6 – 129)	11.5	(8.37 – 16.0)	95.8	(70.0 – 129)	927	(487 – 2,170)	207
12–19 years	120	(104 – 139)	17.5	(13.5 – 20.8)	111	(92.3 – 144)	895	(756 – 1,160)	496
20–39 years	68.4	(53.2 – 88.0)	11.3	(8.37 – 13.1)	50.7	(41.3 – 76.5)	601	(408 – 893)	249
40–59 years	77.2	(59.6 – 99.9)	8.40	(6.24 – 11.2)	75.0	(58.8 – 111)	457	(377 – 839)	231
60 years and older	53.5	(37.7 – 75.8)	7.55	(4.20 – 9.29)	46.9	(28.8 – 78.8)	361	(259 – 823)	160
Males									
Total, 6 years and older	90.2	(75.1 – 108)	12.1	(8.49 – 14.2)	83.6	(64.7 – 110)	724	(584 – 1,050)	661
6–11 years	101	(70.3 – 145)	11.2†	(4.75 – 15.9)	103	(42.5 – 215)	1,050†	(534 – 2,140)	99
12–19 years	132	(107 – 164)	19.4	(11.4 – 24.1)	120	(95.6 – 152)	1,140	(766 – 1,980)	258
20–39 years	94.7	(64.5 – 139)	13.2	(7.79 – 16.6)	67.3	(41.4 – 151)	851	(564 – 1,400)	116
40–59 years	78.7	(54.4 – 114)	8.53	(6.17 – 13.3)	83.2	(58.0 – 134)	390	(368 – 701)	114
60 years and older	53.1	(37.3 – 75.7)	8.34†	(7.92 – 12.2)	40.3	(27.8 – 70.4)	325†	(169 – 1,800)	74
Females									
Total, 6 years and older	69.7	(57.7 – 84.2)	9.41	(7.40 – 11.2)	64.7	(54.2 – 77.9)	476	(427 – 675)	682
6–11 years	103	(74.2 – 142)	11.0†	(7.50 – 24.0)	85.1	(58.3 – 129)	687†	(398 – 7,580)	108
12–19 years	109	(91.8 – 129)	14.3	(9.60 – 22.6)	104	(73.9 – 142)	757	(652 – 1,140)	238
20–39 years	52.7	(37.2 – 74.6)	9.40	(5.61 – 12.1)	43.3	(26.0 – 75.9)	408	(280 – 622)	133
40–59 years	75.9	(51.0 – 113)	7.94	(4.01 – 11.8)	69.9	(47.9 – 109)	462	(369 – 2,070)	117
60 years and older	53.7	(31.4 – 91.7)	6.06†	(2.92 – 9.07)	55.3	(22.5 – 106)	368†	(257 – 1,170)	86

† Estimate is subject to greater uncertainty due to small cell size.

Table 4.3.a.5. Urinary daidzein: Non-Hispanic whites

Geometric mean and selected percentiles of urine concentrations (in µg/L) for non-Hispanic whites in the U.S. population aged 6 years and older, National Health and Nutrition Examination Survey, 2003–2006.

	Geometric mean (95% conf. interval)		Selected percentiles (95% conf. interval)						Sample size
			10th		50th		90th		
Males and Females									
Total, 6 years and older	63.9	(58.7 – 69.6)	8.36	(6.60 – 9.38)	58.5	(52.0 – 65.3)	571	(479 – 684)	2,108
6–11 years	86.5	(70.6 – 106)	16.0	(11.4 – 20.6)	66.6	(56.0 – 93.6)	643	(450 – 985)	193
12–19 years	91.5	(77.3 – 108)	15.2	(10.6 – 17.3)	76.3	(59.5 – 100)	824	(606 – 977)	378
20–39 years	58.5	(47.8 – 71.7)	6.75	(4.48 – 10.3)	53.0	(44.8 – 66.9)	484	(343 – 753)	494
40–59 years	57.9	(50.4 – 66.5)	7.22	(5.29 – 8.66)	50.6	(41.9 – 65.3)	575	(407 – 893)	448
60 years and older	61.6	(52.9 – 71.8)	8.03	(6.59 – 9.36)	61.2	(49.1 – 78.5)	469	(396 – 662)	595
Males									
Total, 6 years and older	70.2	(62.0 – 79.4)	9.34	(7.77 – 12.2)	63.8	(54.1 – 72.9)	680	(509 – 779)	1,035
6–11 years	83.9	(62.4 – 113)	18.4†	(7.93 – 21.7)	63.1	(49.4 – 94.1)	651†	(271 – 1,180)	99
12–19 years	102	(78.3 – 134)	16.6	(12.7 – 23.1)	80.1	(55.1 – 118)	812	(466 – 1,440)	191
20–39 years	63.4	(48.0 – 83.7)	8.03	(3.27 – 14.2)	59.0	(43.8 – 77.0)	575	(341 – 1,010)	217
40–59 years	66.9	(54.2 – 82.7)	8.29	(6.53 – 9.37)	63.4	(42.1 – 83.3)	670	(409 – 970)	229
60 years and older	64.3	(50.0 – 82.9)	9.18	(6.88 – 12.0)	58.7	(42.2 – 88.7)	591	(416 – 762)	299
Females									
Total, 6 years and older	58.3	(52.6 – 64.7)	7.50	(5.79 – 8.68)	53.1	(47.0 – 61.0)	484	(397 – 608)	1,073
6–11 years	89.7	(67.1 – 120)	14.9†	(5.43 – 19.0)	89.1	(50.9 – 141)	583†	(352 – 7,440)	94
12–19 years	81.0	(66.4 – 98.8)	11.8	(7.34 – 15.8)	73.3	(52.3 – 101)	817	(455 – 970)	187
20–39 years	54.0	(42.7 – 68.5)	6.43	(5.19 – 8.74)	51.1	(38.2 – 64.5)	382	(293 – 683)	277
40–59 years	50.0	(42.1 – 59.4)	5.98	(3.46 – 8.36)	43.5	(32.6 – 53.4)	514	(309 – 843)	219
60 years and older	59.6	(49.4 – 71.8)	7.25	(3.83 – 8.51)	61.4	(49.3 – 83.1)	401	(357 – 656)	296

† Estimate is subject to greater uncertainty due to small cell size.

Table 4.3.b. Urinary daidzein: Concentrations by survey cycle

Geometric mean and selected percentiles of urine concentrations (in µg/L) for the U.S. population, National Health and Nutrition Examination Survey, 1999–2006.

	Geometric mean (95% conf. interval)	Selected percentiles (95% conf. interval)			Sample size
		5th	50th	95th	
Total, 6 years and older					
1999–2000	75.1 (61.9 – 91.1)	6.56 (3.36 – 8.12)	69.8 (58.1 – 82.4)	1,310 (1,030 – 1,550)	2,553
2001–2002	51.7 (46.6 – 57.5)	< LOD	52.3 (49.0 – 57.5)	1,240 (919 – 1,850)	2,794
2003–2004	66.7 (60.4 – 73.7)	5.71 (4.00 – 6.43)	62.0 (54.1 – 69.7)	1,070 (924 – 1,330)	2,594
2005–2006	66.5 (59.7 – 74.1)	4.98 (3.70 – 6.58)	58.8 (51.4 – 67.7)	1,180 (1,010 – 1,380)	2,528
Age group					
6–11 years					
1999–2000	90.5 (75.1 – 109)	8.59 (1.43 – 13.6)	100 (71.0 – 129)	1,110 (707 – 1,740)	330
2001–2002	84.9 (71.6 – 101)	11.3 (3.15 – 12.4)	72.1 (56.6 – 96.9)	1,050 (684 – 1,650)	396
2003–2004	84.9 (71.6 – 101)	13.2 (9.77 – 16.2)	65.6 (56.7 – 92.7)	788 (644 – 1,070)	341
2005–2006	94.1 (74.3 – 119)	7.73 (6.35 – 10.8)	73.8 (56.1 – 95.1)	1,870 (1,130 – 6,350)	351
12–19 years					
1999–2000	123 (91.4 – 166)	14.7 (7.23 – 17.6)	124 (85.6 – 165)	1,460 (1,100 – 3,300)	753
2001–2002	69.3 (52.6 – 91.3)	2.63 (< LOD – 6.02)	69.8 (53.2 – 87.5)	1,330 (977 – 2,110)	744
2003–2004	89.0 (75.2 – 105)	9.05 (6.06 – 9.91)	77.9 (60.1 – 104)	1,190 (927 – 1,970)	729
2005–2006	94.4 (76.0 – 117)	9.14 (6.14 – 11.0)	76.9 (59.6 – 102)	1,370 (981 – 2,270)	693
20–39 years					
1999–2000	80.6 (64.3 – 101)	7.55 (3.34 – 9.89)	67.1 (55.6 – 82.5)	1,730 (983 – 4,150)	534
2001–2002	51.5 (42.7 – 62.1)	< LOD	50.7 (40.4 – 64.9)	1,200 (763 – 1,930)	604
2003–2004	59.9 (47.6 – 75.3)	4.82 (3.21 – 6.58)	56.1 (44.9 – 69.0)	1,170 (809 – 1,480)	554
2005–2006	63.4 (51.7 – 77.6)	4.81 (2.19 – 6.27)	52.3 (44.7 – 68.5)	1,360 (737 – 2,240)	583
40–59 years					
1999–2000	55.4 (39.0 – 78.6)	2.50 (< LOD – 7.77)	56.7 (40.8 – 70.7)	1,060 (801 – 1,520)	420
2001–2002	50.6 (40.4 – 63.3)	< LOD	53.1 (39.3 – 68.2)	1,760 (859 – 3,030)	531
2003–2004	67.9 (58.3 – 79.2)	5.13 (3.05 – 6.43)	62.2 (46.1 – 78.7)	1,290 (840 – 3,440)	452
2005–2006	54.9 (47.3 – 63.7)	3.79 (2.99 – 5.86)	50.5 (41.4 – 61.9)	983 (665 – 1,300)	449
60 years and older					
1999–2000	64.6 (53.0 – 78.8)	6.47 (5.61 – 9.10)	61.5 (45.9 – 85.0)	665 (556 – 991)	516
2001–2002	32.0 (26.2 – 39.0)	< LOD	33.8 (28.4 – 40.4)	636 (397 – 1,990)	519
2003–2004	55.7 (44.4 – 69.9)	4.07 (2.51 – 5.72)	56.5 (43.8 – 76.3)	780 (585 – 1,660)	518
2005–2006	66.4 (54.6 – 80.8)	4.76 (1.85 – 8.24)	62.5 (43.9 – 89.5)	952 (707 – 1,600)	452
Gender					
Males					
1999–2000	88.9 (71.4 – 111)	7.75 (5.85 – 10.4)	80.5 (66.9 – 112)	1,540 (1,020 – 2,240)	1,220
2001–2002	49.8 (42.8 – 57.9)	< LOD	50.7 (46.9 – 55.6)	918 (727 – 1,400)	1,375
2003–2004	73.8 (63.4 – 85.9)	6.35 (3.20 – 8.53)	65.2 (56.4 – 76.4)	1,200 (1,020 – 1,370)	1,244
2005–2006	73.9 (65.3 – 83.6)	6.32 (4.02 – 7.91)	66.2 (53.9 – 78.3)	1,180 (1,000 – 1,430)	1,252
Females					
1999–2000	64.1 (52.9 – 77.6)	5.62 (1.86 – 7.80)	57.6 (45.2 – 73.2)	1,210 (652 – 2,010)	1,333
2001–2002	53.6 (48.1 – 59.8)	< LOD	55.4 (49.8 – 62.4)	1,440 (1,190 – 1,990)	1,419
2003–2004	60.7 (53.6 – 68.8)	4.61 (3.50 – 5.95)	57.4 (49.3 – 67.3)	884 (670 – 1,390)	1,350
2005–2006	60.1 (52.5 – 68.9)	4.40 (2.99 – 5.94)	52.4 (45.0 – 61.4)	1,140 (843 – 1,480)	1,276
Race/ethnicity					
Mexican Americans					
1999–2000	78.9 (59.8 – 104)	6.78 (4.37 – 8.83)	66.1 (48.8 – 90.2)	1,340 (977 – 3,000)	816
2001–2002	39.2 (28.5 – 54.0)	< LOD	39.8 (28.8 – 59.7)	880 (633 – 1,770)	679
2003–2004	57.4 (50.2 – 65.7)	4.90 (3.74 – 5.99)	45.4 (35.3 – 53.3)	1,380 (954 – 1,720)	653
2005–2006	60.6 (53.3 – 68.9)	4.35 (2.74 – 5.80)	54.0 (44.1 – 64.5)	1,320 (981 – 1,550)	634
Non-Hispanic Blacks					
1999–2000	91.5 (71.1 – 118)	7.48 (< LOD – 11.2)	102 (84.0 – 131)	1,030 (771 – 1,640)	596
2001–2002	66.3 (47.7 – 91.9)	< LOD	72.9 (52.5 – 96.5)	1,410 (950 – 2,850)	692
2003–2004	75.5 (56.5 – 101)	7.09 (5.71 – 8.69)	67.6 (51.5 – 89.3)	1,150 (699 – 2,380)	681
2005–2006	81.3 (71.6 – 92.4)	6.97 (4.66 – 7.57)	76.5 (69.9 – 94.7)	1,200 (878 – 1,960)	662
Non-Hispanic Whites					
1999–2000	74.7 (61.8 – 90.3)	7.25 (3.27 – 8.95)	66.8 (57.0 – 77.4)	1,360 (990 – 1,730)	901
2001–2002	48.6 (43.8 – 53.9)	< LOD	49.8 (45.8 – 53.1)	1,140 (811 – 1,910)	1,211
2003–2004	65.9 (58.7 – 74.0)	5.10 (3.33 – 6.39)	62.3 (53.0 – 71.3)	1,050 (843 – 1,360)	1,069
2005–2006	62.0 (54.4 – 70.7)	4.55 (3.17 – 6.33)	54.1 (46.9 – 63.9)	1,030 (884 – 1,310)	1,039

< LOD means less than the limit of detection, which may vary for some compounds by year. See Appendix D for LOD.

Figure 4.3.b. Urinary daidzein: Concentrations by survey cycle

Selected percentiles in µg/L (95% confidence intervals), National Health and Nutrition Examination Survey, 1999–2006

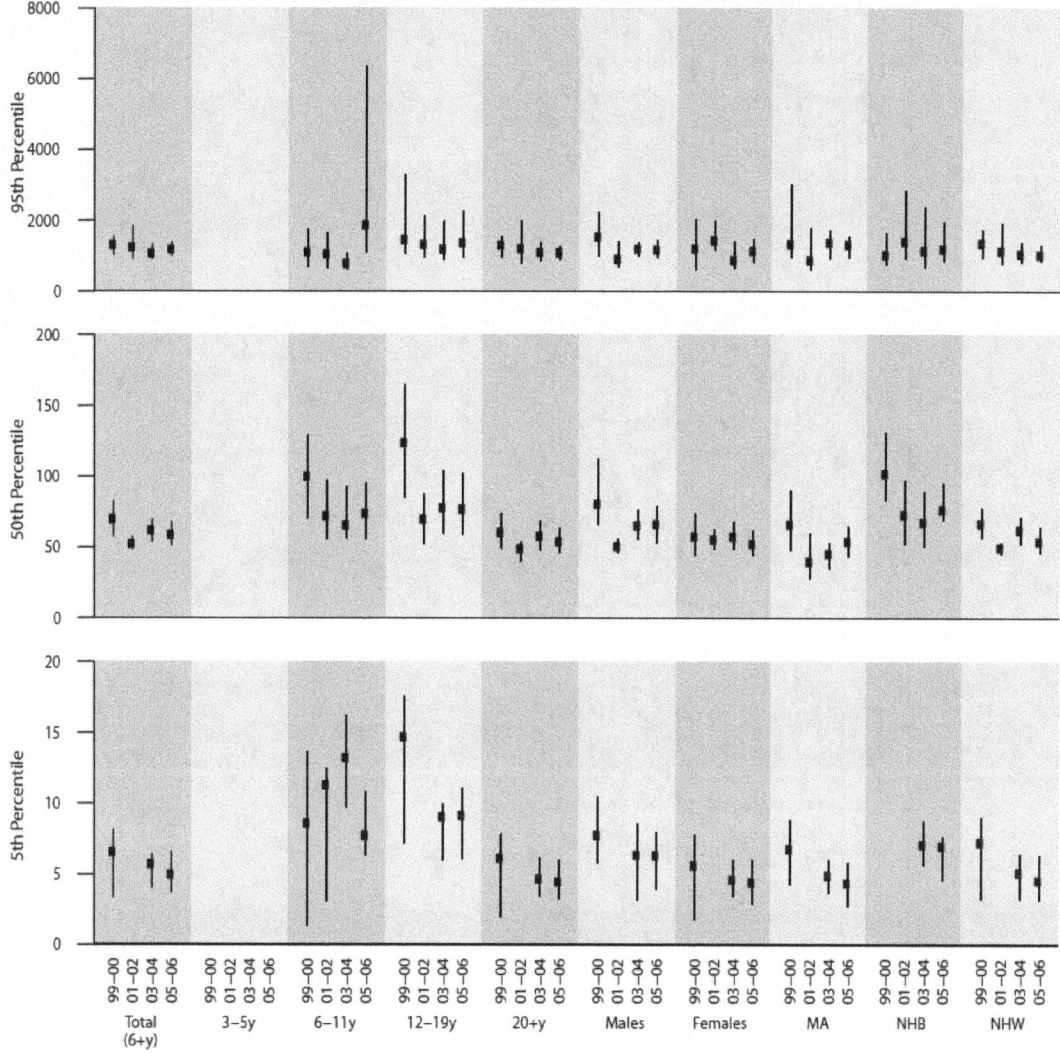

Values in the graph are suppressed if either the point estimate or the lower 95% confidence limit is noted as "< LOD" in the accompanying table.

Table 4.4.a.1. Urinary daidzein (creatinine corrected): Concentrations

Geometric mean and selected percentiles of urine concentrations (in µg/g creatinine) for the total U.S. population aged 6 years and older, National Health and Nutrition Examination Survey, 2003–2006.

	Geometric mean (95% conf. interval)	Selected percentiles (95% conf. interval)					Sample size
		2.5th	5th	50th	95th	97.5th	
Total, 6 years and older	63.7 (60.0 – 67.5)	4.69 (4.17 – 5.11)	6.83 (6.29 – 7.32)	54.6 (50.2 – 58.5)	1,060 (939 – 1,150)	1,890 (1,520 – 2,820)	5,122
Age group							
6–11 years	96.8 (85.1 – 110)	9.11 (7.67 – 11.1)	12.3 (9.30 – 15.7)	72.6 (63.3 – 87.8)	1,630 (1,000 – 2,990)	3,010 (1,860 – 5,360)	692
12–19 years	68.3 (60.0 – 77.7)	5.75 (4.91 – 6.71)	7.91 (6.76 – 9.36)	56.2 (47.3 – 69.0)	910 (755 – 1,210)	1,330 (1,180 – 2,730)	1,422
20–39 years	52.5 (46.6 – 59.3)	3.98 (2.80 – 4.53)	5.88 (4.34 – 6.73)	44.6 (37.9 – 52.2)	878 (685 – 1,100)	1,360 (1,090 – 2,480)	1,137
40–59 years	61.6 (56.1 – 67.8)	4.02 (2.73 – 4.80)	5.99 (4.72 – 7.17)	51.7 (46.0 – 58.2)	1,140 (895 – 2,180)	2,760 (1,510 – 4,990)	901
60 years and older	71.4 (63.3 – 80.5)	5.84 (4.78 – 7.05)	8.24 (7.26 – 9.16)	63.9 (51.3 – 78.0)	1,010 (828 – 1,180)	1,770 (1,120 – 2,940)	970
Gender							
Males	58.6 (53.5 – 64.1)	4.34 (3.58 – 4.79)	6.32 (5.09 – 7.08)	49.9 (45.5 – 55.2)	924 (812 – 1,100)	1,550 (1,190 – 2,640)	2,496
Females	68.9 (63.4 – 74.9)	5.13 (4.29 – 5.94)	7.44 (6.45 – 8.14)	60.0 (51.0 – 68.9)	1,130 (1,010 – 1,510)	2,100 (1,630 – 3,290)	2,626
Race/ethnicity							
Mexican Americans	53.2 (47.7 – 59.3)	3.88 (2.31 – 4.18)	4.66 (4.10 – 5.41)	47.7 (38.6 – 56.1)	973 (859 – 1,170)	1,750 (1,360 – 2,390)	1,287
Non-Hispanic Blacks	55.0 (48.8 – 62.1)	3.99 (3.43 – 4.57)	5.90 (4.51 – 6.56)	48.0 (39.1 – 59.6)	825 (645 – 1,040)	1,360 (1,020 – 2,320)	1,343
Non-Hispanic Whites	65.1 (60.7 – 69.7)	4.86 (4.30 – 5.83)	7.25 (6.49 – 7.90)	56.0 (50.6 – 60.8)	1,080 (940 – 1,200)	1,890 (1,480 – 3,030)	2,108

Figure 4.4.a. Urinary daidzein (creatinine corrected): Concentrations by age group
Geometric mean (95% confidence interval), National Health and Nutrition Examination Survey, 2003–2006

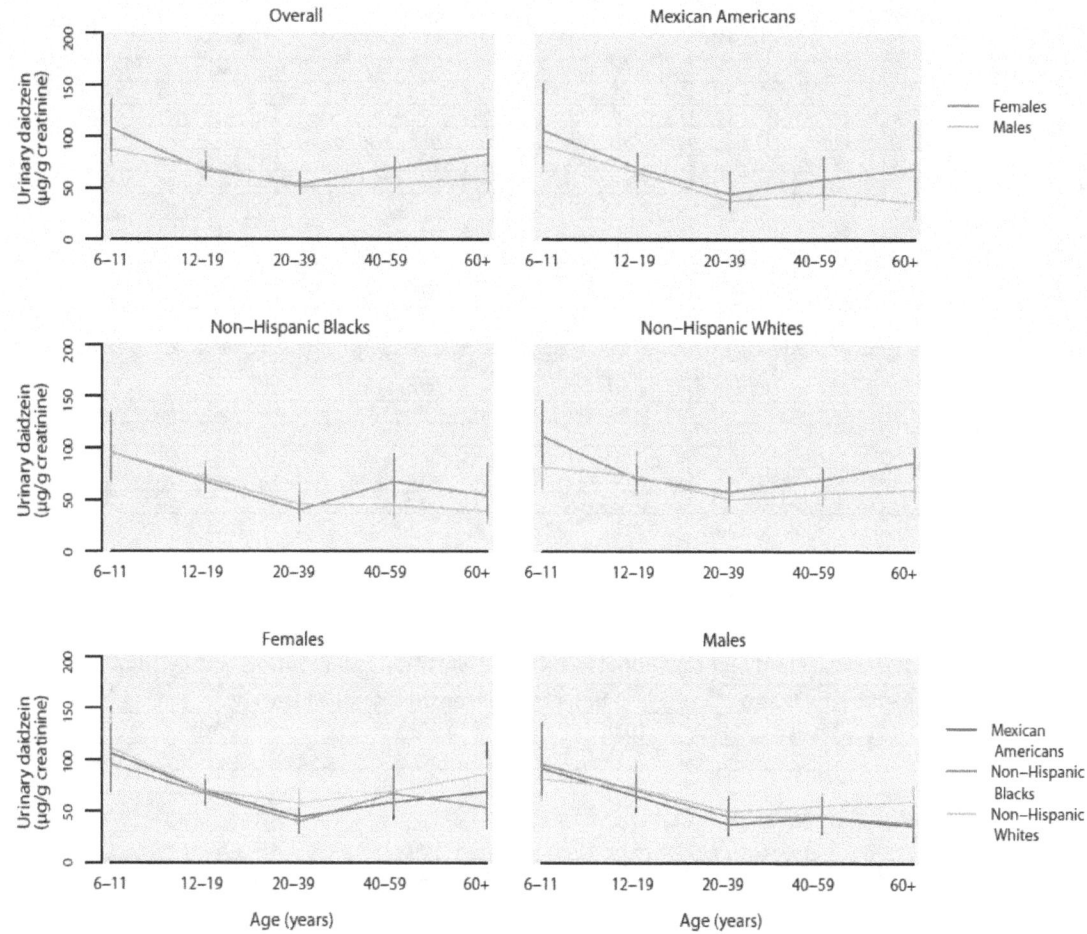

Table 4.4.a.2. Urinary daidzein (creatinine corrected): Total population

Geometric mean and selected percentiles of urine concentrations (in µg/g creatinine) for the total U.S. population aged 6 years and older, National Health and Nutrition Examination Survey, 2003–2006.

	Geometric mean (95% conf. interval)	Selected percentiles (95% conf. interval)			Sample size
		10th	50th	90th	
Males and Females					
Total, 6 years and older	63.7 (60.0 – 67.5)	9.68 (8.96 – 10.5)	54.6 (50.2 – 58.5)	522 (463 – 593)	5,122
6–11 years	96.8 (85.1 – 110)	19.0 (14.8 – 23.0)	72.6 (63.3 – 87.8)	697 (580 – 924)	692
12–19 years	68.3 (60.0 – 77.7)	11.5 (9.80 – 12.7)	56.2 (47.3 – 69.0)	522 (419 – 738)	1,422
20–39 years	52.5 (46.6 – 59.3)	8.66 (7.41 – 9.62)	44.6 (37.9 – 52.2)	424 (338 – 501)	1,137
40–59 years	61.6 (56.1 – 67.8)	8.59 (7.78 – 9.25)	51.7 (46.0 – 58.2)	570 (410 – 894)	901
60 years and older	71.4 (63.3 – 80.5)	11.3 (10.1 – 12.0)	63.9 (51.3 – 78.0)	565 (462 – 702)	970
Males					
Total, 6 years and older	58.6 (53.5 – 64.1)	8.91 (8.16 – 9.82)	49.9 (45.5 – 55.2)	467 (421 – 543)	2,496
6–11 years	87.5 (73.6 – 104)	15.8 (11.8 – 21.6)	68.2 (54.2 – 82.8)	733 (435 – 1,190)	340
12–19 years	69.8 (57.3 – 85.0)	11.6 (9.54 – 13.5)	53.9 (43.2 – 69.7)	580 (404 – 842)	728
20–39 years	51.3 (44.0 – 59.9)	7.55 (6.03 – 9.50)	43.4 (36.9 – 50.3)	451 (379 – 595)	499
40–59 years	54.2 (46.0 – 63.9)	7.88 (6.08 – 8.73)	47.0 (38.7 – 60.1)	458 (305 – 766)	451
60 years and older	59.3 (49.0 – 71.9)	10.0 (8.24 – 11.5)	51.0 (43.3 – 65.7)	423 (370 – 565)	478
Females					
Total, 6 years and older	68.9 (63.4 – 74.9)	10.7 (9.41 – 12.2)	60.0 (51.0 – 68.9)	582 (493 – 702)	2,626
6–11 years	108 (86.1 – 135)	22.3 (14.6 – 27.7)	84.3 (68.0 – 112)	696 (561 – 1,060)	352
12–19 years	66.7 (58.4 – 76.1)	11.4 (9.31 – 13.0)	58.6 (45.9 – 76.2)	514 (379 – 662)	694
20–39 years	53.8 (44.6 – 64.9)	9.21 (7.51 – 10.7)	46.6 (34.7 – 63.9)	349 (237 – 654)	638
40–59 years	69.6 (60.7 – 79.8)	9.63 (7.84 – 12.3)	57.3 (48.8 – 68.7)	699 (459 – 1,130)	450
60 years and older	82.6 (70.8 – 96.4)	12.7 (10.2 – 14.5)	75.0 (58.7 – 92.5)	686 (537 – 965)	492

Table 4.4.a.3. Urinary daidzein (creatinine corrected): Mexican Americans

Geometric mean and selected percentiles of urine concentrations (in µg/g creatinine) for Mexican Americans in the U.S. population aged 6 years and older, National Health and Nutrition Examination Survey, 2003–2006.

	Geometric mean (95% conf. interval)	Selected percentiles (95% conf. interval)			Sample size
		10th	50th	90th	
Males and Females					
Total, 6 years and older	53.2 (47.7 – 59.3)	6.93 (6.05 – 7.61)	47.7 (38.6 – 56.1)	527 (431 – 601)	1,287
6–11 years	98.3 (76.7 – 126)	20.2 (16.6 – 23.2)	80.4 (62.1 – 108)	601 (332 – 1,940)	231
12–19 years	67.5 (56.8 – 80.1)	10.8 (7.46 – 13.3)	57.9 (49.4 – 71.5)	492 (380 – 834)	445
20–39 years	40.7 (33.7 – 49.2)	5.59 (4.19 – 7.06)	30.1 (24.2 – 42.4)	499 (290 – 809)	282
40–59 years	50.7 (39.5 – 65.0)	6.01 (4.56 – 7.76)	45.9 (30.2 – 62.8)	537 (275 – 990)	157
60 years and older	52.0 (36.8 – 73.4)	6.95 (5.30 – 8.24)	49.3 (31.5 – 75.6)	344 (253 – 971)	172
Males					
Total, 6 years and older	48.0 (40.5 – 56.9)	6.05 (5.04 – 7.07)	40.4 (30.2 – 56.1)	469 (355 – 594)	625
6–11 years	91.5 (66.0 – 127)	20.4 (15.5 – 23.2)	74.0 (50.3 – 130)	429 (313 – 1,510)	112
12–19 years	65.2 (50.4 – 84.4)	12.3 (7.04 – 13.8)	55.2 (37.2 – 91.2)	424 (302 – 861)	228
20–39 years	37.8 (27.7 – 51.5)	4.82 (2.22 – 6.78)	27.8 (20.6 – 44.4)	432 (264 – 899)	117
40–59 years	44.3 (29.3 – 67.1)	5.90† (3.67 – 7.61)	29.8 (16.1 – 73.2)	552† (258 – 1,640)	85
60 years and older	36.7 (21.9 – 61.5)	5.57† (4.50 – 6.89)	35.3 (15.0 – 66.2)	309† (110 – 2,740)	83
Females					
Total, 6 years and older	59.6 (50.8 – 69.9)	7.76 (6.39 – 9.44)	53.5 (43.2 – 62.6)	602 (406 – 897)	662
6–11 years	106 (74.4 – 151)	20.1 (13.5 – 27.3)	85.2 (68.2 – 112)	898 (305 – 3,630)	119
12–19 years	69.9 (57.9 – 84.3)	10.1 (6.44 – 13.3)	65.8 (43.1 – 81.9)	736 (477 – 881)	217
20–39 years	44.5 (29.8 – 66.4)	6.66 (4.07 – 8.39)	33.2 (18.7 – 56.2)	569 (207 – 2,670)	165
40–59 years	58.7 (42.8 – 80.4)	6.72† (4.24 – 11.8)	52.7 (40.8 – 75.2)	427† (256 – 924)	72
60 years and older	69.2 (41.2 – 116)	8.25† (3.99 – 13.0)	64.1 (24.7 – 157)	443† (255 – 2,030)	89

† Estimate is subject to greater uncertainty due to small cell size.

Table 4.4.a.4. Urinary daidzein (creatinine corrected): Non-Hispanic blacks

Geometric mean and selected percentiles of urine concentrations (in µg/g creatinine) for non-Hispanic blacks in the U.S. population aged 6 years and older, National Health and Nutrition Examination Survey, 2003–2006.

	Geometric mean (95% conf. interval)	Selected percentiles (95% conf. interval)						Sample size
		10th		50th		90th		
Males and Females								
Total, 6 years and older	55.0 (48.8 – 62.1)	8.72	(7.34 – 9.46)	48.0	(39.1 – 59.6)	437	(389 – 538)	1,343
6–11 years	95.6 (75.9 – 121)	13.3	(11.1 – 18.8)	81.9	(67.4 – 108)	1,010	(647 – 1,910)	207
12–19 years	69.0 (60.5 – 78.8)	9.54	(8.52 – 11.6)	66.5	(51.3 – 85.0)	496	(424 – 640)	496
20–39 years	42.4 (34.5 – 52.2)	6.72	(5.68 – 9.60)	28.1	(23.4 – 44.7)	368	(211 – 702)	249
40–59 years	56.1 (45.9 – 68.6)	8.30	(5.49 – 10.0)	48.7	(38.5 – 66.9)	422	(290 – 614)	231
60 years and older	47.7 (35.0 – 64.9)	9.05	(6.31 – 10.7)	42.0	(25.3 – 67.0)	295	(223 – 603)	160
Males								
Total, 6 years and older	52.7 (44.7 – 62.0)	7.20	(6.40 – 8.99)	44.4	(32.0 – 63.8)	440	(391 – 532)	661
6–11 years	95.5 (67.1 – 136)	11.2†	(8.55 – 13.9)	94.6	(39.1 – 139)	1,210†	(646 – 2,090)	99
12–19 years	70.8 (58.3 – 86.0)	9.79	(7.70 – 11.8)	70.0	(53.8 – 88.7)	584	(426 – 910)	258
20–39 years	45.4 (31.9 – 64.8)	6.49	(3.95 – 8.98)	27.2	(20.2 – 77.0)	410	(234 – 1,360)	116
40–59 years	45.0 (31.4 – 64.5)	6.01	(3.03 – 8.96)	42.1	(29.9 – 58.2)	338	(222 – 684)	114
60 years and older	39.0 (26.7 – 56.8)	7.23†	(4.44 – 11.3)	25.7	(19.2 – 50.9)	238†	(114 – 996)	74
Females								
Total, 6 years and older	57.1 (48.2 – 67.6)	9.36	(7.44 – 11.4)	49.4	(39.9 – 66.3)	419	(330 – 593)	682
6–11 years	95.7 (68.8 – 133)	18.3†	(6.78 – 23.1)	77.5	(61.2 – 95.9)	758†	(307 – 2,820)	108
12–19 years	67.3 (56.6 – 80.0)	9.35	(7.76 – 13.2)	62.7	(46.6 – 85.6)	458	(328 – 895)	238
20–39 years	40.1 (30.2 – 53.3)	7.29	(4.25 – 11.4)	29.9	(23.8 – 42.2)	310	(153 – 668)	133
40–59 years	67.3 (48.1 – 94.2)	9.31	(6.16 – 12.6)	55.0	(35.4 – 90.6)	552	(299 – 922)	117
60 years and older	54.2 (34.6 – 84.9)	9.07†	(4.74 – 11.6)	55.5	(26.1 – 79.8)	312†	(185 – 1,040)	86

† Estimate is subject to greater uncertainty due to small cell size.

Table 4.4.a.5. Urinary daidzein (creatinine corrected): Non-Hispanic whites

Geometric mean and selected percentiles of urine concentrations (in µg/g creatinine) for non-Hispanic whites in the U.S. population aged 6 years and older, National Health and Nutrition Examination Survey, 2003–2006.

	Geometric mean (95% conf. interval)	Selected percentiles (95% conf. interval)						Sample size
		10th		50th		90th		
Males and Females								
Total, 6 years and older	65.1 (60.7 – 69.7)	10.0	(8.80 – 11.4)	56.0	(50.6 – 60.8)	519	(451 – 658)	2,108
6–11 years	93.9 (77.9 – 113)	17.1	(11.9 – 25.8)	70.3	(57.7 – 96.8)	577	(423 – 991)	193
12–19 years	71.8 (60.1 – 85.8)	12.3	(10.4 – 13.6)	57.5	(46.0 – 74.4)	563	(415 – 763)	378
20–39 years	54.0 (45.5 – 64.1)	9.24	(7.14 – 10.8)	46.4	(37.6 – 57.0)	403	(315 – 578)	494
40–59 years	62.2 (55.5 – 69.8)	8.59	(7.54 – 10.0)	52.9	(43.2 – 60.5)	582	(397 – 1,030)	448
60 years and older	73.5 (65.4 – 82.6)	11.4	(10.1 – 12.6)	65.9	(55.2 – 80.0)	548	(459 – 714)	595
Males								
Total, 6 years and older	58.7 (52.2 – 65.9)	9.03	(8.12 – 10.5)	49.9	(43.4 – 57.4)	6456	(369 – 638)	1,035
6–11 years	81.3 (60.7 – 109)	15.6†	(10.8 – 22.6)	60.2	(45.1 – 95.9)	540†	(287 – 2,790)	99
12–19 years	73.1 (55.1 – 97.1)	12.3	(8.32 – 16.7)	54.3	(40.6 – 82.5)	653	(397 – 892)	191
20–39 years	50.3 (39.2 – 64.7)	8.53	(4.63 – 10.7)	41.7	(33.8 – 54.3)	425	(296 – 777)	217
40–59 years	56.0 (46.0 – 68.2)	8.18	(5.53 – 8.99)	46.0	(37.2 – 62.3)	465	(304 – 946)	229
60 years and older	60.0 (48.0 – 74.9)	10.1	(8.07 – 11.6)	54.2	(40.5 – 79.6)	402	(357 – 501)	299
Females								
Total, 6 years and older	71.9 (65.4 – 79.1)	11.6	(9.27 – 13.6)	63.3	(53.8 – 73.5)	589	(484 – 818)	1,073
6–11 years	111 (84.1 – 146)	23.8†	(12.9 – 33.2)	94.0	(66.0 – 124)	578†	(397 – 1,780)	94
12–19 years	70.4 (58.7 – 84.5)	12.2	(7.26 – 16.3)	66.9	(43.9 – 86.4)	520	(372 – 713)	187
20–39 years	57.9 (46.6 – 71.9)	10.1	(7.66 – 13.0)	47.8	(35.8 – 67.5)	385	(237 – 817)	277
40–59 years	69.2 (59.3 – 80.8)	9.16	(7.25 – 13.0)	57.6	(46.3 – 71.7)	894	(410 – 1,310)	219
60 years and older	86.3 (74.3 – 100)	13.4	(10.1 – 15.6)	78.0	(59.8 – 97.1)	656	(519 – 974)	296

† Estimate is subject to greater uncertainty due to small cell size.

Table 4.4.b. Urinary daidzein (creatinine corrected): Concentrations by survey cycle

Geometric mean and selected percentiles of urine concentrations (in µg/g creatinine) for the U.S. population, National Health and Nutrition Examination Survey, 1999–2006.

	Geometric mean (95% conf. interval)	Selected percentiles (95% conf. interval)						Sample size
		5th		50th		95th		
Total, 6 years and older								
1999–2000	68.5	(55.9 – 83.9)	6.25	(2.72 – 8.90)	65.1	(52.8 – 80.8)	943	(838 – 1,150)	2,553
2001–2002	48.5	(43.7 – 54.0)	<LOD		48.3	(43.2 – 56.3)	955	(805 – 1,220)	2,794
2003–2004	62.5	(58.3 – 67.0)	6.82	(5.96 – 7.48)	56.0	(49.9 – 63.5)	1,050	(858 – 1,150)	2,594
2005–2006	64.8	(58.7 – 71.6)	6.88	(6.01 – 7.54)	52.3	(47.9 – 59.7)	1,070	(924 – 1,380)	2,528
Age group								
6–11 years								
1999–2000	92.6	(76.3 – 112)	10.7	(8.22 – 13.1)	93.0	(72.1 – 114)	1,050	(835 – 2,070)	330
2001–2002	96.4	(79.0 – 118)	13.0	(6.07 – 14.7)	85.9	(60.7 – 126)	934	(712 – 1,370)	396
2003–2004	90.4	(77.2 – 106)	15.8	(8.36 – 20.2)	72.4	(58.2 – 99.0)	700	(563 – 1,660)	341
2005–2006	104	(83.1 – 130)	10.8	(8.23 – 13.3)	73.8	(59.5 – 93.5)	2,350	(1,430 – 4,630)	351
12–19 years								
1999–2000	83.1	(58.4 – 118)	7.76	(3.13 – 11.0)	84.8	(54.0 – 123)	991	(725 – 2,680)	753
2001–2002	53.4	(40.8 – 70.0)	2.77	(<LOD – 4.26)	50.8	(38.8 – 77.4)	1,030	(677 – 1,580)	744
2003–2004	66.6	(55.7 – 79.6)	8.31	(6.76 – 9.40)	56.3	(45.0 – 74.4)	873	(667 – 1,270)	729
2005–2006	70.0	(56.9 – 86.2)	7.67	(5.31 – 10.3)	54.7	(42.8 – 74.1)	914	(714 – 1,950)	693
20–39 years								
1999–2000	63.9	(50.7 – 80.6)	5.10	(2.37 – 8.40)	52.8	(41.0 – 81.7)	1,100	(811 – 1,740)	534
2001–2002	41.6	(35.1 – 49.4)	<LOD		43.0	(30.4 – 54.2)	849	(615 – 1,040)	604
2003–2004	50.5	(43.0 – 59.3)	5.95	(4.11 – 7.11)	42.6	(36.1 – 50.6)	870	(570 – 1,360)	554
2005–2006	54.6	(45.0 – 66.4)	5.60	(3.60 – 7.48)	47.0	(34.2 – 65.2)	875	(645 – 1,200)	583
40–59 years								
1999–2000	56.2	(39.7 – 79.6)	3.39	(<LOD – 8.27)	50.3	(39.1 – 71.2)	827	(624 – 1,360)	420
2001–2002	50.2	(40.3 – 62.7)	<LOD		53.3	(40.4 – 67.5)	1,220	(848 – 2,140)	531
2003–2004	65.1	(56.5 – 75.2)	5.51	(4.02 – 7.94)	58.2	(48.9 – 70.6)	1,220	(713 – 4,260)	452
2005–2006	58.5	(50.8 – 67.4)	6.35	(3.70 – 7.64)	46.1	(40.8 – 56.2)	1,090	(714 – 2,890)	449
60 years and older								
1999–2000	77.6	(63.4 – 94.8)	8.64	(5.52 – 12.0)	82.7	(61.7 – 104)	761	(575 – 996)	516
2001–2002	37.9	(31.0 – 46.3)	<LOD		36.0	(25.9 – 44.2)	726	(502 – 1,780)	519
2003–2004	65.9	(55.1 – 78.9)	8.01	(6.03 – 9.02)	61.8	(48.0 – 78.2)	973	(653 – 1,870)	518
2005–2006	77.1	(65.2 – 91.1)	9.10	(6.42 – 11.4)	64.5	(49.7 – 87.6)	1,020	(827 – 1,610)	452
Gender								
Males								
1999–2000	69.7	(54.7 – 88.8)	6.40	(1.93 – 9.19)	69.8	(52.1 – 84.2)	1,040	(908 – 1,180)	1,220
2001–2002	40.5	(34.8 – 47.1)	<LOD		41.6	(34.6 – 47.9)	773	(615 – 969)	1,375
2003–2004	57.7	(49.4 – 67.3)	6.10	(4.73 – 7.35)	48.9	(42.3 – 58.2)	918	(699 – 1,230)	1,244
2005–2006	59.5	(53.3 – 66.3)	6.42	(4.79 – 7.34)	50.7	(43.2 – 57.6)	926	(814 – 1,170)	1,252
Females								
1999–2000	67.4	(54.8 – 82.9)	5.93	(2.71 – 8.38)	62.1	(51.2 – 80.8)	845	(622 – 1,420)	1,333
2001–2002	57.6	(50.8 – 65.2)	<LOD		59.1	(48.2 – 72.9)	1,170	(949 – 1,430)	1,419
2003–2004	67.4	(60.8 – 74.9)	7.43	(6.03 – 8.22)	64.9	(54.7 – 73.3)	1,090	(820 – 1,490)	1,350
2005–2006	70.4	(61.3 – 80.8)	7.47	(5.83 – 8.70)	57.1	(45.2 – 71.2)	1,180	(1,020 – 1,860)	1,276
Race/ethnicity								
Mexican Americans								
1999–2000	72.4	(59.1 – 88.9)	6.47	(3.20 – 8.73)	64.0	(46.9 – 90.9)	1,380	(886 – 3,380)	816
2001–2002	36.9	(27.8 – 49.0)	<LOD		37.0	(24.9 – 57.3)	718	(584 – 1,220)	679
2003–2004	51.8	(45.0 – 59.6)	4.37	(2.94 – 5.89)	47.7	(36.4 – 58.1)	1,120	(870 – 1,380)	653
2005–2006	54.7	(45.6 – 65.7)	4.79	(3.91 – 5.94)	47.2	(36.0 – 60.6)	917	(662 – 1,130)	634
Non-Hispanic Blacks								
1999–2000	58.7	(46.0 – 74.9)	3.74	(<LOD – 6.58)	67.0	(52.1 – 86.0)	797	(598 – 945)	596
2001–2002	46.2	(33.2 – 64.3)	<LOD		49.5	(35.7 – 69.9)	927	(620 – 1,820)	692
2003–2004	53.2	(42.4 – 66.7)	5.94	(3.99 – 6.84)	45.3	(30.0 – 72.1)	706	(564 – 1,030)	681
2005–2006	57.0	(50.3 – 64.5)	5.39	(4.33 – 6.69)	48.5	(42.1 – 59.5)	902	(643 – 1,350)	662
Non-Hispanic Whites								
1999–2000	73.6	(60.7 – 89.2)	8.09	(3.07 – 10.9)	67.9	(57.2 – 81.4)	917	(794 – 1,390)	901
2001–2002	48.0	(43.5 – 53.0)	<LOD		47.0	(42.8 – 55.4)	954	(838 – 1,220)	1,211
2003–2004	64.9	(59.9 – 70.4)	7.20	(6.28 – 8.08)	58.2	(50.9 – 66.8)	1,090	(818 – 1,320)	1,069
2005–2006	65.2	(57.9 – 73.3)	7.34	(5.54 – 8.21)	52.6	(46.5 – 60.6)	1,070	(896 – 1,460)	1,039

< LOD means less than the limit of detection for the uncorrected urine values, which may vary for some compounds by year. See Appendix D for LOD.

Figure 4.4.b. Urinary daidzein (creatinine corrected): Concentrations by survey cycle

Selected percentiles in µg/g creatinine (95% confidence intervals), National Health and Nutrition Examination Survey, 1999–2006

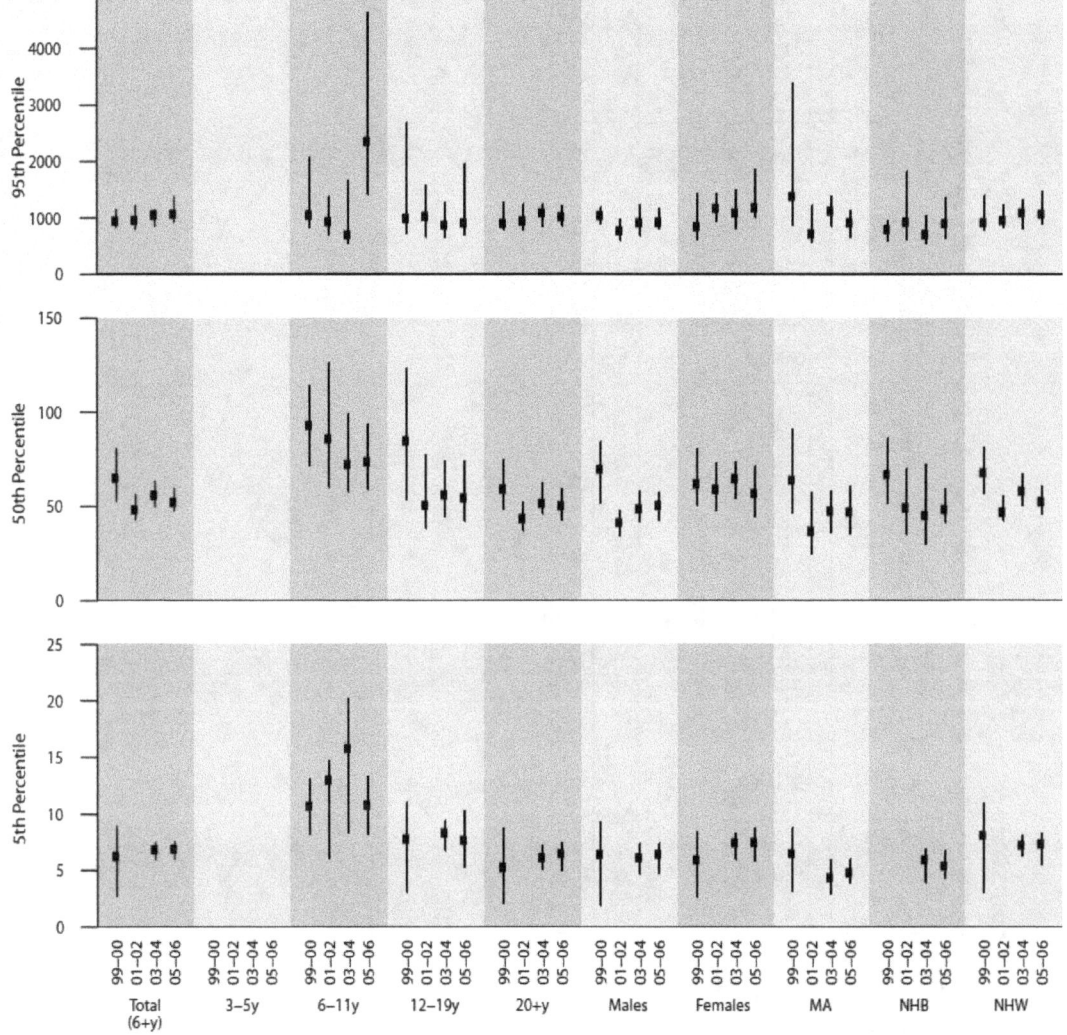

Values in the graph are suppressed if either the point estimate or the lower 95% confidence limit is noted as "< LOD" in the accompanying table.

Table 4.5.a.1. Urinary equol: Concentrations

Geometric mean and selected percentiles of urine concentrations (in µg/L) for the total U.S. population aged 6 years and older, National Health and Nutrition Examination Survey, 2003–2006.

	Geometric mean (95% conf. interval)	Selected percentiles (95% conf. interval)					Sample size
		2.5th	5th	50th	95th	97.5th	
Total, 6 years and older	8.21 (7.61 – 8.85)	.499 (.468 – .593)	.953 (.754 – 1.08)	8.33 (7.59 – 9.06)	64.8 (56.0 – 80.8)	205 (138 – 329)	5,117
Age group							
6-11 years	12.8 (11.1 – 14.8)	1.10 (.794 – 1.49)	1.95 (1.25 – 2.17)	13.2 (10.8 – 16.0)	84.9 (60.3 – 131)	140 (106 – 311)	692
12-19 years	11.1 (10.0 – 12.2)	.996 (.671 – 1.27)	1.62 (1.28 – 1.88)	10.8 (9.61 – 11.7)	72.2 (53.8 – 114)	148 (114 – 287)	1,422
20-39 years	8.39 (7.41 – 9.50)	.594 (.357 – .766)	.897 (.690 – 1.20)	8.80 (7.71 – 9.78)	71.7 (50.4 – 132)	200 (117 – 563)	1,137
40-59 years	6.85 (6.06 – 7.75)	.385 (< LOD – .491)	.559 (.468 – .964)	6.37 (5.36 – 7.63)	56.2 (43.6 – 146)	314 (117 – 1,220)	897
60 years and older	6.96 (6.06 – 8.00)	.393 (< LOD – .621)	.884 (.591 – 1.02)	7.07 (6.06 – 8.03)	51.4 (38.7 – 86.4)	150 (72.5 – 372)	969
Gender							
Males	8.85 (8.10 – 9.66)	.710 (.496 – .967)	1.18 (.986 – 1.28)	9.07 (8.18 – 10.0)	67.2 (55.6 – 93.0)	147 (117 – 246)	2,492
Females	7.65 (6.95 – 8.42)	.450 (.300 – .502)	.715 (.575 – .892)	7.49 (6.81 – 8.27)	64.4 (51.6 – 89.1)	257 (158 – 541)	2,625
Race/ethnicity							
Mexican Americans	6.06 (5.46 – 6.72)	.489 (< LOD – .602)	.793 (.585 – .992)	5.87 (5.28 – 6.69)	46.2 (38.7 – 73.5)	107 (70.7 – 201)	1,287
Non-Hispanic Blacks	7.13 (6.35 – 8.01)	.570 (.343 – .694)	.846 (.693 – 1.02)	6.82 (6.08 – 8.20)	48.5 (40.2 – 61.3)	78.3 (67.8 – 117)	1,340
Non-Hispanic Whites	8.78 (7.99 – 9.65)	.499 (.471 – .580)	.994 (.725 – 1.20)	9.15 (8.27 – 9.99)	69.8 (56.4 – 96.8)	242 (146 – 504)	2,106

< LOD means less than the limit of detection, which may vary for some compounds by year. See Appendix D for LOD.

Figure 4.5.a. Urinary equol: Concentrations by age group

Geometric mean (95% confidence interval), National Health and Nutrition Examination Survey, 2003–2006

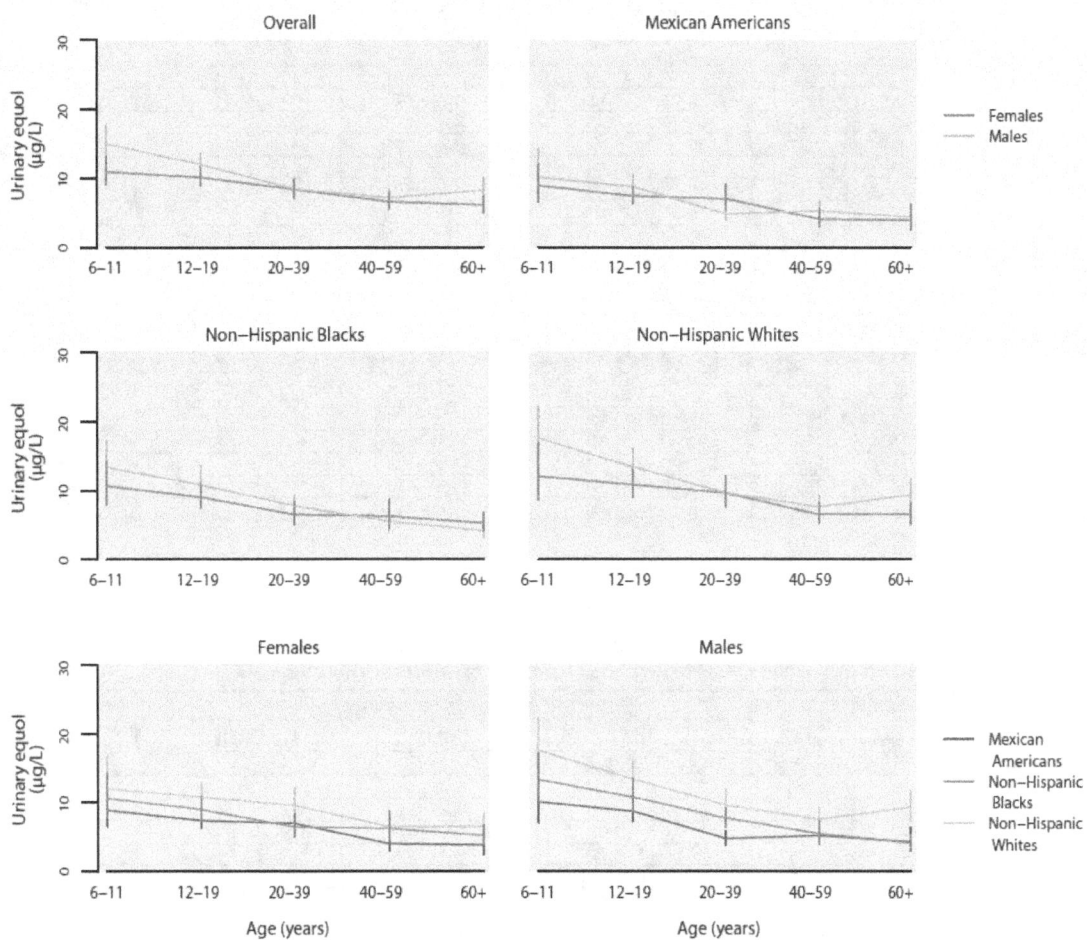

Table 4.5.a.2. Urinary equol: Total population

Geometric mean and selected percentiles of urine concentrations (in µg/L) for the total U.S. population aged 6 years and older, National Health and Nutrition Examination Survey, 2003–2006.

	Geometric mean (95% conf. interval)	Selected percentiles (95% conf. interval) 10th	Selected percentiles (95% conf. interval) 50th	Selected percentiles (95% conf. interval) 90th	Sample size
Males and Females					
Total, 6 years and older	8.21 (7.61 – 8.85)	1.49 (1.30 – 1.60)	8.33 (7.59 – 9.06)	36.7 (33.8 – 39.7)	5,117
6–11 years	12.8 (11.1 – 14.8)	2.75 (2.10 – 3.50)	13.2 (10.8 – 16.0)	45.5 (41.5 – 65.3)	692
12–19 years	11.1 (10.0 – 12.2)	2.61 (2.29 – 2.90)	10.8 (9.61 – 11.7)	42.8 (38.6 – 47.0)	1,422
20–39 years	8.39 (7.41 – 9.50)	1.50 (1.20 – 1.80)	8.80 (7.71 – 9.78)	36.5 (30.8 – 42.8)	1,137
40–59 years	6.85 (6.06 – 7.75)	1.28 (1.07 – 1.41)	6.37 (5.36 – 7.63)	33.3 (29.7 – 37.5)	897
60 years and older	6.96 (6.06 – 8.00)	1.30 (1.09 – 1.51)	7.07 (6.06 – 8.03)	32.0 (24.4 – 39.1)	969
Males					
Total, 6 years and older	8.85 (8.10 – 9.66)	1.60 (1.38 – 1.99)	9.07 (8.18 – 10.0)	38.6 (34.4 – 42.9)	2,492
6–11 years	15.0 (12.6 – 17.8)	3.79 (2.20 – 5.37)	16.4 (13.2 – 19.2)	50.1 (43.4 – 74.2)	340
12–19 years	12.0 (10.5 – 13.7)	2.67 (2.24 – 3.29)	11.7 (10.6 – 12.7)	44.8 (36.9 – 69.0)	728
20–39 years	8.42 (7.10 – 9.99)	1.47 (1.03 – 1.83)	8.70 (7.21 – 10.0)	41.3 (31.1 – 52.6)	499
40–59 years	7.16 (6.07 – 8.44)	1.42 (1.20 – 1.79)	7.44 (5.69 – 8.91)	30.0 (24.3 – 37.4)	447
60 years and older	8.22 (6.78 – 9.98)	1.50 (1.23 – 1.83)	8.44 (7.09 – 10.1)	36.2 (27.5 – 46.9)	478
Females					
Total, 6 years and older	7.65 (6.95 – 8.42)	1.30 (1.19 – 1.50)	7.49 (6.81 – 8.27)	34.8 (32.1 – 38.7)	2,625
6–11 years	10.9 (9.07 – 13.1)	2.43 (1.59 – 2.80)	10.1 (9.16 – 12.5)	43.5 (35.0 – 69.5)	352
12–19 years	10.1 (8.93 – 11.5)	2.49 (1.87 – 2.83)	9.39 (8.03 – 11.4)	40.4 (34.8 – 47.1)	694
20–39 years	8.36 (7.09 – 9.86)	1.50 (1.06 – 1.97)	9.07 (7.09 – 10.6)	32.2 (28.2 – 40.7)	638
40–59 years	6.58 (5.45 – 7.95)	.939 (.529 – 1.29)	5.69 (4.68 – 6.95)	34.5 (30.9 – 45.9)	450
60 years and older	6.10 (5.03 – 7.39)	1.18 (.974 – 1.40)	5.80 (5.20 – 7.32)	26.4 (19.2 – 40.6)	491

Table 4.5.a.3. Urinary equol: Mexican Americans

Geometric mean and selected percentiles of urine concentrations (in µg/L) for Mexican Americans in the U.S. population aged 6 years and older, National Health and Nutrition Examination Survey, 2003–2006.

	Geometric mean (95% conf. interval)	Selected percentiles (95% conf. interval) 10th	Selected percentiles (95% conf. interval) 50th	Selected percentiles (95% conf. interval) 90th	Sample size
Males and Females					
Total, 6 years and older	6.06 (5.46 – 6.72)	1.27 (1.01 – 1.49)	5.87 (5.28 – 6.69)	25.8 (20.9 – 35.4)	1,287
6–11 years	9.49 (7.78 – 11.6)	1.60 (1.05 – 2.47)	9.20 (6.88 – 11.7)	45.5 (37.6 – 85.8)	231
12–19 years	8.07 (7.04 – 9.24)	1.60 (1.44 – 2.01)	7.08 (6.25 – 8.19)	35.7 (27.8 – 49.2)	445
20–39 years	5.71 (4.97 – 6.56)	1.27 (.967 – 1.51)	5.59 (4.49 – 6.42)	21.9 (17.9 – 39.2)	282
40–59 years	4.63 (3.73 – 5.75)	1.08 (< LOD – 1.48)	4.99 (3.92 – 5.86)	19.0 (14.0 – 25.0)	157
60 years and older	4.10 (3.21 – 5.23)	.631 (.379 – .946)	4.73 (3.19 – 6.60)	16.6 (10.8 – 27.3)	172
Males					
Total, 6 years and older	5.92 (5.25 – 6.68)	1.29 (1.04 – 1.57)	5.69 (4.89 – 6.81)	24.6 (19.8 – 32.9)	625
6–11 years	10.1 (7.14 – 14.3)	2.17 (.735 – 3.86)	9.71 (6.15 – 14.4)	40.8 (26.9 – 88.4)	112
12–19 years	8.75 (7.28 – 10.5)	1.83 (1.35 – 2.32)	7.71 (6.15 – 9.42)	41.1 (28.6 – 61.8)	228
20–39 years	4.81 (3.96 – 5.86)	1.15 (.685 – 1.41)	4.55 (3.70 – 6.03)	18.0 (12.6 – 40.6)	117
40–59 years	5.22 (4.05 – 6.72)	1.18† (.707 – 1.98)	5.27 (4.28 – 6.94)	19.5† (12.5 – 31.6)	85
60 years and older	4.36 (3.01 – 6.31)	.600† (< LOD – 1.47)	4.99 (3.05 – 6.89)	17.3† (9.44 – 65.3)	83
Females					
Total, 6 years and older	6.21 (5.35 – 7.22)	1.20 (.793 – 1.51)	6.18 (5.15 – 7.09)	28.0 (20.7 – 39.6)	662
6–11 years	8.89 (6.62 – 11.9)	1.47 (.569 – 2.34)	8.44 (5.75 – 11.4)	57.0 (37.3 – 202)	119
12–19 years	7.41 (6.32 – 8.69)	1.50 (.916 – 2.21)	6.81 (5.51 – 8.03)	28.4 (19.3 – 52.0)	217
20–39 years	6.99 (5.35 – 9.13)	1.37 (.689 – 1.85)	6.79 (4.70 – 9.31)	35.2 (19.6 – 66.9)	165
40–59 years	4.07 (2.94 – 5.64)	.861† (< LOD – 1.36)	3.89 (2.93 – 5.72)	18.3† (14.0 – 34.4)	72
60 years and older	3.90 (2.50 – 6.08)	.671† (< LOD – 1.12)	4.41 (2.15 – 7.53)	14.8† (9.40 – 80.2)	89

< LOD means less than the limit of detection, which may vary for some compounds by year. See Appendix D for LOD.

† Estimate is subject to greater uncertainty due to small cell size.

Table 4.5.a.4. Urinary equol: Non-Hispanic blacks

Geometric mean and selected percentiles of urine concentrations (in µg/L) for non-Hispanic blacks in the U.S. population aged 6 years and older, National Health and Nutrition Examination Survey, 2003–2006.

| | Geometric mean (95% conf. interval) | Selected percentiles (95% conf. interval) | | | Sample size |
		10th	50th	90th	
Males and Females					
Total, 6 years and older	7.13 (6.35 – 8.01)	1.49 (1.28 – 1.70)	6.82 (6.08 – 8.20)	31.3 (27.1 – 36.6)	1,340
6–11 years	11.9 (9.99 – 14.2)	3.00 (2.09 – 3.59)	10.8 (8.53 – 14.0)	54.2 (40.6 – 79.7)	207
12–19 years	9.86 (8.44 – 11.5)	2.40 (1.99 – 2.78)	8.98 (7.83 – 10.3)	42.5 (35.2 – 61.4)	496
20–39 years	7.03 (5.93 – 8.34)	1.50 (1.01 – 2.10)	6.94 (5.91 – 9.58)	24.6 (21.6 – 32.3)	249
40–59 years	5.91 (4.67 – 7.49)	1.19 (.705 – 1.60)	5.49 (4.44 – 7.21)	33.4 (21.8 – 45.8)	228
60 years and older	4.79 (3.89 – 5.91)	.852 (.685 – 1.10)	5.17 (4.14 – 6.24)	21.8 (17.1 – 30.7)	160
Males					
Total, 6 years and older	7.47 (6.72 – 8.30)	1.57 (1.36 – 1.74)	6.78 (5.94 – 8.18)	31.5 (27.0 – 39.4)	658
6–11 years	13.3 (10.4 – 17.1)	3.43† (1.29 – 4.53)	12.7 (9.66 – 14.9)	71.1† (35.1 – 125)	99
12–19 years	10.8 (8.60 – 13.5)	2.73 (1.99 – 3.07)	9.98 (7.56 – 12.6)	40.1 (32.6 – 70.0)	258
20–39 years	7.77 (6.53 – 9.24)	1.46 (1.21 – 2.10)	6.65 (5.38 – 9.46)	27.4 (23.1 – 45.5)	116
40–59 years	5.52 (4.14 – 7.35)	1.46† (1.11 – 1.67)	5.13 (4.01 – 7.66)	24.5† (13.5 – 51.5)	111
60 years and older	4.15 (3.25 – 5.29)	.758† (< LOD – 1.27)	4.28 (3.25 – 5.82)	21.7† (10.8 – 66.2)	74
Females					
Total, 6 years and older	6.87 (5.87 – 8.04)	1.25 (.765 – 1.80)	6.86 (5.92 – 8.46)	30.3 (25.2 – 37.5)	682
6–11 years	10.6 (7.95 – 14.2)	2.52† (1.45 – 3.58)	9.24 (6.86 – 12.6)	47.6† (30.5 – 124)	108
12–19 years	9.01 (7.47 – 10.9)	2.08 (1.31 – 2.78)	8.50 (7.01 – 9.53)	43.6 (31.4 – 71.3)	238
20–39 years	6.49 (5.06 – 8.33)	1.50 (.605 – 2.40)	7.06 (4.83 – 10.1)	22.2 (17.7 – 30.1)	133
40–59 years	6.25 (4.47 – 8.74)	.702 (.318 – 1.88)	5.84 (4.69 – 8.20)	37.0 (24.8 – 63.0)	117
60 years and older	5.26 (4.08 – 6.78)	.872† (.723 – 1.03)	5.43 (3.80 – 8.00)	21.8† (17.4 – 37.7)	86

< LOD means less than the limit of detection, which may vary for some compounds by year. See Appendix D for LOD.

† Estimate is subject to greater uncertainty due to small cell size.

Table 4.5.a.5. Urinary equol: Non-Hispanic whites

Geometric mean and selected percentiles of urine concentrations (in µg/L) for non-Hispanic whites in the U.S. population aged 6 years and older, National Health and Nutrition Examination Survey, 2003–2006.

| | Geometric mean (95% conf. interval) | Selected percentiles (95% conf. interval) | | | Sample size |
		10th	50th	90th	
Males and Females					
Total, 6 years and older	8.78 (7.99 – 9.65)	1.54 (1.30 – 1.80)	9.15 (8.27 – 9.99)	38.2 (34.4 – 43.0)	2,106
6–11 years	14.7 (11.9 – 18.1)	3.40 (2.09 – 5.41)	16.3 (12.7 – 18.8)	44.9 (38.1 – 78.1)	193
12–19 years	12.1 (10.6 – 13.8)	3.09 (2.50 – 3.61)	11.9 (10.6 – 13.6)	42.0 (36.7 – 46.5)	378
20–39 years	9.62 (8.11 – 11.4)	1.57 (1.13 – 2.04)	10.0 (8.77 – 11.7)	42.8 (32.6 – 57.5)	494
40–59 years	7.04 (6.11 – 8.12)	1.29 (.848 – 1.49)	6.87 (5.37 – 8.81)	33.8 (30.8 – 37.4)	447
60 years and older	7.65 (6.47 – 9.04)	1.46 (1.17 – 1.88)	7.66 (6.29 – 8.72)	33.6 (25.9 – 47.8)	594
Males					
Total, 6 years and older	9.68 (8.71 – 10.8)	1.71 (1.40 – 2.10)	10.0 (8.94 – 11.1)	40.1 (36.0 – 45.2)	1,034
6–11 years	17.5 (13.8 – 22.2)	5.59† (2.11 – 6.02)	17.5 (13.5 – 24.4)	44.9† (39.9 – 115)	99
12–19 years	13.4 (11.3 – 16.0)	3.28 (1.89 – 4.54)	12.2 (11.3 – 15.4)	45.0 (36.6 – 79.1)	191
20–39 years	9.63 (7.72 – 12.0)	1.54 (1.00 – 2.07)	10.0 (8.68 – 11.5)	44.3 (32.4 – 82.8)	217
40–59 years	7.61 (6.19 – 9.35)	1.41 (1.08 – 1.91)	7.93 (5.97 – 9.71)	31.4 (26.6 – 42.6)	228
60 years and older	9.32 (7.43 – 11.7)	1.73 (1.27 – 2.50)	9.42 (7.36 – 12.1)	37.6 (30.7 – 55.2)	299
Females					
Total, 6 years and older	7.98 (7.02 – 9.06)	1.45 (1.20 – 1.60)	7.86 (6.93 – 9.16)	35.6 (31.7 – 42.8)	1,072
6–11 years	12.0 (8.61 – 16.7)	2.61† (.948 – 3.85)	12.3 (9.15 – 17.3)	43.2† (27.4 – 91.7)	94
12–19 years	10.8 (8.95 – 13.0)	2.76 (1.92 – 3.64)	11.1 (8.16 – 13.8)	39.9 (32.0 – 45.3)	187
20–39 years	9.60 (7.63 – 12.1)	1.66 (.954 – 2.27)	10.3 (7.50 – 12.8)	37.3 (29.2 – 72.9)	277
40–59 years	6.52 (5.18 – 8.20)	.967 (.492 – 1.32)	6.18 (4.63 – 7.52)	33.9 (30.9 – 47.3)	219
60 years and older	6.54 (5.19 – 8.25)	1.27 (.956 – 1.58)	6.08 (5.27 – 8.01)	29.4 (18.6 – 55.9)	295

† Estimate is subject to greater uncertainty due to small cell size.

Table 4.5.b. Urinary equol: Concentrations by survey cycle

Geometric mean and selected percentiles of urine concentrations (in µg/L) for the U.S. population, National Health and Nutrition Examination Survey, 1999–2006.

	Geometric mean (95% conf. interval)	Selected percentiles (95% conf. interval)						Sample size
		5th		50th		95th		
Total, 6 years and older								
1999–2000	8.37 (7.21 – 9.72)	< LOD		8.00	(6.29 – 9.82)	53.7	(41.6 – 79.6)	2,182
2001–2002	9.17 (7.76 – 10.8)	< LOD		8.94	(7.36 – 10.4)	73.5	(56.4 – 95.8)	2,794
2003–2004	8.02 (7.07 – 9.10)	.934	(.655 – 1.11)	7.98	(6.77 – 9.36)	64.8	(47.0 – 100)	2,590
2005–2006	8.40 (7.63 – 9.24)	.878	(.698 – 1.08)	8.60	(7.91 – 9.17)	64.5	(56.9 – 80.5)	2,527
Age group								
6–11 years								
1999–2000	10.4 (7.65 – 14.3)	< LOD		11.5	(5.76 – 18.5)	55.4	(32.5 – 310)	272
2001–2002	12.2 (10.2 – 14.6)	< LOD		13.7	(11.1 – 16.1)	84.5	(53.6 – 214)	396
2003–2004	12.4 (9.71 – 15.8)	1.92	(1.00 – 2.31)	12.0	(8.45 – 17.6)	85.4	(49.1 – 251)	341
2005–2006	13.3 (11.3 – 15.7)	1.90	(1.02 – 2.49)	13.4	(12.1 – 16.6)	70.3	(54.3 – 228)	351
12–19 years								
1999–2000	10.9 (8.64 – 13.8)	< LOD		10.7	(8.57 – 13.3)	71.6	(51.1 – 235)	657
2001–2002	10.2 (8.50 – 12.1)	< LOD		10.4	(8.27 – 12.5)	68.9	(48.1 – 106)	744
2003–2004	10.6 (8.96 – 12.4)	1.64	(1.05 – 2.11)	10.5	(8.73 – 12.1)	61.8	(46.0 – 113)	729
2005–2006	11.6 (10.3 – 13.0)	1.49	(1.19 – 2.04)	11.2	(9.48 – 12.3)	81.6	(54.9 – 148)	693
20–39 years								
1999–2000	7.66 (6.63 – 8.86)	< LOD		7.55	(5.49 – 9.38)	38.1	(35.6 – 69.4)	439
2001–2002	9.35 (7.40 – 11.8)	< LOD		9.25	(6.95 – 11.3)	67.0	(49.7 – 111)	604
2003–2004	8.81 (7.29 – 10.6)	.980	(.509 – 1.31)	9.11	(7.18 – 10.8)	99.6	(44.4 – 221)	554
2005–2006	8.00 (6.71 – 9.54)	.820	(.587 – 1.18)	8.60	(7.42 – 9.73)	57.1	(45.0 – 95.1)	583
40–59 years								
1999–2000	7.80 (6.17 – 9.84)	< LOD		7.28	(4.97 – 9.09)	53.7	(34.0 – 3,160)	378
2001–2002	8.92 (7.27 – 10.9)	< LOD		8.12	(6.43 – 10.1)	102	(44.7 – 312)	531
2003–2004	6.65 (5.61 – 7.87)	.613	(.372 – 1.04)	6.09	(4.66 – 8.60)	51.6	(38.0 – 140)	448
2005–2006	7.05 (5.83 – 8.54)	.542	(.325 – 1.07)	6.76	(5.33 – 8.36)	63.8	(38.6 – 542)	449
60 years and older								
1999–2000	8.04 (6.93 – 9.33)	< LOD		7.33	(5.55 – 9.70)	54.8	(35.9 – 237)	436
2001–2002	7.18 (5.83 – 8.85)	< LOD		5.68	(3.76 – 8.16)	51.0	(41.8 – 113)	519
2003–2004	6.16 (4.93 – 7.68)	.754	(< LOD – 1.02)	5.88	(4.99 – 7.75)	39.6	(32.2 – 176)	518
2005–2006	7.84 (6.60 – 9.31)	.940	(.599 – 1.16)	7.80	(6.29 – 8.95)	55.5	(42.4 – 326)	451
Gender								
Males								
1999–2000	9.15 (7.37 – 11.4)	< LOD		8.44	(6.38 – 11.2)	68.8	(45.0 – 170)	1,042
2001–2002	9.41 (7.99 – 11.1)	< LOD		9.14	(7.65 – 10.6)	61.4	(52.6 – 87.6)	1,375
2003–2004	8.56 (7.54 – 9.72)	1.07	(.861 – 1.26)	8.70	(7.18 – 10.2)	72.3	(50.8 – 112)	1,240
2005–2006	9.13 (7.99 – 10.4)	1.19	(.892 – 1.29)	9.40	(8.15 – 10.6)	61.7	(53.1 – 94.2)	1,252
Females								
1999–2000	7.70 (6.79 – 8.74)	< LOD		7.56	(5.92 – 8.98)	48.2	(37.6 – 70.9)	1,140
2001–2002	8.94 (7.38 – 10.8)	< LOD		8.54	(6.72 – 10.6)	79.3	(58.9 – 130)	1,419
2003–2004	7.55 (6.44 – 8.84)	.792	(.480 – 1.02)	7.29	(6.12 – 8.96)	60.2	(43.8 – 145)	1,350
2005–2006	7.75 (6.85 – 8.78)	.684	(.486 – .877)	7.56	(6.93 – 8.36)	69.0	(54.8 – 119)	1,275
Race/ethnicity								
Mexican Americans								
1999–2000	5.24 (4.77 – 5.75)	< LOD		4.51	(3.75 – 5.25)	30.3	(22.6 – 62.5)	726
2001–2002	7.22 (6.04 – 8.62)	< LOD		6.49	(4.52 – 8.98)	42.1	(40.1 – 48.7)	679
2003–2004	6.08 (5.08 – 7.28)	.927	(.625 – 1.18)	5.64	(4.65 – 6.77)	43.5	(36.2 – 108)	653
2005–2006	6.04 (5.31 – 6.87)	.663	(.440 – .961)	6.12	(5.32 – 7.09)	47.6	(36.7 – 83.0)	634
Non-Hispanic Blacks								
1999–2000	6.67 (5.16 – 8.63)	< LOD		6.12	(3.87 – 9.88)	36.5	(30.0 – 52.0)	504
2001–2002	7.11 (6.01 – 8.42)	< LOD		6.00	(4.62 – 7.48)	45.2	(40.7 – 99.6)	692
2003–2004	7.32 (6.13 – 8.73)	.753	(.505 – 1.11)	7.85	(6.09 – 9.58)	46.9	(39.8 – 62.3)	678
2005–2006	6.96 (5.89 – 8.22)	.868	(.686 – 1.05)	6.37	(5.48 – 7.85)	48.6	(39.2 – 64.9)	662
Non-Hispanic Whites								
1999–2000	9.38 (7.94 – 11.1)	< LOD		8.98	(6.99 – 11.8)	56.1	(45.4 – 95.5)	744
2001–2002	9.89 (7.90 – 12.4)	< LOD		9.93	(7.31 – 12.5)	74.1	(55.1 – 108)	1,211
2003–2004	8.51 (7.22 – 10.0)	.996	(.618 – 1.19)	8.72	(6.95 – 10.3)	72.9	(46.8 – 120)	1,068
2005–2006	9.05 (8.08 – 10.1)	.965	(.606 – 1.27)	9.48	(8.56 – 10.3)	68.9	(56.9 – 105)	1,038

< LOD means less than the limit of detection, which may vary for some compounds by year. See Appendix D for LOD.

Figure 4.5.b. Urinary equol: Concentrations by survey cycle

Selected percentiles in µg/L (95% confidence intervals), National Health and Nutrition Examination Survey, 1999–2006

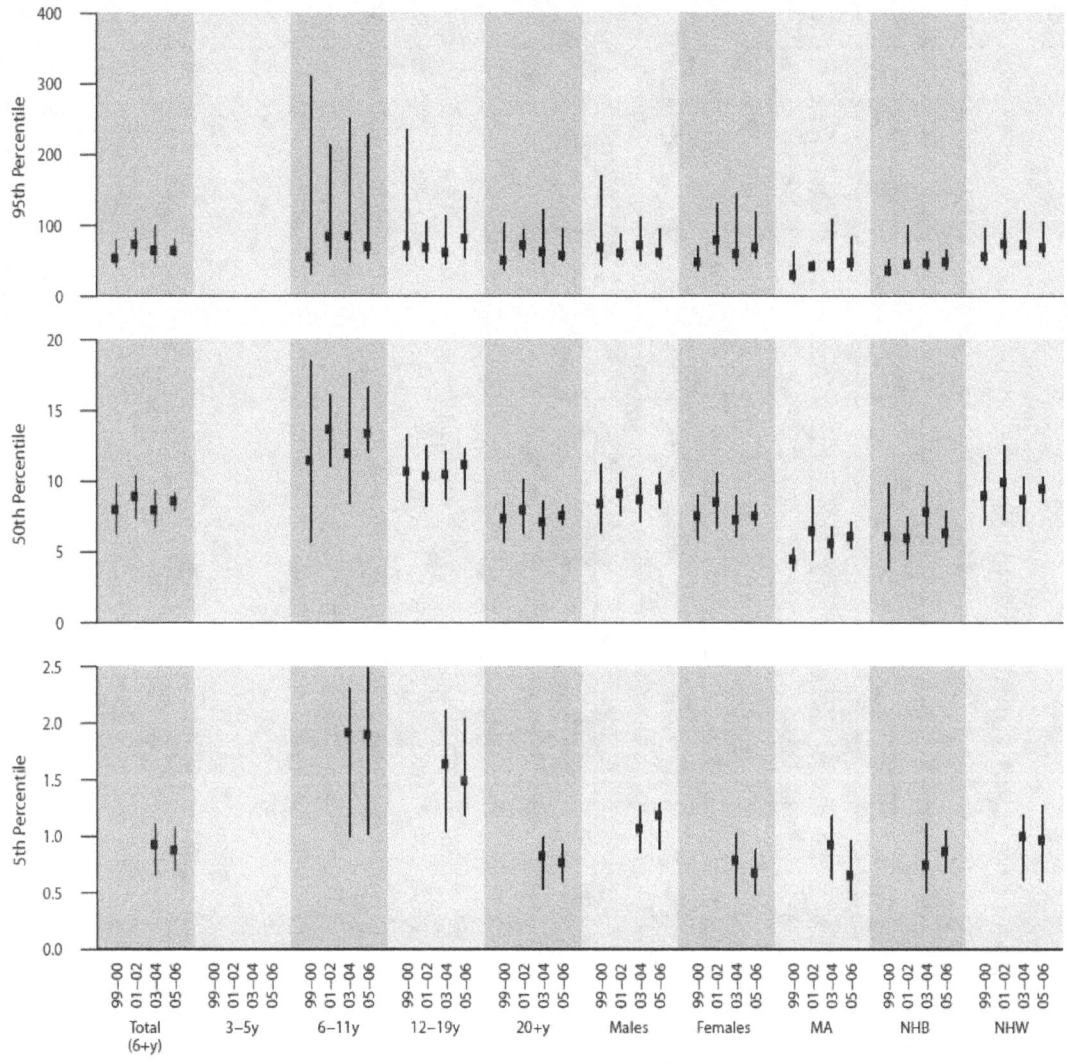

Values in the graph are suppressed if either the point estimate or the lower 95% confidence limit is noted as "< LOD" in the accompanying table.

Table 4.6.a.1. Urinary equol (creatinine corrected): Concentrations

Geometric mean and selected percentiles of urine concentrations (in µg/g creatinine) for the total U.S. population aged 6 years and older, National Health and Nutrition Examination Survey, 2003–2006.

	Geometric mean (95% conf. interval)	Selected percentiles (95% conf. interval)					Sample size
		2.5th	5th	50th	95th	97.5th	
Total, 6 years and older	7.85 (7.31 – 8.43)	.724 (.600 – .799)	1.05 (.898 – 1.18)	7.64 (7.10 – 8.15)	58.1 (48.3 – 78.3)	219 (129 – 356)	5,117
Age group							
6–11 years	13.9 (12.4 – 15.6)	1.45 (1.00 – 2.26)	2.51 (1.79 – 3.00)	14.4 (12.3 – 16.0)	92.0 (59.9 – 129)	136 (117 – 270)	692
12–19 years	8.24 (7.40 – 9.19)	.948 (.501 – 1.34)	1.49 (1.13 – 1.81)	8.04 (7.17 – 8.69)	48.2 (38.2 – 75.3)	118 (80.6 – 216)	1,422
20–39 years	7.15 (6.38 – 8.02)	.675 (.540 – .776)	.901 (.763 – 1.06)	7.06 (6.25 – 7.86)	63.7 (40.1 – 115)	210 (118 – 392)	1,137
40–59 years	6.95 (6.07 – 7.96)	.538 (<LOD – .693)	.792 (.629 – 1.08)	6.57 (5.54 – 7.54)	66.0 (35.1 – 245)	421 (110 – 1,130)	897
60 years and older	8.16 (7.32 – 9.08)	.889 (<LOD – 1.11)	1.33 (1.11 – 1.52)	8.13 (7.12 – 8.80)	45.3 (33.8 – 99.4)	140 (63.1 – 436)	969
Gender							
Males	7.02 (6.46 – 7.64)	.634 (.462 – .769)	.942 (.768 – 1.10)	6.84 (6.27 – 7.53)	51.8 (44.0 – 67.2)	129 (106 – 237)	2,492
Females	8.72 (8.02 – 9.49)	.787 (.705 – .890)	1.18 (.964 – 1.39)	8.36 (7.88 – 8.98)	70.0 (48.3 – 104)	356 (169 – 692)	2,625
Race/ethnicity							
Mexican Americans	5.46 (4.94 – 6.04)	.615 (<LOD – .690)	.867 (.674 – 1.04)	4.84 (4.34 – 5.48)	37.9 (33.4 – 69.8)	129 (83.3 – 192)	1,287
Non-Hispanic Blacks	5.02 (4.48 – 5.62)	.533 (.403 – .669)	.766 (.655 – .917)	4.88 (4.40 – 5.59)	30.5 (26.1 – 42.2)	64.8 (42.5 – 96.6)	1,340
Non-Hispanic Whites	8.94 (8.26 – 9.67)	.792 (.621 – .977)	1.18 (1.07 – 1.38)	8.65 (7.95 – 9.50)	69.4 (48.3 – 107)	267 (155 – 502)	2,106

< LOD means less than the limit of detection for the uncorrected urine values, which may vary for some compounds by year. See Appendix D for LOD.

Figure 4.6.a. Urinary equol (creatinine corrected): Concentrations by age group
Geometric mean (95% confidence interval), National Health and Nutrition Examination Survey, 2003–2006

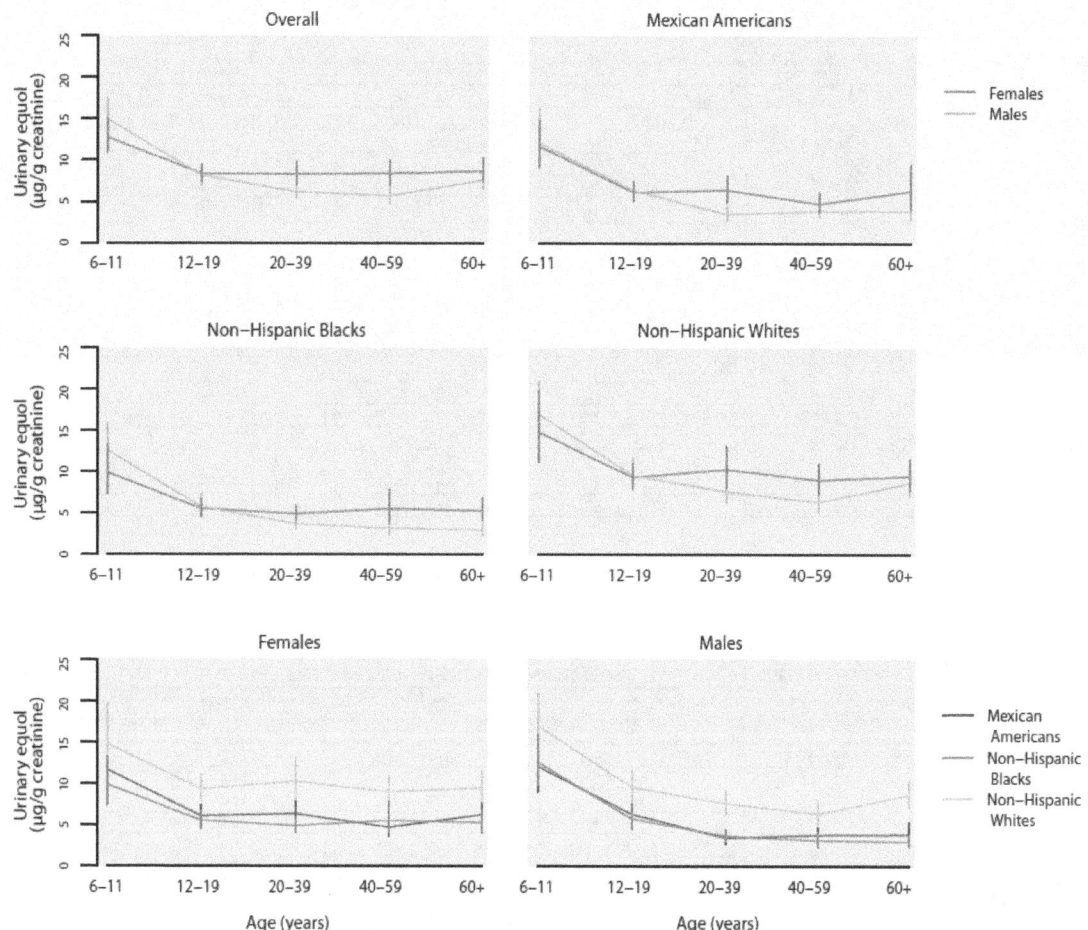

Table 4.6.a.2. Urinary equol (creatinine corrected): Total population

Geometric mean and selected percentiles of urine concentrations (in µg/g creatinine) for the total U.S. population aged 6 years and older, National Health and Nutrition Examination Survey, 2003–2006.

	Geometric mean (95% conf. interval)		Selected percentiles (95% conf. interval)						Sample size
			10th		50th		90th		
Males and Females									
Total, 6 years and older	7.85	(7.31 – 8.43)	1.72	(1.54 – 1.90)	7.64	(7.10 – 8.15)	30.7	(28.8 – 32.6)	5,117
6–11 years	13.9	(12.4 – 15.6)	3.64	(2.88 – 4.34)	14.4	(12.3 – 16.0)	44.9	(40.5 – 57.6)	692
12–19 years	8.24	(7.40 – 9.19)	2.09	(1.87 – 2.39)	8.04	(7.17 – 8.69)	31.3	(26.0 – 35.0)	1,422
20–39 years	7.15	(6.38 – 8.02)	1.45	(1.17 – 1.73)	7.06	(6.25 – 7.86)	29.5	(23.7 – 34.6)	1,137
40–59 years	6.95	(6.07 – 7.96)	1.40	(1.14 – 1.60)	6.57	(5.54 – 7.54)	25.6	(21.3 – 34.3)	897
60 years and older	8.16	(7.32 – 9.08)	2.14	(1.86 – 2.43)	8.13	(7.12 – 8.80)	27.1	(21.6 – 34.0)	969
Males									
Total, 6 years and older	7.02	(6.46 – 7.64)	1.48	(1.28 – 1.76)	6.84	(6.27 – 7.53)	28.8	(25.7 – 31.7)	2,492
6–11 years	15.0	(12.9 – 17.5)	3.84	(3.12 – 4.90)	16.1	(14.7 – 19.0)	45.4	(37.2 – 90.4)	340
12–19 years	8.15	(7.01 – 9.47)	1.92	(1.72 – 2.25)	8.15	(6.93 – 9.51)	31.3	(25.8 – 47.4)	728
20–39 years	6.14	(5.31 – 7.10)	1.26	(.981 – 1.47)	5.83	(4.99 – 6.67)	25.2	(20.0 – 34.6)	499
40–59 years	5.69	(4.78 – 6.77)	1.18	(.790 – 1.58)	5.53	(4.55 – 6.67)	21.8	(15.9 – 33.7)	447
60 years and older	7.58	(6.47 – 8.88)	1.87	(1.37 – 2.25)	7.28	(6.43 – 8.67)	28.8	(20.8 – 34.1)	478
Females									
Total, 6 years and older	8.72	(8.02 – 9.49)	1.95	(1.67 – 2.16)	8.36	(7.88 – 8.98)	32.3	(30.1 – 34.9)	2,625
6–11 years	12.8	(11.0 – 15.0)	3.24	(2.47 – 4.43)	12.8	(10.1 – 14.7)	44.8	(39.8 – 57.7)	352
12–19 years	8.35	(7.44 – 9.37)	2.33	(1.89 – 2.72)	7.94	(7.03 – 8.71)	30.5	(22.8 – 37.1)	694
20–39 years	8.32	(7.03 – 9.84)	1.87	(1.20 – 2.15)	8.08	(7.13 – 9.13)	32.2	(25.0 – 38.8)	638
40–59 years	8.39	(7.05 – 9.98)	1.51	(1.19 – 1.86)	7.92	(6.51 – 9.40)	31.4	(24.1 – 43.1)	450
60 years and older	8.65	(7.36 – 10.2)	2.41	(2.00 – 2.83)	8.44	(7.65 – 9.39)	26.8	(20.4 – 39.8)	491

Table 4.6.a.3. Urinary equol (creatinine corrected): Mexican Americans

Geometric mean and selected percentiles of urine concentrations (in µg/g creatinine) for Mexican Americans in the U.S. population aged 6 years and older, National Health and Nutrition Examination Survey, 2003–2006.

	Geometric mean (95% conf. interval)		Selected percentiles (95% conf. interval)						Sample size
			10th		50th		90th		
Males and Females									
Total, 6 years and older	5.46	(4.94 – 6.04)	1.29	(1.14 – 1.43)	4.84	(4.34 – 5.48)	22.4	(19.7 – 27.6)	1,287
6–11 years	11.9	(10.4 – 13.7)	2.42	(1.84 – 4.06)	10.9	(8.91 – 13.8)	58.9	(30.4 – 121)	231
12–19 years	6.23	(5.49 – 7.07)	1.62	(1.35 – 1.73)	5.57	(4.69 – 6.09)	25.3	(19.7 – 34.5)	445
20–39 years	4.61	(3.91 – 5.42)	1.12	(.736 – 1.37)	4.10	(3.26 – 4.90)	19.6	(15.2 – 31.0)	282
40–59 years	4.24	(3.57 – 5.04)	1.23	(< LOD – 1.43)	4.11	(3.40 – 4.80)	14.0	(11.8 – 27.0)	157
60 years and older	5.06	(4.22 – 6.06)	1.46	(.752 – 1.97)	4.82	(3.84 – 6.04)	19.0	(10.5 – 61.0)	172
Males									
Total, 6 years and older	4.67	(4.08 – 5.35)	1.16	(.883 – 1.34)	4.23	(3.78 – 5.04)	18.9	(16.3 – 21.2)	625
6–11 years	12.1	(9.02 – 16.2)	3.55	(1.73 – 4.93)	10.6	(8.24 – 16.2)	35.9	(27.4 – 108)	112
12–19 years	6.33	(5.37 – 7.48)	1.60	(1.35 – 1.82)	5.58	(4.35 – 6.84)	27.5	(19.6 – 43.7)	228
20–39 years	3.50	(2.79 – 4.38)	.804	(.519 – 1.20)	3.42	(2.99 – 4.15)	11.5	(7.33 – 21.7)	117
40–59 years	3.83	(3.11 – 4.70)	1.27†	(.640 – 1.40)	3.78	(3.16 – 4.90)	11.4†	(8.79 – 26.7)	85
60 years and older	3.88	(2.81 – 5.35)	1.16†	(< LOD – 1.91)	4.17	(3.23 – 5.83)	10.5†	(7.12 – 60.1)	83
Females									
Total, 6 years and older	6.48	(5.83 – 7.21)	1.57	(1.37 – 1.84)	5.75	(4.93 – 6.55)	29.0	(24.0 – 34.5)	662
6–11 years	11.7	(9.26 – 14.8)	2.14	(1.07 – 3.77)	10.9	(8.65 – 13.4)	88.9	(28.8 – 177)	119
12–19 years	6.12	(5.10 – 7.36)	1.59	(1.13 – 1.80)	5.50	(4.49 – 6.06)	24.0	(15.6 – 40.4)	217
20–39 years	6.39	(5.00 – 8.15)	1.62	(1.14 – 2.09)	5.39	(4.01 – 7.25)	30.4	(19.7 – 58.3)	165
40–59 years	4.74	(3.71 – 6.04)	.933†	(< LOD – 1.67)	4.23	(3.33 – 5.37)	21.0†	(13.1 – 31.3)	72
60 years and older	6.28	(4.18 – 9.43)	1.82†	(< LOD – 2.38)	5.43	(3.77 – 8.92)	24.4†	(11.9 – 201)	89

< LOD means less than the limit of detection for the uncorrected urine values, which may vary for some compounds by year. See Appendix D for LOD.

† Estimate is subject to greater uncertainty due to small cell size.

Table 4.6.a.4. Urinary equol (creatinine corrected): Non-Hispanic blacks

Geometric mean and selected percentiles of urine concentrations (in µg/g creatinine) for non-Hispanic blacks in the U.S. population aged 6 years and older, National Health and Nutrition Examination Survey, 2003–2006.

	Geometric mean (95% conf. interval)	Selected percentiles (95% conf. interval)			Sample size
		10th	50th	90th	
Males and Females					
Total, 6 years and older	5.02 (4.48 – 5.62)	1.19 (1.02 – 1.41)	4.88 (4.40 – 5.59)	20.8 (18.2 – 23.7)	1,340
6–11 years	11.2 (9.38 – 13.3)	3.12 (2.54 – 3.56)	9.67 (7.96 – 11.3)	47.8 (34.3 – 64.1)	207
12–19 years	5.66 (4.86 – 6.60)	1.45 (1.14 – 1.68)	5.37 (4.61 – 6.33)	21.5 (16.8 – 27.9)	496
20–39 years	4.36 (3.81 – 4.98)	1.02 (.802 – 1.36)	4.87 (4.24 – 5.64)	12.3 (10.8 – 17.6)	249
40–59 years	4.33 (3.36 – 5.58)	1.02 (.520 – 1.41)	4.06 (2.87 – 5.29)	19.7 (16.8 – 25.8)	228
60 years and older	4.28 (3.53 – 5.19)	1.08 (.798 – 1.38)	4.22 (3.62 – 5.09)	16.7 (13.6 – 23.6)	160
Males					
Total, 6 years and older	4.37 (3.86 – 4.95)	1.01 (.775 – 1.18)	4.24 (3.60 – 4.97)	19.1 (15.2 – 23.4)	658
6–11 years	12.6 (9.98 – 15.9)	3.44† (1.39 – 4.49)	11.0 (8.57 – 14.3)	52.6† (28.7 – 99.7)	99
12–19 years	5.77 (4.53 – 7.34)	1.45 (.957 – 1.76)	5.39 (4.19 – 6.65)	21.7 (15.8 – 36.8)	258
20–39 years	3.73 (3.09 – 4.50)	.892 (.630 – 1.05)	3.82 (3.14 – 5.00)	12.1 (10.5 – 15.9)	116
40–59 years	3.18 (2.40 – 4.21)	.865† (.471 – 1.24)	2.92 (2.24 – 4.31)	11.6† (6.28 – 27.1)	111
60 years and older	3.04 (2.42 – 3.82)	.742† (< LOD – .959)	3.22 (2.07 – 4.15)	13.5† (9.29 – 22.1)	74
Females					
Total, 6 years and older	5.63 (4.95 – 6.40)	1.41 (1.18 – 1.59)	5.45 (4.77 – 6.45)	22.1 (18.5 – 25.5)	682
6–11 years	9.92 (7.41 – 13.3)	2.69† (1.59 – 3.38)	8.60 (6.65 – 11.1)	43.5† (30.1 – 68.7)	108
12–19 years	5.56 (4.61 – 6.70)	1.43 (1.03 – 1.81)	5.30 (4.05 – 7.15)	20.9 (16.0 – 28.0)	238
20–39 years	4.94 (4.12 – 5.92)	1.34 (.768 – 1.89)	5.12 (4.53 – 6.44)	12.3 (10.8 – 20.2)	133
40–59 years	5.55 (3.94 – 7.81)	1.12 (.501 – 1.51)	5.32 (3.42 – 7.37)	24.3 (18.4 – 65.6)	117
60 years and older	5.31 (4.14 – 6.80)	1.51† (1.22 – 1.63)	4.81 (3.98 – 6.91)	19.3† (14.1 – 32.3)	86

< LOD means less than the limit of detection for the uncorrected urine values, which may vary for some compounds by year. See Appendix D for LOD.

† Estimate is subject to greater uncertainty due to small cell size.

Table 4.6.a.5. Urinary equol (creatinine corrected): Non-Hispanic whites

Geometric mean and selected percentiles of urine concentrations (in µg/g creatinine) for non-Hispanic whites in the U.S. population aged 6 years and older, National Health and Nutrition Examination Survey, 2003–2006.

	Geometric mean (95% conf. interval)	Selected percentiles (95% conf. interval)			Sample size
		10th	50th	90th	
Males and Females					
Total, 6 years and older	8.94 (8.26 – 9.67)	2.12 (1.87 – 2.32)	8.65 (7.95 – 9.50)	32.4 (30.4 – 34.8)	2,106
6–11 years	16.0 (13.4 – 19.0)	4.07 (2.54 – 5.84)	17.1 (14.2 – 20.0)	44.8 (39.0 – 81.4)	193
12–19 years	9.48 (8.25 – 10.9)	2.75 (1.97 – 3.28)	9.27 (8.04 – 10.9)	32.1 (26.2 – 38.2)	378
20–39 years	8.87 (7.54 – 10.4)	1.95 (1.28 – 2.31)	8.50 (7.25 – 9.93)	33.2 (26.3 – 55.1)	494
40–59 years	7.58 (6.57 – 8.75)	1.51 (1.15 – 2.02)	7.18 (6.03 – 8.73)	26.5 (21.7 – 35.0)	447
60 years and older	9.12 (8.02 – 10.4)	2.55 (2.13 – 2.94)	8.66 (7.89 – 9.39)	29.1 (22.3 – 38.7)	594
Males					
Total, 6 years and older	8.10 (7.34 – 8.94)	1.91 (1.41 – 2.23)	7.87 (6.92 – 8.89)	30.4 (27.1 – 33.9)	1,034
6–11 years	17.0 (13.8 – 20.9)	4.06† (2.35 – 6.86)	18.4 (15.2 – 21.9)	44.2† (34.9 – 132)	99
12–19 years	9.58 (7.86 – 11.7)	2.18 (1.78 – 3.30)	9.53 (7.67 – 11.5)	32.8 (26.7 – 59.8)	191
20–39 years	7.64 (6.35 – 9.19)	1.59 (1.13 – 2.24)	7.09 (6.21 – 9.30)	28.9 (21.8 – 47.5)	217
40–59 years	6.38 (5.14 – 7.92)	1.17 (.741 – 2.01)	6.44 (4.85 – 7.62)	23.5 (17.7 – 53.0)	228
60 years and older	8.68 (7.23 – 10.4)	2.36 (1.85 – 2.71)	8.31 (6.94 – 9.56)	29.0 (21.6 – 39.1)	299
Females					
Total, 6 years and older	9.84 (8.90 – 10.9)	2.32 (2.00 – 2.77)	9.24 (8.62 – 10.3)	34.0 (30.6 – 39.7)	1,072
6–11 years	14.8 (11.2 – 19.7)	4.05† (.890 – 6.10)	14.1 (11.8 – 18.0)	44.8† (36.8 – 90.7)	94
12–19 years	9.37 (7.98 – 11.0)	3.02 (2.28 – 3.55)	8.70 (7.53 – 11.0)	30.7 (21.3 – 37.5)	187
20–39 years	10.3 (8.07 – 13.1)	2.14 (1.19 – 2.98)	9.09 (8.00 – 11.7)	38.3 (29.8 – 75.9)	277
40–59 years	9.02 (7.44 – 10.9)	1.67 (1.22 – 2.59)	8.68 (6.70 – 12.1)	31.7 (21.7 – 44.0)	219
60 years and older	9.49 (7.84 – 11.5)	2.84 (2.12 – 3.20)	8.89 (8.06 – 10.1)	29.4 (21.0 – 49.8)	295

† Estimate is subject to greater uncertainty due to small cell size.

Table 4.6.b. Urinary equol (creatinine corrected): Concentrations by survey cycle

Geometric mean and selected percentiles of urine concentrations (in µg/g creatinine) for the U.S. population, National Health and Nutrition Examination Survey, 1999–2006.

	Geometric mean (95% conf. interval)	Selected percentiles (95% conf. interval)					Sample size
		5th		50th		95th	
Total, 6 years and older							
1999–2000	7.70 (6.82 – 8.70)	<LOD		7.96 (6.93 – 9.34)		50.0 (43.2 – 67.5)	2,182
2001–2002	8.60 (7.26 – 10.2)	<LOD		7.98 (6.64 – 9.71)		62.5 (52.1 – 87.0)	2,794
2003–2004	7.52 (6.83 – 8.29)	1.01 (.861 – 1.18)		7.29 (6.56 – 8.18)		50.1 (39.9 – 75.5)	2,590
2005–2006	8.18 (7.33 – 9.14)	1.08 (.861 – 1.31)		7.92 (7.01 – 8.75)		67.5 (48.6 – 104)	2,527
Age group							
6–11 years							
1999–2000	10.3 (7.82 – 13.5)	<LOD		11.3 (7.61 – 16.0)		46.6 (33.5 – 151)	272
2001–2002	13.9 (11.2 – 17.2)	<LOD		14.0 (10.6 – 17.0)		80.8 (59.5 – 211)	396
2003–2004	13.2 (10.9 – 15.9)	2.59 (1.57 – 3.11)		12.9 (9.20 – 17.4)		93.4 (49.7 – 134)	341
2005–2006	14.7 (12.6 – 17.1)	2.41 (1.21 – 3.27)		15.3 (13.7 – 17.4)		87.6 (57.6 – 267)	351
12–19 years							
1999–2000	7.61 (6.17 – 9.39)	<LOD		7.94 (6.84 – 9.24)		47.2 (28.6 – 243)	657
2001–2002	7.83 (6.68 – 9.17)	<LOD		7.76 (6.30 – 9.13)		52.6 (36.0 – 160)	744
2003–2004	7.90 (6.59 – 9.49)	1.41 (.856 – 1.87)		8.11 (6.82 – 9.03)		40.4 (32.8 – 100)	729
2005–2006	8.61 (7.53 – 9.83)	1.60 (1.28 – 1.87)		8.03 (7.15 – 9.27)		60.5 (37.4 – 141)	693
20–39 years							
1999–2000	6.20 (5.22 – 7.38)	<LOD		6.32 (5.37 – 7.59)		34.1 (30.5 – 50.5)	439
2001–2002	7.56 (6.16 – 9.27)	<LOD		6.83 (5.60 – 8.78)		53.5 (39.0 – 126)	604
2003–2004	7.42 (6.36 – 8.66)	.902 (.750 – 1.26)		6.88 (5.90 – 7.89)		104 (37.2 – 238)	554
2005–2006	6.90 (5.76 – 8.27)	.887 (.644 – 1.06)		7.09 (5.80 – 8.37)		47.2 (32.9 – 171)	583
40–59 years							
1999–2000	7.84 (6.30 – 9.76)	<LOD		8.06 (6.05 – 9.76)		69.0 (41.9 – 1,680)	378
2001–2002	8.86 (7.19 – 10.9)	<LOD		7.83 (6.18 – 9.71)		81.9 (55.3 – 138)	531
2003–2004	6.40 (5.47 – 7.49)	.777 (.615 – 1.05)		6.54 (5.03 – 7.69)		38.1 (24.2 – 534)	448
2005–2006	7.51 (6.01 – 9.39)	.895 (.343 – 1.34)		6.61 (5.24 – 8.53)		108 (35.1 – 734)	449
60 years and older							
1999–2000	9.72 (8.33 – 11.3)	<LOD		9.63 (7.42 – 11.3)		80.7 (41.1 – 448)	436
2001–2002	8.50 (7.02 – 10.3)	<LOD		7.78 (6.48 – 10.1)		63.7 (38.1 – 161)	519
2003–2004	7.28 (6.19 – 8.56)	1.27 (<LOD – 1.52)		7.63 (6.22 – 8.79)		33.7 (24.8 – 256)	518
2005–2006	9.09 (7.93 – 10.4)	1.38 (1.09 – 1.82)		8.40 (7.49 – 9.42)		51.1 (34.1 – 291)	451
Gender							
Males							
1999–2000	7.01 (5.93 – 8.29)	<LOD		7.31 (5.71 – 8.74)		53.8 (38.9 – 88.4)	1,042
2001–2002	7.66 (6.39 – 9.18)	<LOD		7.43 (5.83 – 9.14)		53.9 (40.7 – 75.8)	1,375
2003–2004	6.71 (6.02 – 7.47)	.912 (.762 – 1.09)		6.62 (5.80 – 7.28)		51.0 (38.7 – 76.6)	1,240
2005–2006	7.35 (6.40 – 8.43)	.984 (.599 – 1.25)		7.02 (5.94 – 8.63)		57.4 (43.3 – 85.6)	1,252
Females							
1999–2000	8.41 (7.33 – 9.66)	<LOD		8.71 (7.52 – 10.2)		46.2 (43.1 – 55.6)	1,140
2001–2002	9.60 (7.99 – 11.5)	<LOD		8.66 (7.02 – 10.6)		84.6 (62.4 – 118)	1,419
2003–2004	8.38 (7.39 – 9.51)	1.15 (.893 – 1.53)		8.29 (7.08 – 9.29)		45.4 (39.0 – 103)	1,350
2005–2006	9.07 (8.04 – 10.2)	1.24 (.885 – 1.41)		8.48 (7.90 – 9.19)		83.5 (53.4 – 165)	1,275
Race/ethnicity							
Mexican Americans							
1999–2000	4.89 (4.36 – 5.47)	<LOD		4.73 (3.90 – 5.23)		37.0 (26.7 – 62.3)	726
2001–2002	6.79 (5.82 – 7.92)	<LOD		6.81 (5.66 – 8.02)		41.2 (34.5 – 54.2)	679
2003–2004	5.48 (4.60 – 6.54)	.932 (.609 – 1.17)		4.69 (4.02 – 5.77)		35.5 (29.2 – 113)	653
2005–2006	5.45 (4.84 – 6.14)	.738 (.548 – 1.02)		4.98 (4.38 – 5.85)		39.4 (31.9 – 81.2)	634
Non-Hispanic Blacks							
1999–2000	4.31 (3.36 – 5.52)	<LOD		4.54 (2.90 – 6.22)		25.8 (20.3 – 33.3)	504
2001–2002	4.96 (4.19 – 5.86)	<LOD		4.37 (3.70 – 5.41)		35.2 (25.4 – 47.4)	692
2003–2004	5.17 (4.38 – 6.10)	.759 (.484 – .958)		5.18 (4.67 – 5.97)		29.7 (24.9 – 51.5)	678
2005–2006	4.88 (4.11 – 5.78)	.769 (.595 – 1.02)		4.72 (3.58 – 5.98)		31.0 (25.4 – 53.3)	662
Non-Hispanic Whites							
1999–2000	9.31 (8.01 – 10.8)	<LOD		9.57 (7.91 – 11.2)		56.2 (46.6 – 73.0)	744
2001–2002	9.77 (7.86 – 12.1)	<LOD		9.14 (7.06 – 12.1)		65.9 (56.8 – 85.0)	1,211
2003–2004	8.39 (7.46 – 9.43)	1.11 (.914 – 1.35)		8.17 (7.13 – 9.23)		56.0 (38.7 – 116)	1,068
2005–2006	9.51 (8.48 – 10.7)	1.31 (1.03 – 1.68)		9.15 (8.06 – 10.5)		77.4 (48.6 – 146)	1,038

< LOD means less than the limit of detection for the uncorrected urine values, which may vary for some compounds by year. See Appendix D for LOD.

Figure 4.6.b. Urinary equol (creatinine corrected): Concentrations by survey cycle

Selected percentiles in µg/g creatinine (95% confidence intervals), National Health and Nutrition Examination Survey, 1999–2006

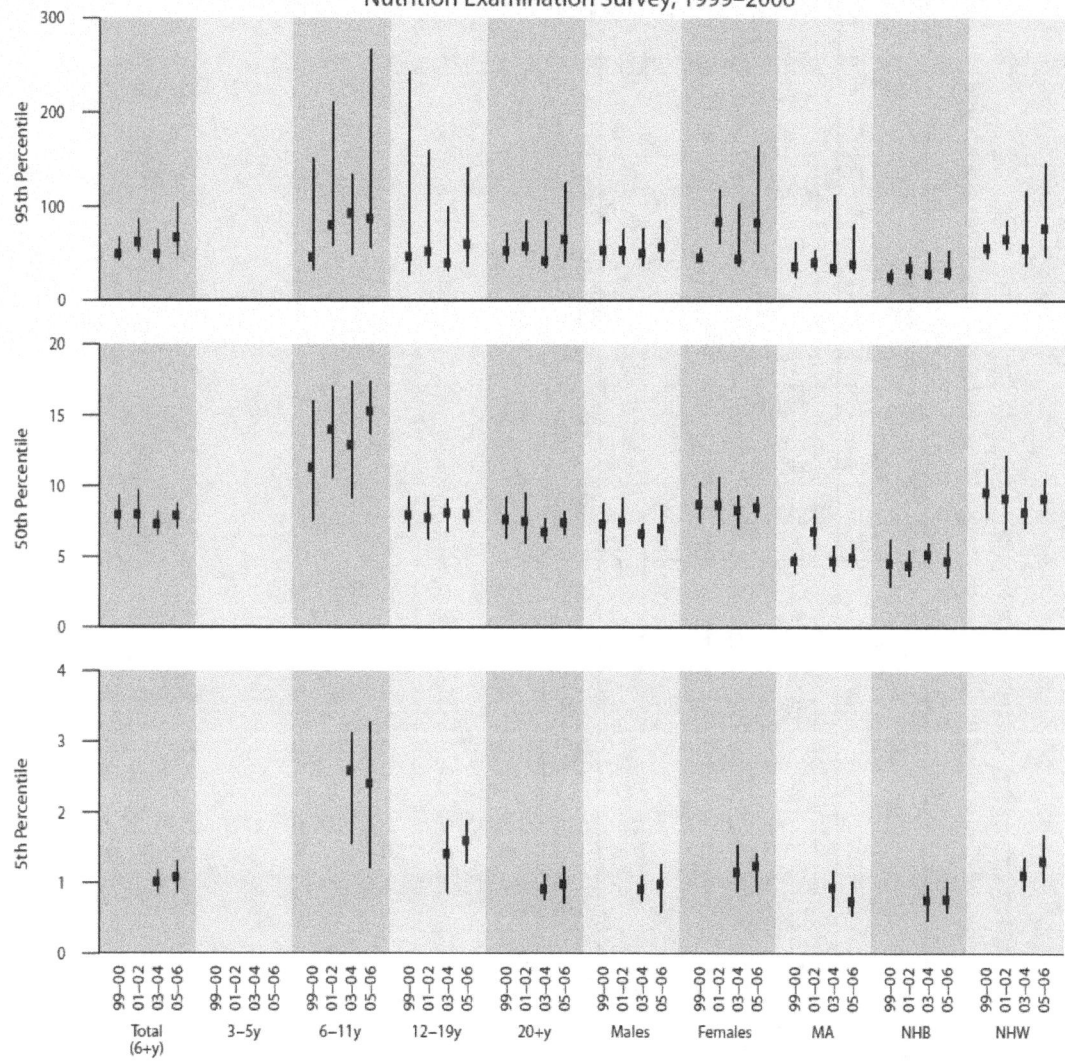

Values in the graph are suppressed if either the point estimate or the lower 95% confidence limit is noted as "< LOD" in the accompanying table.

Table 4.7.a.1. Urinary O-desmethylangolensin: Concentrations

Geometric mean and selected percentiles of urine concentrations (in μg/L) for the total U.S. population aged 6 years and older, National Health and Nutrition Examination Survey, 2003–2006.

	Geometric mean (95% conf. interval)	Selected percentiles (95% conf. interval)					Sample size
		2.5th	5th	50th	95th	97.5th	
Total, 6 years and older	4.80 (4.42 – 5.22)	< LOD	< LOD	4.09 (3.67 – 4.53)	251 (216 – 322)	524 (462 – 612)	5,109
Age group							
6–11 years	6.74 (5.30 – 8.59)	< LOD	.233 (< LOD – .372)	6.17 (4.56 – 8.88)	231 (164 – 371)	445 (361 – 547)	692
12–19 years	7.35 (6.18 – 8.74)	< LOD	< LOD	6.38 (5.25 – 8.33)	285 (229 – 451)	607 (406 – 1,010)	1,422
20–39 years	4.13 (3.52 – 4.86)	< LOD	< LOD	3.32 (2.79 – 3.90)	242 (165 – 400)	485 (402 – 651)	1,129
40–59 years	4.42 (3.81 – 5.13)	< LOD	< LOD	3.88 (2.93 – 5.02)	261 (203 – 481)	657 (385 – 1,150)	899
60 years and older	4.42 (3.69 – 5.30)	< LOD	< LOD	3.71 (2.97 – 4.90)	191 (128 – 404)	455 (341 – 928)	967
Gender							
Males	4.92 (4.29 – 5.63)	< LOD	< LOD	4.21 (3.60 – 5.20)	223 (190 – 299)	476 (383 – 563)	2,492
Females	4.70 (4.26 – 5.18)	< LOD	< LOD	3.92 (3.35 – 4.56)	283 (209 – 406)	649 (455 – 938)	2,617
Race/ethnicity							
Mexican Americans	2.79 (2.29 – 3.39)	< LOD	< LOD	1.93 (1.34 – 2.62)	147 (108 – 226)	304 (227 – 422)	1,286
Non-Hispanic Blacks	5.69 (4.70 – 6.90)	< LOD	< LOD	4.56 (3.88 – 5.72)	279 (208 – 378)	531 (384 – 877)	1,342
Non-Hispanic Whites	4.99 (4.55 – 5.46)	< LOD	< LOD	4.35 (3.90 – 5.12)	245 (201 – 339)	525 (433 – 696)	2,100

< LOD means less than the limit of detection, which may vary for some compounds by year. See Appendix D for LOD.

Figure 4.7.a. Urinary O–desmethylangolensin: Concentrations by age group

Geometric mean (95% confidence interval), National Health and Nutrition Examination Survey, 2003–2006

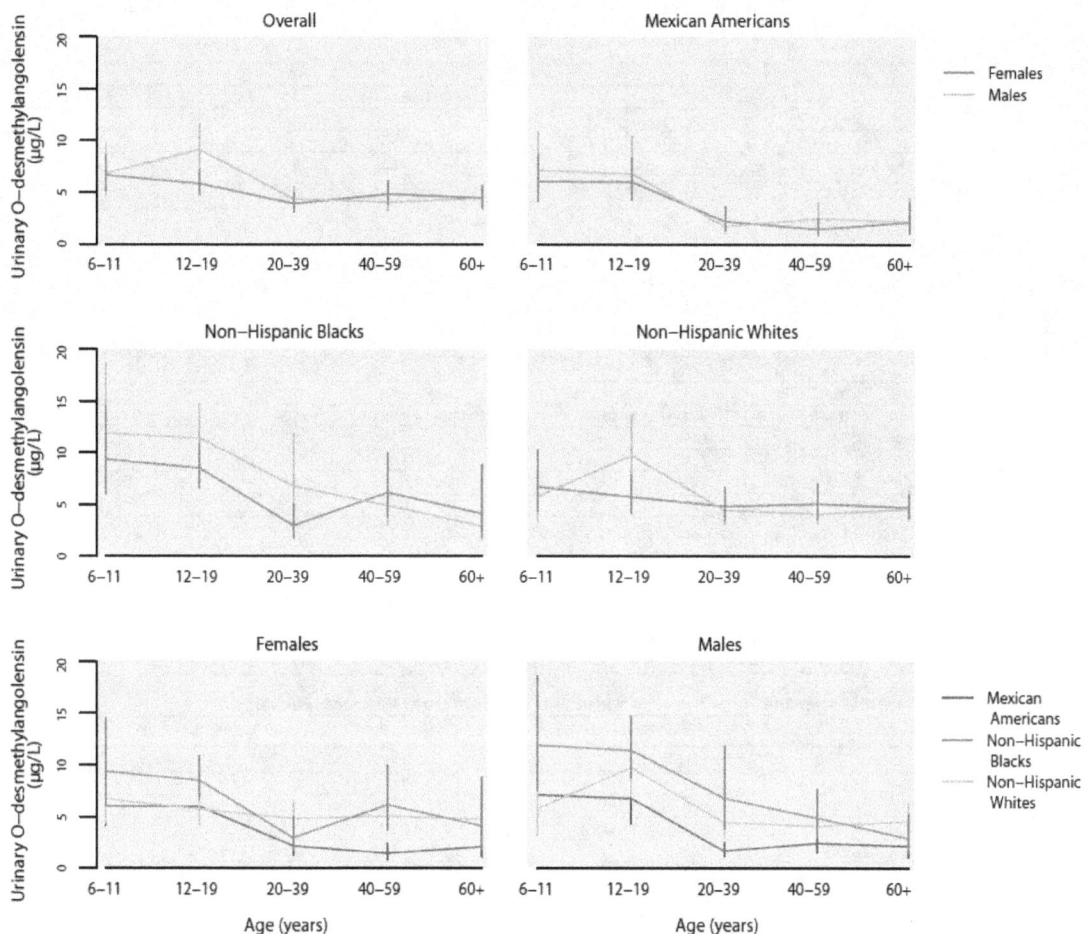

Table 4.7.a.2. Urinary O-desmethylangolensin: Total population

Geometric mean and selected percentiles of urine concentrations (in µg/L) for the total U.S. population aged 6 years and older, National Health and Nutrition Examination Survey, 2003–2006.

	Geometric mean (95% conf. interval)	Selected percentiles (95% conf. interval) 10th		Selected percentiles (95% conf. interval) 50th		Selected percentiles (95% conf. interval) 90th		Sample size
Males and Females								
Total, 6 years and older	4.80 (4.42 – 5.22)	.243	(.210 – .276)	4.09	(3.67 – 4.53)	97.6	(88.0 – 115)	5,109
6–11 years	6.74 (5.30 – 8.59)	.472	(.297 – .655)	6.17	(4.56 – 8.88)	107	(74.1 – 159)	692
12–19 years	7.35 (6.18 – 8.74)	.397	(.300 – .479)	6.38	(5.25 – 8.33)	108	(89.5 – 171)	1,422
20–39 years	4.13 (3.52 – 4.86)	.228	(< LOD – .276)	3.32	(2.79 – 3.90)	86.5	(65.6 – 136)	1,129
40–59 years	4.42 (3.81 – 5.13)	< LOD		3.88	(2.93 – 5.02)	114	(71.0 – 181)	899
60 years and older	4.42 (3.69 – 5.30)	.237	(< LOD – .293)	3.71	(2.97 – 4.90)	84.9	(60.5 – 116)	967
Males								
Total, 6 years and older	4.92 (4.29 – 5.63)	.280	(.231 – .328)	4.21	(3.60 – 5.20)	91.2	(73.4 – 117)	2,492
6–11 years	6.83 (4.77 – 9.78)	.501	(.234 – .705)	5.60	(3.59 – 9.19)	117	(69.6 – 238)	340
12–19 years	9.13 (7.17 – 11.6)	.433	(.341 – .546)	8.73	(6.49 – 11.5)	127	(102 – 253)	728
20–39 years	4.38 (3.41 – 5.61)	.213	(< LOD – .299)	3.63	(3.06 – 4.49)	89.8	(63.3 – 175)	498
40–59 years	4.04 (3.27 – 4.99)	.278	(.207 – .339)	3.34	(2.48 – 4.96)	69.6	(52.0 – 138)	451
60 years and older	4.39 (3.39 – 5.69)	.261	(< LOD – .363)	4.05	(3.01 – 5.43)	75.8	(54.6 – 103)	475
Females								
Total, 6 years and older	4.70 (4.26 – 5.18)	.213	(< LOD – .258)	3.92	(3.35 – 4.56)	105	(80.6 – 151)	2,617
6–11 years	6.65 (5.16 – 8.58)	.392	(.252 – .653)	6.91	(4.76 – 9.15)	100	(60.7 – 158)	352
12–19 years	5.83 (4.79 – 7.10)	.324	(.220 – .480)	4.28	(3.15 – 5.79)	92.9	(71.4 – 104)	694
20–39 years	3.91 (3.12 – 4.89)	.244	(< LOD – .300)	2.83	(2.02 – 3.94)	80.6	(58.4 – 155)	631
40–59 years	4.82 (3.87 – 6.01)	< LOD		4.46	(3.00 – 6.43)	181	(99.3 – 275)	448
60 years and older	4.45 (3.52 – 5.62)	.224	(< LOD – .279)	3.45	(2.71 – 5.36)	88.7	(59.8 – 153)	492

< LOD means less than the limit of detection, which may vary for some compounds by year. See Appendix D for LOD.

Table 4.7.a.3. Urinary O-desmethylangolensin: Mexican Americans

Geometric mean and selected percentiles of urine concentrations (in µg/L) for Mexican Americans in the U.S. population aged 6 years and older, National Health and Nutrition Examination Survey, 2003–2006.

	Geometric mean (95% conf. interval)	Selected percentiles (95% conf. interval) 10th		Selected percentiles (95% conf. interval) 50th		Selected percentiles (95% conf. interval) 90th		Sample size
Males and Females								
Total, 6 years and older	2.79 (2.29 – 3.39)	< LOD		1.93	(1.34 – 2.62)	62.4	(50.0 – 89.5)	1,286
6–11 years	6.57 (4.75 – 9.07)	.446	(.306 – .603)	6.92	(3.88 – 11.0)	103	(58.3 – 189)	231
12–19 years	6.38 (4.66 – 8.73)	.324	(.213 – .396)	5.77	(4.16 – 8.32)	134	(87.6 – 271)	445
20–39 years	1.92 (1.45 – 2.53)	< LOD		1.06	(.693 – 1.53)	58.2	(24.5 – 110)	281
40–59 years	1.91 (1.41 – 2.59)	< LOD		1.21	(.806 – 2.20)	31.7	(21.3 – 70.6)	157
60 years and older	2.15 (1.43 – 3.23)	< LOD		1.47	(.853 – 2.99)	27.9	(17.2 – 50.3)	172
Males								
Total, 6 years and older	2.83 (2.20 – 3.65)	< LOD		1.92	(1.23 – 2.79)	61.5	(47.3 – 89.9)	625
6–11 years	7.12 (4.64 – 10.9)	.506	(.307 – .700)	7.04	(2.90 – 15.9)	115	(61.2 – 275)	112
12–19 years	6.77 (4.40 – 10.4)	.365	(.241 – .462)	6.56	(3.54 – 11.1)	122	(55.4 – 286)	228
20–39 years	1.71 (1.16 – 2.51)	< LOD		.783	(.607 – 1.47)	39.2	(18.1 – 121)	117
40–59 years	2.46 (1.55 – 3.91)	< LOD†		1.80	(.755 – 3.23)	48.1†	(21.9 – 342)	85
60 years and older	2.19 (1.09 – 4.41)	< LOD†		1.39	(.695 – 5.52)	21.6†	(14.0 – 607)	83
Females								
Total, 6 years and older	2.74 (2.17 – 3.45)	< LOD		1.97	(1.27 – 2.85)	64.9	(39.2 – 111)	661
6–11 years	6.03 (4.19 – 8.68)	.378	(.290 – .531)	6.65	(3.89 – 10.5)	81.9	(32.7 – 296)	119
12–19 years	5.99 (4.33 – 8.29)	.302	(< LOD – .381)	4.71	(3.81 – 7.61)	176	(93.4 – 325)	217
20–39 years	2.20 (1.33 – 3.63)	< LOD		1.31	(.772 – 2.43)	63.7	(19.3 – 235)	164
40–59 years	1.45 (.886 – 2.38)	< LOD†		1.06	(.513 – 1.97)	20.7†	(10.1 – 73.1)	72
60 years and older	2.12 (1.13 – 3.98)	< LOD†		1.45	(.808 – 4.19)	38.7†	(11.3 – 1,390)	89

< LOD means less than the limit of detection, which may vary for some compounds by year. See Appendix D for LOD.

† Estimate is subject to greater uncertainty due to small cell size.

Table 4.7.a.4. Urinary O-desmethylangolensin: Non-Hispanic blacks

Geometric mean and selected percentiles of urine concentrations (in µg/L) for non-Hispanic blacks in the U.S. population aged 6 years and older, National Health and Nutrition Examination Survey, 2003–2006.

	Geometric mean (95% conf. interval)	Selected percentiles (95% conf. interval)						Sample size
		10th		**50th**		**90th**		
Males and Females								
Total, 6 years and older	5.69 (4.70 – 6.90)	.267	(.210 – .342)	4.56	(3.88 – 5.72)	113	(89.0 – 157)	1,342
6–11 years	10.6 (7.76 – 14.4)	.639	(.244 – 1.24)	11.1	(7.91 – 16.4)	164	(106 – 338)	207
12–19 years	9.85 (8.13 – 11.9)	.565	(.391 – .896)	10.2	(7.23 – 15.0)	121	(100 – 172)	496
20–39 years	4.31 (3.05 – 6.07)	< LOD		3.25	(2.16 – 4.64)	90.8	(51.6 – 170)	249
40–59 years	5.54 (4.02 – 7.64)	.265	(< LOD – .380)	4.61	(2.91 – 7.10)	124	(80.1 – 220)	231
60 years and older	3.60 (2.02 – 6.39)	.215	(< LOD – .279)	2.57	(1.49 – 4.67)	82.6	(47.3 – 341)	159
Males								
Total, 6 years and older	6.62 (5.17 – 8.47)	.297	(.206 – .458)	5.48	(4.13 – 8.91)	114	(90.2 – 168)	660
6–11 years	11.9 (7.59 – 18.6)	.854†	(.360 – 1.53)	10.8	(5.47 – 20.0)	182†	(106 – 764)	99
12–19 years	11.4 (8.83 – 14.7)	.580	(.376 – .969)	12.7	(7.98 – 17.0)	145	(111 – 241)	258
20–39 years	6.79 (3.90 – 11.8)	.226	(< LOD – .614)	4.57	(2.91 – 12.9)	122	(82.3 – 400)	116
40–59 years	4.89 (3.12 – 7.67)	.244	(< LOD – .474)	4.83	(2.15 – 9.22)	69.3	(46.5 – 216)	114
60 years and older	2.91 (1.60 – 5.30)	.212†	(< LOD – .298)	2.70	(1.05 – 4.21)	48.7†	(20.0 – 868)	73
Females								
Total, 6 years and older	5.01 (3.87 – 6.50)	.246	(< LOD – .334)	4.09	(2.94 – 5.38)	112	(82.0 – 160)	682
6–11 years	9.36 (6.05 – 14.5)	.364†	(< LOD – 1.11)	11.9	(7.46 – 16.4)	121†	(56.0 – 502)	108
12–19 years	8.51 (6.68 – 10.8)	.551	(.259 – .963)	7.87	(5.52 – 14.0)	98.0	(77.3 – 143)	238
20–39 years	2.98 (1.78 – 5.01)	< LOD		2.17	(1.14 – 4.46)	49.2	(27.2 – 160)	133
40–59 years	6.15 (3.81 – 9.90)	.280	(.207 – .388)	4.44	(2.60 – 8.52)	203	(106 – 486)	117
60 years and older	4.11 (1.92 – 8.80)	.217†	(< LOD – .363)	2.45	(1.37 – 8.03)	91.7†	(67.0 – 322)	86

< LOD means less than the limit of detection, which may vary for some compounds by year. See Appendix D for LOD.

† Estimate is subject to greater uncertainty due to small cell size.

Table 4.7.a.5. Urinary O-desmethylangolensin: Non-Hispanic whites

Geometric mean and selected percentiles of urine concentrations (in µg/L) for non-Hispanic whites in the U.S. population aged 6 years and older, National Health and Nutrition Examination Survey, 2003–2006.

	Geometric mean (95% conf. interval)	Selected percentiles (95% conf. interval)						Sample size
		10th		**50th**		**90th**		
Males and Females								
Total, 6 years and older	4.99 (4.55 – 5.46)	.247	(.201 – .293)	4.35	(3.90 – 5.12)	97.9	(86.2 – 123)	2,100
6–11 years	6.20 (4.18 – 9.18)	.443	(< LOD – .679)	5.49	(3.39 – 9.17)	95.4	(60.4 – 203)	193
12–19 years	7.55 (5.92 – 9.63)	.401	(.259 – .571)	6.85	(5.13 – 9.64)	103	(85.0 – 205)	378
20–39 years	4.64 (3.67 – 5.85)	.264	(< LOD – .331)	3.71	(2.94 – 5.33)	104	(65.2 – 161)	488
40–59 years	4.54 (3.75 – 5.51)	< LOD		4.14	(2.91 – 5.62)	121	(67.5 – 185)	447
60 years and older	4.67 (3.89 – 5.60)	.248	(< LOD – .320)	4.09	(3.25 – 5.34)	84.4	(57.6 – 117)	594
Males								
Total, 6 years and older	4.88 (4.11 – 5.80)	.290	(.217 – .350)	4.21	(3.40 – 5.41)	88.8	(67.8 – 120)	1,034
6–11 years	5.78 (3.26 – 10.3)	.445†	(< LOD – .719)	4.99	(1.97 – 10.4)	88.6†	(40.8 – 580)	99
12–19 years	9.72 (7.00 – 13.5)	.429	(.295 – .611)	9.13	(6.14 – 13.6)	125	(88.5 – 365)	191
20–39 years	4.46 (3.13 – 6.36)	.236	(< LOD – .365)	3.56	(2.79 – 5.63)	78.4	(48.1 – 189)	217
40–59 years	4.09 (3.19 – 5.24)	.294	(.201 – .354)	3.02	(2.28 – 5.24)	70.4	(51.0 – 170)	229
60 years and older	4.58 (3.35 – 6.27)	.266	(< LOD – .384)	4.17	(3.21 – 6.29)	72.6	(50.6 – 103)	298
Females								
Total, 6 years and older	5.09 (4.45 – 5.82)	.209	(< LOD – .277)	4.53	(3.79 – 5.58)	112	(74.9 – 175)	1,066
6–11 years	6.72 (4.42 – 10.2)	.438†	(< LOD – .745)	6.05	(3.68 – 12.2)	105†	(48.1 – 310)	94
12–19 years	5.73 (4.21 – 7.80)	.299	(< LOD – .615)	3.99	(2.90 – 8.09)	88.8	(61.2 – 170)	187
20–39 years	4.83 (3.50 – 6.66)	.295	(.221 – .349)	3.90	(2.73 – 6.07)	114	(58.4 – 303)	271
40–59 years	5.06 (3.68 – 6.95)	< LOD		5.51	(2.99 – 7.16)	181	(67.3 – 333)	218
60 years and older	4.74 (3.78 – 5.94)	.237	(< LOD – .311)	3.90	(2.86 – 6.17)	85.9	(53.0 – 168)	296

< LOD means less than the limit of detection, which may vary for some compounds by year. See Appendix D for LOD.

† Estimate is subject to greater uncertainty due to small cell size.

Table 4.7.b. Urinary O-desmethylangolensin: Concentrations by survey cycle

Geometric mean and selected percentiles of urine concentrations (in µg/L) for the U.S. population, National Health and Nutrition Examination Survey, 1999–2006.

	Geometric mean (95% conf. interval)	Selected percentiles (95% conf. interval) 5th	Selected percentiles (95% conf. interval) 50th	Selected percentiles (95% conf. interval) 95th	Sample size
Total, 6 years and older					
1999–2000	4.39 (3.37 – 5.73)	< LOD	4.97 (3.67 – 6.74)	218 (186 – 247)	2,271
2001–2002	4.08 (3.53 – 4.73)	< LOD	3.30 (2.64 – 4.11)	260 (177 – 492)	2,794
2003–2004	4.91 (4.34 – 5.55)	< LOD	4.55 (3.99 – 5.16)	229 (186 – 364)	2,581
2005–2006	4.70 (4.17 – 5.31)	< LOD	3.70 (3.14 – 4.25)	264 (213 – 386)	2,528
Age group					
6–11 years					
1999–2000	5.60 (3.85 – 8.15)	< LOD	7.48 (3.42 – 15.1)	175 (79.4 – 273)	287
2001–2002	6.19 (4.51 – 8.49)	< LOD	5.85 (3.88 – 9.42)	278 (177 – 522)	396
2003–2004	6.32 (4.30 – 9.30)	.319 (< LOD – .590)	6.07 (3.48 – 10.5)	137 (92.3 – 283)	341
2005–2006	7.20 (5.20 – 9.96)	< LOD	6.16 (3.98 – 10.9)	356 (207 – 506)	351
12–19 years					
1999–2000	6.04 (3.76 – 9.70)	< LOD	7.58 (5.18 – 13.2)	194 (136 – 301)	667
2001–2002	5.92 (4.46 – 7.86)	< LOD	5.19 (3.72 – 7.59)	298 (179 – 435)	744
2003–2004	6.36 (4.95 – 8.18)	< LOD	5.27 (3.89 – 8.00)	256 (179 – 416)	729
2005–2006	8.50 (6.48 – 11.2)	.244 (< LOD – .337)	8.06 (5.57 – 11.6)	380 (168 – 869)	693
20–39 years					
1999–2000	4.00 (2.73 – 5.86)	< LOD	4.44 (2.77 – 5.87)	306 (252 – 462)	481
2001–2002	3.36 (2.61 – 4.34)	< LOD	2.48 (1.80 – 3.00)	248 (128 – 680)	604
2003–2004	4.25 (3.24 – 5.58)	< LOD	3.65 (2.74 – 4.89)	317 (154 – 483)	546
2005–2006	4.03 (3.29 – 4.93)	< LOD	3.00 (2.17 – 3.78)	235 (154 – 336)	583
40–59 years					
1999–2000	4.20 (3.13 – 5.62)	< LOD	4.24 (2.78 – 6.11)	171 (119 – 304)	365
2001–2002	5.07 (3.45 – 7.46)	< LOD	4.39 (2.61 – 7.20)	381 (206 – 1,000)	531
2003–2004	5.13 (4.34 – 6.07)	< LOD	5.13 (3.52 – 6.44)	222 (180 – 753)	450
2005–2006	3.84 (2.97 – 4.97)	< LOD	2.92 (1.72 – 4.29)	274 (214 – 587)	449
60 years and older					
1999–2000	3.93 (2.75 – 5.62)	< LOD	4.80 (3.04 – 8.37)	111 (74.5 – 185)	471
2001–2002	2.32 (1.83 – 2.94)	< LOD	1.73 (1.16 – 2.30)	98.3 (70.6 – 464)	519
2003–2004	4.17 (3.09 – 5.63)	< LOD	3.69 (2.71 – 5.88)	203 (129 – 394)	515
2005–2006	4.68 (3.70 – 5.91)	< LOD	3.76 (2.74 – 5.45)	171 (92.6 – 486)	452
Gender					
Males					
1999–2000	4.97 (3.71 – 6.66)	< LOD	5.62 (4.23 – 8.78)	234 (180 – 332)	1,087
2001–2002	3.81 (3.08 – 4.71)	< LOD	3.29 (2.52 – 4.38)	194 (134 – 356)	1,375
2003–2004	4.90 (3.93 – 6.12)	< LOD	4.53 (3.32 – 5.49)	221 (163 – 359)	1,240
2005–2006	4.93 (4.13 – 5.89)	< LOD	3.99 (3.34 – 5.43)	234 (178 – 341)	1,252
Females					
1999–2000	3.92 (2.97 – 5.16)	< LOD	4.22 (3.24 – 5.48)	191 (149 – 245)	1,184
2001–2002	4.36 (3.64 – 5.23)	< LOD	3.34 (2.47 – 4.50)	377 (232 – 750)	1,419
2003–2004	4.91 (4.26 – 5.66)	< LOD	4.59 (3.91 – 5.51)	277 (168 – 450)	1,341
2005–2006	4.50 (3.90 – 5.20)	< LOD	3.29 (2.71 – 4.24)	283 (199 – 499)	1,276
Race/ethnicity					
Mexican Americans					
1999–2000	2.40 (1.55 – 3.73)	< LOD	2.14 (1.40 – 3.43)	191 (128 – 323)	721
2001–2002	2.44 (1.51 – 3.94)	< LOD	1.38 (.501 – 3.33)	151 (80.1 – 498)	679
2003–2004	2.54 (1.86 – 3.48)	< LOD	1.85 (.928 – 3.30)	141 (105 – 272)	652
2005–2006	3.04 (2.29 – 4.05)	< LOD	2.00 (1.36 – 2.84)	151 (95.3 – 271)	634
Non-Hispanic Blacks					
1999–2000	5.75 (4.60 – 7.20)	< LOD	8.78 (5.90 – 10.9)	184 (138 – 320)	527
2001–2002	5.38 (4.01 – 7.21)	< LOD	5.19 (3.04 – 7.31)	308 (193 – 430)	692
2003–2004	5.55 (4.07 – 7.57)	< LOD	4.21 (3.25 – 6.49)	219 (182 – 375)	680
2005–2006	5.83 (4.49 – 7.58)	< LOD	4.84 (3.94 – 6.45)	292 (173 – 471)	662
Non-Hispanic Whites					
1999–2000	4.53 (3.23 – 6.37)	< LOD	4.98 (3.38 – 7.14)	225 (189 – 255)	810
2001–2002	4.13 (3.44 – 4.96)	< LOD	3.35 (2.61 – 4.32)	261 (178 – 546)	1,211
2003–2004	5.28 (4.65 – 5.99)	< LOD	5.23 (4.53 – 5.78)	242 (186 – 407)	1,061
2005–2006	4.72 (4.09 – 5.45)	< LOD	3.72 (3.21 – 4.59)	246 (184 – 391)	1,039

< LOD means less than the limit of detection, which may vary for some compounds by year. See Appendix D for LOD.

Figure 4.7.b. Urinary O–desmethylangolensin: Concentrations by survey cycle

Selected percentiles in µg/L (95% confidence intervals), National Health and Nutrition Examination Survey, 1999–2006

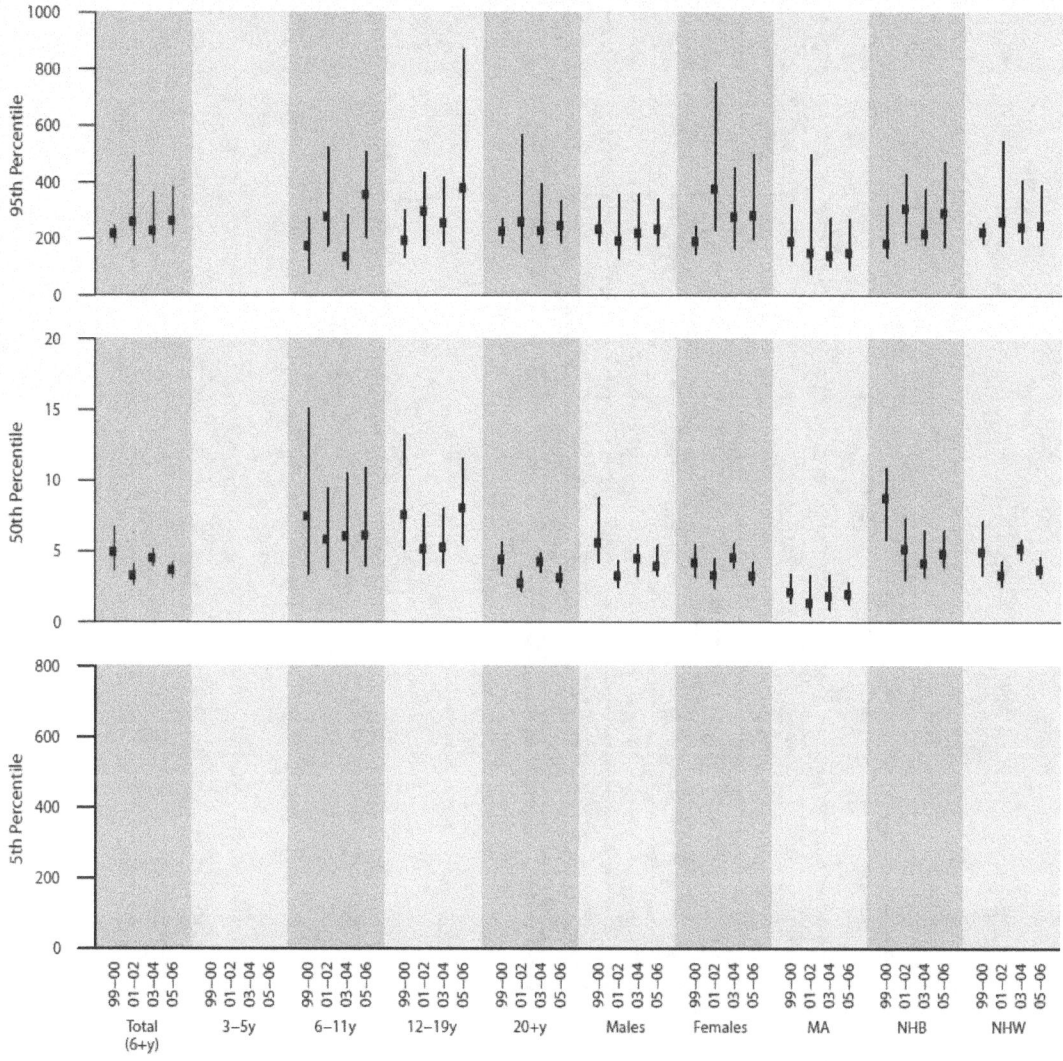

Values in the graph are suppressed if either the point estimate or the lower 95% confidence limit is noted as "< LOD" in the accompanying table.

Table 4.8.a.1. Urinary O-desmethylangolensin (creatinine corrected): Concentrations

Geometric mean and selected percentiles of urine concentrations (in µg/g creatinine) for the total U.S. population aged 6 years and older, National Health and Nutrition Examination Survey, 2003–2006.

	Geometric mean (95% conf. interval)	Selected percentiles (95% conf. interval)					Sample size
		2.5th	5th	50th	95th	97.5th	
Total, 6 years and older	4.58 (4.25 – 4.94)	< LOD	< LOD	3.89 (3.51 – 4.33)	204 (193 – 260)	530 (376 – 725)	5,109
Age group							
6–11 years	7.31 (5.72 – 9.33)	< LOD	.349 (< LOD – .470)	6.11 (4.49 – 8.22)	243 (175 – 349)	362 (317 – 611)	692
12–19 years	5.47 (4.64 – 6.46)	< LOD	< LOD	4.67 (3.74 – 6.52)	201 (136 – 375)	456 (270 – 713)	1,422
20–39 years	3.51 (3.05 – 4.04)	< LOD	< LOD	3.10 (2.38 – 3.74)	181 (144 – 260)	425 (241 – 646)	1,129
40–59 years	4.48 (3.89 – 5.16)	< LOD	< LOD	3.51 (2.96 – 4.33)	243 (194 – 532)	795 (343 – 1,270)	899
60 years and older	5.18 (4.38 – 6.13)	< LOD	< LOD	4.37 (3.42 – 5.80)	239 (140 – 389)	480 (317 – 1,730)	967
Gender							
Males	3.90 (3.42 – 4.44)	< LOD	< LOD	3.41 (2.81 – 4.09)	179 (144 – 227)	325 (256 – 482)	2,492
Females	5.35 (4.85 – 5.91)	< LOD	< LOD	4.40 (3.76 – 5.25)	271 (202 – 396)	738 (548 – 1,020)	2,617
Race/ethnicity							
Mexican Americans	2.51 (2.01 – 3.14)	< LOD	< LOD	1.68 (1.09 – 2.45)	130 (93.0 – 158)	243 (164 – 423)	1,286
Non-Hispanic Blacks	4.00 (3.35 – 4.77)	< LOD	< LOD	3.47 (2.48 – 4.61)	180 (136 – 313)	512 (292 – 876)	1,342
Non-Hispanic Whites	5.07 (4.68 – 5.49)	< LOD	< LOD	4.30 (3.85 – 4.69)	227 (194 – 274)	557 (338 – 824)	2,100

< LOD means less than the limit of detection for the uncorrected urine values, which may vary for some compounds by year. See Appendix D for LOD.

Figure 4.8.a. Urinary O–desmethylangolensin (creatinine corrected): Concentrations by age group

Geometric mean (95% confidence interval), National Health and Nutrition Examination Survey, 2003–2006

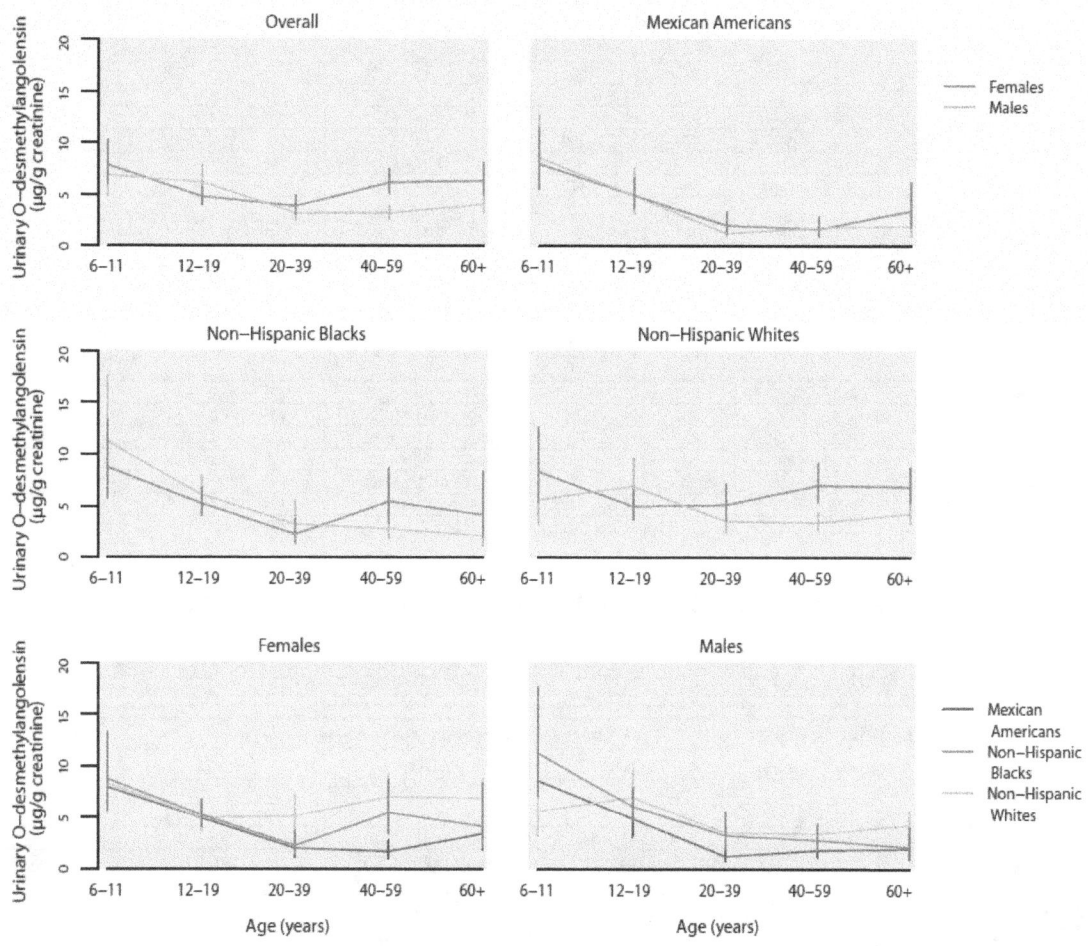

Table 4.8.a.2. Urinary O-desmethylangolensin (creatinine corrected): Total population

Geometric mean and selected percentiles of urine concentrations (in µg/g creatinine) for the total U.S. population aged 6 years and older, National Health and Nutrition Examination Survey, 2003–2006.

	Geometric mean (95% conf. interval)	Selected percentiles (95% conf. interval)						Sample size
		10th		50th		90th		
Males and Females								
Total, 6 years and older	4.58 (4.25 – 4.94)	.312	(.289 – .338)	3.89	(3.51 – 4.33)	93.2	(81.6 – 109)	5,109
6–11 years	7.31 (5.72 – 9.33)	.587	(.389 – .800)	6.11	(4.49 – 8.22)	109	(84.7 – 165)	692
12–19 years	5.47 (4.64 – 6.46)	.320	(.289 – .402)	4.67	(3.74 – 6.52)	86.1	(61.4 – 129)	1,422
20–39 years	3.51 (3.05 – 4.04)	.248	(< LOD – .299)	3.10	(2.38 – 3.74)	78.0	(63.1 – 97.3)	1,129
40–59 years	4.48 (3.89 – 5.16)	< LOD		3.51	(2.96 – 4.33)	138	(76.1 – 190)	899
60 years and older	5.18 (4.38 – 6.13)	.384	(< LOD – .472)	4.37	(3.42 – 5.80)	79.2	(65.8 – 119)	967
Males								
Total, 6 years and older	3.90 (3.42 – 4.44)	.281	(.233 – .323)	3.41	(2.81 – 4.09)	73.1	(58.7 – 85.3)	2,492
6–11 years	6.85 (4.87 – 9.63)	.496	(.308 – .801)	5.45	(3.39 – 8.21)	126	(81.4 – 215)	340
12–19 years	6.19 (4.90 – 7.82)	.315	(.219 – .487)	6.40	(4.16 – 8.62)	94.4	(61.8 – 169)	728
20–39 years	3.19 (2.53 – 4.03)	.196	(< LOD – .283)	2.68	(2.00 – 4.15)	67.3	(46.0 – 93.6)	498
40–59 years	3.20 (2.57 – 3.99)	.251	(.200 – .312)	2.76	(2.03 – 3.84)	51.5	(37.2 – 94.2)	451
60 years and older	4.03 (3.22 – 5.05)	.341	(< LOD – .424)	3.75	(2.54 – 5.01)	64.8	(40.6 – 107)	475
Females								
Total, 6 years and older	5.35 (4.85 – 5.91)	.342	(< LOD – .385)	4.40	(3.76 – 5.25)	131	(95.9 – 158)	2,617
6–11 years	7.83 (6.01 – 10.2)	.682	(.379 – .857)	7.16	(5.34 – 9.21)	100	(77.5 – 164)	352
12–19 years	4.80 (4.03 – 5.72)	.321	(.278 – .392)	4.02	(3.17 – 4.75)	74.9	(54.2 – 120)	694
20–39 years	3.86 (3.08 – 4.83)	.301	(< LOD – .337)	3.44	(2.23 – 4.59)	86.8	(63.3 – 139)	631
40–59 years	6.16 (5.10 – 7.43)	< LOD		5.00	(3.20 – 6.49)	192	(152 – 316)	448
60 years and older	6.31 (4.96 – 8.01)	.426	(< LOD – .643)	5.49	(3.84 – 7.18)	102	(74.4 – 155)	492

< LOD means less than the limit of detection for the uncorrected urine values, which may vary for some compounds by year. See Appendix D for LOD.

Table 4.8.a.3. Urinary O-desmethylangolensin (creatinine corrected): Mexican Americans

Geometric mean and selected percentiles of urine concentrations (in µg/g creatinine) for Mexican Americans in the U.S. population aged 6 years and older, National Health and Nutrition Examination Survey, 2003–2006.

	Geometric mean (95% conf. interval)	Selected percentiles (95% conf. interval)						Sample size
		10th		50th		90th		
Males and Females								
Total, 6 years and older	2.51 (2.01 – 3.14)	< LOD		1.68	(1.09 – 2.45)	52.7	(39.7 – 74.3)	1,286
6–11 years	8.24 (6.07 – 11.2)	.539	(.345 – .845)	7.19	(4.88 – 12.9)	102	(73.3 – 160)	231
12–19 years	4.93 (3.63 – 6.69)	.295	(.240 – .365)	4.46	(3.00 – 6.97)	103	(59.6 – 155)	445
20–39 years	1.55 (1.12 – 2.14)	< LOD		.843	(.692 – 1.16)	33.8	(17.5 – 80.4)	281
40–59 years	1.75 (1.28 – 2.40)	< LOD		1.01	(.818 – 2.03)	27.3	(22.5 – 52.6)	157
60 years and older	2.66 (1.82 – 3.88)	< LOD		1.95	(1.08 – 3.72)	35.9	(25.1 – 63.6)	172
Males								
Total, 6 years and older	2.24 (1.69 – 2.96)	< LOD		1.33	(.935 – 2.07)	45.9	(34.6 – 74.9)	625
6–11 years	8.54 (5.71 – 12.8)	.532	(.307 – 1.03)	7.44	(4.18 – 16.7)	110	(72.7 – 274)	112
12–19 years	4.90 (3.18 – 7.55)	.292	(.208 – .428)	4.55	(2.36 – 10.5)	103	(43.8 – 146)	228
20–39 years	1.24 (.818 – 1.88)	< LOD		.732	(.591 – .930)	28.8	(13.4 – 95.5)	117
40–59 years	1.81 (1.17 – 2.79)	< LOD†		.997	(.601 – 3.02)	36.6†	(16.9 – 156)	85
60 years and older	1.96 (1.00 – 3.82)	< LOD†		1.44	(.646 – 3.16)	20.4†	(12.1 – 159)	83
Females								
Total, 6 years and older	2.86 (2.22 – 3.68)	< LOD		2.16	(1.36 – 3.15)	59.6	(41.4 – 96.0)	661
6–11 years	7.94 (5.56 – 11.4)	.527	(.268 – .811)	6.00	(4.39 – 12.1)	93.0	(62.8 – 156)	119
12–19 years	4.95 (3.71 – 6.60)	.295	(< LOD – .342)	4.20	(2.93 – 6.89)	100	(72.2 – 243)	217
20–39 years	2.01 (1.21 – 3.35)	< LOD		1.01	(.703 – 2.25)	40.5	(13.8 – 203)	164
40–59 years	1.69 (1.02 – 2.80)	< LOD†		1.01	(.870 – 2.39)	27.1†	(16.3 – 66.5)	72
60 years and older	3.41 (1.90 – 6.13)	< LOD†		2.79	(1.08 – 7.40)	45.9†	(23.0 – 803)	89

< LOD means less than the limit of detection for the uncorrected urine values, which may vary for some compounds by year. See Appendix D for LOD.

† Estimate is subject to greater uncertainty due to small cell size.

Table 4.8.a.4. Urinary O-desmethylangolensin (creatinine corrected): Non-Hispanic blacks

Geometric mean and selected percentiles of urine concentrations (in µg/g creatinine) for non-Hispanic blacks in the U.S. population aged 6 years and older, National Health and Nutrition Examination Survey, 2003–2006.

	Geometric mean (95% conf. interval)	Selected percentiles (95% conf. interval)						Sample size
		10th		50th		90th		
Males and Females								
Total, 6 years and older	4.00 (3.35 – 4.77)	.249	(.208 – .295)	3.47	(2.48 – 4.61)	75.6	(60.8 – 97.4)	1,342
6–11 years	9.91 (7.22 – 13.6)	.701	(.469 – .983)	10.1	(7.06 – 15.0)	160	(85.0 – 249)	207
12–19 years	5.66 (4.68 – 6.84)	.336	(.262 – .519)	6.00	(4.57 – 8.05)	72.7	(53.8 – 100)	496
20–39 years	2.67 (1.93 – 3.69)	< LOD		1.99	(1.21 – 3.33)	45.7	(34.3 – 82.1)	249
40–59 years	4.03 (3.01 – 5.39)	.241	(< LOD – .319)	3.60	(1.85 – 6.21)	77.7	(58.0 – 133)	231
60 years and older	3.20 (1.86 – 5.51)	.194	(< LOD – .342)	2.34	(1.45 – 4.24)	73.0	(30.4 – 296)	159
Males								
Total, 6 years and older	3.86 (3.06 – 4.88)	.233	(.157 – .322)	3.81	(2.31 – 4.93)	69.7	(52.6 – 92.1)	660
6–11 years	11.2 (7.16 – 17.6)	.797†	(.574 – 1.50)	10.7	(5.44 – 15.8)	173†	(85.5 – 476)	99
12–19 years	6.09 (4.69 – 7.91)	.324	(.199 – .529)	6.53	(4.50 – 9.81)	81.0	(52.5 – 137)	258
20–39 years	3.26 (1.91 – 5.56)	.157	(< LOD – .342)	2.38	(1.20 – 6.28)	62.5	(41.0 – 133)	116
40–59 years	2.80 (1.83 – 4.28)	.194	(< LOD – .310)	2.10	(1.14 – 5.38)	46.0	(20.8 – 121)	114
60 years and older	2.12 (1.13 – 3.98)	.146†	(< LOD – .217)	1.87	(.716 – 3.04)	28.2†	(12.9 – 664)	73
Females								
Total, 6 years and older	4.11 (3.19 – 5.30)	.265	(< LOD – .330)	3.28	(2.29 – 5.29)	78.9	(62.4 – 126)	682
6–11 years	8.73 (5.75 – 13.3)	.509†	(< LOD – 1.10)	9.53	(5.79 – 15.3)	145†	(55.0 – 522)	108
12–19 years	5.25 (4.09 – 6.74)	.338	(.222 – .575)	5.33	(3.56 – 8.34)	56.7	(46.9 – 78.1)	238
20–39 years	2.27 (1.36 – 3.79)	< LOD		1.83	(.829 – 4.09)	34.9	(21.9 – 122)	133
40–59 years	5.45 (3.42 – 8.68)	.276	(.197 – .411)	4.28	(1.91 – 7.76)	148	(74.5 – 835)	117
60 years and older	4.15 (2.06 – 8.34)	.334†	(< LOD – .461)	2.59	(1.22 – 6.75)	88.1†	(36.1 – 366)	86

< LOD means less than the limit of detection for the uncorrected urine values, which may vary for some compounds by year. See Appendix D for LOD.

† Estimate is subject to greater uncertainty due to small cell size.

Table 4.8.a.5. Urinary O-desmethylangolensin (creatinine corrected): Non-Hispanic whites

Geometric mean and selected percentiles of urine concentrations (in µg/g creatinine) for non-Hispanic whites in the U.S. population aged 6 years and older, National Health and Nutrition Examination Survey, 2003–2006.

	Geometric mean (95% conf. interval)	Selected percentiles (95% conf. interval)						Sample size
		10th		50th		90th		
Males and Females								
Total, 6 years and older	5.07 (4.68 – 5.49)	.347	(.312 – .382)	4.30	(3.85 – 4.69)	100	(86.1 – 136)	2,100
6–11 years	6.72 (4.52 – 9.99)	.515	(< LOD – .823)	5.35	(3.55 – 8.26)	126	(75.5 – 219)	193
12–19 years	5.92 (4.64 – 7.57)	.342	(.259 – .492)	4.83	(3.42 – 8.22)	91.6	(59.4 – 149)	378
20–39 years	4.25 (3.40 – 5.30)	.321	(< LOD – .376)	3.90	(3.10 – 4.89)	86.6	(67.4 – 129)	488
40–59 years	4.89 (4.13 – 5.79)	< LOD		3.75	(3.03 – 4.81)	160	(88.4 – 194)	447
60 years and older	5.57 (4.72 – 6.57)	.417	(< LOD – .498)	4.76	(3.87 – 6.27)	78.8	(65.6 – 120)	594
Males								
Total, 6 years and older	4.08 (3.45 – 4.83)	.304	(.237 – .370)	3.57	(2.90 – 4.35)	73.4	(58.4 – 88.8)	1,034
6–11 years	5.60 (3.23 – 9.71)	.403†	(< LOD – .810)	4.09	(2.17 – 8.47)	109†	(43.9 – 358)	99
12–19 years	6.94 (4.98 – 9.67)	.311	(.186 – .652)	6.78	(3.52 – 13.0)	103	(58.5 – 260)	191
20–39 years	3.54 (2.51 – 5.00)	.257	(< LOD – .350)	3.16	(2.22 – 4.91)	69.1	(40.0 – 95.7)	217
40–59 years	3.42 (2.66 – 4.40)	.278	(.191 – .389)	2.96	(2.16 – 3.95)	55.5	(36.3 – 150)	229
60 years and older	4.27 (3.25 – 5.62)	.354	(< LOD – .493)	3.86	(2.76 – 5.25)	60.7	(37.5 – 117)	298
Females								
Total, 6 years and older	6.27 (5.53 – 7.11)	.400	(< LOD – .428)	5.31	(4.37 – 6.35)	141	(108 – 183)	1,066
6–11 years	8.31 (5.47 – 12.6)	.803†	(< LOD – 1.05)	6.95	(4.34 – 11.5)	132†	(75.9 – 259)	94
12–19 years	4.99 (3.73 – 6.67)	.347	(< LOD – .484)	4.27	(3.11 – 5.86)	74.7	(47.4 – 131)	187
20–39 years	5.12 (3.67 – 7.15)	.359	(.304 – .418)	4.61	(3.37 – 6.48)	103	(66.8 – 197)	271
40–59 years	7.01 (5.37 – 9.15)	< LOD		5.48	(3.20 – 7.60)	194	(157 – 323)	218
60 years and older	6.86 (5.44 – 8.66)	.484	(< LOD – .719)	5.96	(4.28 – 7.84)	104	(73.9 – 167)	296

< LOD means less than the limit of detection for the uncorrected urine values, which may vary for some compounds by year. See Appendix D for LOD.

† Estimate is subject to greater uncertainty due to small cell size.

Table 4.8.b. Urinary O-desmethylangolensin (creatinine corrected): Concentrations by survey cycle

Geometric mean and selected percentiles of urine concentrations (in µg/g creatinine) for the U.S. population, National Health and Nutrition Examination Survey, 1999–2006.

	Geometric mean (95% conf. interval)	Selected percentiles (95% conf. interval) 5th	Selected percentiles (95% conf. interval) 50th	Selected percentiles (95% conf. interval) 95th	Sample size
Total, 6 years and older					
1999–2000	4.03 (2.97 – 5.45)	<LOD	4.44 (3.11 – 6.27)	165 (143 – 220)	2,271
2001–2002	3.83 (3.32 – 4.42)	<LOD	3.23 (2.56 – 4.12)	281 (157 – 433)	2,794
2003–2004	4.58 (4.19 – 5.01)	<LOD	4.09 (3.55 – 4.58)	201 (185 – 271)	2,581
2005–2006	4.59 (4.04 – 5.21)	<LOD	3.66 (3.12 – 4.41)	211 (182 – 326)	2,528
Age group					
6–11 years					
1999–2000	6.00 (4.04 – 8.91)	<LOD	7.13 (4.26 – 16.0)	172 (98.0 – 264)	287
2001–2002	7.03 (5.05 – 9.77)	<LOD	6.47 (4.28 – 11.4)	302 (155 – 468)	396
2003–2004	6.73 (4.55 – 9.97)	.389 (<LOD – .743)	5.92 (4.10 – 8.22)	146 (88.9 – 382)	341
2005–2006	7.93 (5.73 – 11.0)	<LOD	7.15 (3.86 – 11.3)	340 (253 – 495)	351
12–19 years					
1999–2000	4.13 (2.33 – 7.35)	<LOD	5.68 (2.94 – 11.0)	117 (77.3 – 337)	667
2001–2002	4.57 (3.44 – 6.07)	<LOD	3.86 (2.87 – 5.32)	249 (134 – 331)	744
2003–2004	4.76 (3.71 – 6.11)	<LOD	4.25 (3.22 – 6.13)	182 (119 – 269)	729
2005–2006	6.30 (4.89 – 8.13)	.274 (<LOD – .304)	5.67 (3.60 – 8.37)	251 (127 – 705)	693
20–39 years					
1999–2000	3.18 (2.13 – 4.76)	<LOD	3.53 (2.09 – 5.26)	226 (165 – 272)	481
2001–2002	2.72 (2.10 – 3.51)	<LOD	2.06 (1.55 – 2.97)	152 (99.5 – 442)	604
2003–2004	3.55 (2.86 – 4.40)	<LOD	2.98 (2.24 – 3.75)	214 (114 – 434)	546
2005–2006	3.47 (2.84 – 4.25)	<LOD	3.22 (2.11 – 4.37)	166 (136 – 207)	583
40–59 years					
1999–2000	4.26 (3.27 – 5.56)	<LOD	3.57 (2.42 – 6.26)	156 (133 – 261)	365
2001–2002	5.04 (3.50 – 7.26)	<LOD	4.39 (2.65 – 7.23)	473 (212 – 885)	531
2003–2004	4.93 (4.19 – 5.80)	<LOD	4.29 (3.06 – 6.30)	227 (190 – 612)	450
2005–2006	4.09 (3.19 – 5.24)	<LOD	3.01 (2.16 – 4.19)	259 (189 – 800)	449
60 years and older					
1999–2000	4.66 (3.13 – 6.94)	<LOD	6.37 (3.15 – 11.3)	104 (81.6 – 172)	471
2001–2002	2.75 (2.14 – 3.52)	<LOD	1.86 (1.30 – 2.79)	150 (78.7 – 449)	519
2003–2004	4.93 (3.88 – 6.28)	<LOD	4.37 (3.20 – 6.17)	239 (136 – 418)	515
2005–2006	5.42 (4.19 – 7.02)	<LOD	4.31 (2.90 – 7.08)	244 (111 – 754)	452
Gender					
Males					
1999–2000	3.95 (2.79 – 5.58)	<LOD	4.50 (2.96 – 6.47)	209 (130 – 265)	1,087
2001–2002	3.10 (2.48 – 3.86)	<LOD	2.87 (2.00 – 3.89)	152 (101 – 334)	1,375
2003–2004	3.83 (3.10 – 4.73)	<LOD	3.33 (2.45 – 4.35)	193 (128 – 255)	1,240
2005–2006	3.97 (3.33 – 4.72)	<LOD	3.48 (2.75 – 4.33)	165 (144 – 230)	1,252
Females					
1999–2000	4.10 (3.00 – 5.60)	<LOD	4.17 (3.10 – 6.33)	155 (119 – 341)	1,184
2001–2002	4.68 (3.87 – 5.68)	<LOD	3.74 (2.78 – 4.87)	398 (199 – 741)	1,419
2003–2004	5.45 (4.71 – 6.30)	<LOD	4.81 (4.08 – 5.89)	243 (194 – 318)	1,341
2005–2006	5.27 (4.56 – 6.09)	<LOD	3.98 (3.07 – 5.49)	323 (201 – 683)	1,276
Race/ethnicity					
Mexican Americans					
1999–2000	2.19 (1.49 – 3.24)	<LOD	1.87 (1.16 – 3.04)	135 (96.7 – 290)	721
2001–2002	2.30 (1.48 – 3.57)	<LOD	1.45 (.769 – 3.15)	107 (59.9 – 303)	679
2003–2004	2.30 (1.68 – 3.15)	<LOD	1.65 (.847 – 3.02)	125 (89.4 – 171)	652
2005–2006	2.75 (1.92 – 3.93)	<LOD	1.68 (1.06 – 2.91)	134 (74.9 – 204)	634
Non-Hispanic Blacks					
1999–2000	3.65 (2.92 – 4.57)	<LOD	5.21 (3.70 – 6.74)	117 (83.6 – 283)	527
2001–2002	3.75 (2.75 – 5.11)	<LOD	3.54 (2.13 – 5.48)	217 (102 – 371)	692
2003–2004	3.90 (3.02 – 5.04)	<LOD	3.13 (1.94 – 5.59)	146 (127 – 231)	680
2005–2006	4.09 (3.13 – 5.34)	<LOD	4.20 (2.48 – 5.69)	207 (113 – 454)	662
Non-Hispanic Whites					
1999–2000	4.48 (3.11 – 6.47)	<LOD	4.72 (2.91 – 7.48)	178 (148 – 227)	810
2001–2002	4.08 (3.41 – 4.88)	<LOD	3.51 (2.46 – 4.57)	300 (158 – 505)	1,211
2003–2004	5.18 (4.71 – 5.70)	<LOD	4.58 (4.15 – 5.31)	225 (189 – 308)	1,061
2005–2006	4.96 (4.33 – 5.69)	<LOD	3.96 (3.28 – 4.67)	227 (184 – 333)	1,039

< LOD means less than the limit of detection for the uncorrected urine values, which may vary for some compounds by year. See Appendix D for LOD.

Figure 4.8.b. Urinary O–desmethylangolensin (creatinine corrected): Concentrations by survey cycle

Selected percentiles in µg/g creatinine (95% confidence intervals), National Health and Nutrition Examination Survey, 1999–2006

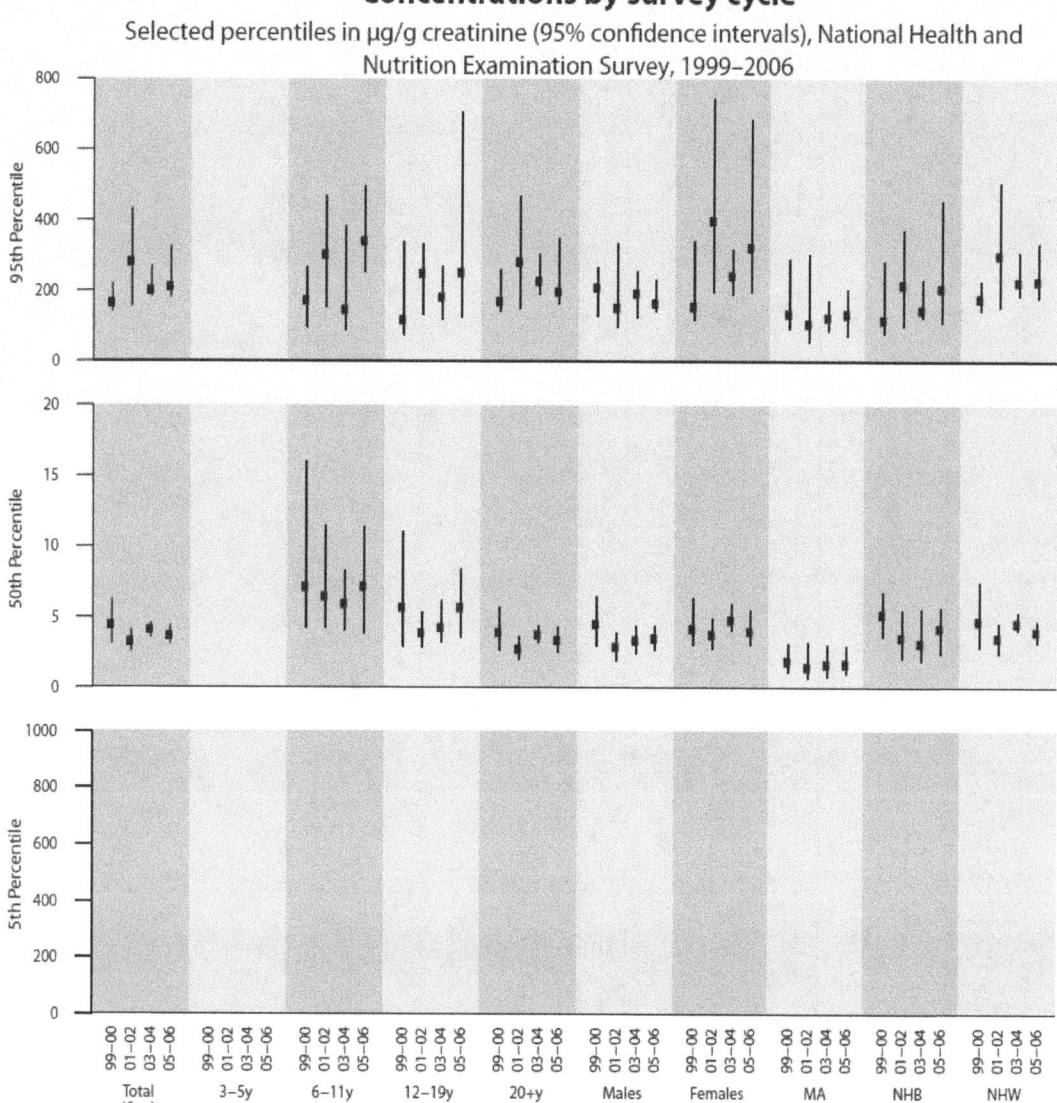

Values in the graph are suppressed if either the point estimate or the lower 95% confidence limit is noted as "< LOD" in the accompanying table.

Table 4.9.a.1. Urinary enterodiol: Concentrations

Geometric mean and selected percentiles of urine concentrations (in µg/L) for the total U.S. population aged 6 years and older, National Health and Nutrition Examination Survey, 2003–2006.

	Geometric mean (95% conf. interval)	Selected percentiles (95% conf. interval)						Sample size
		2.5th	5th	50th	95th	97.5th		
Total, 6 years and older	38.6 (35.8 – 41.6)	.745 (.399 – 1.29)	2.48 (1.79 – 3.01)	43.9 (41.1 – 47.2)	377 (335 – 414)	579 (496 – 683)		5,122
Age group								
6–11 years	37.4 (32.2 – 43.3)	2.24 (.856 – 4.39)	5.43 (2.74 – 6.96)	40.2 (35.8 – 45.4)	265 (199 – 357)	387 (335 – 558)		692
12–19 years	42.0 (38.3 – 46.1)	2.23 (.927 – 3.06)	5.16 (2.97 – 6.05)	44.2 (39.5 – 50.3)	295 (267 – 354)	462 (374 – 656)		1,422
20–39 years	39.2 (34.7 – 44.2)	.763 (.392 – 1.50)	2.70 (1.49 – 3.87)	43.7 (39.7 – 49.9)	365 (314 – 494)	651 (493 – 1,350)		1,137
40–59 years	37.2 (31.3 – 44.1)	< LOD	1.72 (.528 – 2.44)	44.8 (37.6 – 51.6)	423 (330 – 512)	658 (462 – 1,250)		901
60 years and older	38.5 (34.3 – 43.2)	.478 (< LOD – 1.61)	2.42 (1.28 – 3.37)	44.9 (38.9 – 52.6)	362 (301 – 475)	620 (442 – 1,140)		970
Gender								
Males	40.1 (35.9 – 44.7)	.697 (< LOD – 1.29)	2.49 (1.47 – 3.72)	45.9 (41.2 – 49.2)	382 (308 – 453)	585 (457 – 1,060)		2,496
Females	37.2 (33.7 – 41.1)	.813 (< LOD – 1.60)	2.44 (1.59 – 3.02)	42.3 (39.6 – 45.9)	356 (307 – 446)	561 (464 – 712)		2,626
Race/ethnicity								
Mexican Americans	35.6 (31.2 – 40.5)	.899 (< LOD – 1.78)	2.41 (1.70 – 2.94)	39.9 (35.5 – 44.6)	359 (287 – 434)	457 (392 – 890)		1,287
Non-Hispanic Blacks	37.4 (33.8 – 41.3)	1.02 (< LOD – 1.65)	2.90 (2.15 – 3.51)	43.1 (38.4 – 47.4)	275 (249 – 348)	438 (372 – 517)		1,343
Non-Hispanic Whites	38.7 (34.9 – 42.8)	.640 (< LOD – 1.36)	2.44 (1.49 – 3.41)	44.2 (40.2 – 49.6)	367 (310 – 423)	575 (480 – 701)		2,108

< LOD means less than the limit of detection, which may vary for some compounds by year. See Appendix D for LOD.

Figure 4.9.a. Urinary enterodiol: Concentrations by age group

Geometric mean (95% confidence interval), National Health and Nutrition Examination Survey, 2003–2006

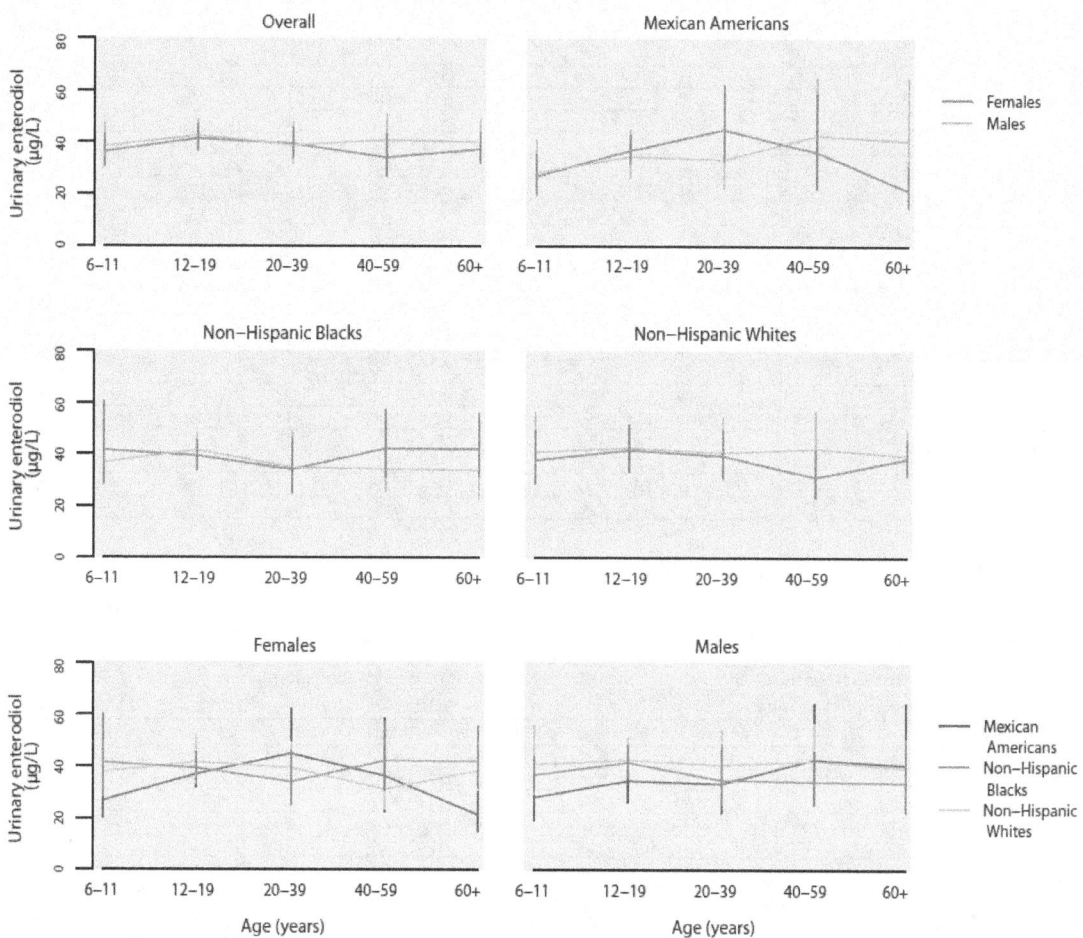

Table 4.9.a.2. Urinary enterodiol: Total population

Geometric mean and selected percentiles of urine concentrations (in µg/L) for the total U.S. population aged 6 years and older, National Health and Nutrition Examination Survey, 2003–2006.

	Geometric mean (95% conf. interval)	Selected percentiles (95% conf. interval)			Sample size
		10th	50th	90th	
Males and Females					
Total, 6 years and older	38.6 (35.8 – 41.6)	5.86 (4.78 – 6.69)	43.9 (41.1 – 47.2)	243 (231 – 260)	5,122
6–11 years	37.4 (32.2 – 43.3)	8.10 (6.48 – 9.64)	40.2 (35.8 – 45.4)	150 (126 – 204)	692
12–19 years	42.0 (38.3 – 46.1)	8.12 (6.76 – 9.75)	44.2 (39.5 – 50.3)	192 (168 – 229)	1,422
20–39 years	39.2 (34.7 – 44.2)	5.37 (4.41 – 6.89)	43.7 (39.7 – 49.9)	237 (216 – 267)	1,137
40–59 years	37.2 (31.3 – 44.1)	3.96 (2.46 – 6.11)	44.8 (37.6 – 51.6)	266 (250 – 284)	901
60 years and older	38.5 (34.3 – 43.2)	5.80 (3.81 – 6.96)	44.9 (38.9 – 52.6)	256 (219 – 280)	970
Males					
Total, 6 years and older	40.1 (35.9 – 44.7)	6.59 (5.15 – 7.44)	45.9 (41.2 – 49.2)	255 (228 – 269)	2,496
6–11 years	38.4 (31.1 – 47.5)	8.71 (5.91 – 13.1)	39.7 (34.8 – 47.9)	144 (119 – 267)	340
12–19 years	42.6 (37.3 – 48.7)	8.25 (6.58 – 10.2)	48.4 (38.5 – 56.4)	196 (170 – 250)	728
20–39 years	38.9 (31.6 – 47.9)	5.61 (3.56 – 7.73)	43.8 (36.7 – 50.8)	236 (202 – 293)	499
40–59 years	40.8 (32.8 – 50.7)	5.03 (2.54 – 8.69)	47.7 (38.3 – 54.0)	279 (261 – 332)	451
60 years and older	40.1 (33.1 – 48.7)	6.13 (4.41 – 7.48)	50.2 (41.1 – 56.3)	256 (210 – 307)	478
Females					
Total, 6 years and older	37.2 (33.7 – 41.1)	5.09 (4.12 – 6.40)	42.3 (39.6 – 45.9)	237 (211 – 262)	2,626
6–11 years	36.3 (30.5 – 43.1)	7.66 (5.98 – 9.58)	40.7 (32.9 – 49.6)	157 (120 – 220)	352
12–19 years	41.4 (36.8 – 46.6)	8.00 (5.89 – 10.0)	41.9 (37.7 – 46.4)	181 (155 – 221)	694
20–39 years	39.4 (34.2 – 45.5)	4.90 (4.25 – 6.75)	43.7 (39.8 – 53.3)	243 (209 – 301)	638
40–59 years	34.1 (27.1 – 42.9)	3.31 (1.49 – 5.80)	41.6 (34.4 – 51.5)	244 (205 – 278)	450
60 years and older	37.3 (31.9 – 43.6)	4.59 (2.99 – 6.98)	42.3 (33.7 – 51.7)	255 (204 – 302)	492

Table 4.9.a.3. Urinary enterodiol: Mexican Americans

Geometric mean and selected percentiles of urine concentrations (in µg/L) for Mexican Americans in the U.S. population aged 6 years and older, National Health and Nutrition Examination Survey, 2003–2006.

	Geometric mean (95% conf. interval)	Selected percentiles (95% conf. interval)			Sample size
		10th	50th	90th	
Males and Females					
Total, 6 years and older	35.6 (31.2 – 40.5)	4.89 (4.22 – 5.85)	39.9 (35.5 – 44.6)	227 (182 – 294)	1,287
6–11 years	27.4 (21.8 – 34.5)	2.79 (1.96 – 5.28)	33.0 (24.6 – 40.2)	166 (130 – 245)	231
12–19 years	35.6 (30.9 – 41.1)	5.80 (3.99 – 8.54)	42.0 (34.8 – 48.2)	178 (141 – 203)	445
20–39 years	38.2 (29.5 – 49.6)	5.52 (3.85 – 7.09)	41.8 (31.6 – 52.4)	245 (183 – 438)	282
40–59 years	39.5 (28.6 – 54.5)	5.19 (1.73 – 11.5)	41.1 (31.9 – 53.6)	272 (192 – 385)	157
60 years and older	28.4 (22.0 – 36.8)	3.31 (1.54 – 5.74)	35.1 (22.0 – 49.2)	165 (111 – 340)	172
Males					
Total, 6 years and older	34.9 (28.8 – 42.2)	4.34 (3.14 – 6.04)	43.3 (35.6 – 49.9)	206 (165 – 288)	625
6–11 years	28.1 (19.2 – 40.9)	2.97 (.785 – 7.94)	34.7 (22.8 – 48.2)	135 (92.4 – 185)	112
12–19 years	34.5 (26.5 – 45.0)	4.74 (2.34 – 9.50)	41.5 (30.3 – 52.8)	189 (126 – 266)	228
20–39 years	33.4 (22.2 – 50.1)	4.48 (.741 – 7.36)	42.6 (24.6 – 55.0)	204 (135 – 414)	117
40–59 years	42.7† (28.2 – 64.6)	4.04† (< LOD – 14.4)	51.2 (32.8 – 64.8)	256† (170 – 404)	85
60 years and older	40.6 (25.5 – 64.6)	4.67† (2.24 – 6.33)	42.7 (19.6 – 89.1)	222† (160 – 2,850)	83
Females					
Total, 6 years and older	36.3 (32.0 – 41.2)	5.48 (4.68 – 6.52)	37.1 (31.4 – 42.1)	238 (185 – 325)	662
6–11 years	26.7 (20.1 – 35.4)	2.49 (1.71 – 4.92)	30.5 (20.3 – 43.1)	196 (136 – 335)	119
12–19 years	36.9 (32.0 – 42.4)	7.51 (5.16 – 9.36)	42.2 (35.0 – 53.7)	162 (118 – 195)	217
20–39 years	44.9 (32.5 – 62.1)	6.26 (3.86 – 9.31)	41.4 (27.8 – 61.5)	306 (193 – 937)	165
40–59 years	36.3 (22.5 – 58.5)	5.97† (< LOD – 11.6)	31.7 (19.0 – 59.2)	274† (189 – 476)	72
60 years and older	21.3 (15.0 – 30.3)	2.49† (.826 – 4.86)	28.1 (16.1 – 45.6)	115† (67.5 – 254)	89

< LOD means less than the limit of detection, which may vary for some compounds by year. See Appendix D for LOD.

† Estimate is subject to greater uncertainty due to small cell size.

Table 4.9.a.4. Urinary enterodiol: Non-Hispanic blacks

Geometric mean and selected percentiles of urine concentrations (in µg/L) for non-Hispanic blacks in the U.S. population aged 6 years and older, National Health and Nutrition Examination Survey, 2003–2006.

	Geometric mean (95% conf. interval)	Selected percentiles (95% conf. interval)						Sample size
		10th		50th		90th		
Males and Females								
Total, 6 years and older	37.4 (33.8 – 41.3)	6.94	(5.78 – 8.13)	43.1	(38.4 – 47.4)	202	(164 – 241)	1,343
6–11 years	39.0 (32.6 – 46.6)	8.75	(7.57 – 10.9)	38.5	(32.6 – 47.4)	144	(113 – 222)	207
12–19 years	40.4 (35.4 – 45.5)	7.82	(6.32 – 10.2)	45.9	(40.2 – 53.4)	203	(158 – 252)	496
20–39 years	34.4 (28.9 – 40.8)	4.70	(2.73 – 9.26)	43.1	(30.9 – 49.3)	182	(138 – 247)	249
40–59 years	38.3 (31.0 – 47.3)	6.45	(3.55 – 9.50)	42.9	(34.8 – 56.0)	229	(159 – 306)	231
60 years and older	38.6 (29.7 – 50.2)	5.01	(2.37 – 11.3)	41.5	(33.1 – 54.2)	213	(143 – 308)	160
Males								
Total, 6 years and older	35.8 (31.0 – 41.4)	7.23	(5.38 – 9.93)	41.2	(37.1 – 44.8)	199	(145 – 256)	661
6–11 years	36.7 (30.6 – 44.0)	8.71†	(5.22 – 12.3)	37.6	(32.5 – 45.6)	130†	(93.9 – 271)	99
12–19 years	41.5 (35.7 – 48.2)	8.60	(6.42 – 10.6)	46.0	(36.3 – 56.7)	220	(161 – 274)	258
20–39 years	34.8 (25.0 – 48.5)	9.49	(1.28 – 12.7)	42.3	(28.4 – 49.0)	194	(117 – 649)	116
40–59 years	34.2 (25.5 – 45.8)	6.41	(.424 – 11.2)	40.1	(31.0 – 51.0)	181	(103 – 339)	114
60 years and older	33.8 (22.6 – 50.5)	3.16†	(< LOD – 9.91)	38.8	(22.4 – 60.4)	235†	(178 – 506)	74
Females								
Total, 6 years and older	38.8 (33.8 – 44.5)	6.71	(4.70 – 8.09)	45.3	(36.5 – 52.9)	209	(159 – 246)	682
6–11 years	41.5 (28.5 – 60.3)	8.80†	(5.57 – 12.1)	38.5	(25.1 – 63.3)	162†	(105 – 734)	108
12–19 years	39.3 (34.1 – 45.3)	7.36	(4.62 – 10.8)	45.8	(38.4 – 54.9)	181	(148 – 227)	238
20–39 years	34.0 (25.1 – 45.9)	4.44	(1.93 – 7.72)	43.6	(29.2 – 57.8)	163	(129 – 250)	133
40–59 years	42.1 (31.0 – 57.1)	6.38	(3.20 – 9.27)	47.1	(30.4 – 65.8)	241	(167 – 440)	117
60 years and older	42.0 (31.7 – 55.6)	8.15†	(2.80 – 14.6)	44.5	(31.8 – 61.6)	173†	(120 – 404)	86

< LOD means less than the limit of detection, which may vary for some compounds by year. See Appendix D for LOD.

† Estimate is subject to greater uncertainty due to small cell size.

Table 4.9.a.5. Urinary enterodiol: Non-Hispanic whites

Geometric mean and selected percentiles of urine concentrations (in µg/L) for non-Hispanic whites in the U.S. population aged 6 years and older, National Health and Nutrition Examination Survey, 2003–2006.

	Geometric mean (95% conf. interval)	Selected percentiles (95% conf. interval)						Sample size
		10th		50th		90th		
Males and Females								
Total, 6 years and older	38.7 (34.9 – 42.8)	5.87	(4.61 – 6.90)	44.2	(40.2 – 49.6)	244	(228 – 264)	2,108
6–11 years	39.3 (30.9 – 50.1)	8.74	(6.52 – 13.2)	40.4	(34.8 – 48.0)	139	(115 – 232)	193
12–19 years	42.1 (36.3 – 48.8)	8.80	(6.91 – 10.6)	42.8	(36.5 – 54.4)	176	(154 – 230)	378
20–39 years	40.0 (33.4 – 47.9)	5.42	(4.12 – 7.14)	43.8	(36.4 – 55.7)	238	(207 – 296)	494
40–59 years	36.3 (29.2 – 45.1)	3.71	(2.29 – 6.10)	45.2	(35.6 – 54.8)	264	(243 – 281)	448
60 years and older	38.8 (34.2 – 43.9)	5.91	(3.70 – 7.29)	46.0	(38.9 – 56.1)	258	(213 – 280)	595
Males								
Total, 6 years and older	41.1 (35.5 – 47.6)	6.75	(5.23 – 8.72)	46.4	(40.6 – 52.7)	259	(222 – 275)	1,035
6–11 years	40.8 (29.6 – 56.1)	9.08†	(4.58 – 17.3)	39.9	(32.8 – 49.3)	129†	(109 – 356)	99
12–19 years	42.5 (35.6 – 50.7)	9.11	(6.18 – 11.8)	48.2	(36.1 – 57.6)	176	(148 – 252)	191
20–39 years	40.6 (30.3 – 54.3)	5.50	(3.34 – 9.65)	43.8	(33.6 – 59.1)	238	(184 – 394)	217
40–59 years	42.2 (31.6 – 56.5)	5.30	(2.37 – 10.1)	48.1	(36.7 – 58.2)	280	(259 – 415)	229
60 years and older	39.4 (31.3 – 49.4)	6.58	(4.37 – 8.47)	50.3	(40.5 – 56.9)	246	(182 – 286)	299
Females								
Total, 6 years and older	36.4 (31.6 – 41.9)	4.79	(3.03 – 6.57)	42.3	(38.0 – 49.9)	240	(201 – 273)	1,073
6–11 years	37.7 (28.8 – 49.2)	7.98†	(2.17 – 11.7)	41.0	(29.3 – 54.4)	155†	(94.9 – 369)	94
12–19 years	41.6 (33.6 – 51.6)	8.15	(5.01 – 13.4)	40.1	(34.9 – 51.0)	174	(131 – 278)	187
20–39 years	39.4 (31.4 – 49.4)	4.87	(3.72 – 7.60)	46.0	(34.2 – 56.9)	236	(183 – 332)	277
40–59 years	31.2 (23.5 – 41.4)	2.52	(.780 – 5.15)	40.5	(31.0 – 55.4)	242	(189 – 276)	219
60 years and older	38.3 (32.0 – 45.8)	4.66	(2.91 – 7.14)	44.6	(33.4 – 58.2)	263	(207 – 309)	296

† Estimate is subject to greater uncertainty due to small cell size.

Table 4.9.b. Urinary enterodiol: Concentrations by survey cycle

Geometric mean and selected percentiles of urine concentrations (in µg/L) for the U.S. population, National Health and Nutrition Examination Survey, 1999–2006.

	Geometric mean (95% conf. interval)	Selected percentiles (95% conf. interval) 5th		Selected percentiles (95% conf. interval) 50th		Selected percentiles (95% conf. interval) 95th		Sample size
Total, 6 years and older								
1999–2000	26.6 (21.9 – 32.3)	< LOD		33.9 (29.5 – 38.7)		263 (219 – 338)		2,527
2001–2002	35.7 (32.5 – 39.3)	2.10 (< LOD – 3.07)		39.3 (36.4 – 43.1)		253 (225 – 307)		2,794
2003–2004	39.5 (36.1 – 43.3)	2.45 (1.76 – 2.91)		44.8 (40.7 – 50.3)		367 (318 – 424)		2,594
2005–2006	37.7 (33.2 – 42.9)	2.47 (.884 – 3.82)		42.4 (39.3 – 47.2)		378 (316 – 447)		2,528
Age group								
6–11 years								
1999–2000	26.5 (17.1 – 41.0)	< LOD		29.3 (21.2 – 43.4)		272 (203 – 477)		327
2001–2002	33.6 (29.8 – 37.8)	3.40 (1.90 – 5.06)		35.5 (29.4 – 43.5)		202 (170 – 333)		396
2003–2004	42.0 (34.5 – 51.1)	6.62 (2.92 – 8.30)		42.0 (34.6 – 49.1)		311 (230 – 523)		341
2005–2006	33.2 (26.1 – 42.3)	2.86 (1.71 – 6.66)		38.5 (34.7 – 44.3)		178 (136 – 377)		351
12–19 years								
1999–2000	29.8 (23.8 – 37.2)	< LOD		34.0 (27.8 – 42.0)		252 (193 – 357)		744
2001–2002	35.3 (30.5 – 40.9)	3.30 (2.02 – 5.23)		37.6 (34.8 – 42.9)		235 (172 – 344)		744
2003–2004	45.1 (39.4 – 51.6)	5.28 (3.63 – 6.65)		46.2 (38.8 – 56.8)		324 (276 – 416)		729
2005–2006	39.1 (34.0 – 45.0)	4.19 (1.72 – 6.24)		41.0 (36.8 – 46.4)		264 (232 – 367)		693
20–39 years								
1999–2000	27.4 (22.1 – 34.1)	< LOD		36.0 (29.9 – 41.3)		230 (177 – 401)		535
2001–2002	35.3 (29.5 – 42.3)	< LOD		42.5 (36.6 – 47.6)		244 (213 – 371)		604
2003–2004	39.7 (33.2 – 47.5)	2.69 (1.32 – 3.59)		44.5 (37.7 – 53.9)		372 (308 – 654)		554
2005–2006	38.6 (32.3 – 46.2)	3.01 (1.16 – 4.28)		43.5 (34.5 – 53.8)		352 (289 – 519)		583
40–59 years								
1999–2000	26.1 (21.4 – 31.8)	< LOD		34.6 (28.9 – 41.2)		280 (249 – 406)		414
2001–2002	37.3 (29.2 – 47.7)	< LOD		40.5 (34.5 – 50.9)		289 (232 – 488)		531
2003–2004	35.3 (28.6 – 43.6)	1.36 (< LOD – 2.16)		42.6 (36.3 – 50.6)		418 (283 – 712)		452
2005–2006	39.0 (29.4 – 51.8)	2.30 (< LOD – 4.32)		45.9 (34.1 – 59.0)		445 (287 – 651)		449
60 years and older								
1999–2000	23.7 (18.8 – 30.0)	< LOD		29.7 (21.9 – 37.4)		264 (167 – 479)		507
2001–2002	35.4 (30.0 – 41.8)	2.87 (1.55 – 4.49)		36.5 (30.2 – 46.0)		224 (195 – 364)		519
2003–2004	41.7 (36.7 – 47.4)	2.84 (1.82 – 4.35)		50.8 (43.2 – 58.3)		309 (265 – 615)		518
2005–2006	35.6 (29.0 – 43.8)	1.66 (< LOD – 3.05)		39.9 (31.1 – 51.8)		415 (322 – 614)		452
Gender								
Males								
1999–2000	25.3 (19.5 – 32.7)	< LOD		33.0 (28.0 – 37.9)		258 (179 – 324)		1,206
2001–2002	35.2 (31.8 – 39.1)	< LOD		40.4 (36.8 – 44.2)		263 (225 – 351)		1,375
2003–2004	39.7 (36.2 – 43.6)	2.43 (.998 – 3.97)		45.1 (40.6 – 50.6)		360 (275 – 515)		1,244
2005–2006	40.4 (32.8 – 49.8)	2.64 (.957 – 4.13)		46.1 (39.1 – 52.0)		413 (291 – 544)		1,252
Females								
1999–2000	27.9 (23.4 – 33.3)	< LOD		36.0 (29.9 – 40.2)		280 (228 – 397)		1,321
2001–2002	36.2 (32.2 – 40.7)	3.20 (< LOD – 4.75)		38.5 (35.3 – 43.4)		246 (222 – 286)		1,419
2003–2004	39.3 (33.8 – 45.5)	2.60 (1.33 – 3.36)		44.8 (38.5 – 52.7)		396 (313 – 485)		1,350
2005–2006	35.4 (30.3 – 41.2)	2.43 (.524 – 3.72)		41.0 (35.7 – 45.3)		338 (272 – 477)		1,276
Race/ethnicity								
Mexican Americans								
1999–2000	21.7 (19.5 – 24.1)	< LOD		27.9 (24.6 – 34.6)		212 (171 – 258)		791
2001–2002	30.5 (25.7 – 36.3)	1.62 (< LOD – 2.79)		33.8 (29.0 – 39.1)		240 (198 – 304)		679
2003–2004	33.1 (26.4 – 41.6)	1.90 (< LOD – 3.68)		38.5 (31.7 – 47.1)		298 (201 – 4,230)		653
2005–2006	38.1 (32.2 – 45.1)	2.60 (1.91 – 3.84)		40.5 (35.4 – 47.5)		382 (295 – 514)		634
Non-Hispanic Blacks								
1999–2000	25.7 (21.5 – 30.6)	< LOD		31.2 (24.4 – 35.9)		266 (219 – 356)		597
2001–2002	35.1 (28.8 – 42.8)	2.08 (< LOD – 3.42)		38.8 (33.3 – 49.8)		222 (178 – 386)		692
2003–2004	40.3 (34.7 – 46.8)	3.23 (1.48 – 4.64)		47.2 (40.7 – 54.4)		284 (244 – 442)		681
2005–2006	34.7 (30.1 – 40.1)	2.73 (2.01 – 3.30)		38.4 (33.3 – 45.1)		268 (248 – 382)		662
Non-Hispanic Whites								
1999–2000	29.1 (24.2 – 35.1)	< LOD		37.5 (31.6 – 43.7)		271 (219 – 401)		899
2001–2002	35.6 (31.8 – 40.0)	1.82 (< LOD – 3.21)		40.4 (36.5 – 44.7)		254 (219 – 341)		1,211
2003–2004	40.1 (35.6 – 45.1)	2.64 (1.59 – 3.48)		45.9 (38.9 – 55.3)		368 (305 – 441)		1,069
2005–2006	37.3 (31.2 – 44.6)	2.36 (.472 – 3.81)		42.6 (37.1 – 49.6)		366 (286 – 456)		1,039

< LOD means less than the limit of detection, which may vary for some compounds by year. See Appendix D for LOD.

Figure 4.9.b. Urinary enterodiol: Concentrations by survey cycle

Selected percentiles in μg/L (95% confidence intervals), National Health and
Nutrition Examination Survey, 1999–2006

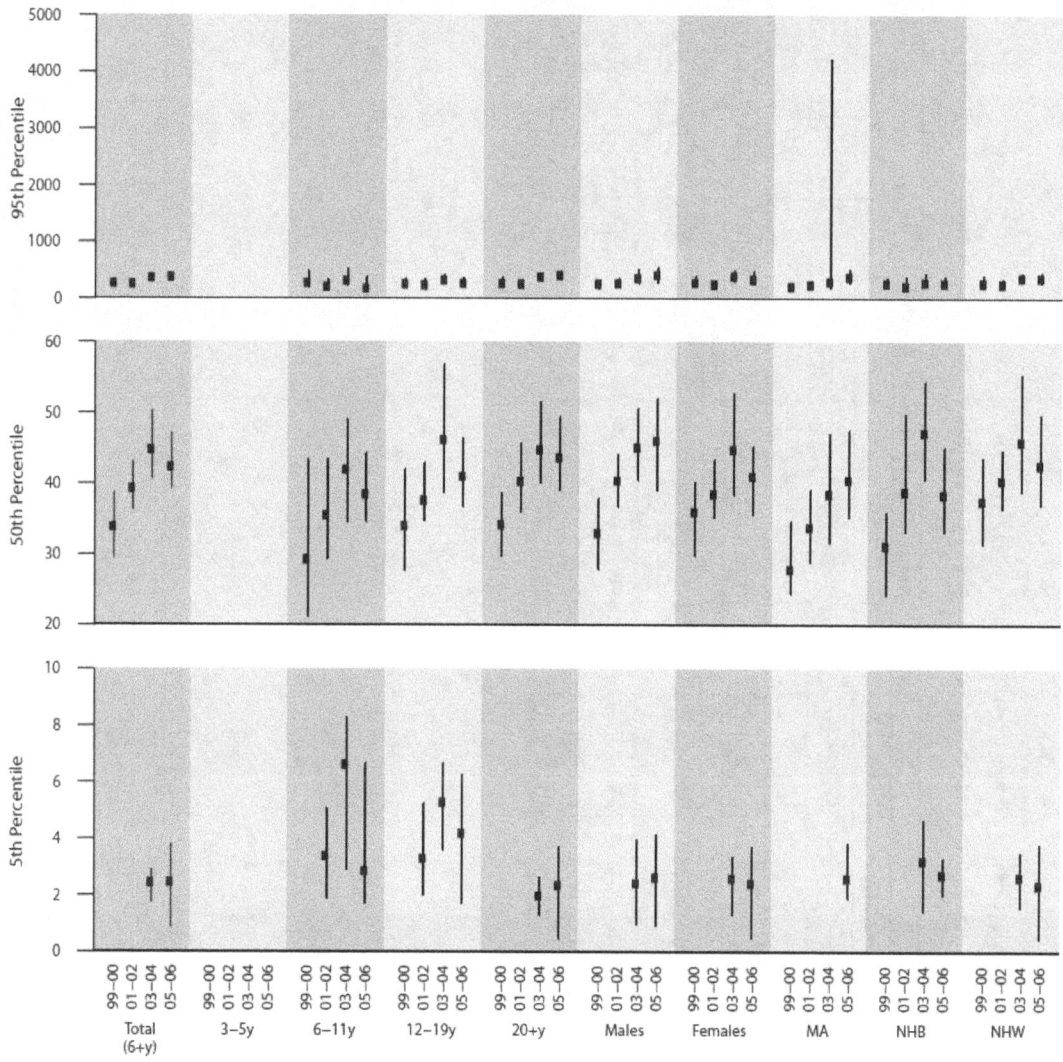

Values in the graph are suppressed if either the point estimate or the lower 95% confidence limit is noted as "< LOD" in the accompanying table.

Table 4.10.a.1. Urinary enterodiol (creatinine corrected): Concentrations

Geometric mean and selected percentiles of urine concentrations (in µg/g creatinine) for the total U.S. population aged 6 years and older, National Health and Nutrition Examination Survey, 2003–2006.

	Geometric mean (95% conf. interval)	Selected percentiles (95% conf. interval)						Sample size
		2.5th	5th	50th	95th	97.5th	
Total, 6 years and older	36.9 (34.3 – 39.7)	.909 (.427 – 1.35)	2.69 (1.93 – 3.70)	41.1 (38.2 – 44.1)	309 (283 – 360)	501 (440 – 716)	5,122
Age group							
6–11 years	40.5 (35.1 – 46.7)	3.41 (1.25 – 4.93)	6.16 (3.95 – 7.30)	43.6 (38.1 – 48.1)	216 (198 – 311)	367 (267 – 589)	692
12–19 years	31.3 (28.7 – 34.1)	1.87 (.883 – 2.78)	3.58 (2.79 – 4.68)	33.6 (31.9 – 36.1)	186 (163 – 232)	278 (220 – 542)	1,422
20–39 years	33.4 (29.3 – 38.1)	.793 (.250 – 1.49)	2.29 (1.52 – 2.99)	34.9 (31.6 – 43.0)	301 (244 – 400)	492 (366 – 808)	1,137
40–59 years	37.6 (31.8 – 44.5)	< LOD	1.75 (.889 – 3.41)	42.7 (36.6 – 50.2)	376 (286 – 491)	686 (438 – 1,530)	901
60 years and older	45.1 (39.9 – 50.9)	.610 (< LOD – 1.82)	4.15 (1.05 – 5.93)	51.0 (47.1 – 55.6)	386 (290 – 539)	556 (469 – 1,500)	970
Gender							
Males	31.8 (28.5 – 35.5)	.588 (< LOD – 1.30)	2.25 (1.31 – 3.67)	34.6 (32.0 – 38.0)	280 (233 – 338)	445 (331 – 789)	2,496
Females	42.5 (38.9 – 46.4)	.975 (< LOD – 1.86)	2.95 (2.22 – 4.19)	48.4 (45.0 – 54.6)	375 (296 – 432)	563 (445 – 852)	2,626
Race/ethnicity							
Mexican Americans	32.1 (27.9 – 36.9)	1.20 (< LOD – 1.87)	2.67 (1.62 – 3.47)	35.1 (30.5 – 39.3)	305 (239 – 375)	431 (337 – 876)	1,287
Non-Hispanic Blacks	26.3 (23.5 – 29.3)	.859 (< LOD – 1.10)	2.60 (1.56 – 3.18)	27.8 (24.9 – 31.4)	196 (165 – 218)	276 (224 – 353)	1,343
Non-Hispanic Whites	39.4 (35.5 – 43.6)	.849 (< LOD – 1.40)	2.87 (1.86 – 4.12)	45.4 (40.8 – 49.6)	315 (287 – 375)	508 (438 – 736)	2,108

< LOD means less than the limit of detection for the uncorrected urine values, which may vary for some compounds by year. See Appendix D for LOD.

Figure 4.10.a. Urinary enterodiol (creatinine corrected): Concentrations by age group

Geometric mean (95% confidence interval), National Health and Nutrition Examination Survey, 2003–2006

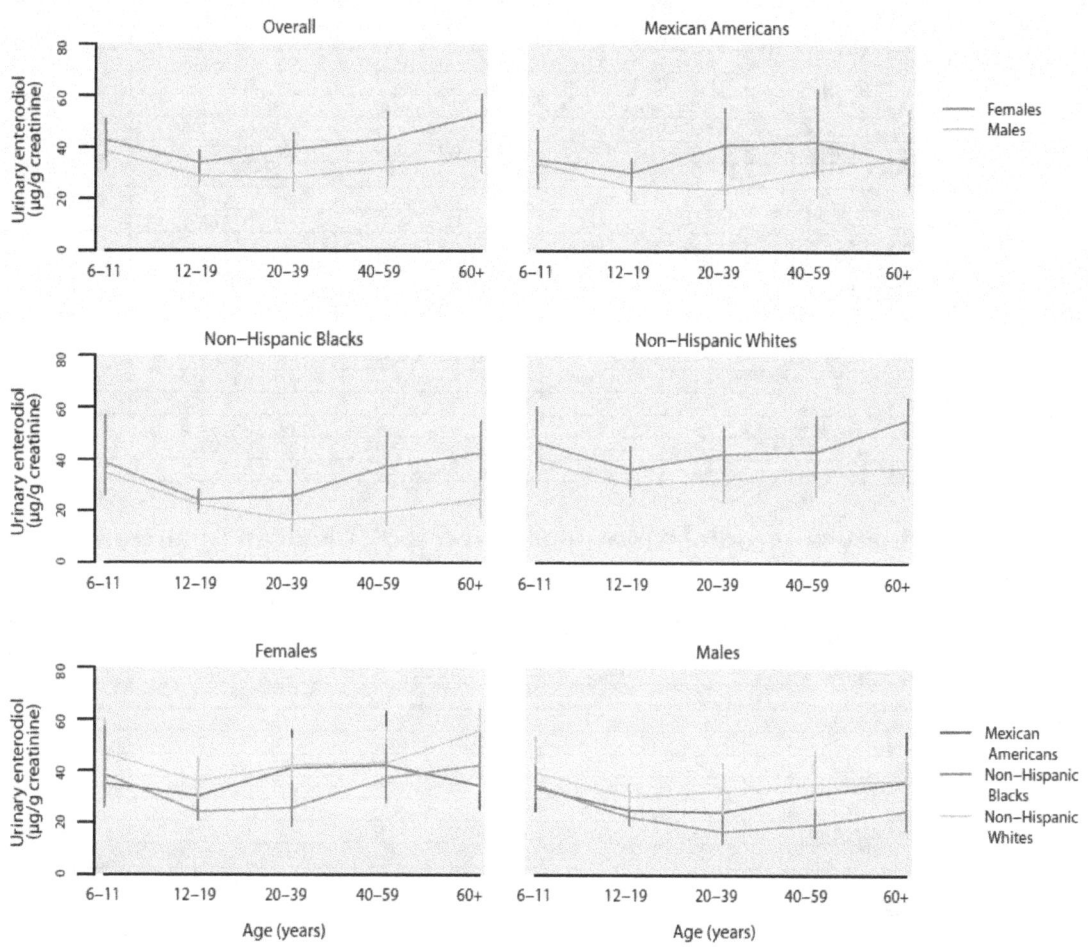

Table 4.10.a.2. Urinary enterodiol (creatinine corrected): Total population

Geometric mean and selected percentiles of urine concentrations (in μg/g creatinine) for the total U.S. population aged 6 years and older, National Health and Nutrition Examination Survey, 2003–2006.

	Geometric mean (95% conf. interval)		Selected percentiles (95% conf. interval)						Sample size
			10th		50th		90th		
Males and Females									
Total, 6 years and older	36.9	(34.3 – 39.7)	6.26	(5.53 – 7.25)	41.1	(38.2 – 44.1)	202	(185 – 213)	5,122
6–11 years	40.5	(35.1 – 46.7)	8.85	(6.90 – 12.2)	43.6	(38.1 – 48.1)	166	(134 – 201)	692
12–19 years	31.3	(28.7 – 34.1)	6.90	(5.55 – 8.00)	33.6	(31.9 – 36.1)	130	(117 – 154)	1,422
20–39 years	33.4	(29.3 – 38.1)	5.04	(4.01 – 6.33)	34.9	(31.6 – 43.0)	185	(156 – 230)	1,137
40–59 years	37.6	(31.8 – 44.5)	5.64	(3.76 – 7.61)	42.7	(36.6 – 50.2)	217	(201 – 275)	901
60 years and older	45.1	(39.9 – 50.9)	7.91	(6.45 – 9.98)	51.0	(47.1 – 55.6)	228	(198 – 290)	970
Males									
Total, 6 years and older	31.8	(28.5 – 35.5)	5.68	(4.73 – 6.43)	34.6	(32.0 – 38.0)	176	(150 – 210)	2,496
6–11 years	38.5	(31.7 – 46.9)	8.54	(6.17 – 13.0)	38.3	(33.3 – 46.1)	144	(117 – 205)	340
12–19 years	28.9	(25.7 – 32.5)	5.59	(5.19 – 7.40)	32.6	(28.5 – 34.9)	123	(113 – 134)	728
20–39 years	28.3	(23.0 – 34.9)	4.69	(3.28 – 5.94)	29.9	(25.6 – 35.5)	152	(128 – 253)	499
40–59 years	32.3	(25.6 – 40.8)	5.53	(3.19 – 7.12)	33.7	(28.4 – 43.1)	207	(158 – 305)	451
60 years and older	36.9	(30.3 – 45.1)	6.29	(4.32 – 8.00)	43.8	(38.4 – 51.5)	204	(169 – 240)	478
Females									
Total, 6 years and older	42.5	(38.9 – 46.4)	7.53	(5.73 – 8.57)	48.4	(45.0 – 54.6)	210	(198 – 234)	2,626
6–11 years	42.7	(35.9 – 50.8)	9.12	(6.71 – 12.6)	48.1	(40.3 – 57.8)	177	(140 – 218)	352
12–19 years	34.1	(30.1 – 38.5)	8.29	(4.44 – 9.54)	36.0	(32.2 – 39.7)	144	(119 – 165)	694
20–39 years	39.2	(33.9 – 45.5)	5.48	(3.87 – 7.78)	46.3	(35.7 – 57.4)	203	(165 – 243)	638
40–59 years	43.4	(35.2 – 53.6)	5.72	(2.41 – 9.51)	52.6	(42.7 – 63.1)	231	(207 – 301)	450
60 years and older	52.8	(46.0 – 60.6)	9.89	(7.70 – 11.6)	57.4	(50.4 – 65.3)	249	(201 – 407)	492

Table 4.10.a.3. Urinary enterodiol (creatinine corrected): Mexican Americans

Geometric mean and selected percentiles of urine concentrations (in μg/g creatinine) for Mexican Americans in the U.S. population aged 6 years and older, National Health and Nutrition Examination Survey, 2003–2006.

	Geometric mean (95% conf. interval)		Selected percentiles (95% conf. interval)						Sample size
			10th		50th		90th		
Males and Females									
Total, 6 years and older	32.1	(27.9 – 36.9)	4.54	(3.80 – 6.35)	35.1	(30.5 – 39.3)	185	(145 – 226)	1,287
6–11 years	34.4	(27.9 – 42.4)	5.18	(3.71 – 6.71)	37.2	(33.9 – 44.9)	178	(135 – 226)	231
12–19 years	27.5	(23.8 – 31.9)	4.55	(3.18 – 7.34)	33.6	(28.0 – 37.6)	123	(96.1 – 147)	445
20–39 years	30.9	(23.4 – 40.7)	4.02	(2.24 – 6.39)	31.1	(27.4 – 39.6)	203	(126 – 343)	282
40–59 years	36.1	(27.6 – 47.3)	5.14	(2.37 – 11.4)	35.2	(27.5 – 43.1)	234	(172 – 328)	157
60 years and older	35.1	(29.0 – 42.6)	5.53	(5.00 – 7.33)	40.9	(32.0 – 50.3)	171	(127 – 206)	172
Males									
Total, 6 years and older	27.6	(22.7 – 33.4)	3.88	(2.69 – 5.22)	33.1	(27.7 – 39.2)	145	(125 – 188)	625
6–11 years	33.6	(24.5 – 46.3)	5.54	(1.57 – 10.7)	39.3	(30.6 – 49.5)	136	(109 – 223)	112
12–19 years	25.0	(19.6 – 31.9)	3.94	(1.46 – 7.15)	31.8	(22.5 – 38.9)	128	(88.0 – 179)	228
20–39 years	24.2	(16.6 – 35.3)	3.11	(.554 – 5.48)	27.9	(20.7 – 38.8)	126	(93.7 – 316)	117
40–59 years	31.3	(21.1 – 46.5)	4.37†	(< LOD – 9.03)	36.9	(24.4 – 56.4)	151†	(125 – 326)	85
60 years and older	36.1	(23.6 – 55.3)	5.32†	(1.31 – 7.57)	42.1	(24.2 – 74.3)	180†	(111 – 3,470)	83
Females									
Total, 6 years and older	37.9	(33.8 – 42.5)	6.60	(4.51 – 9.67)	35.9	(33.1 – 40.5)	214	(182 – 310)	662
6–11 years	35.2	(26.6 – 46.6)	5.04	(3.18 – 6.59)	36.4	(28.5 – 45.9)	189	(140 – 434)	119
12–19 years	30.4	(26.0 – 35.7)	6.37	(3.16 – 9.37)	36.5	(29.2 – 40.5)	111	(87.0 – 153)	217
20–39 years	41.1	(30.3 – 55.6)	6.65	(2.66 – 10.7)	34.6	(28.4 – 43.7)	225	(156 – 1,900)	165
40–59 years	42.2	(28.5 – 62.7)	10.9†	(< LOD – 15.6)	34.7	(24.5 – 42.5)	322†	(224 – 401)	72
60 years and older	34.4	(25.4 – 46.4)	7.20†	(1.42 – 12.2)	39.5	(30.7 – 49.7)	134†	(114 – 219)	89

< LOD means less than the limit of detection for the uncorrected urine values, which may vary for some compounds by year. See Appendix D for LOD.

† Estimate is subject to greater uncertainty due to small cell size.

Table 4.10.a.4. Urinary enterodiol (creatinine corrected): Non-Hispanic blacks

Geometric mean and selected percentiles of urine concentrations (in µg/g creatinine) for non-Hispanic blacks in the U.S. population aged 6 years and older, National Health and Nutrition Examination Survey, 2003–2006.

	Geometric mean (95% conf. interval)		Selected percentiles (95% conf. interval)						Sample size
			10th		50th		90th		
Males and Females									
Total, 6 years and older	26.3	(23.5 – 29.3)	5.31	(4.24 – 6.34)	27.8	(24.9 – 31.4)	125	(110 – 152)	1,343
6–11 years	36.6	(30.6 – 43.8)	9.75	(7.92 – 11.3)	34.5	(25.8 – 45.8)	136	(108 – 215)	207
12–19 years	23.2	(20.8 – 25.8)	4.63	(3.25 – 5.70)	26.0	(23.5 – 29.3)	97.7	(86.3 – 107)	496
20–39 years	21.3	(17.7 – 25.7)	3.72	(2.11 – 6.01)	23.0	(17.8 – 28.7)	114	(101 – 145)	249
40–59 years	27.8	(22.9 – 33.9)	4.81	(3.72 – 6.10)	31.2	(25.2 – 42.5)	138	(98.2 – 207)	231
60 years and older	34.4	(27.2 – 43.5)	6.11	(3.63 – 7.83)	40.0	(25.1 – 53.3)	158	(126 – 211)	160
Males									
Total, 6 years and older	20.9	(17.8 – 24.6)	4.17	(3.10 – 5.70)	23.1	(21.0 – 25.9)	103	(84.9 – 141)	661
6–11 years	34.7	(28.7 – 41.9)	9.17†	(6.49 – 13.8)	27.8	(23.6 – 42.1)	133†	(87.7 – 254)	99
12–19 years	22.2	(19.3 – 25.5)	3.94	(2.80 – 5.30)	25.8	(22.0 – 30.4)	98.2	(78.0 – 114)	258
20–39 years	16.7	(12.1 – 23.1)	3.28	(.958 – 7.92)	15.6	(13.4 – 23.1)	98.0	(48.0 – 228)	116
40–59 years	19.5	(14.7 – 25.9)	3.83	(.303 – 5.78)	24.4	(19.1 – 30.5)	88.7	(62.6 – 143)	114
60 years and older	24.8	(17.4 – 35.3)	2.85†	(< LOD – 5.98)	29.4	(16.7 – 46.4)	154†	(105 – 375)	74
Females									
Total, 6 years and older	31.8	(27.2 – 37.1)	6.96	(4.95 – 7.88)	34.8	(28.3 – 44.5)	145	(124 – 183)	682
6–11 years	38.7	(26.3 – 56.9)	9.48†	(5.62 – 11.4)	36.2	(23.8 – 63.6)	138†	(104 – 671)	108
12–19 years	24.3	(21.1 – 27.9)	5.67	(2.69 – 8.07)	26.0	(22.5 – 31.5)	97.2	(83.9 – 118)	238
20–39 years	25.8	(18.5 – 36.1)	4.01	(1.38 – 6.49)	28.5	(21.8 – 40.2)	122	(104 – 202)	133
40–59 years	37.3	(27.8 – 50.0)	7.65	(4.05 – 10.2)	45.8	(26.5 – 61.7)	186	(131 – 262)	117
60 years and older	42.4	(32.8 – 54.7)	7.78†	(3.31 – 15.1)	42.5	(29.1 – 68.6)	157†	(127 – 219)	86

< LOD means less than the limit of detection for the uncorrected urine values, which may vary for some compounds by year. See Appendix D for LOD.
† Estimate is subject to greater uncertainty due to small cell size.

Table 4.10.a.5. Urinary enterodiol (creatinine corrected): Non-Hispanic whites

Geometric mean and selected percentiles of urine concentrations (in µg/g creatinine) for non-Hispanic whites in the U.S. population aged 6 years and older, National Health and Nutrition Examination Survey, 2003–2006.

	Geometric mean (95% conf. interval)		Selected percentiles (95% conf. interval)						Sample size
			10th		50th		90th		
Males and Females									
Total, 6 years and older	39.4	(35.5 – 43.6)	6.60	(5.58 – 8.19)	45.4	(40.8 – 49.6)	205	(186 – 224)	2,108
6–11 years	42.6	(34.0 – 53.4)	11.1	(5.34 – 16.8)	46.1	(37.0 – 52.0)	151	(121 – 226)	193
12–19 years	33.0	(28.8 – 37.8)	7.53	(5.66 – 9.35)	34.6	(31.7 – 40.5)	132	(117 – 163)	378
20–39 years	36.9	(30.1 – 45.0)	5.49	(3.01 – 7.72)	42.6	(32.9 – 54.0)	187	(154 – 248)	494
40–59 years	39.0	(31.5 – 48.3)	5.69	(3.16 – 8.27)	46.7	(37.1 – 56.0)	217	(195 – 290)	448
60 years and older	46.2	(40.4 – 52.9)	8.98	(6.44 – 11.1)	52.2	(47.7 – 56.5)	234	(199 – 291)	595
Males									
Total, 6 years and older	34.4	(29.6 – 40.0)	6.14	(4.80 – 7.62)	37.5	(32.7 – 42.5)	186	(150 – 238)	1,035
6–11 years	39.5	(29.3 – 53.4)	12.2†	(1.42 – 18.9)	38.4	(31.5 – 49.8)	127†	(93.3 – 328)	99
12–19 years	30.3	(26.1 – 35.3)	6.16	(5.29 – 8.96)	33.2	(27.5 – 40.5)	123	(111 – 139)	191
20–39 years	32.2	(23.7 – 43.7)	5.54	(2.27 – 8.17)	32.5	(23.0 – 47.3)	185	(128 – 338)	217
40–59 years	35.4	(26.0 – 48.1)	5.70	(2.28 – 9.38)	37.4	(28.6 – 50.0)	213	(158 – 341)	229
60 years and older	36.7	(29.0 – 46.4)	6.56	(2.03 – 10.7)	44.0	(38.4 – 52.2)	195	(164 – 241)	299
Females									
Total, 6 years and older	44.9	(39.5 – 51.0)	7.63	(5.36 – 9.36)	55.6	(47.8 – 60.8)	216	(199 – 251)	1,073
6–11 years	46.6	(36.2 – 60.0)	10.2†	(4.05 – 15.4)	53.8	(41.4 – 64.6)	171†	(131 – 302)	94
12–19 years	36.2	(29.2 – 44.9)	8.91	(4.19 – 10.9)	39.1	(31.4 – 46.2)	151	(117 – 216)	187
20–39 years	42.2	(33.9 – 52.5)	4.89	(2.69 – 8.91)	56.3	(40.0 – 66.8)	203	(159 – 275)	277
40–59 years	43.1	(32.8 – 56.7)	5.49	(1.59 – 9.39)	58.2	(42.5 – 71.1)	217	(204 – 305)	219
60 years and older	55.5	(48.1 – 64.0)	10.2	(7.90 – 12.2)	60.5	(51.3 – 67.3)	291	(203 – 469)	296

† Estimate is subject to greater uncertainty due to small cell size.

Table 4.10.b. Urinary enterodiol (creatinine corrected): Concentrations by survey cycle

Geometric mean and selected percentiles of urine concentrations (in µg/g creatinine) for the U.S. population, National Health and Nutrition Examination Survey, 1999–2006.

	Geometric mean (95% conf. interval)	Selected percentiles (95% conf. interval) 5th	Selected percentiles (95% conf. interval) 50th	Selected percentiles (95% conf. interval) 95th	Sample size
Total, 6 years and older					
1999–2000	24.2 (20.3 – 28.9)	<LOD	29.9 (25.1 – 34.7)	239 (203 – 320)	2,527
2001–2002	33.5 (30.7 – 36.7)	2.54 (<LOD – 2.96)	37.6 (33.0 – 42.0)	224 (201 – 249)	2,794
2003–2004	37.0 (33.6 – 40.7)	2.45 (1.86 – 3.57)	41.7 (38.0 – 45.4)	293 (249 – 376)	2,594
2005–2006	36.8 (32.7 – 41.4)	2.95 (1.16 – 4.43)	40.9 (36.0 – 46.1)	323 (283 – 421)	2,528
Age group					
6–11 years					
1999–2000	27.0 (18.6 – 39.3)	<LOD	33.5 (22.1 – 43.6)	278 (199 – 534)	327
2001–2002	38.1 (32.5 – 44.7)	3.88 (2.45 – 5.14)	39.3 (31.0 – 53.1)	303 (244 – 390)	396
2003–2004	44.7 (37.4 – 53.5)	6.38 (3.61 – 8.72)	46.5 (38.6 – 58.0)	213 (184 – 414)	341
2005–2006	36.6 (28.9 – 46.4)	4.69 (1.80 – 7.52)	37.8 (33.0 – 46.5)	221 (186 – 349)	351
12–19 years					
1999–2000	20.1 (16.7 – 24.2)	<LOD	24.0 (19.9 – 30.1)	157 (125 – 176)	744
2001–2002	27.2 (23.3 – 31.8)	2.75 (1.30 – 4.91)	28.7 (25.0 – 34.8)	150 (116 – 316)	744
2003–2004	33.8 (30.3 – 37.7)	4.69 (2.38 – 5.62)	34.7 (33.3 – 38.2)	216 (155 – 344)	729
2005–2006	29.0 (25.2 – 33.3)	3.01 (2.13 – 3.60)	31.1 (28.0 – 36.1)	165 (160 – 214)	693
20–39 years					
1999–2000	21.7 (17.1 – 27.6)	<LOD	26.4 (21.4 – 32.4)	232 (149 – 371)	535
2001–2002	28.5 (23.7 – 34.3)	<LOD	30.2 (25.2 – 39.4)	187 (156 – 277)	604
2003–2004	33.5 (27.4 – 40.9)	2.26 (1.63 – 2.71)	33.8 (27.9 – 46.2)	299 (245 – 425)	554
2005–2006	33.3 (27.5 – 40.3)	2.39 (.618 – 4.04)	36.2 (30.4 – 47.2)	318 (207 – 523)	583
40–59 years					
1999–2000	26.4 (21.9 – 31.9)	<LOD	31.8 (27.4 – 38.7)	293 (217 – 358)	414
2001–2002	37.1 (30.0 – 45.7)	<LOD	44.2 (37.7 – 51.2)	246 (180 – 305)	531
2003–2004	33.8 (27.6 – 41.5)	1.16 (<LOD – 2.44)	40.8 (33.6 – 47.8)	369 (241 – 719)	452
2005–2006	41.6 (31.7 – 54.5)	2.95 (<LOD – 5.29)	46.6 (34.2 – 61.6)	375 (276 – 802)	449
60 years and older					
1999–2000	28.6 (23.0 – 35.6)	<LOD	33.5 (29.2 – 43.9)	258 (186 – 430)	507
2001–2002	41.9 (35.8 – 49.2)	3.67 (2.14 – 6.71)	46.3 (41.8 – 50.8)	238 (220 – 360)	519
2003–2004	49.4 (42.8 – 57.0)	5.75 (1.73 – 6.45)	57.1 (51.9 – 63.1)	309 (230 – 697)	518
2005–2006	41.3 (33.4 – 51.1)	2.15 (<LOD – 5.47)	45.4 (38.7 – 52.1)	418 (290 – 798)	452
Gender					
Males					
1999–2000	19.8 (15.4 – 25.4)	<LOD	25.3 (20.6 – 31.1)	198 (153 – 287)	1,206
2001–2002	28.7 (26.0 – 31.7)	<LOD	31.4 (27.0 – 36.7)	212 (184 – 259)	1,375
2003–2004	31.1 (27.5 – 35.0)	2.03 (1.17 – 3.66)	34.8 (32.2 – 38.4)	249 (195 – 368)	1,244
2005–2006	32.5 (26.7 – 39.5)	2.46 (.565 – 4.41)	34.2 (29.5 – 41.0)	310 (229 – 493)	1,252
Females					
1999–2000	29.3 (25.0 – 34.4)	<LOD	35.3 (29.6 – 41.6)	320 (233 – 370)	1,321
2001–2002	38.9 (34.9 – 43.3)	3.35 (<LOD – 4.62)	43.8 (39.3 – 48.7)	234 (185 – 305)	1,419
2003–2004	43.6 (38.3 – 49.7)	2.76 (2.24 – 4.15)	49.0 (43.4 – 57.7)	375 (280 – 464)	1,350
2005–2006	41.4 (36.1 – 47.4)	3.10 (.952 – 5.10)	48.2 (41.8 – 55.7)	372 (277 – 473)	1,276
Race/ethnicity					
Mexican Americans					
1999–2000	19.6 (17.3 – 22.2)	<LOD	23.2 (19.8 – 28.6)	193 (164 – 233)	791
2001–2002	28.7 (24.5 – 33.7)	2.60 (<LOD – 3.88)	31.0 (27.0 – 36.9)	220 (157 – 338)	679
2003–2004	29.9 (23.8 – 37.4)	1.88 (<LOD – 2.68)	33.8 (26.7 – 42.4)	240 (211 – 401)	653
2005–2006	34.4 (28.3 – 41.8)	3.45 (2.15 – 3.97)	35.3 (30.9 – 39.6)	314 (245 – 578)	634
Non-Hispanic Blacks					
1999–2000	16.5 (13.9 – 19.5)	<LOD	18.4 (14.4 – 22.8)	173 (136 – 311)	597
2001–2002	24.5 (19.4 – 30.8)	1.76 (<LOD – 3.48)	27.0 (22.6 – 33.4)	157 (127 – 387)	692
2003–2004	28.4 (24.2 – 33.3)	3.18 (2.04 – 3.81)	30.1 (26.1 – 36.0)	202 (158 – 230)	681
2005–2006	24.3 (20.5 – 28.9)	1.66 (.980 – 2.91)	25.3 (22.1 – 30.3)	186 (147 – 251)	662
Non-Hispanic Whites					
1999–2000	28.7 (24.5 – 33.6)	<LOD	34.4 (28.9 – 39.3)	252 (210 – 366)	899
2001–2002	35.2 (31.5 – 39.4)	2.50 (<LOD – 2.90)	40.8 (34.4 – 46.8)	225 (198 – 276)	1,211
2003–2004	39.5 (34.5 – 45.3)	2.71 (2.21 – 3.73)	45.5 (38.4 – 53.4)	299 (249 – 402)	1,069
2005–2006	39.2 (33.3 – 46.1)	2.99 (.537 – 5.09)	45.0 (39.4 – 50.2)	330 (284 – 441)	1,039

< LOD means less than the limit of detection for the uncorrected urine values, which may vary for some compounds by year. See Appendix D for LOD.

Figure 4.10.b. Urinary enterodiol (creatinine corrected): Concentrations by survey cycle

Selected percentiles in µg/g creatinine (95% confidence intervals), National Health and Nutrition Examination Survey, 1999–2006

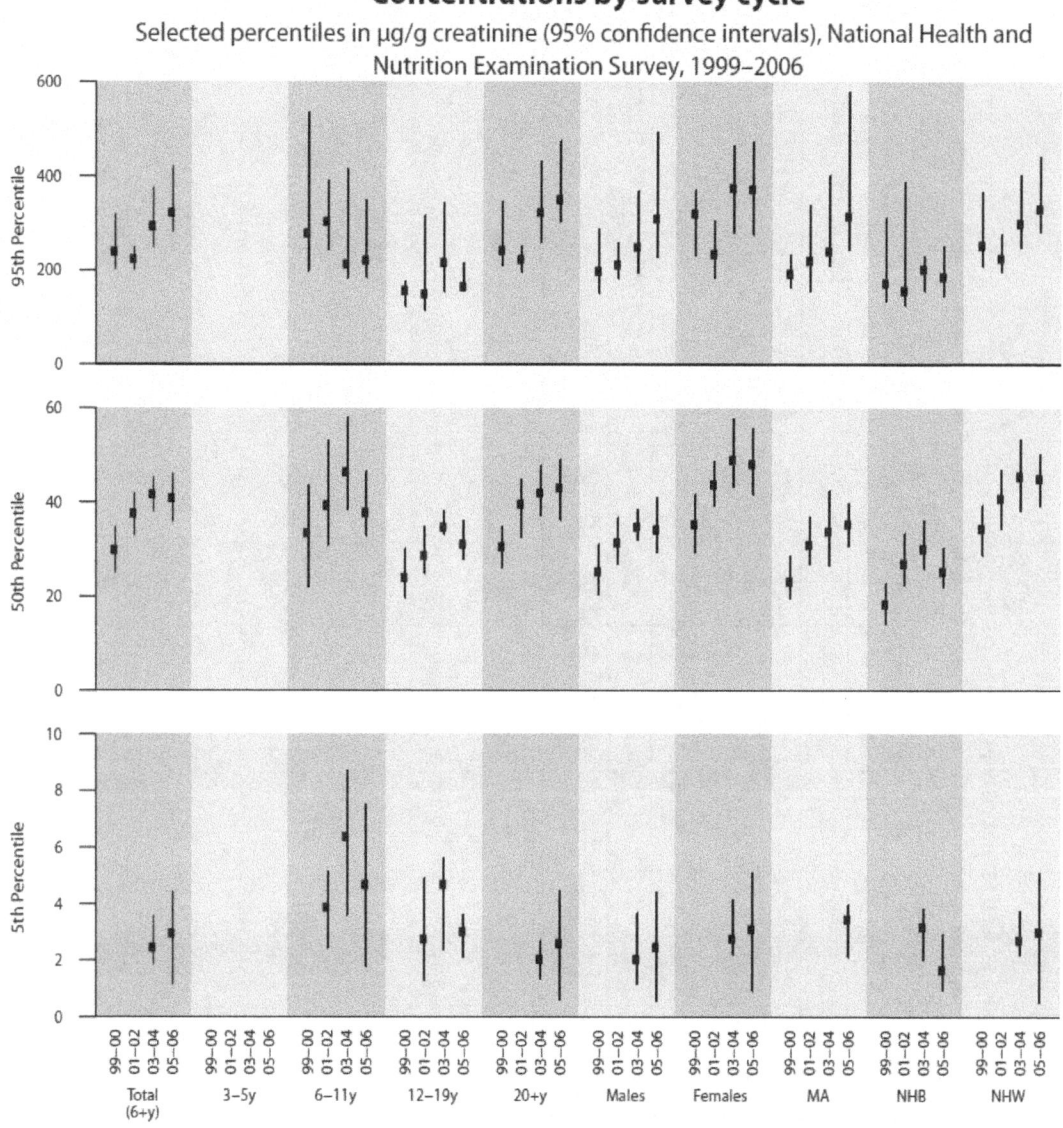

Values in the graph are suppressed if either the point estimate or the lower 95% confidence limit is noted as "< LOD" in the accompanying table.

Table 4.11.a.1. Urinary enterolactone: Concentrations

Geometric mean and selected percentiles of urine concentrations (in µg/L) for the total U.S. population aged 6 years and older, National Health and Nutrition Examination Survey, 2003–2006.

	Geometric mean (95% conf. interval)	Selected percentiles (95% conf. interval)					Sample size
		2.5th	5th	50th	95th	97.5th	
Total, 6 years and older	290 (266 – 317)	5.51 (3.93 – 6.69)	10.9 (9.27 – 14.5)	390 (350 – 435)	2,740 (2,560 – 2,980)	3,800 (3,390 – 4,340)	5,122
Age group							
6–11 years	340 (287 – 403)	11.4 (3.72 – 23.1)	25.6 (13.5 – 35.2)	413 (334 – 503)	2,150 (1,770 – 2,590)	2,670 (2,250 – 4,230)	692
12–19 years	303 (270 – 339)	5.99 (4.82 – 9.04)	14.0 (8.09 – 18.1)	394 (363 – 445)	2,560 (2,020 – 2,900)	3,290 (2,860 – 4,900)	1,422
20–39 years	272 (236 – 314)	6.15 (2.81 – 9.09)	10.8 (7.26 – 17.6)	349 (307 – 413)	2,810 (2,460 – 3,380)	3,930 (3,330 – 6,420)	1,137
40–59 years	271 (231 – 317)	3.90 (2.39 – 5.55)	7.59 (4.89 – 12.1)	389 (310 – 461)	3,050 (2,470 – 3,640)	4,130 (3,220 – 5,180)	901
60 years and older	327 (288 – 371)	5.82 (1.91 – 9.57)	14.1 (8.96 – 17.7)	476 (396 – 559)	2,690 (2,360 – 3,330)	3,460 (2,960 – 5,610)	970
Gender							
Males	307 (275 – 343)	5.60 (3.53 – 8.21)	12.5 (9.00 – 15.7)	424 (378 – 468)	2,850 (2,600 – 3,150)	3,790 (3,210 – 4,530)	2,496
Females	275 (242 – 313)	5.15 (3.46 – 6.73)	10.3 (8.69 – 14.3)	364 (321 – 422)	2,630 (2,360 – 3,070)	3,780 (3,190 – 5,400)	2,626
Race/ethnicity							
Mexican Americans	315 (282 – 352)	6.62 (5.35 – 9.21)	16.7 (8.05 – 25.3)	402 (364 – 435)	2,410 (2,040 – 2,940)	3,300 (2,670 – 4,760)	1,287
Non-Hispanic Blacks	299 (270 – 331)	5.73 (2.54 – 6.66)	11.0 (6.72 – 15.2)	421 (365 – 469)	2,300 (2,210 – 2,670)	3,140 (2,820 – 3,770)	1,343
Non-Hispanic Whites	287 (256 – 322)	5.56 (3.56 – 7.65)	11.0 (8.84 – 16.5)	387 (336 – 447)	2,740 (2,510 – 3,130)	3,850 (3,350 – 4,520)	2,108

Figure 4.11.a. Urinary enterolactone: Concentrations by age group

Geometric mean (95% confidence interval), National Health and Nutrition Examination Survey, 2003–2006

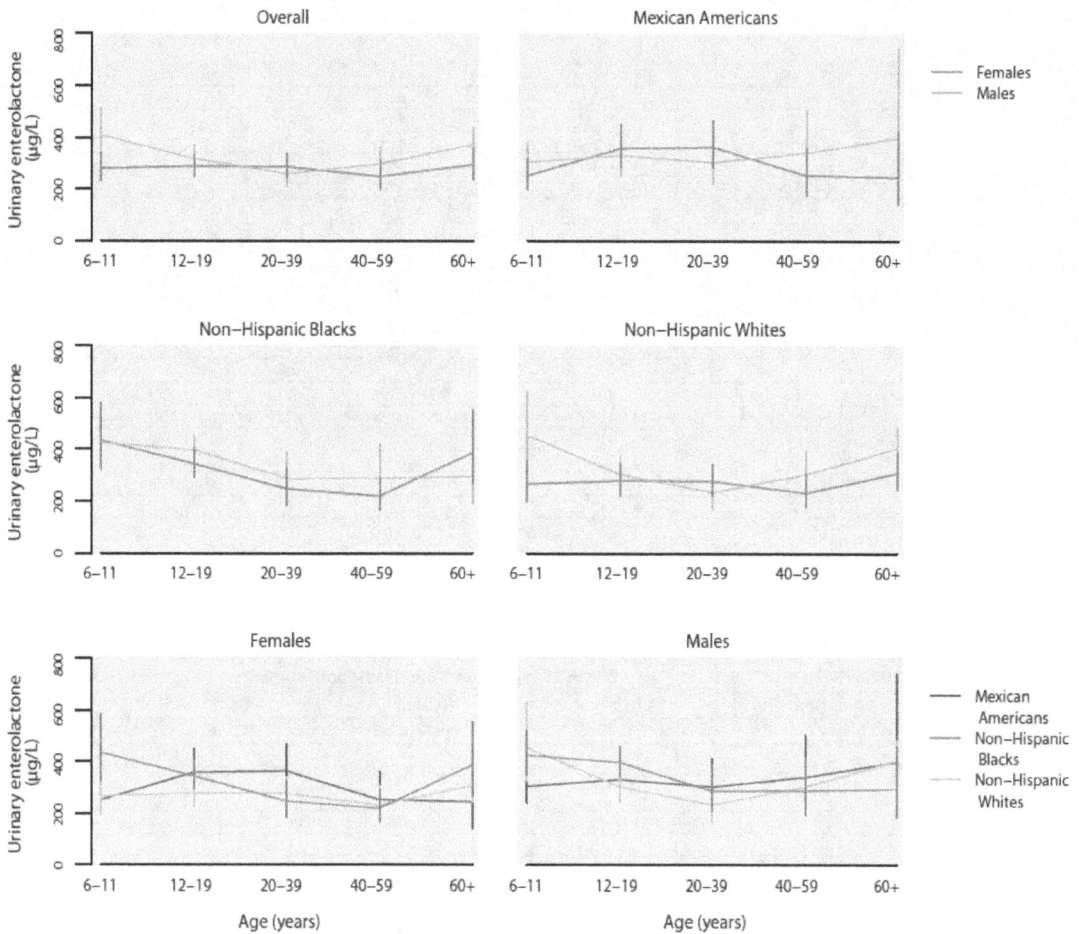

Table 4.11.a.2. Urinary enterolactone: Total population

Geometric mean and selected percentiles of urine concentrations (in µg/L) for the total U.S. population aged 6 years and older, National Health and Nutrition Examination Survey, 2003–2006.

	Geometric mean (95% conf. interval)		Selected percentiles (95% conf. interval)						Sample size
			10th		50th		90th		
Males and Females									
Total, 6 years and older	290	(266 – 317)	26.5	(23.0 – 30.9)	390	(350 – 435)	1,810	(1,700 – 1,970)	5,122
6–11 years	340	(287 – 403)	56.2	(32.4 – 76.6)	413	(334 – 503)	1,490	(1,200 – 1,880)	692
12–19 years	303	(270 – 339)	27.3	(19.2 – 44.1)	394	(363 – 445)	1,680	(1,490 – 1,910)	1,422
20–39 years	272	(236 – 314)	26.5	(20.2 – 35.4)	349	(307 – 413)	1,780	(1,540 – 2,060)	1,137
40–59 years	271	(231 – 317)	19.8	(14.2 – 26.7)	389	(310 – 461)	1,950	(1,560 – 2,430)	901
60 years and older	327	(288 – 371)	30.1	(18.9 – 42.3)	476	(396 – 559)	2,020	(1,790 – 2,300)	970
Males									
Total, 6 years and older	307	(275 – 343)	28.8	(23.3 – 36.5)	424	(378 – 468)	1,910	(1,730 – 2,060)	2,496
6–11 years	408	(324 – 514)	79.9	(45.3 – 126)	481	(381 – 582)	1,520	(1,140 – 2,130)	340
12–19 years	318	(272 – 371)	28.6	(20.1 – 51.1)	418	(369 – 495)	1,800	(1,530 – 2,240)	728
20–39 years	259	(211 – 318)	26.2	(16.7 – 37.4)	334	(244 – 427)	1,790	(1,530 – 2,320)	499
40–59 years	297	(241 – 365)	21.7	(12.8 – 32.5)	427	(309 – 537)	2,050	(1,530 – 2,950)	451
60 years and older	373	(318 – 438)	38.9	(20.7 – 59.7)	551	(441 – 651)	2,040	(1,690 – 2,720)	478
Females									
Total, 6 years and older	275	(242 – 313)	24.6	(19.9 – 28.9)	364	(321 – 422)	1,770	(1,540 – 2,000)	2,626
6–11 years	280	(233 – 336)	32.3	(24.1 – 57.3)	346	(260 – 445)	1,420	(1,080 – 2,230)	352
12–19 years	288	(250 – 331)	23.3	(16.5 – 47.6)	372	(320 – 421)	1,520	(1,370 – 1,730)	694
20–39 years	286	(242 – 337)	27.3	(20.2 – 38.7)	354	(311 – 443)	1,760	(1,360 – 2,500)	638
40–59 years	248	(197 – 313)	19.3	(10.8 – 26.6)	349	(271 – 421)	1,840	(1,450 – 2,330)	450
60 years and older	294	(239 – 362)	26.8	(16.3 – 41.8)	424	(323 – 541)	2,010	(1,700 – 2,280)	492

Table 4.11.a.3. Urinary enterolactone: Mexican Americans

Geometric mean and selected percentiles of urine concentrations (in µg/L) for Mexican Americans in the U.S. population aged 6 years and older, National Health and Nutrition Examination Survey, 2003–2006.

	Geometric mean (95% conf. interval)		Selected percentiles (95% conf. interval)						Sample size
			10th		50th		90th		
Males and Females									
Total, 6 years and older	315	(282 – 352)	39.4	(28.0 – 48.8)	402	(364 – 435)	1,630	(1,460 – 1,930)	1,287
6–11 years	278	(238 – 325)	53.7	(36.8 – 70.2)	348	(265 – 403)	1,100	(898 – 1,510)	231
12–19 years	344	(288 – 411)	54.9	(36.7 – 77.6)	447	(386 – 526)	1,590	(1,280 – 2,050)	445
20–39 years	329	(276 – 393)	38.9	(21.1 – 56.1)	389	(334 – 471)	1,900	(1,470 – 2,650)	282
40–59 years	295	(220 – 396)	28.5	(12.0 – 43.9)	411	(286 – 578)	1,510	(1,260 – 2,150)	157
60 years and older	305	(192 – 484)	29.7	(6.75 – 60.8)	438	(204 – 673)	1,800	(1,270 – 5,730)	172
Males									
Total, 6 years and older	320	(276 – 372)	38.3	(25.0 – 51.0)	423	(362 – 501)	1,700	(1,490 – 2,030)	625
6–11 years	305	(243 – 382)	55.3	(34.8 – 94.5)	367	(243 – 433)	1,210	(862 – 1,960)	112
12–19 years	331	(249 – 440)	46.6	(31.6 – 67.2)	441	(325 – 562)	1,660	(1,180 – 2,480)	228
20–39 years	303	(224 – 411)	25.1	(6.52 – 63.5)	390	(276 – 518)	1,890	(1,350 – 2,780)	117
40–59 years	340	(230 – 504)	28.6†	(12.2 – 44.6)	540	(286 – 673)	1,500†	(1,250 – 3,450)	85
60 years and older	399	(215 – 739)	38.2†	(4.50 – 106)	521	(205 – 1,080)	2,030†	(1,350 – 6,680)	83
Females									
Total, 6 years and older	309	(268 – 356)	43.0	(21.6 – 57.0)	366	(317 – 436)	1,560	(1,280 – 1,960)	662
6–11 years	252	(201 – 316)	46.3	(32.3 – 56.2)	319	(243 – 407)	1,010	(776 – 1,740)	119
12–19 years	358	(286 – 449)	65.0	(31.6 – 94.3)	446	(356 – 567)	1,460	(1,160 – 2,040)	217
20–39 years	363	(283 – 466)	45.0	(14.8 – 74.7)	383	(310 – 566)	1,900	(1,260 – 3,510)	165
40–59 years	253	(177 – 360)	21.0†	(5.66 – 44.2)	317	(192 – 525)	1,440†	(920 – 3,070)	72
60 years and older	245	(142 – 423)	18.4†	(5.17 – 52.4)	267	(149 – 676)	1,690†	(994 – 3,320)	89

† Estimate is subject to greater uncertainty due to small cell size.

Table 4.11.a.4. Urinary enterolactone: Non-Hispanic blacks

Geometric mean and selected percentiles of urine concentrations (in µg/L) for non-Hispanic blacks in the U.S. population aged 6 years and older, National Health and Nutrition Examination Survey, 2003–2006.

	Geometric mean (95% conf. interval)		Selected percentiles (95% conf. interval)						Sample size
			10th		50th		90th		
Males and Females									
Total, 6 years and older	299	(270 – 331)	26.0	(21.3 – 43.2)	421	(365 – 469)	1,580	(1,450 – 1,790)	1,343
6–11 years	429	(362 – 509)	117	(55.9 – 164)	419	(348 – 565)	1,560	(1,350 – 2,070)	207
12–19 years	370	(335 – 408)	46.6	(30.1 – 64.8)	523	(472 – 569)	1,640	(1,460 – 1,970)	496
20–39 years	264	(215 – 326)	23.0	(10.3 – 45.2)	437	(305 – 538)	1,410	(1,210 – 2,230)	249
40–59 years	248	(195 – 316)	19.8	(7.86 – 31.8)	326	(239 – 423)	1,630	(1,390 – 2,210)	231
60 years and older	349	(267 – 455)	39.2	(14.7 – 66.3)	551	(368 – 611)	1,760	(1,270 – 2,330)	160
Males									
Total, 6 years and older	320	(272 – 375)	30.8	(17.1 – 56.8)	439	(339 – 549)	1,740	(1,480 – 2,210)	661
6–11 years	425	(348 – 519)	123†	(89.3 – 164)	363	(303 – 558)	1,460†	(1,320 – 2,160)	99
12–19 years	397	(345 – 457)	58.9	(34.1 – 79.3)	502	(412 – 605)	1,770	(1,420 – 2,810)	258
20–39 years	287	(212 – 389)	24.9	(6.85 – 46.6)	444	(248 – 595)	1,860	(1,430 – 3,290)	116
40–59 years	288	(198 – 419)	16.4	(2.90 – 78.2)	344	(236 – 698)	1,880	(1,380 – 2,860)	114
60 years and older	295	(191 – 456)	17.8†	(4.36 – 60.4)	520	(287 – 646)	1,290†	(1,080 – 2,200)	74
Females									
Total, 6 years and older	282	(253 – 315)	23.9	(18.9 – 43.7)	418	(356 – 464)	1,470	(1,310 – 1,750)	682
6–11 years	434	(324 – 582)	94.1†	(22.9 – 174)	531	(364 – 624)	1,590†	(1,140 – 2,390)	108
12–19 years	344	(294 – 402)	33.9	(15.3 – 59.8)	530	(439 – 596)	1,590	(1,350 – 1,910)	238
20–39 years	247	(187 – 327)	18.0	(8.47 – 45.5)	421	(246 – 540)	1,180	(934 – 1,760)	133
40–59 years	220	(166 – 291)	21.5	(6.67 – 39.7)	303	(178 – 410)	1,530	(1,140 – 2,250)	117
60 years and older	387	(271 – 553)	44.3†	(10.3 – 109)	575	(365 – 666)	1,770†	(1,430 – 2,340)	86

† Estimate is subject to greater uncertainty due to small cell size.

Table 4.11.a.5. Urinary enterolactone: Non-Hispanic whites

Geometric mean and selected percentiles of urine concentrations (in µg/L) for non-Hispanic whites in the U.S. population aged 6 years and older, National Health and Nutrition Examination Survey, 2003–2006.

	Geometric mean (95% conf. interval)		Selected percentiles (95% conf. interval)						Sample size
			10th		50th		90th		
Males and Females									
Total, 6 years and older	287	(256 – 322)	26.3	(22.3 – 31.2)	387	(336 – 447)	1,810	(1,650 – 2,010)	2,108
6–11 years	355	(279 – 452)	56.3	(25.8 – 99.3)	456	(279 – 562)	1,480	(1,100 – 2,250)	193
12–19 years	292	(248 – 344)	27.1	(17.2 – 54.8)	369	(325 – 424)	1,660	(1,390 – 1,950)	378
20–39 years	254	(207 – 312)	26.3	(18.2 – 35.4)	313	(235 – 389)	1,640	(1,410 – 2,290)	494
40–59 years	266	(219 – 323)	19.1	(12.2 – 26.9)	393	(300 – 480)	1,850	(1,510 – 2,440)	448
60 years and older	347	(301 – 401)	33.4	(20.6 – 45.2)	495	(427 – 588)	2,060	(1,800 – 2,400)	595
Males									
Total, 6 years and older	308	(265 – 358)	29.4	(22.9 – 38.0)	434	(374 – 489)	1,900	(1,660 – 2,160)	1,035
6–11 years	454	(328 – 629)	97.2†	(29.3 – 181)	528	(338 – 805)	1,560†	(1,070 – 2,670)	99
12–19 years	304	(245 – 379)	27.8	(10.6 – 56.7)	391	(337 – 493)	1,760	(1,360 – 2,340)	191
20–39 years	234	(173 – 316)	25.4	(9.45 – 38.0)	269	(194 – 400)	1,570	(1,300 – 2,460)	217
40–59 years	303	(232 – 397)	22.0	(9.47 – 38.6)	437	(304 – 578)	2,130	(1,580 – 2,880)	229
60 years and older	404	(339 – 482)	40.6	(21.8 – 72.4)	596	(454 – 697)	2,080	(1,700 – 2,780)	299
Females									
Total, 6 years and older	268	(227 – 316)	24.6	(19.0 – 29.0)	350	(294 – 415)	1,760	(1,450 – 2,090)	1,073
6–11 years	267	(199 – 358)	26.4†	(12.5 – 71.6)	278	(207 – 488)	1,390†	(1,040 – 3,010)	94
12–19 years	279	(224 – 347)	21.0	(14.5 – 64.0)	336	(257 – 404)	1,540	(1,020 – 1,990)	187
20–39 years	277	(224 – 342)	26.9	(19.5 – 35.1)	335	(264 – 408)	1,770	(1,230 – 2,790)	277
40–59 years	232	(177 – 305)	17.1	(8.39 – 26.9)	348	(220 – 423)	1,730	(1,250 – 2,200)	219
60 years and older	308	(245 – 388)	29.2	(17.2 – 42.6)	434	(323 – 570)	2,040	(1,690 – 2,360)	296

† Estimate is subject to greater uncertainty due to small cell size.

Table 4.11.b. Urinary enterolactone: Concentrations by survey cycle

Geometric mean and selected percentiles of urine concentrations (in µg/L) for the U.S. population, National Health and Nutrition Examination Survey, 1999–2006.

	Geometric mean (95% conf. interval)	Selected percentiles (95% conf. interval) 5th	Selected percentiles (95% conf. interval) 50th	Selected percentiles (95% conf. interval) 95th	Sample size
Total, 6 years and older					
1999–2000	239 (200 – 286)	8.77 (4.68 – 13.0)	315 (246 – 380)	2,800 (2,520 – 3,200)	2,548
2001–2002	259 (233 – 287)	9.27 (6.84 – 11.8)	350 (314 – 389)	2,720 (1,970 – 3,440)	2,794
2003–2004	298 (265 – 334)	13.9 (10.0 – 17.9)	395 (332 – 462)	2,620 (2,370 – 2,980)	2,594
2005–2006	283 (245 – 327)	9.40 (5.54 – 14.3)	384 (339 – 456)	2,880 (2,540 – 3,170)	2,528
Age group					
6–11 years					
1999–2000	308 (219 – 432)	34.7 (< LOD – 45.9)	354 (243 – 473)	2,790 (1,850 – 4,390)	331
2001–2002	288 (245 – 339)	23.4 (12.0 – 41.1)	329 (275 – 405)	2,190 (1,520 – 2,610)	396
2003–2004	384 (287 – 513)	36.1 (8.67 – 75.5)	414 (303 – 557)	2,300 (1,750 – 3,760)	341
2005–2006	300 (242 – 373)	19.6 (4.34 – 30.0)	390 (279 – 544)	1,890 (1,420 – 2,630)	351
12–19 years					
1999–2000	250 (191 – 327)	10.0 (3.06 – 16.5)	316 (244 – 408)	2,920 (2,270 – 4,630)	746
2001–2002	267 (231 – 308)	16.1 (10.1 – 20.0)	318 (256 – 398)	2,170 (1,620 – 3,480)	744
2003–2004	314 (267 – 369)	18.4 (6.64 – 26.0)	399 (335 – 461)	2,620 (2,120 – 3,080)	729
2005–2006	292 (245 – 348)	9.91 (5.93 – 14.9)	393 (350 – 490)	2,320 (1,830 – 3,090)	693
20–39 years					
1999–2000	231 (182 – 293)	8.06 (1.33 – 17.0)	303 (228 – 380)	2,660 (2,310 – 4,310)	535
2001–2002	242 (196 – 301)	8.89 (6.56 – 10.9)	335 (263 – 419)	2,890 (1,870 – 4,740)	604
2003–2004	279 (224 – 349)	14.1 (6.47 – 23.0)	372 (289 – 474)	2,500 (1,830 – 3,330)	554
2005–2006	265 (218 – 322)	9.63 (4.72 – 19.0)	337 (276 – 381)	3,130 (2,410 – 7,470)	583
40–59 years					
1999–2000	211 (161 – 278)	2.50 (.690 – 7.44)	297 (229 – 401)	2,970 (2,250 – 5,070)	420
2001–2002	250 (187 – 333)	7.35 (3.98 – 11.5)	369 (278 – 429)	2,880 (1,870 – 4,820)	531
2003–2004	271 (231 – 319)	10.2 (7.40 – 12.5)	372 (281 – 429)	2,720 (2,350 – 4,400)	452
2005–2006	270 (203 – 360)	5.04 (2.73 – 13.3)	397 (299 – 539)	3,060 (2,260 – 4,030)	449
60 years and older					
1999–2000	261 (205 – 331)	10.3 (4.10 – 18.7)	315 (238 – 417)	2,680 (2,240 – 4,580)	516
2001–2002	288 (247 – 334)	8.74 (3.09 – 17.8)	386 (311 – 451)	2,450 (1,710 – 3,460)	519
2003–2004	327 (287 – 372)	17.3 (9.92 – 21.1)	457 (367 – 547)	2,690 (2,360 – 3,170)	518
2005–2006	327 (260 – 410)	11.9 (6.63 – 17.1)	507 (374 – 632)	2,680 (2,070 – 4,400)	452
Gender					
Males					
1999–2000	254 (212 – 304)	10.4 (6.45 – 12.8)	351 (266 – 417)	2,720 (2,460 – 3,480)	1,219
2001–2002	262 (233 – 295)	9.23 (6.76 – 10.9)	339 (314 – 386)	3,040 (2,310 – 4,570)	1,375
2003–2004	314 (280 – 351)	17.8 (10.7 – 21.9)	424 (375 – 474)	2,610 (2,120 – 3,340)	1,244
2005–2006	301 (247 – 368)	9.40 (4.26 – 14.9)	421 (347 – 512)	3,110 (2,750 – 3,520)	1,252
Females					
1999–2000	226 (180 – 284)	6.64 (.711 – 16.8)	287 (237 – 340)	2,810 (2,280 – 4,450)	1,329
2001–2002	255 (226 – 288)	9.25 (5.66 – 13.9)	356 (298 – 397)	2,190 (1,720 – 3,140)	1,419
2003–2004	283 (233 – 343)	10.5 (9.33 – 15.6)	369 (282 – 464)	2,620 (2,270 – 3,420)	1,350
2005–2006	267 (220 – 324)	9.18 (6.13 – 15.1)	357 (318 – 444)	2,650 (2,210 – 3,340)	1,276
Race/ethnicity					
Mexican Americans					
1999–2000	212 (169 – 265)	6.58 (.710 – 13.4)	281 (232 – 338)	2,690 (2,430 – 3,350)	813
2001–2002	275 (221 – 342)	12.6 (4.92 – 26.8)	347 (313 – 395)	2,320 (1,650 – 3,490)	679
2003–2004	275 (239 – 316)	9.35 (6.08 – 15.6)	375 (316 – 434)	2,240 (1,920 – 3,170)	653
2005–2006	359 (311 – 415)	26.7 (18.2 – 38.6)	418 (363 – 514)	2,640 (2,010 – 3,390)	634
Non-Hispanic Blacks					
1999–2000	262 (194 – 352)	8.91 (.671 – 17.0)	360 (293 – 449)	2,480 (1,990 – 4,170)	594
2001–2002	279 (224 – 347)	7.85 (3.49 – 15.7)	420 (339 – 488)	1,980 (1,690 – 2,530)	692
2003–2004	324 (282 – 372)	15.5 (6.01 – 26.1)	425 (358 – 525)	2,230 (1,960 – 2,630)	681
2005–2006	276 (237 – 322)	7.55 (5.86 – 11.4)	410 (346 – 483)	2,560 (2,210 – 3,030)	662
Non-Hispanic Whites					
1999–2000	247 (196 – 312)	8.26 (2.25 – 15.6)	317 (241 – 401)	2,990 (2,530 – 4,070)	901
2001–2002	268 (236 – 305)	9.30 (6.94 – 11.8)	356 (308 – 398)	2,780 (1,960 – 3,810)	1,211
2003–2004	301 (256 – 355)	16.3 (10.1 – 19.8)	397 (307 – 490)	2,650 (2,340 – 3,340)	1,069
2005–2006	274 (228 – 329)	9.17 (4.29 – 14.8)	372 (318 – 459)	2,900 (2,420 – 3,340)	1,039

< LOD means less than the limit of detection, which may vary for some compounds by year. See Appendix D for LOD.

Figure 4.11.b. Urinary enterolactone: Concentrations by survey cycle

Selected percentiles in µg/L (95% confidence intervals), National Health and Nutrition Examination Survey, 1999–2006

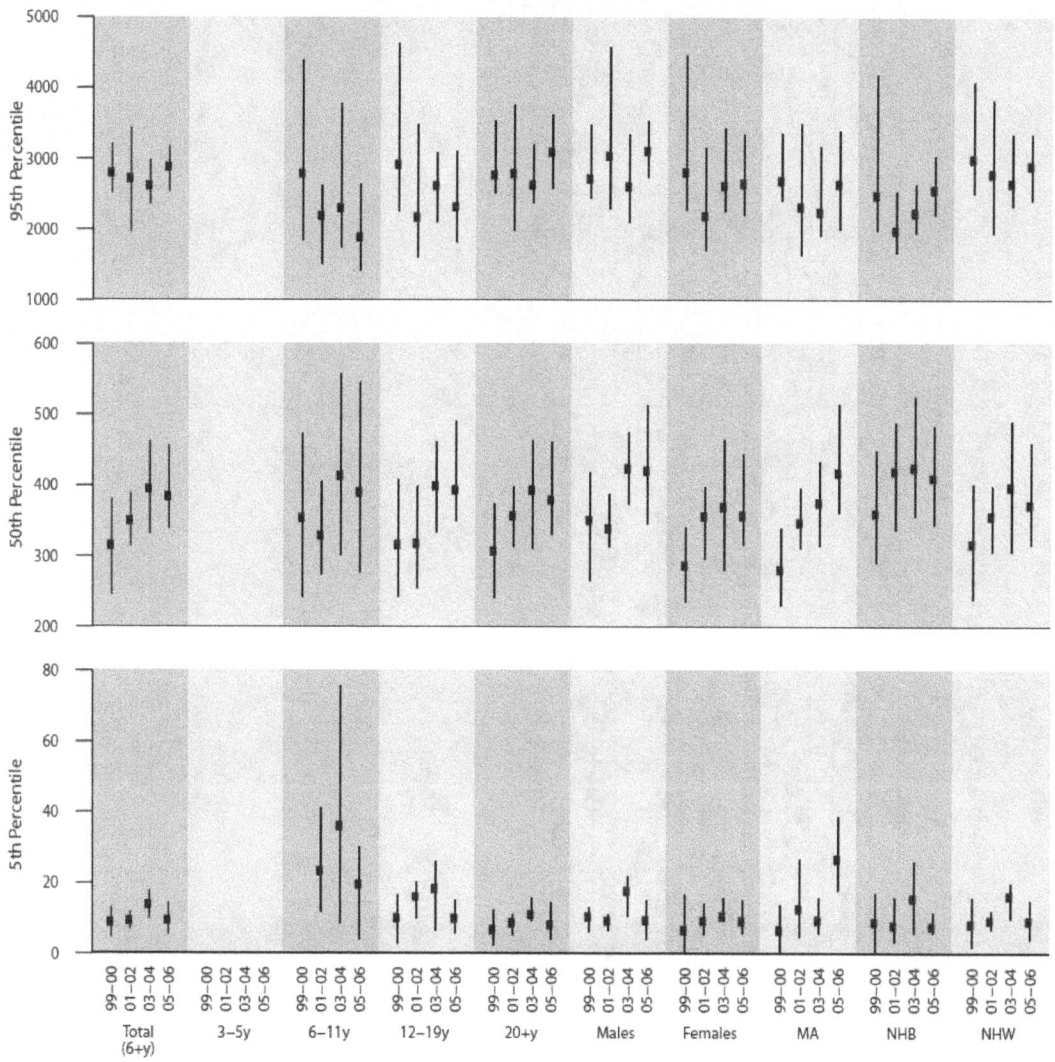

Values in the graph are suppressed if either the point estimate or the lower 95% confidence limit is noted as "< LOD" in the accompanying table.

Table 4.12.a.1. Urinary enterolactone (creatinine corrected): Concentrations

Geometric mean and selected percentiles of urine concentrations (in µg/g creatinine) for the total U.S. population aged 6 years and older, National Health and Nutrition Examination Survey, 2003–2006.

	Geometric mean (95% conf. interval)	Selected percentiles (95% conf. interval)					Sample size
		2.5th	5th	50th	95th	97.5th	
Total, 6 years and older	277 (252 – 305)	5.55 (4.13 – 6.95)	11.2 (9.15 – 13.5)	375 (341 – 418)	2,500 (2,250 – 2,890)	3,780 (3,380 – 4,390)	5,122
Age group							
6-11 years	368 (312 – 434)	14.6 (7.65 – 30.5)	33.6 (21.0 – 47.1)	463 (382 – 535)	2,120 (1,770 – 2,530)	2,630 (2,300 – 3,430)	692
12-19 years	225 (203 – 250)	6.79 (4.71 – 8.45)	11.3 (7.51 – 14.7)	290 (271 – 307)	1,470 (1,330 – 1,790)	2,180 (1,580 – 3,540)	1,422
20-39 years	232 (200 – 269)	4.10 (2.40 – 8.49)	9.56 (6.42 – 13.7)	314 (273 – 363)	2,440 (1,860 – 3,750)	3,780 (2,880 – 5,890)	1,137
40-59 years	274 (231 – 326)	4.59 (2.61 – 6.17)	8.62 (5.64 – 13.1)	366 (323 – 468)	2,870 (2,260 – 4,000)	4,880 (3,470 – 6,600)	901
60 years and older	383 (334 – 438)	6.04 (2.51 – 9.36)	13.5 (8.69 – 18.9)	582 (502 – 671)	2,780 (2,480 – 3,620)	4,110 (3,400 – 5,060)	970
Gender							
Males	244 (216 – 275)	4.80 (2.78 – 6.36)	10.7 (6.43 – 13.5)	336 (298 – 371)	2,110 (1,930 – 2,310)	2,930 (2,440 – 3,460)	2,496
Females	313 (275 – 357)	6.82 (4.83 – 8.44)	11.3 (9.39 – 15.4)	418 (360 – 481)	2,890 (2,560 – 3,740)	4,590 (3,880 – 5,900)	2,626
Race/ethnicity							
Mexican Americans	284 (251 – 322)	5.88 (3.39 – 8.31)	14.6 (9.01 – 21.8)	366 (331 – 417)	1,920 (1,670 – 2,260)	2,350 (2,110 – 3,390)	1,287
Non-Hispanic Blacks	210 (189 – 233)	4.37 (2.46 – 5.15)	7.91 (5.58 – 10.8)	294 (274 – 325)	1,480 (1,340 – 1,670)	2,020 (1,690 – 2,300)	1,343
Non-Hispanic Whites	292 (258 – 331)	5.97 (3.88 – 8.66)	12.6 (9.39 – 14.6)	406 (350 – 469)	2,730 (2,330 – 3,370)	4,180 (3,430 – 5,250)	2,108

Figure 4.12.a. Urinary enterolactone (creatinine corrected): Concentrations by age group

Geometric mean (95% confidence interval), National Health and Nutrition Examination Survey, 2003–2006

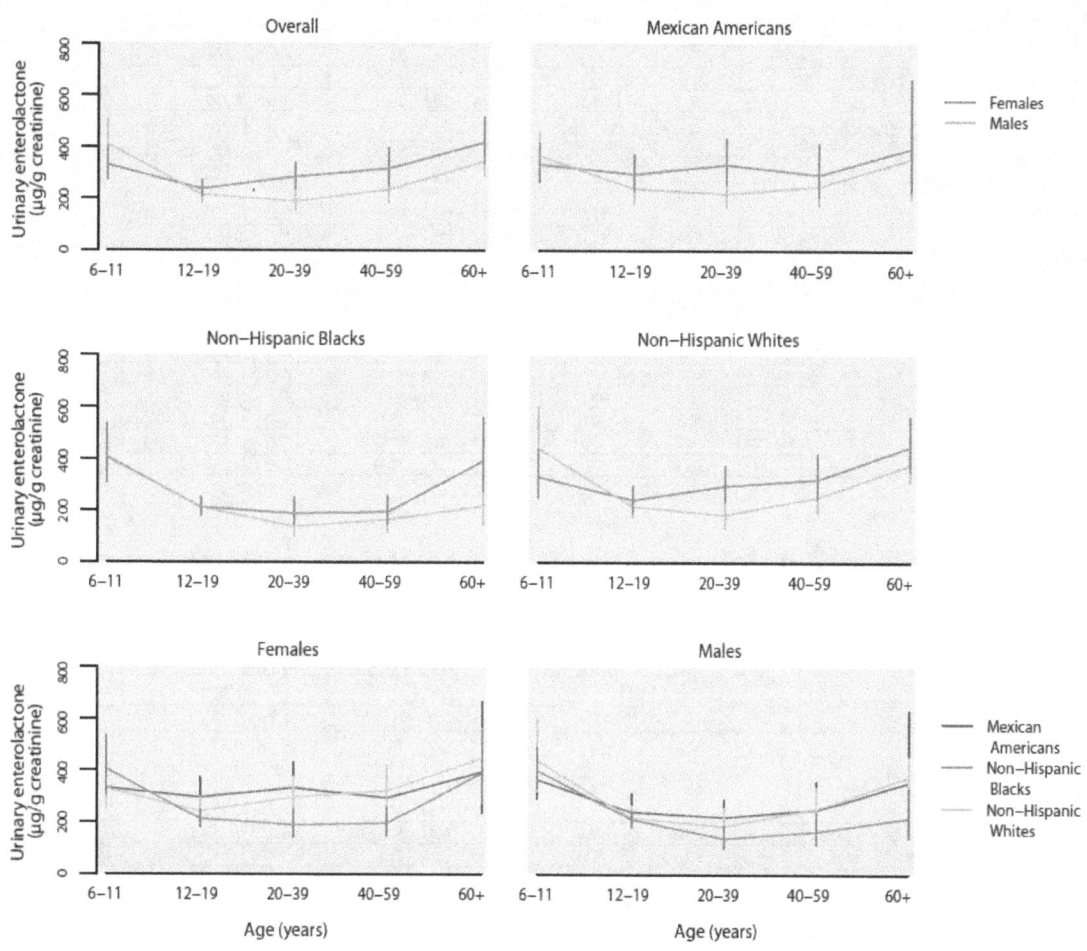

Table 4.12.a.2. Urinary enterolactone (creatinine corrected): Total population

Geometric mean and selected percentiles of urine concentrations (in µg/g creatinine) for the total U.S. population aged 6 years and older, National Health and Nutrition Examination Survey, 2003–2006.

	Geometric mean (95% conf. interval)	Selected percentiles (95% conf. interval)						Sample size
		10th		50th		90th		
Males and Females								
Total, 6 years and older	277	(252 – 305)	26.1	(20.3 – 31.3)	375	(341 – 418)	1,620 (1,480 – 1,800)	5,122
6–11 years	368	(312 – 434)	79.9	(44.5 – 104)	463	(382 – 535)	1,480 (1,200 – 1,900)	692
12–19 years	225	(203 – 250)	22.6	(18.0 – 36.1)	290	(271 – 307)	1,140 (996 – 1,220)	1,422
20–39 years	232	(200 – 269)	20.0	(15.1 – 28.5)	314	(273 – 363)	1,460 (1,250 – 1,720)	1,137
40–59 years	274	(231 – 326)	21.1	(15.4 – 28.7)	366	(323 – 468)	1,720 (1,510 – 2,100)	901
60 years and older	383	(334 – 438)	33.8	(22.8 – 46.9)	582	(502 – 671)	2,130 (1,840 – 2,310)	970
Males								
Total, 6 years and older	244	(216 – 275)	21.0	(16.3 – 28.5)	336	(298 – 371)	1,400 (1,290 – 1,580)	2,496
6–11 years	409	(329 – 508)	91.0	(45.7 – 127)	471	(395 – 622)	1,380 (1,190 – 2,000)	340
12–19 years	215	(188 – 247)	20.9	(13.6 – 34.9)	292	(258 – 312)	1,150 (924 – 1,390)	728
20–39 years	189	(152 – 234)	16.8	(11.7 – 21.7)	257	(209 – 315)	1,290 (1,050 – 1,610)	499
40–59 years	235	(187 – 296)	18.5	(12.7 – 30.6)	328	(267 – 417)	1,450 (1,230 – 1,930)	451
60 years and older	344	(289 – 409)	35.8	(16.2 – 57.6)	522	(452 – 576)	1,720 (1,490 – 2,210)	478
Females								
Total, 6 years and older	313	(275 – 357)	30.0	(22.8 – 35.5)	418	(360 – 481)	1,840 (1,640 – 2,210)	2,626
6–11 years	329	(271 – 399)	56.3	(31.6 – 89.2)	431	(324 – 515)	1,660 (1,080 – 2,310)	352
12–19 years	237	(208 – 270)	25.5	(14.5 – 43.8)	285	(251 – 320)	1,080 (918 – 1,230)	694
20–39 years	284	(237 – 340)	30.8	(15.9 – 42.8)	377	(315 – 431)	1,640 (1,360 – 2,360)	638
40–59 years	316	(253 – 395)	23.7	(15.5 – 32.1)	424	(334 – 585)	2,130 (1,580 – 2,940)	450
60 years and older	417	(336 – 517)	28.3	(19.4 – 53.4)	636	(511 – 784)	2,290 (2,020 – 2,730)	492

Table 4.12.a.3. Urinary enterolactone (creatinine corrected): Mexican Americans

Geometric mean and selected percentiles of urine concentrations (in µg/g creatinine) for Mexican Americans in the U.S. population aged 6 years and older, National Health and Nutrition Examination Survey, 2003–2006.

	Geometric mean (95% conf. interval)	Selected percentiles (95% conf. interval)						Sample size
		10th		50th		90th		
Males and Females								
Total, 6 years and older	284	(251 – 322)	37.6	(27.2 – 48.7)	366	(331 – 417)	1,410 (1,240 – 1,620)	1,287
6–11 years	349	(304 – 400)	79.6	(57.9 – 113)	404	(338 – 472)	1,330 (1,020 – 1,670)	231
12–19 years	266	(225 – 315)	40.1	(26.8 – 56.0)	343	(286 – 397)	1,160 (986 – 1,320)	445
20–39 years	266	(218 – 324)	29.6	(14.6 – 47.7)	328	(257 – 408)	1,480 (1,210 – 1,940)	282
40–59 years	270	(203 – 358)	25.4	(10.6 – 46.6)	400	(291 – 589)	1,190 (898 – 1,770)	157
60 years and older	376	(246 – 576)	29.4	(8.02 – 89.3)	487	(332 – 761)	1,800 (1,550 – 2,210)	172
Males								
Total, 6 years and older	253	(219 – 291)	31.0	(22.9 – 44.1)	334	(287 – 401)	1,210 (1,020 – 1,480)	625
6–11 years	365	(292 – 457)	88.4	(58.8 – 127)	403	(290 – 494)	1,390 (956 – 1,970)	112
12–19 years	240	(185 – 312)	31.2	(18.5 – 42.9)	289	(241 – 375)	1,170 (928 – 1,530)	228
20–39 years	220	(167 – 290)	27.2	(3.66 – 48.2)	257	(222 – 396)	1,270 (930 – 1,900)	117
40–59 years	249	(174 – 358)	23.3†	(6.34 – 49.2)	399	(235 – 603)	898† (841 – 1,530)	85
60 years and older	355	(200 – 631)	37.2†	(3.60 – 128)	503	(322 – 714)	1,540† (1,100 – 6,820)	83
Females								
Total, 6 years and older	322	(275 – 378)	40.7	(28.9 – 66.8)	382	(331 – 484)	1,600 (1,330 – 1,870)	662
6–11 years	332	(267 – 413)	64.3	(34.7 – 110)	401	(311 – 538)	1,130 (861 – 1,830)	119
12–19 years	296	(235 – 372)	57.9	(30.5 – 99.0)	378	(316 – 443)	1,100 (860 – 1,350)	217
20–39 years	332	(257 – 430)	39.7	(17.2 – 71.6)	361	(292 – 548)	1,630 (1,300 – 3,210)	165
40–59 years	294	(209 – 414)	28.5†	(3.25 – 64.6)	374	(215 – 655)	1,390† (1,090 – 2,590)	72
60 years and older	395	(235 – 663)	25.8†	(5.58 – 112)	487	(197 – 1,220)	1,880† (1,590 – 4,100)	89

† Estimate is subject to greater uncertainty due to small cell size.

Table 4.12.a.4. Urinary enterolactone (creatinine corrected): Non-Hispanic blacks

Geometric mean and selected percentiles of urine concentrations (in µg/g creatinine) for non-Hispanic blacks in the U.S. population aged 6 years and older, National Health and Nutrition Examination Survey, 2003–2006.

	Geometric mean (95% conf. interval)		Selected percentiles (95% conf. interval)						Sample size
			10th		50th		90th		
Males and Females									
Total, 6 years and older	210	(189 – 233)	20.2	(13.8 – 30.9)	294	(274 – 325)	1,080	(995 – 1,210)	1,343
6–11 years	403	(342 – 476)	126	(82.0 – 147)	469	(378 – 550)	1,300	(1,080 – 1,660)	207
12–19 years	212	(194 – 232)	30.8	(19.9 – 38.3)	282	(251 – 313)	843	(755 – 1,010)	496
20–39 years	164	(133 – 201)	15.8	(10.5 – 22.2)	263	(194 – 306)	914	(741 – 1,040)	249
40–59 years	180	(143 – 228)	11.8	(5.52 – 24.1)	264	(207 – 321)	1,080	(933 – 1,390)	231
60 years and older	311	(242 – 399)	25.1	(12.7 – 61.0)	489	(325 – 693)	1,430	(1,210 – 1,770)	160
Males									
Total, 6 years and older	187	(157 – 222)	20.0	(11.2 – 31.3)	267	(223 – 305)	1,050	(940 – 1,200)	661
6–11 years	401	(329 – 489)	122†	(69.6 – 153)	417	(332 – 523)	1,220†	(1,020 – 1,730)	99
12–19 years	212	(186 – 243)	31.8	(19.4 – 44.2)	264	(222 – 301)	923	(767 – 1,320)	258
20–39 years	138	(103 – 185)	12.2	(2.62 – 27.1)	192	(113 – 291)	969	(657 – 1,180)	116
40–59 years	165	(114 – 238)	10.2	(3.65 – 35.8)	233	(167 – 305)	1,040	(711 – 1,440)	114
60 years and older	217	(142 – 330)	14.8†	(3.29 – 51.0)	329	(249 – 440)	1,090†	(842 – 3,370)	74
Females									
Total, 6 years and older	231	(207 – 259)	20.3	(13.3 – 35.8)	317	(286 – 349)	1,150	(974 – 1,410)	682
6–11 years	405	(308 – 532)	127†	(20.6 – 163)	512	(386 – 585)	1,360†	(898 – 2,610)	108
12–19 years	212	(180 – 250)	26.0	(11.1 – 39.8)	299	(249 – 360)	814	(727 – 927)	238
20–39 years	188	(144 – 246)	16.1	(7.55 – 32.9)	276	(197 – 347)	820	(619 – 1,360)	133
40–59 years	195	(147 – 258)	11.4	(5.89 – 33.6)	289	(205 – 392)	1,170	(928 – 1,600)	117
60 years and older	391	(275 – 557)	40.6†	(9.12 – 96.7)	707	(327 – 822)	1,620†	(1,380 – 2,090)	86

† Estimate is subject to greater uncertainty due to small cell size.

Table 4.12.a.5. Urinary enterolactone (creatinine corrected): Non-Hispanic whites

Geometric mean and selected percentiles of urine concentrations (in µg/g creatinine) for non-Hispanic whites in the U.S. population aged 6 years and older, National Health and Nutrition Examination Survey, 2003–2006.

	Geometric mean (95% conf. interval)		Selected percentiles (95% conf. interval)						Sample size
			10th		50th		90th		
Males and Females									
Total, 6 years and older	292	(258 – 331)	26.3	(20.0 – 31.5)	406	(350 – 469)	1,680	(1,510 – 2,020)	2,108
6–11 years	385	(305 – 486)	80.8	(35.3 – 113)	467	(367 – 615)	1,380	(1,170 – 2,000)	193
12–19 years	229	(196 – 267)	22.7	(14.2 – 39.5)	277	(247 – 318)	1,150	(959 – 1,320)	378
20–39 years	234	(188 – 292)	18.7	(12.5 – 29.1)	319	(258 – 417)	1,550	(1,200 – 2,350)	494
40–59 years	286	(232 – 352)	22.5	(14.8 – 30.7)	379	(323 – 500)	1,810	(1,500 – 2,210)	448
60 years and older	415	(358 – 480)	38.5	(23.7 – 57.9)	611	(529 – 717)	2,210	(1,850 – 2,610)	595
Males									
Total, 6 years and older	258	(219 – 304)	20.6	(16.0 – 30.1)	360	(309 – 418)	1,490	(1,320 – 1,680)	1,035
6–11 years	440	(322 – 602)	111†	(32.6 – 149)	478	(380 – 740)	1,330†	(1,150 – 2,850)	99
12–19 years	217	(178 – 265)	20.8	(13.2 – 36.5)	295	(230 – 345)	1,150	(843 – 1,400)	191
20–39 years	185	(134 – 256)	16.1	(5.82 – 20.9)	263	(176 – 362)	1,330	(1,010 – 2,350)	217
40–59 years	254	(190 – 338)	18.8	(12.8 – 34.3)	338	(267 – 497)	1,570	(1,270 – 2,040)	229
60 years and older	377	(313 – 454)	38.1	(18.3 – 61.4)	551	(467 – 666)	1,820	(1,480 – 2,430)	299
Females									
Total, 6 years and older	330	(280 – 389)	31.3	(23.1 – 39.4)	447	(375 – 526)	1,990	(1,660 – 2,530)	1,073
6–11 years	330	(250 – 436)	57.0†	(24.7 – 98.5)	427	(257 – 554)	1,690†	(1,010 – 2,420)	94
12–19 years	242	(198 – 296)	28.8	(12.4 – 75.4)	264	(238 – 320)	1,180	(909 – 1,350)	187
20–39 years	296	(236 – 373)	30.0	(13.3 – 48.8)	417	(312 – 470)	1,690	(1,250 – 3,260)	277
40–59 years	322	(247 – 419)	25.9	(15.8 – 32.6)	445	(323 – 614)	2,130	(1,500 – 3,470)	219
60 years and older	447	(355 – 562)	35.6	(21.3 – 69.1)	662	(529 – 845)	2,400	(2,090 – 3,040)	296

† Estimate is subject to greater uncertainty due to small cell size.

Table 4.12.b. Urinary enterolactone (creatinine corrected): Concentrations by survey cycle

Geometric mean and selected percentiles of urine concentrations (in µg/g creatinine) for the U.S. population, National Health and Nutrition Examination Survey, 1999–2006.

	Geometric mean (95% conf. interval)	Selected percentiles (95% conf. interval)			Sample size
		5th	50th	95th	
Total, 6 years and older					
1999–2000	218 (184 – 260)	7.15 (4.06 – 9.89)	284 (247 – 336)	2,250 (1,890 – 2,930)	2,548
2001–2002	243 (220 – 268)	7.63 (5.19 – 10.3)	323 (293 – 360)	2,120 (1,790 – 2,460)	2,794
2003–2004	279 (245 – 317)	12.3 (9.27 – 14.5)	371 (325 – 430)	2,400 (2,030 – 2,890)	2,594
2005–2006	276 (237 – 321)	9.89 (6.76 – 13.8)	382 (330 – 447)	2,640 (2,260 – 3,380)	2,528
Age group					
6–11 years					
1999–2000	315 (238 – 416)	38.6 (<LOD – 66.8)	380 (269 – 431)	2,040 (1,640 – 3,510)	331
2001–2002	327 (274 – 391)	27.3 (10.5 – 59.2)	349 (264 – 477)	1,980 (1,570 – 3,360)	396
2003–2004	409 (310 – 540)	41.0 (11.1 – 79.7)	469 (356 – 628)	2,300 (1,750 – 3,390)	341
2005–2006	331 (268 – 408)	23.4 (8.67 – 46.6)	456 (326 – 526)	1,820 (1,580 – 2,970)	351
12–19 years					
1999–2000	169 (133 – 214)	6.86 (2.00 – 13.6)	209 (172 – 263)	1,820 (1,340 – 2,460)	746
2001–2002	206 (178 – 239)	12.2 (7.63 – 14.1)	254 (224 – 292)	1,500 (1,240 – 2,730)	744
2003–2004	235 (202 – 273)	14.7 (6.78 – 20.2)	285 (256 – 307)	1,510 (1,310 – 2,700)	729
2005–2006	216 (184 – 254)	9.50 (5.93 – 13.1)	296 (254 – 335)	1,410 (1,170 – 1,890)	693
20–39 years					
1999–2000	183 (143 – 235)	5.46 (.836 – 8.94)	248 (199 – 291)	1,900 (1,480 – 3,890)	535
2001–2002	196 (160 – 240)	4.83 (2.86 – 9.88)	298 (251 – 334)	1,670 (1,430 – 2,450)	604
2003–2004	235 (186 – 299)	10.0 (4.07 – 14.8)	324 (250 – 422)	2,140 (1,640 – 3,890)	554
2005–2006	229 (187 – 279)	9.40 (4.07 – 16.0)	299 (256 – 348)	2,630 (1,680 – 6,020)	583
40–59 years					
1999–2000	215 (165 – 279)	4.14 (1.49 – 8.85)	282 (244 – 375)	2,520 (2,030 – 4,780)	420
2001–2002	248 (191 – 321)	5.90 (3.49 – 10.7)	335 (266 – 435)	2,450 (1,600 – 4,940)	531
2003–2004	260 (218 – 310)	8.64 (6.33 – 13.5)	354 (300 – 444)	2,450 (2,010 – 4,240)	452
2005–2006	288 (213 – 389)	8.45 (3.84 – 13.9)	394 (306 – 602)	3,380 (2,280 – 4,890)	449
60 years and older					
1999–2000	313 (227 – 432)	14.0 (3.73 – 20.9)	431 (312 – 611)	2,530 (1,940 – 4,500)	516
2001–2002	341 (296 – 392)	9.15 (4.22 – 17.6)	432 (383 – 476)	2,550 (2,130 – 3,030)	519
2003–2004	387 (330 – 453)	18.4 (10.5 – 21.5)	547 (439 – 682)	2,690 (2,340 – 3,340)	518
2005–2006	379 (300 – 478)	11.9 (6.12 – 17.7)	597 (495 – 730)	3,030 (2,250 – 4,480)	452
Gender					
Males					
1999–2000	199 (170 – 234)	7.25 (3.82 – 9.99)	262 (231 – 309)	2,020 (1,810 – 2,480)	1,219
2001–2002	213 (191 – 238)	6.70 (4.49 – 9.78)	287 (256 – 317)	1,960 (1,620 – 2,660)	1,375
2003–2004	245 (215 – 280)	12.8 (9.17 – 14.8)	330 (289 – 372)	2,030 (1,770 – 2,390)	1,244
2005–2006	243 (196 – 300)	8.40 (4.08 – 13.6)	336 (280 – 416)	2,200 (1,930 – 2,640)	1,252
Females					
1999–2000	238 (191 – 297)	7.08 (2.40 – 14.0)	303 (263 – 378)	2,550 (2,010 – 3,520)	1,329
2001–2002	274 (241 – 312)	9.46 (5.43 – 13.8)	356 (314 – 405)	2,140 (1,970 – 2,430)	1,419
2003–2004	314 (257 – 385)	11.2 (8.54 – 17.0)	414 (330 – 501)	2,810 (2,290 – 3,940)	1,350
2005–2006	313 (261 – 375)	12.4 (9.39 – 15.7)	419 (342 – 527)	3,080 (2,520 – 4,780)	1,276
Race/ethnicity					
Mexican Americans					
1999–2000	194 (165 – 228)	3.78 (2.01 – 15.3)	253 (224 – 282)	2,020 (1,700 – 2,810)	813
2001–2002	259 (213 – 314)	13.0 (3.24 – 23.2)	361 (298 – 409)	1,630 (1,320 – 3,010)	679
2003–2004	248 (217 – 282)	6.88 (4.10 – 14.5)	349 (310 – 397)	1,800 (1,470 – 2,260)	653
2005–2006	324 (267 – 393)	26.3 (13.0 – 36.2)	378 (321 – 471)	2,030 (1,680 – 2,770)	634
Non-Hispanic Blacks					
1999–2000	168 (124 – 226)	3.12 (.422 – 9.24)	215 (175 – 276)	1,590 (1,220 – 3,280)	594
2001–2002	195 (153 – 248)	6.71 (4.02 – 9.33)	303 (257 – 334)	1,460 (1,110 – 1,730)	692
2003–2004	228 (194 – 268)	10.8 (4.54 – 17.1)	300 (274 – 341)	1,460 (1,220 – 2,110)	681
2005–2006	193 (167 – 223)	6.32 (4.70 – 8.61)	285 (249 – 330)	1,490 (1,290 – 1,660)	662
Non-Hispanic Whites					
1999–2000	243 (194 – 304)	7.71 (3.26 – 11.8)	324 (280 – 389)	2,490 (2,010 – 3,540)	901
2001–2002	265 (232 – 302)	7.97 (5.19 – 11.8)	340 (299 – 393)	2,400 (1,980 – 2,900)	1,211
2003–2004	297 (248 – 356)	13.5 (9.57 – 17.5)	409 (331 – 492)	2,590 (2,040 – 3,380)	1,069
2005–2006	288 (238 – 347)	11.0 (5.96 – 14.9)	403 (329 – 497)	2,910 (2,310 – 4,180)	1,039

< LOD means less than the limit of detection for the uncorrected urine values, which may vary for some compounds by year. See Appendix D for LOD.

Figure 4.12.b. Urinary enterolactone (creatinine corrected): Concentrations by survey cycle

Selected percentiles in μg/g creatinine (95% confidence intervals), National Health and Nutrition Examination Survey, 1999–2006

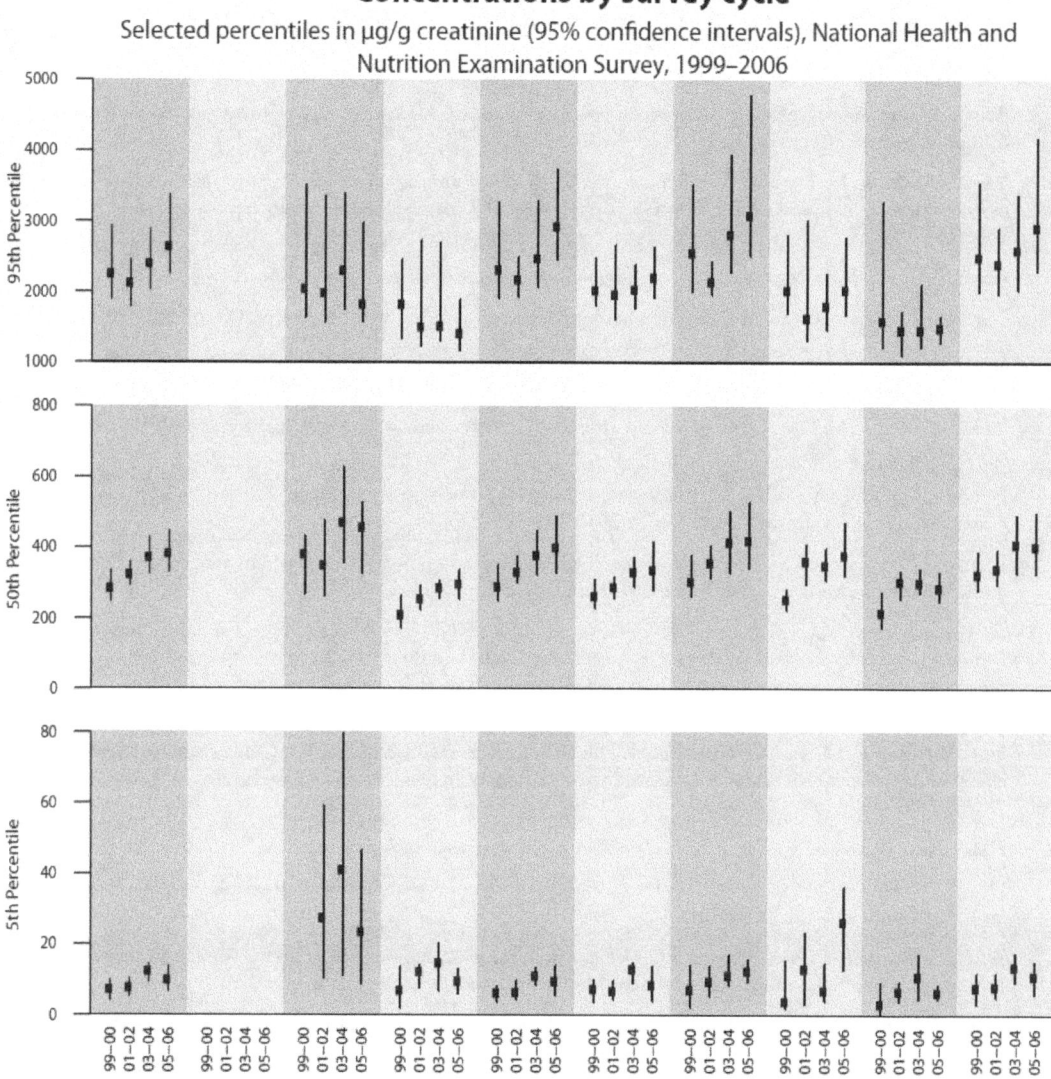

Values in the graph are suppressed if either the point estimate or the lower 95% confidence limit is noted as "< LOD" in the accompanying table.

References

Balk E, Chung M, Chew P, Raman G, Kupelnick B, Tatsioni A, et al. Tufts-New England Medical Center Evidence-based Practice Center. Effects of soy on health outcomes. Summary. Rockville (MD): Agency for Healthcare Research and Quality; July 2005. Evidence Report/Technology Assessment No. 126. Contract No. 290-02-0022.) AHRQ Publication No. 05-E024-1.

Buck K, Zaineddin AK, Vrieling A, Linselsen J, Chang-Claude J. Meta-analyses of lignans and enterolignans in relation to breast cancer risk. Am J Clin Nutr. 2010;92:141–153.

Cassidy A, Brown JE, Hawdon A, Faughnan MA, King LJ, Millward J, et al. Factors affecting the bioavailability of soy isoflavones in humans after ingestion of physiologically relevant levels from different soy foods. J Nutr. 2006;136:45–51.

Clavel T, Doré J, Blaut M. Bioavailability of lignans in human subjects. Nutr Res Rev. 2006;19:187–196.

Cornwell T, Cohick W, Raskin I. Dietary phytoestrogens and health. Phytochemistry. 2004;65:995–1016.

Doerge DR, Chang HC, Churchwell MI, Holder CL. Analysis of soy isoflavone conjugation in vitro and in human blood using liquid chromatography-mass spectrometry. Drug Metab Disp. 2000;283:298–307.

Doerge DR, Sheehan DM. Goitrogenic and estrogenic activity of soy isoflavones. Environ Health Perspect. 2002;110(Suppl 3):349–353.

Dong JY, Qin LQ. Soy isoflavones consumption and risk of breast cancer incidence or recurrency: a meta-analysis of prospective studies. Breast Cancer Res Tr. 2010;125:315–323.

Erdman JW Jr, Badger TM, Lampe JW, Setchell KDR, Messina M. Not all soy products are created equal: caution needed in interpretation of research results. J Nutr. 2004;134:1229S–1233S.

Grace PB, Taylor JI, Low Y, Luben RN, Mulligan AA, Botting NP, et al. Phytoestrogen concentrations in serum and spot urine as biomarkers for dietary phytoestrogen intake and their relation to breast cancer risk in European prospective investigation of cancer and nutrition—Norfolk. Cancer Epidemiol Biomarkers and Prev. 2004;13:698–708.

Hamilton-Reeves JM, Vazquez G, Duval SJ, Phipps WR, Kurzer MS, Messina MJ. Clinical studies show no effects of soy protein or isoflavones on reproductive hormones in men: results of a meta-analysis. Fertil Steril. 2010;94:997–1007.

Hoikkala AA, Schiavoni E, Wähälä K. Analyis of phyto-oestrogens in biological matrices. Brit J Nutr. 2003;89:S5–S18.

Howes LG, Howes JB, Knight DC. Isoflavone therapy for menopausal flushes: a systematic review and meta-analysis. Maturitas. 2006;55:203–211.

Jacobs A, Wegewitz U, Sommerfeld C, Grossklaus R, Lampen A. Efficacy of isoflavones in relieving vasomotor menopausal symptoms – A systematic review. Mol Nutr Food Res. 2009;53:1084–1097.

Klein KO. Isoflavones, soy-based infant formulas, and relevance to endocrine function. Nutr Rev. 1998;56:193–204.

Lampe JW, Gustafson DR, Hutchins AM, Martini MG, Li S, Wahala K, et al. Urinary isoflavonoid and lignan excretion on a western diet: relation to soy, vegetable and fruit intake. Cancer Epidemiol Biomarkers and Prev. 1999;8:699–707.

Liu J, Ho SC, Su XY, Chen WQ, Zhang CX, Chen YM. Effect of long-term intervention of soy isoflavones on bone mineral density in women: A meta-analysis of randomized controlled trials. Bone. 2010;44:948–953.

McCarver G, Bhatia J, Chambers C, Clarke R, Etzel R, Foster W, et al. NTP-CERHR expert panel report on the developmental toxicity of soy infant formula. Birth Defects Res. (Part B) 2011;92:421–468.

Mortensen A, Kulling SE, Schwartz H, Rowland I, Ruefer CE, Rimbach G, et al. Analytical and compositional aspects of isoflavones in food and their biological effects. Mol Nutr Food Res. 2009;59:S266–S309.

Nagel SC, vomSaal FS, Welshons WV. The effective free fraction of estradiol and xenoestrogens in human serum measured by whole cell uptake assays: physiology of delivery modifies estrogenic activity. Proc Soc Exp Biol Med. 1998;217:300–309.

Nesbitt PD, Lam Y, Thompson LU. Human metabolism of mammalian lignan precursors in raw and processed flaxseed. Am J Clin Nutr. 1999;69:549–555.

Nielsen ILF, Williamson G. Review of the factors affecting bioavailability of soy isoflavones in humans. Nutr Cancer. 2007;57:1–10.

Pan A, Yu D, Demark-Wahnefried W, Franco OH, Lin X. Meta-analysis of the effects of flaxseed interventions on blood lipids. Am J Clin Nutr. 2009;90:288–297.

Parker DL, Rybak ME, Pfeiffer CM. Phytoestrogen biomonitoring: an extractionless LC-MS/MS method for measuring urinary isoflavones and lignans using atmospheric pressure photoionization (APPI). Anal Bioanal Chem. 2012;402:1123–1136.

Pérez-Jiménez J, Hubert J, Hooper L, Cassidy A, Manach C, Williamson G, Scalbert A. Urinary metabolites as biomarkers of polyphenol intake in humans: a systematic review. Am J Clin Nutr. 2010;92:801–809.

Peterson J, Dwyer J, Adlercreutz A, Scalbert A, Jacques P, Mccullough ML. Dietary lignans: physiology and potential for cardiovascular disease risk reduction. Nutr Rev. 2010;68:571–603.

Rowland IR, Wiseman H, Sanders TAB, Adlercreutz H, Bowey EA. Interindividual variation in metabolism of soy isoflavones and lignans: influence of habitual diet on equol production by the gut microflora. Nutr Cancer. 2000;36:27–32.

Rowland I, Faughnan M, Hoey L, Wahala K, Williamson G, Cassidy A. Bioavailability of phyto-estrogens. Br J Nutr. 2003;89(Suppl 1):S45–S58.

Rozman KK, Bhatia J, Calafat AM, Chambers C, Culty M, Etzel RA, et al. NTP-CERHR expert panel report on the reproductive and developmental toxicity of soy formula. Birth Defects Res. (Part B) 2006*a*;77:280–397.

Rozman KK, Bhatia J, Calafat AM, Chambers C, Culty M, Etzel RA, et al. NTP-CERHR expert panel report on the reproductive and developmental toxicity of genistein. Birth Defects Res. (Part B) 2006*b*;77:485–638.

Rybak ME, Parker DL, Pfeiffer CM. Determination of urinary phytoestrogens by HPLC-MS/MS: a comparison of atmospheric pressure chemical ionization (APCl) and electrospray ionization (ESI). J Chromatogr B. 2008;861:145–150.

Setchell KD, Zimmer-Nechemias L, Cai J, Heubi JE. Exposure of infants to phyto-oestrogens from soy-based infant formula. Lancet. 1997;350:23–27.

Setchell KD, Briwb NM, Lydeking-Olsen E. The clinical importance of the metabolite equol a clue to the effectiveness of soy and its isoflavones. J Nutr. 2002;132:3577–3584.

Setchell KDR, Brown NM, Desai PB, Zimmer-Nechimias L, Wolfe B, Jakate AS, et al. Bioavailability, disposition, and dose-response effects of soy isoflavones when consumed by healthy women at physiologically typical dietary intakes. J Nutr. 2003*a*; 133:1027–1035.

Setchell KDR, Faughnan MS, Acades T, Zimmer-Nechemias L, Brown NM, Wolfe BE, et al. Comparing the pharmacokinetics of daidzein and genistein with the use of 13C-labeled tracers in premenopausal women. Am J Clin Nutr. 2003*b*;77:411–419.

Setchell KD, Cole SJ. Method of defining equol-producer status and its frequency among vegetarians. J Nutr. 2006;136:2188–2193.

Strom BL, Schinnar R, Ziegler EE, Barnhart KT, Sammel MD, Macones GA, et al. Exposure to soy-based formula in infancy and endocrinological and reproductive outcomes in young adulthood. JAMA. 2001;286:807–814.

U.S. Centers for Disease Control and Prevention. Fourth National Report on Human Exposure to Environmental Chemicals. Atlanta (GA): CDC; 2009. [cited 2011]. Available at: http://www.cdc.gov/exposurereport.

U.S. Centers for Disease Control and Prevention. Analytic note for urinary phytoestrogens 2005-2006. Hyattsville (MD): CDC; 2011 (in press). [cited 2011]. Available at: http://www.cdc.gov/nchs/nhanes/nhanes2005-2006/L54PHY_D.htm.

U.S. Department of Agriculture and U.S. Department of Health and Human Services. Dietary Guidelines for Americans, 2010. 7th Edition, Washington, DC: U.S. Government Printing Office, December 2010. [cited 2011]. Available at: http://www.cnpp.usda.gov/DGAs2010-PolicyDocument.htm.

Vafeiadou K, Hall WL, Williams CM. Does genotype and equol-production status affect response to isoflavones? Data from a pan-European study on the effects of isoflavones on cardiovascular risk markers in post-menopausal women. Proc Nutr Soc. 2006;65:106–115.

Valentin-Blasini L, Sadowski MA, Walden D, Caltabiano L, Needham LL, Barr DB. Urinary phytoestrogen concentrations in the U.S. population (1999–2000). J Exposure Anal Environ Epidemiol. 2005;15:509–523.

Yan L, Spitznagel EL. Soy consumption and prostate cancer risk in men: a revisit of a meta-analysis. Am J Clin Nutr. 2009;89:1155–1163.

5. Acrylamide Hemoglobin Adducts

- Acrylamide
- Glycidamide
- Glycidamide-to-acrylamide ratio

Acrylamide Hemoglobin Adducts

Background Information

Sources. Acrylamide is a chemical naturally found in starchy foods that are cooked at high temperatures (above 120°C) and low-moisture conditions, such as those used for baking or frying. There are also several foods in which acrylamide appears to form in high-moisture conditions at lower temperatures, such as prune juice and canned ripe black olives (Robin 2007). Acrylamide is formed in food mainly due to a reaction between the amino acid asparagine and reducing sugars, such as glucose and fructose (Stadler 2002, Mottram 2002). The formation of acrylamide is part of the Maillard reaction, which leads to browning and flavor changes in cooked foods. Foods that contain high acrylamide levels include potato chips, crackers, snacks, and coffee (U.S. Food and Drug Administration 2006, Dybing 2005). Most people consume foods containing acrylamide on a daily basis. Acrylamide is present in tobacco smoke (Smith 2000), and it is an industrial chemical used in products for water purification, grouts, packaging, cosmetics, and scientific research (U.S. Environmental Protection Agency 1994).

Health Effects. High levels of acrylamide can be neurotoxic in both humans and animals and carcinogenic in animals. Acrylamide has been categorized by the International Agency for Research on Cancer as a suspected human carcinogen (IARC 1995). In the most recent edition of the National Toxicology Program Report on Carcinogens, acrylamide has been categorized as *"reasonably anticipated to be a human carcinogen* based on sufficient evidence of carcinogenicity from studies in experimental animals" (U.S. National Toxicology Program 2011). The U.S. Environmental Protection Agency has characterized acrylamide as "likely to be carcinogenic to humans" (U.S. Environmental Protection Agency 2010). In the body, some acrylamide is metabolized to glycidamide, an epoxide of acrylamide, through action of cytochrome P450 2E1. In contrast to acrylamide, glycidamide reacts with DNA in the body and is therefore considered the genotoxic agent. Acrylamide and glycidamide are cleared through the body mainly by formation of glutathione adducts and excretion in urine. Neither compound accumulates in the body.

Intake. The estimated intake of acrylamide from food in the general U.S. population (ages 2 and older) is on average 0.44 microgram per kilogram bodyweight per day (μg/kg bw/day), with a 90th percentile of 0.95 μg/kg bw/day. Children 2–5 years of age consume about twice the amount that adults consume (U.S. Food and Drug Administration 2006, Tran 2010). These levels are about 100 times below those known to cause neurotoxic effects or cancer in animals. The lifelong exposure of most of the population to acrylamide through food and smoking has, however, raised concerns about its potential health effects at these low levels of intake. Initial studies using food intake questionnaires to investigate possible associations between acrylamide intake and various cancers mostly did not find any associations (Hogervorst 2010). To obtain more information about the actual acrylamide exposure in the body, further investigations using biomarkers of acrylamide exposure were recommended.

Biochemical Indicators and Methods. Hemoglobin adducts of acrylamide and glycidamide reliably reflect the internal dose of acrylamide during the preceding two to four months (Bergmark 1991, Törnqvist 2002). The measured hemoglobin adduct levels reflect a time-weighted average of exposure over the lifetime of the erythrocyte (Fennell 1992). Hemoglobin adducts show a high within-person correlation over time, suggesting that a single blood measurement is a relatively good indicator of long-term acrylamide intake (Wilson 2009). Hemoglobin adducts, however, are not specific with regard to the source of acrylamide intake or exposure. Therefore, studies using these biomarkers to investigate acrylamide intake from foods need to control for exposures from other sources, such as smoking. Persons who smoke tobacco products have higher acrylamide exposure than those not smoking (Vesper 2007). Exposure to second hand smoke seems to have a small but significant effect on hemoglobin adduct levels in non-smokers (Vesper 2010).

Analytical methods measuring hemoglobin adducts of acrylamide determine the adducts at the N-terminal valine of the hemoglobin protein chains. Initial methods employed gas chromatography coupled with mass spectrometry; these methods were based on a modified Edman reaction, which was first described for measuring N-terminal hemoglobin adducts of ethylene oxide, propylene oxide, and styrene oxide (Mowrer 1986). These initial methods were further developed and optimized to measure hemoglobin adducts of acrylamide and glycidamide (Törnqvist 1986, Vesper 2006).

Data in NHANES. No data exist on acrylamide hemoglobin adduct concentrations in NHANES prior to 2003. This report shows first-time NHANES data for hemoglobin adducts of acrylamide and glycidamide. Data presented in this report were generated by use of high-performance liquid chromatography coupled to tandem mass spectrometry (LC-MS/MS); this method uses stable isotope labeled peptide adducts (same amino acid sequence as hemoglobin) of acrylamide and glycidamide as internal standards (Vesper 2008).

Highlights

The first-time acrylamide hemoglobin adduct concentrations in the U.S. population showed the following demographic patterns and characteristics:

- Hemoglobin adduct concentrations were detectable in 98% of all blood samples measured.

- We found demographic differences for the glycidamide-to-acrylamide hemoglobin adduct ratios, but no consistent age, gender, or race/ethnicity patterns for the hemoglobin adduct concentrations.

New data from NHANES 2003–2004 allow us for the first time to assess the exposure of the U.S. population to acrylamide. Measurement of hemoglobin adducts provides information both about acrylamide exposure and metabolism. The glycidamide-to-acrylamide hemoglobin adduct ratio can be used as an indicator of the extent of acrylamide metabolism and thus as an indicator of formation of the genotoxic metabolite glycidamide in the body and its detoxification. Children had higher glycidamide-to-acrylamide hemoglobin adduct ratios compared to adolescents and adults (Figure H.5.a), suggesting differences in acrylamide metabolism or metabolic rate among age groups (Vesper 2010). Non-Hispanic blacks (NHB) had lower hemoglobin adduct ratios compared to non-Hispanic whites (NHW) and Mexican Americans (MA), which may indicate differences in polymorphisms of the genes involved in phase II detoxification of acrylamide and glycidamide (Vesper 2010). More research is needed to better understand factors influencing acrylamide metabolism and the relationship between acrylamide exposure and health risks.

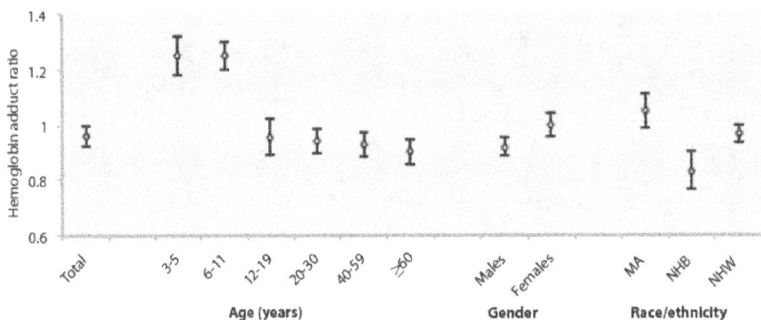

Figure H.5.a. Geometric mean of glycidamide-to-acrylamide hemoglobin adduct ratio in the U.S. population aged 3 years and older, National Health and Nutrition Examination Survey, 2003–2004.

Error bars represent 95 percent confidence intervals.

Detailed Observations

The selected observations mentioned below are derived from the tables and figures presented next. Statements about categorical differences between demographic groups noted below are based on non-overlapping confidence limits from univariate analysis without adjusting for demographic variables (e.g., age, sex, race/ethnicity) or other blood concentration determinants (e.g., dietary intake, supplement usage, smoking, BMI). A multivariate analysis may alter the size and statistical significance of these categorical differences. Furthermore, additional significant differences of smaller magnitude may be present despite their lack of mention here (e.g., if confidence limits slightly overlap or if differences are not statistically significant before covariate adjustment has occurred). For a selection of citations of descriptive NHANES papers related to these biochemical indicators of diet and nutrition, see **Appendix G.**

Geometric mean concentrations (NHANES 2003–2004):

- Acrylamide and glycidamide hemoglobin adduct concentrations were comparable across age groups except for older persons, who had lower concentrations (Tables 5.1.a.1 and 5.2.a.1; Figures 5.1.a and 5.2.a).

- Acrylamide (Table 5.1.a.1) and glycidamide hemoglobin adduct concentrations (Table 5.2.a.1) were comparable for males and females.

- Acrylamide hemoglobin adduct concentrations were comparable across the three race/ethnic groups (Table 5.1.a). Non-Hispanic blacks had lower glycidamide hemoglobin adduct concentrations than both non-Hispanic whites and Mexican Americans (Table 5.2.a.1).

- Glycidamide-to-acrylamide hemoglobin adduct ratios were higher in children (3-5 and 6-11 years of age) compared to adolescents and adults, higher in females compared to males, and lower in non-Hispanic blacks compared to both non-Hispanic whites and Mexican Americans (Table 5.3.a.1 and Figure 5.3.a).

Table 5.1.a.1. Acrylamide hemoglobin adduct: Concentrations

Geometric mean and selected percentiles of whole blood concentrations (in pmol/g Hb) for the total U.S. population aged 3 years and older, National Health and Nutrition Examination Survey, 2003–2004.

	Geometric mean (95% conf. interval)	Selected percentiles (95% conf. interval)						Sample size
		2.5th	5th	50th	95th	97.5th	
Total, 3 years and older	61.2 (58.1 – 64.4)	25.7 (23.7 – 26.8)	29.2 (27.6 – 30.5)	54.7 (52.8 – 57.6)	192 (170 – 219)	236 (219 – 277)	7,101
Age group							
3–5 years	59.4 (53.6 – 65.7)	30.9† (28.9 – 34.0)	35.9 (29.7 – 38.0)	58.2 (52.5 – 64.7)	108 (90.3 – 229)	115† (107 – 238)	350
6–11 years	58.6 (56.1 – 61.2)	31.5 (27.2 – 35.1)	36.1 (32.2 – 38.7)	57.3 (55.1 – 59.6)	98.7 (91.3 – 103)	106 (101 – 137)	769
12–19 years	57.4 (54.4 – 60.5)	28.4 (25.7 – 29.8)	31.4 (30.0 – 32.6)	54.4 (52.1 – 57.3)	132 (118 – 156)	173 (147 – 214)	1,889
20–39 years	68.5 (64.1 – 73.3)	26.5 (23.9 – 28.4)	30.3 (28.0 – 31.7)	59.8 (57.0 – 63.9)	225 (200 – 254)	270 (237 – 341)	1,406
40–59 years	64.0 (59.9 – 68.4)	24.1 (22.2 – 27.0)	29.1 (26.1 – 31.2)	55.1 (52.1 – 59.1)	219 (189 – 250)	256 (227 – 328)	1,164
60 years and older	50.1 (47.9 – 52.3)	21.6 (19.1 – 23.3)	26.0 (23.2 – 27.2)	46.5 (44.1 – 49.1)	140 (126 – 153)	175 (151 – 211)	1,523
Gender							
Males	63.9 (60.2 – 67.9)	26.0 (23.0 – 28.0)	29.0 (27.2 – 31.1)	56.9 (53.6 – 60.0)	219 (195 – 237)	257 (236 – 305)	3,509
Females	58.7 (55.9 – 61.5)	25.0 (23.3 – 26.2)	29.4 (27.9 – 30.3)	53.3 (51.8 – 55.8)	164 (149 – 196)	213 (179 – 253)	3,592
Race/ethnicity							
Mexican Americans	61.7 (58.7 – 64.9)	33.4 (29.4 – 35.5)	36.5 (34.5 – 38.3)	57.4 (54.4 – 60.3)	149 (127 – 186)	211 (186 – 244)	1,792
Non-Hispanic Blacks	63.8 (57.1 – 71.2)	23.9 (23.1 – 24.7)	27.3 (26.0 – 29.1)	57.0 (51.9 – 64.0)	217 (181 – 285)	285 (233 – 357)	1,818
Non-Hispanic Whites	62.3 (58.9 – 65.9)	26.5 (24.1 – 27.7)	29.6 (28.2 – 31.3)	55.2 (52.9 – 58.5)	196 (175 – 223)	235 (222 – 276)	2,958

† Estimate is subject to greater uncertainty due to small cell size.

Figure 5.1.a. Acrylamide hemoglobin adduct: Concentrations by age group
Geometric mean (95% confidence interval), National Health and Nutrition Examination Survey, 2003–2004

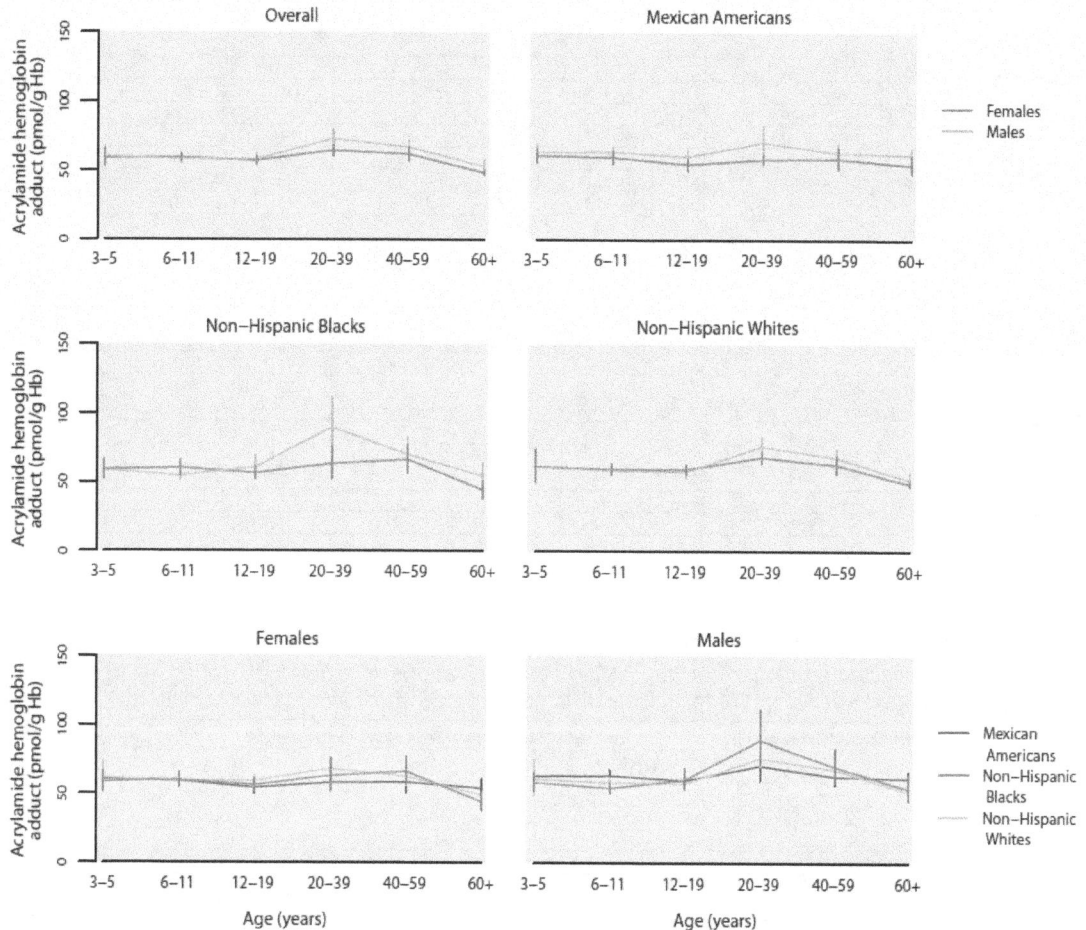

Table 5.1.a.2. Acrylamide hemoglobin adduct: Total population

Geometric mean and selected percentiles of whole blood concentrations (in pmol/g Hb) for the total U.S. population aged 3 years and older, National Health and Nutrition Examination Survey, 2003–2004.

	Geometric mean (95% conf. interval)	Selected percentiles (95% conf. interval)						Sample size
		10th		50th		90th		
Males and Females								
Total, 3 years and older	61.2	(58.1 – 64.4)	33.7	(32.4 – 35.1)	54.7	(52.8 – 57.6)	140 (125 – 155)	7,101
3–5 years	59.4	(53.6 – 65.7)	38.5	(33.3 – 42.9)	58.2	(52.5 – 64.7)	90.2 (83.2 – 108)	350
6–11 years	58.6	(56.1 – 61.2)	39.6	(37.9 – 42.7)	57.3	(55.1 – 59.6)	86.7 (81.9 – 93.0)	769
12–19 years	57.4	(54.4 – 60.5)	35.6	(33.8 – 37.1)	54.4	(52.1 – 57.3)	99.9 (91.0 – 115)	1,889
20–39 years	68.5	(64.1 – 73.3)	35.1	(32.5 – 37.7)	59.8	(57.0 – 63.9)	164 (153 – 195)	1,406
40–59 years	64.0	(59.9 – 68.4)	33.5	(31.9 – 35.3)	55.1	(52.1 – 59.1)	160 (142 – 190)	1,164
60 years and older	50.1	(47.9 – 52.3)	29.6	(27.7 – 31.2)	46.5	(44.1 – 49.1)	96.1 (90.2 – 107)	1,523
Males								
Total, 3 years and older	63.9	(60.2 – 67.9)	33.6	(31.3 – 35.6)	56.9	(53.6 – 60.0)	152 (140 – 177)	3,509
3–5 years	59.8	(53.2 – 67.2)	38.8	(30.3 – 43.5)	57.8	(49.4 – 65.8)	91.4 (82.7 – 115)	189
6–11 years	58.1	(55.2 – 61.1)	39.6	(35.4 – 41.9)	56.6	(54.7 – 59.3)	86.5 (81.2 – 91.3)	370
12–19 years	57.8	(53.7 – 62.3)	35.0	(32.0 – 37.2)	53.9	(51.1 – 57.7)	107 (94.6 – 127)	976
20–39 years	73.0	(66.9 – 79.7)	35.0	(30.8 – 38.7)	63.8	(59.3 – 68.6)	209 (168 – 228)	655
40–59 years	66.7	(62.2 – 71.6)	33.4	(29.3 – 36.0)	57.3	(51.0 – 64.1)	177 (150 – 205)	572
60 years and older	52.6	(47.8 – 57.9)	29.1	(27.4 – 31.3)	48.0	(42.9 – 52.8)	117 (96.9 – 143)	747
Females								
Total, 3 years and older	58.7	(55.9 – 61.5)	33.9	(32.7 – 35.1)	53.3	(51.8 – 55.8)	125 (112 – 143)	3,592
3–5 years	58.9	(52.9 – 65.5)	37.6	(22.3 – 43.7)	59.5	(53.1 – 63.3)	86.1 (79.4 – 134)	161
6–11 years	59.1	(56.5 – 61.8)	40.4	(36.7 – 44.2)	57.4	(55.2 – 60.2)	86.9 (81.0 – 97.5)	399
12–19 years	56.9	(54.5 – 59.5)	36.9	(33.7 – 37.9)	55.3	(53.0 – 57.7)	97.5 (87.4 – 109)	913
20–39 years	64.3	(60.5 – 68.3)	35.2	(33.0 – 37.5)	56.8	(54.4 – 59.5)	152 (131 – 163)	751
40–59 years	61.6	(56.6 – 67.0)	33.4	(32.1 – 35.4)	53.8	(50.2 – 58.9)	151 (125 – 186)	592
60 years and older	48.1	(46.7 – 49.6)	29.8	(27.2 – 31.7)	45.4	(44.3 – 46.9)	84.0 (77.5 – 93.6)	776

Table 5.1.a.3. Acrylamide hemoglobin adduct: Mexican Americans

Geometric mean and selected percentiles of whole blood concentrations (in pmol/g Hb) for Mexican Americans in the U.S. population aged 3 years and older, National Health and Nutrition Examination Survey, 2003–2004.

	Geometric mean (95% conf. interval)	Selected percentiles (95% conf. interval)						Sample size
		10th		50th		90th		
Males and Females								
Total, 3 years and older	61.7	(58.7 – 64.9)	40.0	(38.2 – 42.1)	57.4	(54.4 – 60.3)	101 (95.4 – 115)	1,792
3–5 years	62.0	(57.8 – 66.6)	45.6†	(39.5 – 48.1)	59.6	(56.9 – 65.0)	87.4† (78.8 – 104)	90
6–11 years	61.6	(58.2 – 65.3)	44.3	(40.9 – 45.6)	61.4	(55.9 – 67.0)	88.3 (84.0 – 96.4)	250
12–19 years	57.3	(53.8 – 61.0)	38.7	(37.4 – 40.1)	55.2	(51.4 – 59.8)	86.9 (79.6 – 96.5)	590
20–39 years	64.5	(59.9 – 69.5)	40.7	(38.6 – 42.6)	57.5	(54.6 – 60.4)	118 (96.2 – 191)	321
40–59 years	60.9	(55.2 – 67.1)	38.7	(33.8 – 42.2)	56.1	(48.4 – 63.9)	117 (91.6 – 153)	208
60 years and older	57.5	(53.9 – 61.4)	36.5	(31.9 – 38.3)	53.9	(50.0 – 57.9)	108 (91.3 – 120)	333
Males								
Total, 3 years and older	65.7	(60.9 – 70.9)	41.4	(38.6 – 43.4)	58.2	(55.0 – 62.6)	122 (103 – 185)	882
3–5 years	63.2	(57.5 – 69.5)	47.3†	(40.5 – 48.8)	59.8	(57.1 – 65.5)	88.0† (74.1 – 122)	47
6–11 years	63.5	(59.7 – 67.6)	44.5	(40.8 – 48.3)	62.5	(59.6 – 68.1)	92.0 (84.2 – 102)	117
12–19 years	60.1	(55.8 – 64.8)	39.4	(36.8 – 41.5)	56.8	(53.7 – 61.0)	96.3 (85.5 – 124)	301
20–39 years	70.8	(60.5 – 82.9)	42.1	(37.6 – 44.7)	59.4	(53.2 – 66.6)	176 (111 – 353)	146
40–59 years	63.0	(57.3 – 69.3)	39.2†	(25.0 – 44.2)	54.8	(50.1 – 59.7)	124† (92.9 – 193)	109
60 years and older	61.6	(57.0 – 66.5)	36.7	(32.5 – 38.2)	58.0	(51.6 – 64.0)	118 (101 – 151)	162
Females								
Total, 3 years and older	57.6	(54.8 – 60.6)	39.0	(36.5 – 40.8)	55.4	(52.0 – 59.4)	89.0 (82.5 – 96.2)	910
3–5 years	60.7	(55.9 – 65.8)	43.4†	(36.4 – 48.5)	59.5	(49.3 – 68.0)	82.5† (77.2 – 102)	43
6–11 years	59.5	(55.3 – 64.1)	44.0	(39.6 – 45.0)	58.4	(52.3 – 65.7)	82.2 (79.6 – 96.2)	133
12–19 years	54.5	(50.1 – 59.3)	38.1	(35.0 – 39.7)	53.1	(47.3 – 60.0)	79.4 (72.0 – 93.5)	289
20–39 years	58.2	(54.6 – 62.0)	39.1	(34.9 – 41.9)	55.1	(50.8 – 60.9)	94.5 (81.1 – 108)	175
40–59 years	58.6	(51.4 – 66.7)	38.7†	(35.6 – 39.6)	57.8	(45.5 – 66.9)	94.9† (82.2 – 138)	99
60 years and older	54.2	(48.2 – 60.9)	35.7	(19.3 – 40.4)	50.5	(46.3 – 57.3)	85.6 (79.3 – 110)	171

† Estimate is subject to greater uncertainty due to small cell size.

Table 5.1.a.4. Acrylamide hemoglobin adduct: Non-Hispanic blacks

Geometric mean and selected percentiles of whole blood concentrations (in pmol/g Hb) for non-Hispanic blacks in the U.S. population aged 3 years and older, National Health and Nutrition Examination Survey, 2003–2004.

	Geometric mean (95% conf. interval)		Selected percentiles (95% conf. interval)						Sample size
			10th		50th		90th		
Males and Females									
Total, 3 years and older	63.8	(57.1 – 71.2)	32.3	(30.6 – 33.9)	57.0	(51.9 – 64.0)	156	(123 – 210)	1,818
3–5 years	58.7	(53.4 – 64.5)	39.9	(34.1 – 44.1)	56.0	(53.0 – 62.9)	87.1	(74.3 – 156)	126
6–11 years	57.1	(53.6 – 60.8)	38.6	(33.8 – 41.1)	56.7	(52.3 – 60.4)	85.6	(77.4 – 97.8)	277
12–19 years	58.6	(53.3 – 64.3)	34.4	(31.6 – 36.7)	55.2	(52.3 – 58.9)	110	(97.5 – 138)	667
20–39 years	73.8	(60.9 – 89.4)	33.2	(29.8 – 37.8)	64.4	(53.5 – 80.8)	209	(155 – 293)	290
40–59 years	67.9	(59.3 – 77.8)	32.3	(28.5 – 34.5)	59.4	(49.7 – 69.9)	182	(152 – 250)	259
60 years and older	48.1	(42.3 – 54.6)	24.5	(21.4 – 26.1)	43.1	(39.3 – 50.7)	106	(94.7 – 133)	199
Males									
Total, 3 years and older	68.7	(60.8 – 77.6)	32.1	(29.1 – 34.8)	61.7	(55.2 – 68.2)	194	(140 – 241)	918
3–5 years	58.5	(52.4 – 65.4)	37.0†	(25.8 – 45.7)	55.7	(52.2 – 65.1)	88.3†	(74.7 – 158)	70
6–11 years	54.5	(51.1 – 58.1)	37.7	(31.8 – 40.3)	55.5	(48.5 – 59.4)	75.3	(70.6 – 97.3)	133
12–19 years	60.7	(53.5 – 68.9)	35.2	(30.8 – 37.2)	55.8	(50.8 – 63.8)	121	(102 – 161)	356
20–39 years	89.4	(72.1 – 111)	34.0	(29.9 – 40.4)	86.5	(66.6 – 110)	240	(202 – 361)	142
40–59 years	70.0	(59.3 – 82.6)	29.0	(20.9 – 33.2)	63.9	(51.4 – 72.9)	207	(158 – 290)	123
60 years and older	54.2	(45.8 – 64.2)	25.4†	(21.5 – 28.9)	46.2	(40.9 – 61.0)	116†	(98.5 – 230)	94
Females									
Total, 3 years and older	59.8	(53.4 – 66.8)	32.4	(30.2 – 34.4)	54.5	(48.3 – 60.5)	133	(106 – 171)	900
3–5 years	58.9	(52.3 – 66.3)	43.6†	(32.2 – 45.3)	56.2	(48.4 – 67.3)	82.9†	(67.1 – 129)	56
6–11 years	60.1	(55.2 – 65.4)	39.4	(35.3 – 43.2)	58.1	(52.1 – 68.0)	95.1	(85.5 – 106)	144
12–19 years	56.5	(52.2 – 61.0)	33.5	(30.4 – 36.7)	53.7	(51.3 – 57.4)	106	(86.0 – 136)	311
20–39 years	63.2	(52.5 – 75.9)	32.8	(27.1 – 37.6)	56.4	(45.3 – 69.7)	153	(106 – 290)	148
40–59 years	66.3	(57.0 – 77.1)	35.1	(24.1 – 39.3)	56.5	(47.1 – 71.0)	173	(147 – 228)	136
60 years and older	44.2	(38.2 – 51.2)	23.7†	(19.4 – 26.0)	41.1	(37.8 – 46.9)	92.1†	(69.4 – 143)	105

† Estimate is subject to greater uncertainty due to small cell size.

Table 5.1.a.5. Acrylamide hemoglobin adduct: Non-Hispanic whites

Geometric mean and selected percentiles of whole blood concentrations (in pmol/g Hb) for non-Hispanic whites in the U.S. population aged 3 years and older, National Health and Nutrition Examination Survey, 2003–2004.

	Geometric mean (95% conf. interval)		Selected percentiles (95% conf. interval)						Sample size
			10th		50th		90th		
Males and Females									
Total, 3 years and older	62.3	(58.9 – 65.9)	34.0	(32.5 – 35.7)	55.2	(52.9 – 58.5)	145	(130 – 165)	2,958
3–5 years	61.1	(51.7 – 72.2)	39.0†	(20.8 – 44.7)	58.5	(47.7 – 78.2)	98.7†	(82.6 – 118)	93
6–11 years	59.0	(56.2 – 62.0)	39.9	(35.1 – 44.6)	58.0	(55.2 – 60.3)	85.9	(80.4 – 91.5)	178
12–19 years	58.6	(55.3 – 62.2)	36.3	(33.3 – 38.5)	54.9	(52.7 – 57.9)	105	(95.0 – 120)	505
20–39 years	72.2	(67.6 – 77.0)	35.7	(31.4 – 39.4)	63.5	(59.2 – 68.5)	174	(157 – 198)	663
40–59 years	65.3	(60.6 – 70.4)	33.7	(32.1 – 36.1)	56.2	(52.1 – 61.1)	167	(143 – 206)	606
60 years and older	50.4	(47.9 – 53.0)	30.6	(28.5 – 31.9)	46.8	(43.9 – 49.7)	92.3	(84.1 – 113)	913
Males									
Total, 3 years and older	64.7	(60.6 – 69.0)	33.9	(31.4 – 36.3)	57.4	(53.1 – 60.9)	155	(141 – 187)	1,441
3–5 years	60.9	(49.4 – 75.0)	41.3†	(31.0 – 45.6)	57.3	(44.2 – 82.0)	103†	(81.4 – 118)	50
6–11 years	58.6	(55.5 – 61.9)	40.0†	(30.1 – 46.5)	56.6	(54.7 – 59.1)	85.9†	(77.4 – 94.8)	84
12–19 years	57.8	(53.5 – 62.5)	34.4	(31.7 – 37.0)	52.9	(50.2 – 57.0)	109	(94.7 – 134)	257
20–39 years	76.3	(70.4 – 82.8)	36.1	(30.0 – 41.0)	67.0	(60.9 – 73.8)	213	(166 – 228)	293
40–59 years	68.0	(62.5 – 74.0)	34.6	(29.3 – 38.0)	58.2	(50.8 – 66.1)	183	(150 – 213)	302
60 years and older	52.0	(46.7 – 57.8)	29.8	(27.5 – 31.5)	47.8	(42.4 – 52.5)	110	(87.5 – 136)	455
Females									
Total, 3 years and older	60.2	(57.0 – 63.5)	34.3	(32.8 – 35.5)	54.0	(52.1 – 57.1)	135	(119 – 154)	1,517
3–5 years	61.4	(51.2 – 73.6)	37.6†	(20.8 – 44.2)	62.2	(47.4 – 75.7)	91.2†	(79.5 – 238)	43
6–11 years	59.4	(55.7 – 63.4)	39.7†	(28.6 – 44.8)	58.5	(55.3 – 61.2)	84.6†	(78.2 – 141)	94
12–19 years	59.5	(56.1 – 63.2)	38.1	(34.4 – 40.4)	57.4	(54.1 – 59.9)	100	(92.2 – 117)	248
20–39 years	68.3	(64.0 – 72.9)	35.4	(30.6 – 39.3)	59.6	(54.7 – 65.8)	160	(147 – 182)	370
40–59 years	62.8	(56.9 – 69.2)	33.3	(32.2 – 35.2)	54.5	(50.3 – 60.7)	155	(129 – 217)	304
60 years and older	49.2	(47.8 – 50.6)	31.3	(29.5 – 33.2)	45.7	(45.0 – 47.4)	84.3	(74.6 – 103)	458

† Estimate is subject to greater uncertainty due to small cell size.

Table 5.2.a.1. Glycidamide hemoglobin adduct: Concentrations

Geometric mean and selected percentiles of whole blood concentrations (in pmol/g Hb) for the total U.S. population aged 3 years and older, National Health and Nutrition Examination Survey, 2003–2004.

	Geometric mean (95% conf. interval)	Selected percentiles (95% conf. interval)						Sample size
		2.5th	5th	50th	95th	97.5th	
Total, 3 years and older	59.3 (56.7 – 62.1)	17.5 (< LOD – 20.9)	24.1 (21.4 – 25.8)	59.9 (57.5 – 62.4)	167 (155 – 183)	205 (193 – 235)	7,278
Age group							
3–5 years	71.6 (66.9 – 76.7)	35.3† (27.7 – 37.8)	38.9 (33.4 – 46.3)	71.1 (67.0 – 79.1)	126 (121 – 136)	135† (128 – 166)	411
6–11 years	74.1 (70.3 – 78.2)	36.8 (33.0 – 38.6)	41.2 (36.8 – 44.6)	75.0 (70.9 – 77.9)	140 (128 – 158)	157 (144 – 201)	784
12–19 years	55.4 (51.1 – 60.1)	< LOD	23.3 (< LOD – 27.0)	59.2 (56.1 – 62.0)	145 (126 – 171)	173 (152 – 230)	1,931
20–39 years	65.0 (61.4 – 68.9)	20.6 (< LOD – 23.8)	26.9 (23.8 – 28.9)	64.0 (60.1 – 68.8)	195 (175 – 220)	244 (221 – 282)	1,446
40–59 years	60.1 (56.8 – 63.5)	17.8 (< LOD – 22.8)	24.1 (18.8 – 27.2)	58.8 (55.1 – 61.1)	179 (158 – 201)	210 (194 – 265)	1,177
60 years and older	45.5 (42.8 – 48.3)	< LOD	18.6 (12.1 – 21.1)	46.8 (44.8 – 49.2)	129 (115 – 145)	163 (141 – 199)	1,529
Gender							
Males	59.5 (56.9 – 62.3)	17.8 (11.3 – 20.7)	24.0 (21.5 – 25.7)	59.3 (56.9 – 61.7)	174 (158 – 199)	219 (193 – 292)	3,604
Females	59.1 (56.0 – 62.5)	14.3 (< LOD – 21.4)	24.5 (19.2 – 27.3)	60.4 (57.5 – 63.9)	158 (146 – 175)	197 (183 – 212)	3,674
Race/ethnicity							
Mexican Americans	64.7 (61.2 – 68.4)	22.5 (< LOD – 30.5)	32.8 (25.7 – 36.1)	65.4 (61.1 – 69.8)	152 (138 – 171)	199 (167 – 246)	1,841
Non-Hispanic Blacks	53.6 (50.6 – 56.7)	< LOD	17.4 (9.74 – 20.9)	55.5 (51.9 – 59.2)	159 (134 – 216)	206 (162 – 315)	1,900
Non-Hispanic Whites	61.1 (57.6 – 64.9)	19.6 (8.65 – 23.2)	25.5 (23.3 – 26.9)	60.6 (57.8 – 64.2)	172 (158 – 195)	213 (196 – 249)	3,008

< LOD means less than the limit of detection, which may vary for some compounds by year. See Appendix D for LOD.

† Estimate is subject to greater uncertainty due to small cell size.

Figure 5.2.a. Glycidamide hemoglobin adduct: Concentrations by age group

Geometric mean (95% confidence interval), National Health and Nutrition Examination Survey, 2003–2004

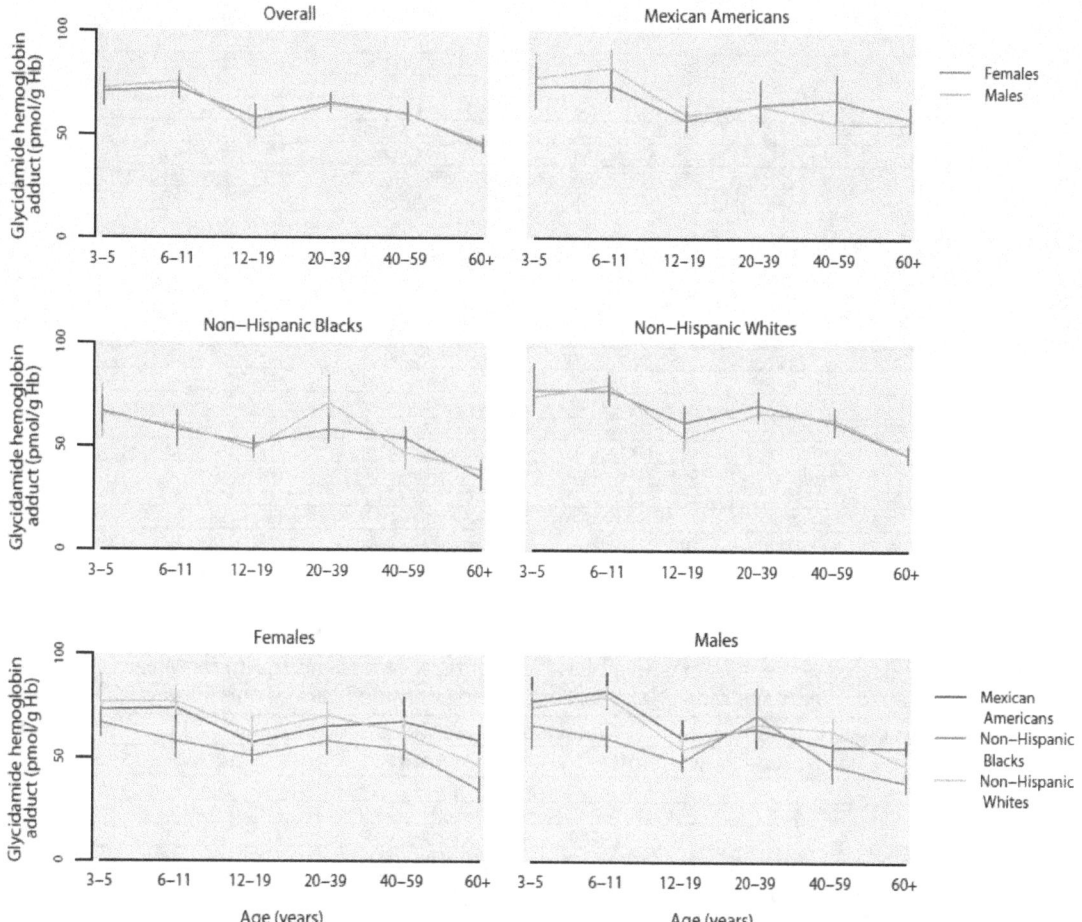

Table 5.2.a.2. Glycidamide hemoglobin adduct: Total population

Geometric mean and selected percentiles of whole blood concentrations (in pmol/g Hb) for the total U.S. population aged 3 years and older, National Health and Nutrition Examination Survey, 2003–2004.

	Geometric mean (95% conf. interval)		Selected percentiles (95% conf. interval)						Sample size
			10th		50th		90th		
Males and Females									
Total, 3 years and older	59.3	(56.7 – 62.1)	30.6	(28.7 – 32.4)	59.9	(57.5 – 62.4)	130	(120 – 140)	7,278
3–5 years	71.6	(66.9 – 76.7)	47.8	(39.0 – 51.4)	71.1	(67.0 – 79.1)	118	(107 – 126)	411
6–11 years	74.1	(70.3 – 78.2)	47.5	(43.8 – 49.4)	75.0	(70.9 – 77.9)	121	(113 – 135)	784
12–19 years	55.4	(51.1 – 60.1)	31.5	(27.3 – 33.8)	59.2	(56.1 – 62.0)	113	(96.8 – 141)	1,931
20–39 years	65.0	(61.4 – 68.9)	33.0	(29.9 – 35.4)	64.0	(60.1 – 68.8)	149	(136 – 167)	1,446
40–59 years	60.1	(56.8 – 63.5)	30.6	(27.7 – 32.8)	58.8	(55.1 – 61.1)	139	(124 – 158)	1,177
60 years and older	45.5	(42.8 – 48.3)	24.4	(22.6 – 25.6)	46.8	(44.8 – 49.2)	96.2	(90.6 – 103)	1,529
Males									
Total, 3 years and older	59.5	(56.9 – 62.3)	29.8	(27.6 – 32.0)	59.3	(56.9 – 61.7)	136	(124 – 148)	3,604
3–5 years	72.4	(67.5 – 77.7)	47.9	(38.4 – 52.2)	70.7	(66.8 – 76.6)	117	(99.9 – 145)	215
6–11 years	75.7	(71.8 – 79.9)	48.2	(45.6 – 50.3)	75.7	(69.9 – 79.6)	118	(112 – 140)	381
12–19 years	52.8	(48.2 – 57.8)	29.3	(24.5 – 32.7)	57.0	(53.2 – 61.0)	111	(97.5 – 134)	1,000
20–39 years	64.6	(60.9 – 68.6)	32.0	(28.6 – 33.8)	60.6	(57.6 – 65.9)	163	(149 – 174)	681
40–59 years	59.9	(56.3 – 63.8)	29.6	(26.1 – 32.8)	58.9	(54.3 – 62.2)	140	(128 – 164)	577
60 years and older	46.3	(42.8 – 50.1)	24.4	(22.2 – 25.7)	45.8	(41.6 – 48.6)	106	(95.4 – 129)	750
Females									
Total, 3 years and older	59.1	(56.0 – 62.5)	31.3	(29.1 – 33.4)	60.4	(57.5 – 63.9)	125	(116 – 135)	3,674
3–5 years	70.8	(63.8 – 78.7)	45.8	(34.1 – 53.1)	72.1	(65.7 – 82.0)	118	(104 – 130)	196
6–11 years	72.4	(67.2 – 77.9)	46.3	(43.6 – 48.3)	73.7	(69.6 – 77.9)	122	(106 – 142)	403
12–19 years	58.3	(52.8 – 64.5)	33.7	(28.7 – 35.7)	60.9	(56.5 – 65.8)	114	(95.9 – 160)	931
20–39 years	65.5	(61.4 – 69.8)	35.2	(31.0 – 38.2)	67.7	(61.4 – 73.7)	136	(123 – 160)	765
40–59 years	60.2	(55.3 – 65.6)	30.7	(27.8 – 34.3)	58.6	(53.1 – 64.8)	137	(115 – 160)	600
60 years and older	44.8	(41.8 – 48.1)	24.4	(21.3 – 26.3)	47.7	(45.2 – 50.8)	87.0	(81.1 – 93.8)	779

Table 5.2.a.3. Glycidamide hemoglobin adduct: Mexican Americans

Geometric mean and selected percentiles of whole blood concentrations (in pmol/g Hb) for Mexican Americans in the U.S. population aged 3 years and older, National Health and Nutrition Examination Survey, 2003–2004.

	Geometric mean (95% conf. interval)		Selected percentiles (95% conf. interval)						Sample size
			10th		50th		90th		
Males and Females									
Total, 3 years and older	64.7	(61.2 – 68.4)	39.4	(38.4 – 40.5)	65.4	(61.1 – 69.8)	118	(111 – 130)	1,841
3–5 years	75.5	(67.6 – 84.3)	49.6	(40.2 – 55.0)	74.4	(65.9 – 87.3)	114	(103 – 164)	117
6–11 years	78.5	(72.8 – 84.6)	52.1	(46.5 – 55.3)	78.5	(76.0 – 81.4)	126	(116 – 140)	256
12–19 years	58.7	(53.3 – 64.5)	37.0	(32.2 – 40.3)	62.3	(55.8 – 67.0)	99.7	(93.8 – 115)	601
20–39 years	64.7	(58.2 – 72.0)	39.0	(35.1 – 42.2)	63.9	(59.4 – 70.5)	128	(108 – 168)	324
40–59 years	61.2	(52.8 – 71.0)	38.4	(17.5 – 41.0)	60.5	(52.9 – 73.0)	115	(103 – 144)	212
60 years and older	57.1	(53.8 – 60.5)	33.1	(29.3 – 36.1)	55.8	(50.6 – 61.9)	107	(97.6 – 117)	331
Males									
Total, 3 years and older	64.2	(60.0 – 68.7)	38.3	(33.3 – 39.7)	63.6	(59.3 – 68.4)	129	(114 – 160)	909
3–5 years	77.6	(67.7 – 89.1)	52.5†	(35.6 – 58.5)	75.7	(68.5 – 87.5)	124†	(101 – 187)	58
6–11 years	82.6	(74.3 – 91.7)	55.2	(48.0 – 60.9)	79.7	(77.4 – 88.6)	128	(115 – 161)	125
12–19 years	60.0	(52.4 – 68.6)	36.4	(28.3 – 40.4)	63.4	(56.3 – 68.4)	115	(91.4 – 159)	306
20–39 years	64.4	(55.9 – 74.2)	38.2	(29.2 – 40.6)	60.1	(54.5 – 67.4)	161	(107 – 279)	146
40–59 years	56.0	(47.0 – 66.6)	32.8†	(4.98 – 39.7)	56.5	(49.9 – 62.8)	111†	(94.7 – 157)	111
60 years and older	55.6	(52.4 – 59.0)	30.3	(17.5 – 35.1)	54.6	(51.7 – 58.5)	110	(97.4 – 141)	163
Females									
Total, 3 years and older	65.2	(60.7 – 70.0)	41.9	(39.3 – 44.1)	67.7	(61.8 – 73.7)	111	(106 – 120)	932
3–5 years	73.2	(63.2 – 84.9)	46.6†	(42.6 – 49.5)	72.9	(58.1 – 88.9)	108†	(91.8 – 155)	59
6–11 years	73.8	(66.6 – 81.8)	47.4	(43.0 – 52.2)	74.0	(66.4 – 81.5)	119	(108 – 144)	131
12–19 years	57.3	(52.7 – 62.4)	37.1	(33.5 – 40.9)	61.2	(54.4 – 67.2)	94.5	(88.0 – 102)	295
20–39 years	65.1	(55.1 – 76.8)	42.4	(28.4 – 46.4)	68.9	(63.2 – 77.5)	114	(104 – 131)	178
40–59 years	67.4	(57.3 – 79.3)	39.8†	(34.4 – 43.6)	67.4	(54.8 – 81.6)	118†	(105 – 156)	101
60 years and older	58.4	(52.1 – 65.5)	36.0	(27.3 – 39.4)	56.8	(46.6 – 65.2)	104	(87.4 – 124)	168

† Estimate is subject to greater uncertainty due to small cell size.

Table 5.2.a.4. Glycidamide hemoglobin adduct: Non-Hispanic blacks

Geometric mean and selected percentiles of whole blood concentrations (in pmol/g Hb) for non-Hispanic blacks in the U.S. population aged 3 years and older, National Health and Nutrition Examination Survey, 2003–2004.

	Geometric mean (95% conf. interval)	Selected percentiles (95% conf. interval)						Sample size
		10th		50th		90th		
Males and Females								
Total, 3 years and older	53.6	(50.6 – 56.7)	27.1	(24.4 – 29.8)	55.5	(51.9 – 59.2)	121	(110 – 142)	1,900
3–5 years	66.3	(58.9 – 74.6)	41.3	(26.9 – 48.6)	70.0	(58.0 – 79.8)	101	(96.2 – 112)	141
6–11 years	58.7	(54.5 – 63.2)	35.8	(27.2 – 41.1)	63.0	(57.3 – 69.2)	108	(96.7 – 126)	282
12–19 years	49.7	(47.0 – 52.5)	27.0	(24.8 – 29.3)	52.6	(49.5 – 56.1)	106	(87.7 – 124)	690
20–39 years	63.5	(56.8 – 71.1)	33.4	(26.9 – 35.7)	63.7	(55.8 – 73.8)	144	(120 – 228)	311
40–59 years	50.6	(45.2 – 56.7)	23.5	(17.5 – 29.4)	50.9	(46.2 – 56.4)	133	(95.3 – 186)	265
60 years and older	36.3	(32.9 – 40.1)	15.4	(10.4 – 19.4)	39.7	(36.6 – 42.9)	84.6	(79.9 – 98.7)	211
Males								
Total, 3 years and older	54.8	(49.8 – 60.4)	26.5	(23.5 – 28.6)	56.4	(52.2 – 61.8)	134	(114 – 162)	956
3–5 years	65.8	(54.8 – 79.0)	40.1†	(< LOD – 49.0)	70.8	(54.1 – 84.2)	100†	(95.0 – 130)	77
6–11 years	59.5	(53.9 – 65.7)	35.7	(4.48 – 43.5)	62.9	(54.4 – 68.5)	108	(92.6 – 141)	133
12–19 years	48.5	(44.4 – 53.0)	25.3	(21.2 – 27.8)	51.0	(46.6 – 56.0)	113	(90.4 – 141)	369
20–39 years	71.1	(60.0 – 84.3)	33.3	(27.7 – 36.6)	70.1	(57.1 – 83.5)	152	(121 – 309)	154
40–59 years	46.9	(39.1 – 56.2)	17.5	(4.35 – 20.9)	50.3	(43.7 – 56.6)	156	(101 – 207)	124
60 years and older	38.8	(34.7 – 43.3)	19.9†	(9.71 – 22.2)	41.2	(33.6 – 47.1)	81.8†	(74.1 – 120)	99
Females								
Total, 3 years and older	52.5	(49.6 – 55.5)	28.0	(22.2 – 32.1)	55.0	(50.3 – 60.1)	114	(101 – 132)	944
3–5 years	66.9	(60.4 – 74.1)	40.4†	(30.2 – 55.7)	68.3	(58.2 – 79.8)	100†	(89.7 – 109)	64
6–11 years	57.9	(49.9 – 67.1)	35.7	(< LOD – 41.3)	63.5	(54.0 – 74.1)	106	(96.3 – 120)	149
12–19 years	50.8	(47.2 – 54.7)	30.7	(24.9 – 33.1)	54.1	(50.7 – 57.8)	98.7	(83.2 – 122)	321
20–39 years	58.0	(51.8 – 64.9)	33.3	(< LOD – 35.7)	60.3	(52.6 – 69.8)	130	(111 – 183)	157
40–59 years	53.9	(49.1 – 59.1)	29.8	(22.5 – 33.3)	50.9	(46.1 – 57.8)	115	(90.7 – 169)	141
60 years and older	34.7	(29.2 – 41.2)	14.1	(< LOD – 19.4)	38.7	(34.4 – 42.9)	87.3	(74.8 – 103)	112

< LOD means less than the limit of detection, which may vary for some compounds by year. See Appendix D for LOD.

† Estimate is subject to greater uncertainty due to small cell size.

Table 5.2.a.5. Glycidamide hemoglobin adduct: Non-Hispanic whites

Geometric mean and selected percentiles of whole blood concentrations (in pmol/g Hb) for non-Hispanic whites in the U.S. population aged 3 years and older, National Health and Nutrition Examination Survey, 2003–2004.

	Geometric mean (95% conf. interval)	Selected percentiles (95% conf. interval)						Sample size
		10th		50th		90th		
Males and Females								
Total, 3 years and older	61.1	(57.6 – 64.9)	31.1	(28.9 – 32.8)	60.6	(57.8 – 64.2)	135	(124 – 149)	3,008
3–5 years	75.5	(67.8 – 84.1)	50.7†	(37.9 – 53.7)	72.3	(65.8 – 88.4)	121†	(114 – 133)	110
6–11 years	78.5	(73.8 – 83.6)	51.3	(43.2 – 55.7)	76.0	(74.1 – 79.5)	123	(109 – 150)	183
12–19 years	57.9	(52.8 – 63.5)	33.4	(27.6 – 34.9)	60.4	(57.1 – 62.9)	115	(97.9 – 148)	512
20–39 years	68.5	(63.9 – 73.5)	32.9	(29.7 – 37.3)	67.5	(61.1 – 72.9)	160	(142 – 176)	682
40–59 years	62.8	(58.4 – 67.5)	31.9	(29.1 – 34.2)	60.4	(56.8 – 64.4)	143	(129 – 164)	610
60 years and older	46.6	(43.1 – 50.5)	25.0	(23.3 – 26.6)	47.7	(45.1 – 50.9)	96.7	(89.9 – 106)	911
Males								
Total, 3 years and older	61.0	(57.6 – 64.6)	30.2	(28.2 – 32.5)	60.1	(57.3 – 62.8)	140	(125 – 155)	1,473
3–5 years	74.2	(66.5 – 82.7)	48.0†	(37.9 – 55.0)	68.7	(60.3 – 88.3)	118†	(98.8 – 195)	58
6–11 years	79.8	(74.8 – 85.1)	55.5†	(47.5 – 57.9)	75.8	(70.9 – 84.9)	116†	(108 – 156)	87
12–19 years	54.4	(48.8 – 60.7)	30.4	(24.0 – 34.3)	57.3	(53.2 – 60.5)	102	(93.6 – 143)	264
20–39 years	66.7	(62.4 – 71.3)	31.9	(28.5 – 35.3)	62.9	(58.3 – 67.8)	170	(154 – 182)	308
40–59 years	63.7	(58.1 – 69.8)	32.3	(26.5 – 35.6)	60.6	(56.6 – 64.6)	141	(129 – 168)	303
60 years and older	46.9	(42.4 – 51.7)	24.5	(21.1 – 26.4)	45.9	(41.5 – 49.1)	106	(95.5 – 128)	453
Females								
Total, 3 years and older	61.2	(57.1 – 65.7)	31.7	(29.1 – 34.3)	61.1	(57.9 – 65.8)	132	(120 – 147)	1,535
3–5 years	77.1	(66.0 – 90.1)	51.9†	(< LOD – 60.9)	78.6	(62.4 – 100)	124†	(101 – 135)	52
6–11 years	77.2	(70.7 – 84.2)	48.7†	(39.3 – 53.1)	76.6	(71.9 – 80.3)	125†	(99.1 – 197)	96
12–19 years	62.0	(54.9 – 70.0)	34.4	(27.2 – 41.5)	63.0	(57.9 – 69.5)	119	(99.0 – 168)	248
20–39 years	70.5	(64.4 – 77.1)	36.5	(28.0 – 42.6)	71.2	(63.9 – 78.3)	142	(130 – 191)	374
40–59 years	61.9	(55.7 – 68.9)	30.9	(27.7 – 35.5)	60.0	(54.1 – 68.0)	144	(116 – 182)	307
60 years and older	46.5	(42.7 – 50.6)	25.7	(23.9 – 26.9)	49.3	(46.3 – 51.5)	87.1	(80.4 – 97.9)	458

< LOD means less than the limit of detection, which may vary for some compounds by year. See Appendix D for LOD.

† Estimate is subject to greater uncertainty due to small cell size.

Table 5.3.a.1. Glycidamide-to-acrylamide hemoglobin adduct ratio

Geometric mean and selected percentiles of ratio (no units) of whole blood concentrations (in pmol/g Hb) for the total U.S. population aged 3 years and older, National Health and Nutrition Examination Survey, 2003–2004.

	Geometric mean (95% conf. interval)	Selected percentiles (95% conf. interval)					Sample size
		2.5th	5th	50th	95th	97.5th	
Total, 3 years and older	.958 (.923 – .995)	.406 (< LOD – .477)	.529 (.489 – .562)	1.01 (.984 – 1.03)	1.65 (1.57 – 1.81)	1.88 (1.75 – 2.21)	6,844
Age group							
3–5 years	1.25 (1.18 – 1.32)	.715† (.097 – .835)	.836 (.435 – .881)	1.28 (1.23 – 1.38)	1.77 (1.64 – 2.02)	2.00† (1.73 – 2.30)	336
6–11 years	1.25 (1.20 – 1.30)	.691 (.555 – .772)	.807 (.700 – .852)	1.28 (1.23 – 1.33)	2.02 (1.88 – 2.47)	2.51 (2.02 – 4.24)	742
12–19 years	.952 (.889 – 1.02)	< LOD	.560 (< LOD – .625)	1.01 (.987 – 1.04)	1.72 (1.52 – 2.47)	2.14 (1.72 – 3.88)	1,817
20–39 years	.939 (.896 – .985)	.419 (< LOD – .492)	.537 (.474 – .585)	.988 (.939 – 1.03)	1.62 (1.53 – 1.77)	1.84 (1.66 – 2.19)	1,364
40–59 years	.926 (.883 – .970)	.400 (< LOD – .469)	.507 (.466 – .540)	.974 (.935 – 1.01)	1.58 (1.49 – 1.76)	1.75 (1.63 – 2.42)	1,124
60 years and older	.900 (.855 – .948)	< LOD	.475 (.359 – .528)	.961 (.928 – .984)	1.57 (1.48 – 1.73)	1.78 (1.63 – 2.34)	1,461
Gender							
Males	.918 (.886 – .951)	.410 (.313 – .470)	.514 (.487 – .537)	.955 (.926 – .990)	1.58 (1.52 – 1.69)	1.79 (1.66 – 2.09)	3,389
Females	.999 (.956 – 1.04)	.402 (< LOD – .493)	.566 (.464 – .622)	1.06 (1.02 – 1.09)	1.72 (1.62 – 1.93)	1.97 (1.79 – 2.59)	3,455
Race/ethnicity							
Mexican Americans	1.05 (.987 – 1.11)	.513 (< LOD – .603)	.616 (.554 – .684)	1.09 (1.03 – 1.16)	1.73 (1.60 – 2.17)	1.99 (1.77 – 2.57)	1,739
Non-Hispanic Blacks	.830 (.762 – .904)	.098 (.042 – .343)	.397 (.141 – .447)	.893 (.845 – .949)	1.62 (1.46 – 1.96)	1.82 (1.64 – 2.94)	1,736
Non-Hispanic Whites	.967 (.932 – 1.00)	< LOD	.548 (.507 – .591)	1.01 (.984 – 1.03)	1.63 (1.54 – 1.80)	1.85 (1.71 – 2.18)	2,859

< LOD means less than the limit of detection for either the whole blood acrylamide adduct or the glycidamide adduct, which may vary for some compounds by year. See Appendix D for LOD.

† Estimate is subject to greater uncertainty due to small cell size.

Figure 5.3.a. Glycidamide–to–acrylamide hemoglobin adduct ratio: By age group

Geometric mean (95% confidence interval), National Health and Nutrition Examination Survey, 2003–2004

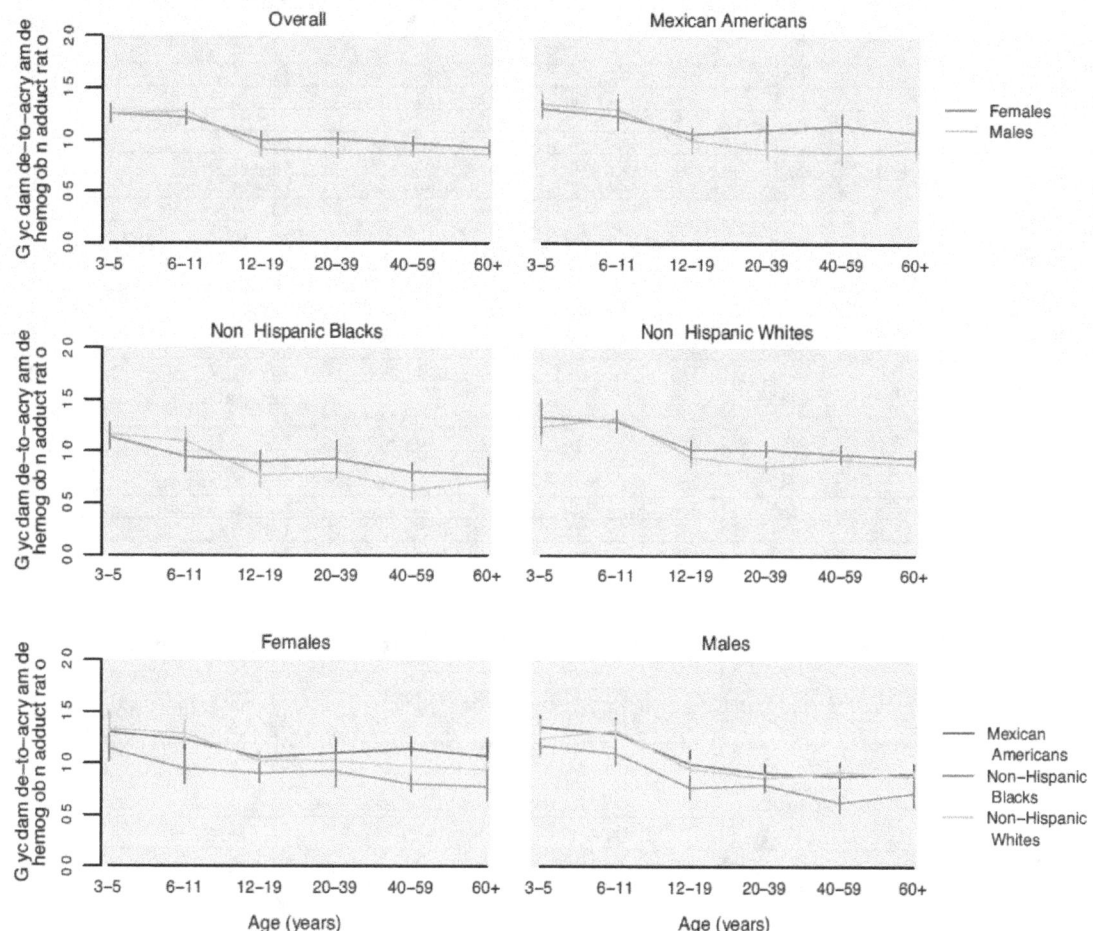

Table 5.3.a.2. Glycidamide-to-acrylamide hemoglobin adduct ratio: Total population

Geometric mean and selected percentiles of ratio (no units) of whole blood concentrations (in pmol/g Hb) for the total U.S. population aged 3 years and older, National Health and Nutrition Examination Survey, 2003–2004.

	Geometric mean (95% conf. interval)	Selected percentiles (95% conf. interval)			Sample size
		10th	50th	90th	
Males and Females					
Total, 3 years and older	.958 (.923 – .995)	.642 (.620 – .661)	1.01 (.984 – 1.03)	1.48 (1.42 – 1.54)	6,844
3–5 years	1.25 (1.18 – 1.32)	.944 (.647 – 1.05)	1.28 (1.23 – 1.38)	1.61 (1.57 – 1.78)	336
6–11 years	1.25 (1.20 – 1.30)	.899 (.853 – .923)	1.28 (1.23 – 1.33)	1.72 (1.61 – 1.96)	742
12–19 years	.952 (.889 – 1.02)	.670 (.609 – .719)	1.01 (.987 – 1.04)	1.45 (1.37 – 1.62)	1,817
20–39 years	.939 (.896 – .985)	.643 (.606 – .668)	.988 (.939 – 1.03)	1.43 (1.38 – 1.51)	1,364
40–59 years	.926 (.883 – .970)	.618 (.561 – .643)	.974 (.935 – 1.01)	1.41 (1.36 – 1.51)	1,124
60 years and older	.900 (.855 – .948)	.607 (.550 – .649)	.961 (.928 – .984)	1.39 (1.32 – 1.49)	1,461
Males					
Total, 3 years and older	.918 (.886 – .951)	.610 (.585 – .632)	.955 (.926 – .990)	1.41 (1.35 – 1.49)	3,389
3–5 years	1.25 (1.16 – 1.35)	.863 (.621 – 1.06)	1.26 (1.22 – 1.38)	1.60 (1.54 – 1.86)	181
6–11 years	1.28 (1.22 – 1.35)	.899 (.846 – .983)	1.31 (1.22 – 1.39)	1.72 (1.66 – 1.97)	359
12–19 years	.908 (.842 – .980)	.651 (.599 – .677)	.984 (.952 – 1.01)	1.38 (1.34 – 1.47)	944
20–39 years	.874 (.832 – .918)	.607 (.562 – .641)	.895 (.862 – .939)	1.25 (1.20 – 1.34)	638
40–59 years	.883 (.848 – .920)	.573 (.537 – .618)	.933 (.895 – .979)	1.34 (1.23 – 1.49)	549
60 years and older	.865 (.823 – .908)	.558 (.508 – .629)	.905 (.860 – .943)	1.35 (1.26 – 1.47)	718
Females					
Total, 3 years and older	.999 (.956 – 1.04)	.679 (.641 – .711)	1.06 (1.02 – 1.09)	1.52 (1.47 – 1.61)	3,455
3–5 years	1.25 (1.17 – 1.34)	.971 (.811 – 1.04)	1.29 (1.22 – 1.45)	1.64 (1.51 – 2.07)	155
6–11 years	1.22 (1.15 – 1.29)	.898 (.833 – .923)	1.27 (1.20 – 1.29)	1.71 (1.58 – 2.00)	383
12–19 years	1.00 (.928 – 1.08)	.730 (.635 – .776)	1.04 (1.00 – 1.10)	1.57 (1.41 – 1.84)	873
20–39 years	1.01 (.958 – 1.07)	.690 (.651 – .701)	1.08 (1.02 – 1.13)	1.55 (1.47 – 1.70)	726
40–59 years	.967 (.904 – 1.03)	.639 (.563 – .706)	1.01 (.957 – 1.07)	1.47 (1.39 – 1.59)	575
60 years and older	.929 (.865 – .998)	.647 (.534 – .710)	.998 (.969 – 1.04)	1.41 (1.35 – 1.52)	743

Table 5.3.a.3. Glycidamide-to-acrylamide hemoglobin adduct ratio: Mexican Americans

Geometric mean and selected percentiles of ratio (no units) of whole blood concentrations (in pmol/g Hb) for Mexican Americans in the U.S. population aged 3 years and older, National Health and Nutrition Examination Survey, 2003–2004.

	Geometric mean (95% conf. interval)	Selected percentiles (95% conf. interval)			Sample size
		10th	50th	90th	
Males and Females					
Total, 3 years and older	1.05 (.987 – 1.11)	.748 (.697 – .780)	1.09 (1.03 – 1.16)	1.57 (1.46 – 1.75)	1,739
3–5 years	1.32 (1.26 – 1.40)	1.06† (.957 – 1.11)	1.33 (1.25 – 1.41)	1.59† (1.54 – 1.88)	89
6–11 years	1.27 (1.17 – 1.37)	.953 (.923 – .989)	1.25 (1.19 – 1.34)	1.76 (1.57 – 2.53)	244
12–19 years	1.03 (.965 – 1.09)	.767 (.717 – .822)	1.05 (.999 – 1.12)	1.50 (1.42 – 1.73)	568
20–39 years	.997 (.904 – 1.10)	.689 (.608 – .755)	1.06 (.972 – 1.14)	1.56 (1.42 – 1.77)	312
40–59 years	.999 (.918 – 1.09)	.718 (.616 – .772)	1.04 (.988 – 1.12)	1.51 (1.36 – 2.60)	202
60 years and older	.989 (.908 – 1.08)	.716 (.561 – .774)	.996 (.936 – 1.05)	1.38 (1.28 – 1.62)	324
Males					
Total, 3 years and older	.977 (.916 – 1.04)	.689 (.616 – .722)	1.01 (.949 – 1.07)	1.52 (1.41 – 1.60)	858
3–5 years	1.35 (1.25 – 1.46)	1.09† (1.02 – 1.15)	1.33 (1.14 – 1.54)	1.60† (1.55 – 1.95)	46
6–11 years	1.29 (1.16 – 1.44)	.984 (.102 – 1.06)	1.26 (1.19 – 1.38)	1.85 (1.57 – 4.24)	117
12–19 years	.996 (.880 – 1.13)	.750 (.602 – .813)	1.03 (.948 – 1.12)	1.49 (1.42 – 1.67)	290
20–39 years	.907 (.823 – 1.00)	.660 (.532 – .708)	.930 (.877 – 1.02)	1.39 (1.19 – 1.64)	141
40–59 years	.886 (.775 – 1.01)	.611† (.197 – .722)	.946 (.872 – 1.01)	1.34† (1.24 – 1.60)	106
60 years and older	.906 (.820 – 1.00)	.642 (.087 – .750)	.937 (.877 – 1.00)	1.28 (1.23 – 1.36)	158
Females					
Total, 3 years and older	1.12 (1.06 – 1.19)	.847 (.801 – .890)	1.17 (1.10 – 1.25)	1.62 (1.49 – 1.96)	881
3–5 years	1.30 (1.22 – 1.38)	.993† (.905 – 1.11)	1.32 (1.25 – 1.40)	1.58† (1.45 – 1.76)	43
6–11 years	1.23 (1.10 – 1.38)	.926 (.860 – .977)	1.25 (1.16 – 1.33)	1.68 (1.57 – 1.95)	127
12–19 years	1.06 (1.01 – 1.11)	.820 (.716 – .870)	1.08 (1.02 – 1.16)	1.54 (1.39 – 2.11)	278
20–39 years	1.10 (.980 – 1.24)	.871 (.658 – .936)	1.17 (1.10 – 1.27)	1.70 (1.50 – 2.10)	171
40–59 years	1.14 (1.04 – 1.25)	.823† (.754 – .889)	1.16 (1.04 – 1.36)	1.54† (1.43 – 2.60)	96
60 years and older	1.07 (.919 – 1.24)	.777 (.486 – .881)	1.05 (.881 – 1.28)	1.48 (1.32 – 3.87)	166

† Estimate is subject to greater uncertainty due to small cell size.

Table 5.3.a.4. Glycidamide-to-acrylamide hemoglobin adduct ratio: Non-Hispanic blacks

Geometric mean and selected percentiles of ratio (no units) of whole blood concentrations (in pmol/g Hb) for non-Hispanic blacks in the U.S. population aged 3 years and older, National Health and Nutrition Examination Survey, 2003–2004.

| | Geometric mean (95% conf. interval) | | Selected percentiles (95% conf. interval) | | | | | | Sample size |
			10th		50th		90th		
Males and Females									
Total, 3 years and older	.830	(.762 – .904)	.526	(.440 – .588)	.893	(.845 – .949)	1.39	(1.27 – 1.60)	1,736
3–5 years	1.15	(1.08 – 1.23)	.865	(.697 – .961)	1.15	(1.07 – 1.24)	1.53	(1.37 – 1.83)	122
6–11 years	1.02	(.927 – 1.13)	.708	(.563 – .793)	1.10	(1.00 – 1.20)	1.74	(1.58 – 1.92)	265
12–19 years	.834	(.752 – .925)	.582	(.484 – .635)	.893	(.858 – .931)	1.38	(1.26 – 1.66)	637
20–39 years	.865	(.768 – .975)	.547	(.424 – .604)	.900	(.827 – .974)	1.39	(1.24 – 1.64)	277
40–59 years	.720	(.642 – .807)	.427	(.340 – .509)	.805	(.746 – .874)	1.19	(1.11 – 1.35)	248
60 years and older	.752	(.652 – .868)	.458	(.184 – .542)	.822	(.743 – .915)	1.24	(1.15 – 1.62)	187
Males									
Total, 3 years and older	.782	(.721 – .847)	.512	(.429 – .546)	.830	(.784 – .878)	1.31	(1.20 – 1.53)	875
3–5 years	1.17	(1.10 – 1.24)	.940†	(< LOD – .985)	1.14	(1.08 – 1.24)	1.57†	(1.39 – 1.82)	68
6–11 years	1.10	(.985 – 1.23)	.711	(.560 – .831)	1.12	(1.02 – 1.20)	1.78	(1.66 – 2.11)	126
12–19 years	.770	(.666 – .890)	.554	(.420 – .613)	.833	(.808 – .859)	1.30	(1.12 – 1.64)	341
20–39 years	.797	(.739 – .860)	.490	(.431 – .537)	.808	(.741 – .880)	1.18	(1.06 – 1.77)	136
40–59 years	.628	(.532 – .741)	.413	(.073 – .483)	.727	(.643 – .809)	1.11	(1.02 – 1.24)	115
60 years and older	.717	(.592 – .869)	.457†	(.046 – .565)	.766	(.691 – .853)	1.15†	(1.02 – 2.25)	89
Females									
Total, 3 years and older	.875	(.788 – .972)	.581	(.412 – .643)	.951	(.885 – 1.00)	1.42	(1.31 – 1.62)	861
3–5 years	1.14	(1.02 – 1.27)	.792†	(.716 – .967)	1.16	(1.03 – 1.26)	1.48†	(1.32 – 2.00)	54
6–11 years	.947	(.807 – 1.11)	.690	(< LOD – .784)	1.08	(.955 – 1.21)	1.55	(1.32 – 2.11)	139
12–19 years	.905	(.815 – 1.00)	.603	(.447 – .701)	.983	(.921 – 1.05)	1.44	(1.31 – 1.82)	296
20–39 years	.924	(.778 – 1.10)	.602	(< LOD – .726)	.974	(.885 – 1.12)	1.52	(1.36 – 1.89)	141
40–59 years	.802	(.728 – .885)	.463	(.380 – .602)	.870	(.805 – .926)	1.24	(1.15 – 1.48)	133
60 years and older	.778	(.643 – .941)	.425†	(< LOD – .574)	.831	(.766 – 1.00)	1.32†	(1.15 – 3.57)	98

< LOD means less than the limit of detection for either the whole blood acrylamide adduct or the glycidamide adduct, which may vary for some compounds by year. See Appendix D for LOD.

† Estimate is subject to greater uncertainty due to small cell size.

Table 5.3.a.5. Glycidamide-to-acrylamide hemoglobin adduct ratio: Non-Hispanic whites

Geometric mean and selected percentiles of ratio (no units) of whole blood concentrations (in pmol/g Hb) for non-Hispanic whites in the U.S. population aged 3 years and older, National Health and Nutrition Examination Survey, 2003–2004.

	Geometric mean (95% conf. interval)	Selected percentiles (95% conf. interval)			Sample size
		10th	50th	90th	
Males and Females					
Total, 3 years and older	.967 (.932 – 1.00)	.651 (.629 – .675)	1.01 (.984 – 1.03)	1.47 (1.41 – 1.53)	2,859
3–5 years	1.28 (1.15 – 1.43)	.863† (.097 – 1.18)	1.32 (1.23 – 1.47)	1.61† (1.56 – 2.05)	89
6–11 years	1.31 (1.23 – 1.38)	.939 (.852 – .989)	1.32 (1.27 – 1.38)	1.72 (1.55 – 2.41)	172
12–19 years	.979 (.901 – 1.06)	.699 (.642 – .748)	1.02 (.981 – 1.07)	1.42 (1.36 – 1.61)	490
20–39 years	.939 (.896 – .984)	.645 (.610 – .678)	.984 (.924 – 1.02)	1.42 (1.37 – 1.51)	648
40–59 years	.948 (.910 – .988)	.629 (.591 – .658)	.986 (.954 – 1.02)	1.41 (1.34 – 1.50)	586
60 years and older	.914 (.859 – .972)	.631 (.553 – .669)	.966 (.935 – .989)	1.40 (1.33 – 1.55)	874
Males					
Total, 3 years and older	.927 (.898 – .958)	.627 (.605 – .649)	.955 (.922 – .993)	1.39 (1.33 – 1.48)	1,400
3–5 years	1.24 (1.07 – 1.43)	.842† (.621 – 1.10)	1.27 (1.10 – 1.46)	1.57† (1.48 – 2.06)	48
6–11 years	1.32 (1.24 – 1.41)	.944† (.748 – 1.03)	1.33 (1.27 – 1.42)	1.70† (1.57 – 2.25)	82
12–19 years	.947 (.862 – 1.04)	.669 (.609 – .722)	1.01 (.940 – 1.04)	1.37 (1.32 – 1.41)	254
20–39 years	.862 (.820 – .905)	.609 (.549 – .644)	.886 (.852 – .930)	1.24 (1.20 – 1.30)	289
40–59 years	.922 (.891 – .954)	.619 (.557 – .649)	.945 (.910 – .987)	1.33 (1.23 – 1.44)	291
60 years and older	.880 (.835 – .929)	.570 (.512 – .636)	.922 (.862 – .953)	1.38 (1.27 – 1.49)	436
Females					
Total, 3 years and older	1.01 (.961 – 1.05)	.681 (.648 – .706)	1.06 (1.02 – 1.09)	1.52 (1.45 – 1.62)	1,459
3–5 years	1.33 (1.17 – 1.51)	1.01† (<LOD – 1.19)	1.46 (1.26 – 1.48)	1.72† (1.51 – 2.09)	41
6–11 years	1.29 (1.19 – 1.40)	.923† (.777 – .995)	1.28 (1.20 – 1.39)	1.79† (1.54 – 2.97)	90
12–19 years	1.02 (.929 – 1.11)	.743 (.636 – .786)	1.05 (.996 – 1.13)	1.57 (1.37 – 1.87)	236
20–39 years	1.02 (.954 – 1.10)	.691 (.654 – .700)	1.06 (1.00 – 1.14)	1.55 (1.46 – 1.77)	359
40–59 years	.975 (.899 – 1.06)	.639 (.513 – .736)	1.02 (.969 – 1.08)	1.43 (1.38 – 1.63)	295
60 years and older	.942 (.866 – 1.02)	.658 (.528 – .724)	1.00 (.968 – 1.05)	1.43 (1.35 – 1.56)	438

< LOD means less than the limit of detection for either the whole blood acrylamide adduct or the glycidamide adduct, which may vary for some compounds by year. See Appendix D for LOD.

† Estimate is subject to greater uncertainty due to small cell size.

References

Bergmark E, Calleman CJ, Costa LG. Formation of hemoglobin adducts of acrylamide and its epoxide metabolite glycidamide in the rat. Toxicol Appl Pharmacol. 1991;111:352–363.

Dybing E, Farmer PB, Andersen M, Fennell TR, Lalljie SPD, Müller DJ, et al. Human exposure and internal dose assessments of acrylamide in food. Food Chem Toxicol. 2005;43:365–410.

Fennell TR, Sumner SC, Walker VE. A model for the formation and removal of hemoglobin adducts. Cancer Epidemiol Biomarkers Prev. 1992;1:213–219.

Hogervorst JG, Baars BJ, Schouten LJ, Konings EJ, Goldbohm RA, van den Brandt PA. The carcinogenicity of dietary acrylamide intake: a comparative discussion of epidemiological and experimental animal research. Crit Rev Toxicol. 2010;40:485–512.

International Agency for Research on Cancer. Acrylamide. IARC Monogr Eval Carcinog Risk Hum. 1995;60:1–45.

Mottram DS, Wedzicha BL, Dodson AT. Acrylamide is formed in the Maillard reaction. Nature. 2002;419:448–449.

Mowrer J, Törnqvist M, Jensen S, Ehrenberg L. Modified Edman degradation applied to hemoglobin for monitoring occupational exposure to alkylating agents. Toxicol Environ Chem. 1986;11:215–231.

Robin LP, Cianci S. June/July 2007 Ask the Regulators: Acrylamide, Furan, and the FDA. Available at: http://www.fda.gov/Food/FoodSafety/FoodContaminantsAdulteration/ChemicalContaminants/Acrylamide/ucm194482.htm.

Smith J, Perfetty TA, Rumple MA, Rodgam A, Doolittle D. "IARC group 2A carcinogens" reported in cigarette mainstream smoke. Food Chem Toxicol. 2000;38:371–378.

Stadler RH, Blank I, Varga N, Robert F, Hau J, Guy PA, et al. Acrylamide from Maillard reaction products. Nature. 2002;419:449–450.

Törnqvist M, Fred C, Haglund J, Helleberg H, Paulsson B, Rydberg P. Protein adducts: quantitative and qualitative aspects of their formation, analysis and applications. J Chromatogr B. 2002;778:279–308.

Törnqvist M, Mowrer J, Jensen S, Ehrenberg L. Monitoring environmental cancer initiators through hemoglobin adducts by a modified Edman degradation method. Anal. Biochem. 1986;154:255–266.

Tran NL, Barraj LM, Murphy MM, Bi X. Dietary acrylamide exposure and hemoglobin adducts—National Health and Nutrition Examination Survey (2003–04). Food Chem Tox. 2010;48:3098–3108.

U.S. Environmental Protection Agency. Chemical summary for acrylamide. 1994. Available at: http://www.epa.gov/chemfact/s_acryla.txt.

U.S. Environmental Protection Agency. Toxicological review of acrylamide. 2010. Available at: http://www.epa.gov/iris/toxreviews/0286tr.pdf.

U.S. Food and Drug Administration. The 2006 exposure assessment for acrylamide. 2006. Available at: http://www.fda.gov/downloads/Food/FoodSafety/FoodContaminantsAdulteration/ChemicalContaminants/Acrylamide/UCM197239.pdf.

U.S. National Toxicology Program. Report on Carcinogens. Twelfth edition. 2011. Available at: http://ntp.niehs.nih.gov/ntp/roc/twelfth/roc12.pdf.

Vesper HW, Ospina M, Meyers T, Ingham L, Smith A, Gray JG, Myers GL. Automated method for measuring globin adducts of acrylamide and glycidamide at optimized Edman reaction conditions. Rapid Commun Mass Spectrom. 2006;20:959–964.

Vesper HW, Bernert JT, Ospina M, Meyers T, Ingham L, Smith A, et al. Assessment of the relation between biomarkers for smoking and biomarkers for acrylamide exposure in humans. Cancer Epidemiol Biomarkers Prev. 2007;16:2471–2478.

Vesper HW, Slimani N, Hallmans G, Tjonneland A, Agudo A, Benetou V, et al. Cross-sectional study on acrylamide hemoglobin adducts in subpopulations from the European Prospective Investigation into Cancer and Nutrition (EPIC) Study. J Agric Food Chem. 2008;56:6046–6053.

Vesper HW, Caudill SP, Osterloh JD, Meyers T, Scott D, Myers GL. 2009. Exposure of the U.S. Population to acrylamide in the National Health and Nutrition Examination Survey 2003–2004. Environ Health Perspect. 2010;118:278–283.

Wilson KM, Vesper HW, Tocco P, Sampson L, Rosén J, Hellenäs KE, et al. Validation of a food frequency questionnaire measurement of dietary acrylamide intake using hemoglobin adducts of acrylamide and glycidamide. Cancer Causes Control. 2009;20:269–278.

Appendices

Appendix A
NHANES Reports Related to Nutritional Status

National Center for Health Statistics (NCHS) Data Briefs

http://www.cdc.gov/nchs/products/databriefs.htm

Looker AC, Johnson CL, Lacher DA, Pfeiffer CM, Schleicher RL, Sempos CT. Vitamin D status: United States, 2001–2006. NCHS Data Brief, No 59. Hyattsville, MD: National Center for Health Statistics. 2011.

McDowell MA, Lacher DA, Pfeiffer CM, Mulinare J, Picciano MF, Rader JI, et al. Blood Folate Levels: The Latest NHANES Results. NCHS Data Brief, No 6. Hyattsville, MD: National Center for Health Statistics. 2008.

National Center for Health Statistics (NCHS) Advance Data Reports

http://www.cdc.gov/nchs/products/ad.htm

Advance Data No. 349. Prevalence of leading types of dietary supplements used in the Third National Health and Nutrition Examination Survey, 1988–94. 8 pp. (PHS) 2005–1250.

Advance Data No. 348. Dietary intake of fats and fatty acids for the United States population: 1999-2000. 7 pp. (PHS) 2005–1250.

Advance Data No. 341. Dietary intake of selected minerals for the United States population: 1999–2000. 6 pp. (PHS) 2004–1250.

Advance Data No. 339. Dietary intake of selected vitamins for the United States population: 1999–2000. 5 pp. (PHS) 2004–1250.

Advance Data No. 334. Dietary intake of ten key nutrients for public health, United States: 1999–2000. 4 pp. (PHS) 2003–1250.

National Center for Health Statistics (NCHS) Series 11 Reports

http://www.cdc.gov/nchs/products/series/series11.htm

Hollowell JG, van Assendelft OW, Gunter EW, Lewis BG, Najjar M, Pfeiffer C. Hematological and iron-related analytes—Reference data for persons aged 1 year and over: United States, 1988–1994. National Center for Health Statistics. Vital Health Stat Series No. 11(247), 2005.

Bialostosky K, Wright JD, Kennedy-Stephenson J, McDowell M, Johnson CL. Dietary intake of macronutrients, micronutrients, and other dietary constituents: United States 1988–1994. National Center for Health Statistics. Vital Health Stat Series No. 11(245), 2002.

Ervin RB, Wright JD, Kennedy-Stephenson J. Use of dietary supplements in the United States, 1988-1994. National Center for Health Statistics. Vital Health Stat Series No. 11(244), 1999.

Wright JD, Bialostosky K, Gunter EW, Carroll MD, Najjar MF, Bowman BA, Johnson CL. Blood folate and vitamin B12: United States, 1988–1994. National Center for Health Statistics. Vital Health Stat Series No. 11(243), 1998.

Fulwood R, Johnson CL, Bryner JD, Gunter EW, McGrath CR. Hematological and nutritional biochemistry reference data for persons 6 months–74 years of age: United States, 1976–1980. National Center for Health Statistics. Vital Health Stat Series No. 11(232), 1982.

National Center for Health Statistics (NCHS) Series 2 Reports

http://www.cdc.gov/nchs/products/series/series02.htm

Looker AC, Gunter EW, Cook JD, Green R, Harris JW. Comparing serum ferritin values from different population surveys. National Center for Health Statistics. Vital Health Stat Series No. 2(111), 1991.

Life Sciences Research Office (LSRO) Reports

Pilch SM. Assessment of the vitamin A nutritional status of the U.S. population based on data collected in the Health and Nutrition Examination Surveys. Bethesda (MD): Federation of American Societies for Experimental Biology; 1985.

Senti FR, Pilch SM. Analysis of the folate nutritional status of the U.S. population based on data collected in the Second National Health and Nutrition Examination Survey, 1976–1980. Bethesda (MD): Federation of American Societies for Experimental Biology; 1984.

Pilch SM, Senti FR. Assessment of iron nutritional status of the U.S. population based on data collected in the Second National Health and Nutrition Examination Survey, 1976–1980. Bethesda (MD): Federation of American Societies for Experimental Biology; 1984.

Pilch SM, Senti FR. Assessment of zinc nutritional status of the U.S. population based on data collected in the Second National Health and Nutrition Examination Survey, 1976–1980. Bethesda (MD): Federation of American Societies for Experimental Biology; 1984.

Life Sciences Research Office. 1989. An update report on nutrition monitoring in the United States. Prepared for the U.S. Department of Agriculture and the U.S. Department of Health and Human Services. DHHS Publication No. (PHS) 89–1255. Available from U.S. Government Printing Office, Washington, D.C.

Life Sciences Research Office. 1994. Assessment of folate methodology used in the Third National Health and Nutrition Survey (NHANES 1988-1994). Prepared for the Center for Food Safety and Applied Nutrition, Food and Drug Administration, Department of Health and Human Services. Washington, D.C.

Appendix B
Information Presented in the Report

The table below provides information on the type of data included for each indicator and the years of NHANES covered.

Indicator	Table: Concentrations	Figure: Concentrations by age group	Tables: Concentrations by race/ethnic group	Table and Figure: Concentrations by survey cycle	Table(s): Prevalence (Deficiency/Excess)	Table(s): Prevalence by survey cycle (Deficiency/Excess)
Water-Soluble Vitamins						
B Vitamins and Related Biochemical Compounds						
Serum folate	2003-2006	2003-2006	2003-2006	1999-2006	not shown*/none	not shown*/none
Red blood cell folate	2003-2006	2003-2006	2003-2006	1999-2006	2003-2006/none	1999-2006/none
Serum pyridoxal-5'-phosphate	2005-2006	2005-2006	2005-2006	none	2005-2006/none	none/none
Serum 4-pyridoxic acid	2005-2006	2005-2006	2005-2006	none	none/none	none/none
Serum vitamin B12	2003-2006	2003-2006	2003-2006	1999-2006	2003-2006/none	1999-2006/none
Plasma homocysteine	2003-2006	2003-2006	2003-2006	1999-2006	2003-2006/none	1999-2006/none
Plasma methylmalonic acid	2003-2004	2003-2004	2003-2004	1999-2004	2003-2004/none	1999-2004/none
Serum vitamin C	2003-2006	2003-2006	2003-2006	2003-2006	2003-2006/none	2003-2006/none
Fat-Soluble Vitamins and Nutrients						
Vitamins A and E and Carotenoids						
Serum vitamin A	2005-2006	2005-2006	2005-2006	1999-2002; 2005-2006	2005-2006/2005-2006	1999-2002; 2005-2006/ 1999-2002; 2005-2006
Serum retinyl palmitate	2005-2006	2005-2006	2005-2006	none	none/none	none/none
Serum retinyl stearate	2005-2006	not shown*	2005-2006	none	none/none	none/none
Serum vitamin E	2005-2006	2005-2006	2005-2006	1999-2002; 2005-2006	2005-2006/not shown*	1999-2002; 2005-2006/ not shown*
Serum *gamma*-tocopherol	2005-2006	2005-2006	2005-2006	1999-2002; 2005-2006	none/none	none/none
Serum *alpha*-carotene	2005-2006	2005-2006	2005-2006	2001-2002; 2005-2006	none/none	none/none
Serum *trans*-beta-carotene	2005-2006	2005-2006	2005-2006	2001-2002; 2005-2006	none/none	none/none
Serum *cis*-beta-carotene	2005-2006	not shown*	2005-2006	2001-2002; 2005-2006	none/none	none/none
Serum *beta*-cryptoxanthin	2005-2006	2005-2006	2005-2006	2001-2002; 2005-2006	none/none	none/none
Serum lutein and zeaxanthin	2005-2006	2005-2006	2005-2006	2001-2002; 2005-2006	none/none	none/none
Serum *trans*-lycopene	2005-2006	2005-2006	2005-2006	2001-2002; 2005-2006	none/none	none/none
Serum total lycopene	2005-2006	2005-2006	2005-2006	none	none/none	none/none
Serum 25-hydroxyvitamin D	2003-2006	2003-2006	2003-2006	2001-2006	2003-2006/2003-2006	2001-2006/2001-2006
Fatty Acids - Saturated						
Plasma myristic acid (14:0)	2003-2004	2003-2004	2003-2004	none	none/none	none/none
Plasma palmitic acid (16:0)	2003-2004	2003-2004	2003-2004	none	none/none	none/none
Plasma stearic acid (18:0)	2003-2004	2003-2004	2003-2004	none	none/none	none/none
Plasma arachidic acid (20:0)	2003-2004	2003-2004	2003-2004	none	none/none	none/none
Plasma docosanoic acid (22:0)	2003-2004	2003-2004	2003-2004	none	none/none	none/none
Plasma lignoceric acid (24:0)	2003-2004	2003-2004	2003-2004	none	none/none	none/none

Indicator	Table: Concentrations	Figure: Concentrations by age group	Tables: Concentrations by race/ethnic group	Table and Figure: Concentrations by survey cycle	Table(s): Prevalence (Deficiency/Excess)	Table(s): Prevalence by survey cycle (Deficiency/Excess)
Fatty Acids - Monounsaturated						
Plasma myristoleic acid (14:1n-5)	2003-2004	2003-2004	2003-2004	none	none/none	none/none
Plasma palmitoleic acid (16:1n-7)	2003-2004	2003-2004	2003-2004	none	none/none	none/none
Plasma cis-vaccenic acid (18:1n-7)	2003-2004	2003-2004	2003-2004	none	none/none	none/none
Plasma oleic acid (18:1n-9)	2003-2004	2003-2004	2003-2004	none	none/none	none/none
Plasma eicosenoic acid (20:1n-9)	2003-2004	2003-2004	2003-2004	none	none/none	none/none
Plasma docosenoic acid (22:1n-9)	2003-2004	2003-2004	2003-2004	none	none/none	none/none
Plasma nervonic acid (24:1n-9)	2003-2004	2003-2004	2003-2004	none	none/none	none/none
Fatty Acids - Polyunsaturated						
Plasma linoleic acid (18:2n-6)	2003-2004	2003-2004	2003-2004	none	none/none	none/none
Plasma alpha-linolenic acid (18:3n-3)	2003-2004	2003-2004	2003-2004	none	none/none	none/none
Plasma gamma-linolenic acid (18:3n-6)	2003-2004	2003-2004	2003-2004	none	none/none	none/none
Plasma eicosadienoic acid (20:2n-6)	2003-2004	2003-2004	2003-2004	none	none/none	none/none
Plasma homo-gamma-linolenic acid (20:3n-6)	2003-2004	2003-2004	2003-2004	none	none/none	none/none
Plasma arachidonic acid (20:4n-6)	2003-2004	2003-2004	2003-2004	none	none/none	none/none
Plasma eicosapentaenoic acid (20:5n-3)	2003-2004	2003-2004	2003-2004	none	none/none	none/none
Plasma docosatetraenoic acid (22:4n-6)	2003-2004	2003-2004	2003-2004	none	none/none	none/none
Plasma docosapentaenoic acid (22:5n-3)	2003-2004	2003-2004	2003-2004	none	none/none	none/none
Plasma docosapentaenoic acid (22:5n-6)	2003-2004	2003-2004	2003-2004	none	none/none	none/none
Plasma docosahexaenoic acid (22:6n-3)	2003-2004	2003-2004	2003-2004	none	none/none	none/none
Trace Elements						
Iron-Status Indicators						
Serum ferritin	2003-2006	2003-2006	2003-2006	1999-2006	2003-2006/2003-2006	1999-2006/1999-2006
Serum soluble transferrin receptor	2003-2006	2003-2006	2003-2006	2003-2006	2003-2006/none	2003-2006/none
Body iron	2003-2006	2003-2006	2003-2006	2003-2006	2003-2006/none	2003-2006/none
Urinary iodine	2003-2006	2003-2006	2003-2006	2001-2006	none/none	none/none
Isoflavones & Lignans						
Urinary genistein	2003-2006	2003-2006	2003-2006	1999-2006	none/none	none/none
Urinary daidzein	2003-2006	2003-2006	2003-2006	1999-2006	none/none	none/none
Urinary equol	2003-2006	2003-2006	2003-2006	1999-2006	none/none	none/none
Urinary O-desmethylangolensin	2003-2006	2003-2006	2003-2006	1999-2006	none/none	none/none
Urinary enterodiol	2003-2006	2003-2006	2003-2006	1999-2006	none/none	none/none
Urinary enterolactone	2003-2006	2003-2006	2003-2006	1999-2006	none/none	none/none
Acrylamide Hemoglobin Adducts						
Acrylamide hemoglobin adduct	2003-2004	2003-2004	2003-2004	none	none/none	none/none
Glycidamide hemoglobin adduct	2003-2004	2003-2004	2003-2004	none	none/none	none/none
Glycidamide-to-acrylamide hemoglobin adduct ratio	2003-2004	2003-2004	2003-2004	none	none/none	none/none

* Prevalence table is not shown if most or all estimates have been suppressed because of the RSE being ≥ 40%.

Appendix C
Cutoff Points used to Generate Prevalence Estimates

The table below presents the cutoff values used to calculate prevalence estimates of low or high concentrations of biochemical indicators for various population groups and the years for which NHANES data were available. The clinical interpretation of the cutoff values is described in the text that accompanies each chapter.

Indicator	Units	Cutoff value	Population described	NHANES years available
Water-Soluble Vitamins				
Serum folate	ng/mL	< 2	≥ 3 years	1999–2002
			≥ 1 years	2003–2006
Red blood cell folate	ng/mL	< 95	≥ 3 years	1999–2002
			≥ 1 years	2003–2006
Serum pyridoxal-5'-phosphate	nmol/L	< 20	≥ 1 years	2005–2006
Serum vitamin B12	pg/mL	< 200	≥ 3 years	1999–2002
			≥ 1 years	2003–2006
Plasma homocysteine	μmol/L	> 13	≥ 3 years	1999–2004
			≥ 20 years	2005–2006
Plasma methylmalonic acid	nmol/L	> 271	≥ 3 years	1999–2004
Serum vitamin C	μmol/L	< 11.4	≥ 6 years	2003–2006
Fat-Soluble Vitamins				
Serum vitamin A	μg/dL	< 20	≥ 6 years	1999–2002; 2005–2006
	μg/dL	> 100	≥ 6 years	1999–2002; 2005–2006
Serum vitamin E	μg/dL	< 500	≥ 6 years	1999–2002; 2005–2006
	μg/dL	> 20,000	≥ 6 years	1999–2002; 2005–2006
Serum 25-hydroxyvitamin D	nmol/L	< 30	≥ 6 years or ≥ 1 year*	2001–2006
	nmol/L	30–< 50	≥ 6 years or ≥ 1 year*	2001–2006
	nmol/L	< 40	≥ 6 years or ≥ 1 year*	2001–2006
	nmol/L	> 125	≥ 6 years or ≥ 1 year*	2001–2006
Iron-Status Indicators				
Serum ferritin	ng/mL	< 12	1-5 years	1999–2006
	ng/mL	< 15	Females 12-49 years	1999–2006
	ng/mL	< 15	Males ≥ 6 years	1999–2002
	ng/mL	> 150	Females 12-49 years	1999–2006
	ng/mL	> 200	Males ≥ 12 years	1999–2002
Serum soluble transferrin receptor	mg/L	> 4.4	Females 12-49 years	2003–2006
Body iron	mg/kg	< 0	1-5 years	2003–2006
	mg/kg	< 0	Females 12-49 years	2003–2006

*2001–2002: ≥ 6 years; 2003–2006: ≥ 1 year

Appendix D
References for Analytical Methods for Biochemical Indicators

Detailed Laboratory Procedure Manuals for Each Analytical Method:

- NHANES 2003–2004: http://www.cdc.gov/nchs/nhanes/nhanes2003-2004/lab_methods_03_04.htm.

- NHANES 2005–2006: http://www.cdc.gov/nchs/nhanes/nhanes2005-2006/lab_methods_05_06.htm.

Additional Useful Analytical Method References:

Water-Soluble Vitamins

Gunter EW, Bowman BA, Caudill SP, Twite DB, Adams MJ, Sampson EJ. Results of an international round robin for serum folate and whole-blood folate. Clin Chem. 1996;42:1689–1694.

Life Sciences Research Office. Assessment of folate methodology used in the Third National Health and Nutrition Survey (NHANES 1988-1994). Washington, D.C.: Center for Food Safety and Applied Nutrition, Food and Drug Administration, Department of Health and Human Services; 1994.

McCoy LF, Bowen MB, Xu M, Chen H, Schleicher RL. Improved HPLC assay for measuring serum vitamin C with 1-methyluric acid used as an electrochemically active internal standard. Clin Chem. 2005;51:1062–1064.

Pfeiffer CM, Twite D, Shih J, Holets-McCormack SR, Gunter EW. Method comparison for total plasma homocysteine between the Abbott IMx analyzer and an HPLC assay with internal standardization. Clin Chem. 1999;45(1):152–153.

Pfeiffer CM, Huff DL, Smith SJ, Miller DT, Gunter EW. Comparison of plasma total homocysteine measurements in 14 laboratories: an international study. Clin Chem. 1999;45(8):1261–1268.

Pfeiffer CM, Smith SJ, Miller DT, Gunter EW. Comparison of serum and plasma methylmalonic acid measurements in 13 laboratories: an international study. Clin Chem. 1999;45:2236–2242.

Pfeiffer CM, Caudill SP, Gunter EW, Bowman BA, Jacques PF, Selhub J, et al. Discussion of critical issues related to the comparison of homocysteine values between the Third National Health and Nutrition Examination Survey (NHANES) and NHANES 1999+. J Nutr. 2000;130:2850–2854.

Rybak ME, Pfeiffer CM. Clinical analysis of vitamin B6: Determination of pyridoxal 5'-phosphate and 4-pyridoxic acid in human serum by reversed-phase high-performance liquid chromatography with chlorite postcolumn derivatization. Anal Biochem. 2004;333:336–344.

Rybak ME, Jain RB, Pfeiffer CM. Clinical vitamin B_6 analysis: an inter-laboratory comparison of pyridoxal 5'-phosphate measurements in serum. Clin Chem. 2005;51:1223–1231.

Rybak ME, Pfeiffer CM. A simplified protein precipitation and filtration procedure for determining serum vitamin B6 by high-performance liquid chromatography. Anal Biochem. 2009;388:175–177.

Fat-Soluble Vitamins and Nutrients

Sowell AL, Huff DL, Yeager PR, Caudill SP, Gunter EW. Retinol, alpha-tocopherol, lutein/zeaxanthin, beta-cryptoxanthin, lycopene, alpha-carotene, trans-beta-carotene, and four retinyl esters in serum determined simultaneously by reversed-phase HPLC with multi-wavelength detection. Clin Chem. 1994;40:411–416.

Trace Elements

Looker AC, Gunter EW, Johnson CL. Methods to assess iron status in various NHANES surveys. Nutr Rev. 1995;53:246–254.

Pfeiffer CM, Cook JD, Mei Z, Cogswell ME, Looker AC, Lacher DA. Evaluation of an automated soluble transferrin receptor (sTfR) assay on the Roche Hitachi analyzer and its comparison to two ELISA assays. Clin Chim Acta 2007;382:112–116.

Caldwell KL, Maxwell CB, Makhmudov A, Pino S, Braverman LE, Jones RL, et al. Use of inductively coupled plasma mass spectrometry to measure urinary iodine in NHANES 2000: comparison with previous method. Clin Chem. 2003;49:1019–1021.

Isoflavones and Lignans

Valentin-Blasini L, Blount BC, Rogers HS, Needham LL. HPLC-MS/MS method for the measurement of seven phytoestrogens in human serum and urine. J Expo Anal Environ Epidemiol. 2000;10:799–807.

Kuklenyik Z, Ye X, Reich JA, Needham LL, Calafat AM. Automated on-line and off-line solid phase extraction methods for measuring isoflavones and lignans in urine. J Chromatogr Sci. 2004;42:495–500.

Rybak ME, Parker DL, Pfeiffer CM. Determination of urinary phytoestrogens by HPLC-MS/MS: a comparison of atmospheric pressure chemical ionization (APCI) and electrospray ionization (ESI). J Chromatogr B. 2008;861:145–150.

Parker DL, Rybak ME, Pfeiffer CM. Phytoestrogen biomonitoring: an extractionless LC-MS/MS method for measuring urinary isoflavones and lignans using atmospheric pressure photoionization (APPI). Anal Bioanal Chem. 2012;402:1123-1136.

Acrylamide Hemoglobin Adducts

Vesper HW, Ospina M, Meyers T, Ingham L, Smith A, Gray JG, Myers GL. Automated method for measuring globin adducts of acrylamide and glycidamide at optimized Edman reaction conditions. Rapid Commun Mass Spectrom. 2006;20:959–964.

Appendix E
Confidence Interval Estimation for Percentiles

A large body of literature describes various methods to estimate percentiles and to derive the variance and confidence intervals for complex survey data. Highlighted in the literature are the following methods: Woodruff method (Woodruff 1952), "test inversion" method (Francisco and Fuller 1991), the Normal transformation method (Korn and Graubard 1999), and Replication methods (Kovar 1988, Rogers 2003).

Confidence intervals for percentiles in this report were calculated with the Woodruff method. This method uses the standard error of the empirical distribution function at the selected percentile and constructs a 95% confidence interval, followed by back transformation using the inverse of the empirical distribution. The previous National Report on Biochemical Indicators of Diet and Nutrition in the U.S. Population, 1999–2002 used a variation of the Woodruff method by combining it with the method of Clopper and Pearson proposed by Korn and Graubard (1999) for complex surveys. This approach was used previously because large-sample normal approximations used to calculate confidence intervals for proportions close to zero or 1 can lead to confidence intervals with poor coverage properties. However, a paper by Sitter and Wu (2001) concluded that despite the fact that confidence intervals around the empirical distribution function at tail regions perform poorly, the Woodruff confidence intervals obtained by inverting these poorly behaved intervals perform very well for percentiles. Therefore, the confidence intervals presented in this report are based on the Woodruff approach with no further modifications, as described in the steps below.

Background

Define an arbitrary percentile X_p, such that $F(X) = P(X \leq X_p) = p$. This is pictured in Figure 1, where the y-axis displays the empirical distribution function (cdf) over a set of hypothetical values. In this example, $p = 0.5$ and so $X_{0.5}$ is the median. Both SAS (version 9.2) and SUDAAN (version 10.0) find X_p through linear interpolation. Let $\hat{F}(x_j)$ be an estimate of the empirical distribution function at x and assume data $x_1, x_2, \ldots x_n$ are a rank ordered listing of the sampled values, such that x_1 is the minimum value and x_n is the maximum value; then the estimated percentile by use of linear interpolation is calculated as:

$$\hat{X}_p = x_j + \frac{p - \hat{F}(x_j)}{\hat{F}(x_{j+1}) - \hat{F}(x_j)}\left(x_{j+1} - x_j\right) \quad \hat{F}(x_j) \leq p < \hat{F}(x_{j+1}).$$

To find the percentiles and confidence intervals in this report, we used results derived from SUDAAN's PROC DESCRIPT (DESIGN=WR) PERCENTILE statement and results from the Histogram output group.

Figure 1: Definition of a percentile

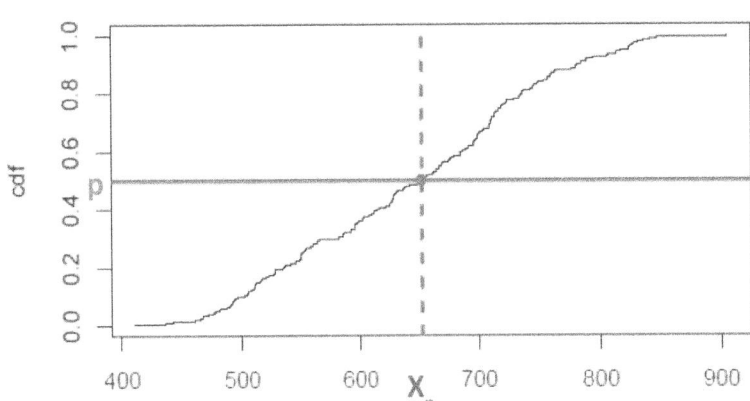

Analyte Value

Step 1

Use SUDAAN (DESIGN=WR) to estimate the percentiles, the empirical distribution, and the standard error of the empirical distribution function at each point. SUDAAN uses a Horowitz-Thompson estimator of the empirical distribution function at each value. The estimated empirical distribution function can be outputted into a dataset using the HISTPCT statement in conjunction with an OUTPUT statement in PROC DESCRIPT. By default, SUDAAN estimates the empirical distribution function by using a maximum of 100 equally spaced percentages to divide the population into bins. We used the option /NPCT in the HISTPCT statement to change this default to allow a jump in the empirical distribution function at every unique data value, up to 2950 unique values. An output file is generated by SUDAAN to contain: the upper endpoint of the current bin in the histogram, the cumulative percent less than or equal to the upper endpoint of the current bin and the respective estimated standard error of the cumulative percent. This file is used to obtain 95% confidence intervals of the empirical distribution function at the selected percentile. In some rare cases, using the values of the upper endpoint available in this file may differ slightly from a rank order list of the weighted sampled values if there are more than 2950 distinct values. This difference may lead to very small differences when comparing the confidence limits to other software which uses Woodruff confidence limits based on the weighted sample values. Sample SUDAAN code for serum folate (FOL) is as follows:

PROC DESCRIPT DATA=NHANES03_06 FILETYPE=SAS DESIGN=WR ;

    NEST SDMVSTRA SDMVPSU/MISSUNIT;

    WEIGHT WTMEC4YR;

    VAR   LBXFOL;

    PERCENTILES 5 10 90 95 /MEDIAN ;

    HISPCT /NPCT=2950;

    OUTPUT QTILE /FILENAME=PCTILES

FILETYPE=SAS REPLACE ;

OUTPUT UPPEREND CUMPCT SECUMPCT   /FILENAME=HIST FILETYPE=SAS

REPLACE;

If you change the first OUTPUT statement in the above program to

OUTPUT QTILE LOWQTILE UPQTILE /FILENAME=PCTILES FILETYPE=SAS
REPLACE ;

SUDAAN will provide the upper and lower confidence limits based on the "test inversion" method of Francisco and Fuller. However, as mentioned earlier, this report does not use SUDAAN's default method to generate confidence intervals for percentiles.

Step 2

Using SAS DATA steps to manipulate the output files from Step 1, find the value of the estimated cumulative distribution function that is less than or equal to **p** using the values of the cumulative percent produced by SUDAAN in the output file HIST:

Save $\hat{F}(x_j)$ and the corresponding standard error (SE) estimate at $\hat{F}(x_j)$ and proceed to step 3.

$$\hat{F}(x_j) \leq p < \hat{F}(x_{j+1})$$

Step 3

Using **p (the desired percentile)** and the standard error of the estimate of $\hat{F}(x_j)$, compute the 95% confidence interval for p: (p_L, p_U) as $p \pm t_{0.025,DF} SE$, where the degrees of freedom (DF) are the number of primary sampling units minus the number of strata and SE is the standard error from step 2. To get the appropriate degrees of freedom for each subgroup use the ATLEVEL1 and ATLEVEL2 options in SUDAAN's PROC DESCRIPT to count up the number of strata and PSUs with valid data. This must be done in a separate call to PROC DESCRIPT than the one that calculates the percentiles because the HISTPCT statement is not available with ATLEVEL. Note: SAS (version 9.2) uses the empirical point estimate at the desired percentile, $\hat{p} = \hat{F}(x_j)$, in order to calculate the 95% confidence interval as $\hat{p} \pm t_{0.025,DF} SE$.

Step 4

Map the lower (p_L) and upper (p_U) confidence intervals of the empirical distribution function at the desired percentile using the inverse of the empirical distribution function (see Figure 2) and linear interpolation to get the confidence interval for the percentile of interest.

Let $\hat{L}_p$ be the lower confidence limit of the estimated percentile and $\hat{U}_p$ be the upper confidence limit of the estimated percentile. $x_1, x_2, \ldots x_n$ are a rank ordered listing of the values as produced by SUDAAN using HISTPCT, such that x_1 is the minimum value and x_n is the maximum value; then these can be found from the following expressions:

$$\hat{L}_p = \begin{cases} x_1 & p_L < \hat{F}(x_1) \\[2ex] x_j + \dfrac{p_L - \hat{F}(x_j)}{\hat{F}(x_{j+1}) - \hat{F}(x_j)}(x_{j+1} - x_j) & \hat{F}(x_j) \le p_L < \hat{F}(x_{j+1}) \\[2ex] x_n & p_L = 1 \end{cases}$$

$$\hat{U}_p = \begin{cases} x_1 & p_U < \hat{F}(x_1) \\[2ex] x_j + \dfrac{p_U - \hat{F}(x_j)}{\hat{F}(x_{j+1}) - \hat{F}(x_j)}(x_{j+1} - x_j) & \hat{F}(x_j) \le p_U < \hat{F}(x_{j+1}) \\[2ex] x_n & p_U = 1 \end{cases}$$

Figure 2

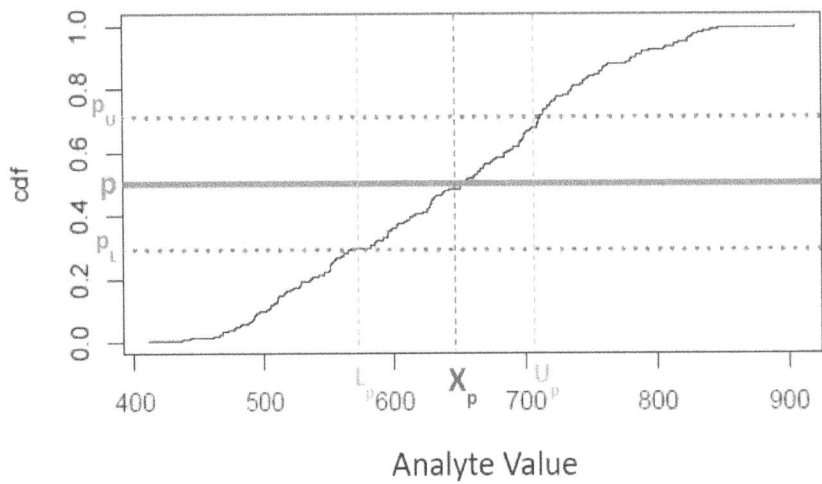

Analyte Value

Commercial Software

PROC DESRIPT in SUDAAN (version 8.0 and higher) calculates confidence limits for the percentiles using the "test-inversion" method by Fransisco and Fuller, as noted in Step 1.

PROC SURVEYMEANS (SAS version 9.1 and higher) can be used to obtain Woodruff like confidence intervals for percentiles. However, the SURVEYMEANS method differs slightly from the traditional Woodruff method as noted in Step 3.

References

Francisco CA, Fuller WA. Quantile estimation with a complex survey design. Annals Statist. 1991;19:454–469.

Korn EL, Graubard BI. Analysis of Health Surveys. Wiley: New York, 1999.

Kovar JG, Rao JNK, Wu CFL. Bootstrap and other methods to measure errors in survey estimated. Can J Statist. 1988;16S:25–45.

Research Triangle Institute (2008). *SUDAAN Language Manual, Release 10.0* Research Triangle Park, NC: Research Triangle Institute.

Rogers JW. Estimating the variance of percentiles using replicate weights. Proceedings of the Section on Survey Research Methods. 2003.

Sitter RR, Wu C. A note on Woodruff confidence intervals for quantiles. Statist Probabil Letters. 2001;52:353–358.

Woodruff RS. Confidence intervals for medians and other position measures. J Am Statist Assoc. 1952;57:622–627.

U.S. Centers for Disease Control and Prevention. NHANES Analytic guidelines, the Third National Health and Nutrition Examination Survey, NHANES III (1988–94). Hyattsville (MD): National Center for Health Statistics; October 1996 [cited 2008]. Available from: http://www.cdc.gov/nchs/data/nhanes/nhanes3/nh3gui.pdf.

Appendix F
Limit of Detection Table

The table below presents the analytical limit of detection (LOD) for each indicator. The LOD is the level at which the measurement has a 95 percent probability of being greater than zero (Taylor 1987). For the same indicator, LOD values may change over time as a result of changes to analytical methods. This was the case for serum ferritin and urinary phytoestrogens. We used the highest LOD value when multi-year data were combined. The information provided in parentheses specifies what proportion of results was below the LOD for each indicator and survey cycle.

Indicator	Units	1999-2000	2001-2002	2003-2004	2005-2006
Water-Soluble Vitamins					
B Vitamins and Related Biochemical Compounds					
Serum folate	ng/mL	0.1 (0%)	0.1 (0%)	0.1 (0%)	0.1 (0%)
Red blood cell folate	ng/mL	20 (0%)	20 (0%)	20 (< 1%)	20 (0%)
Serum pyridoxal-5'-phosphate	nmol/L	no data	no data	no data	0.3 (0%)
Serum 4-pyridoxic acid	nmol/L	no data	no data	no data	0.3 (0%)
Serum vitamin B12	pg/mL	20 (0%)	20 (0%)	20 (0%)	20 (0%)
Plasma homocysteine	µmol/L	0.35 (0%)	0.35 (0%)	0.35 (0%)	0.35 (0%)
Plasma methylmalonic acid	nmol/L	50 (1%)	50 (1%)	50 (< 1%)	no data
Serum vitamin C	µmol/L	no data	no data	0.68 (< 1%)	0.68 (< 1%)
Fat-Soluble Vitamins and Nutrients					
Vitamins A and E and Carotenoids					
Serum vitamin A (retinol)	µg/dL	1.03 (0%)	1.03 (0%)	no data	1.03 (< 1%)
Serum vitamin E (*alpha*-tocopherol)	µg/dL	40.7 (0%)	40.7 (0%)	no data	40.7 (0%)
Serum *gamma*-tocopherol	µg/dL	10.7 (< 1%)	10.7 (< 1%)	no data	10.7 (0%)
Serum *alpha*-carotene	µg/dL	no data	0.7 (9%)	no data	0.7 (7%)
Serum *trans-beta*-carotene	µg/dL	no data	0.8 (< 1%)	no data	0.8 (< 1%)
Serum *cis-beta*-carotene	µg/dL	no data	0.7 (52%)	no data	0.7 (51%)
Serum *beta*-cryptoxanthin	µg/dL	no data	0.9 (< 1%)	no data	0.9 (< 1%)
Serum lutein and zeaxanthin	µg/dL	no data	2.4 (< 1%)	no data	2.4 (< 1%)
Serum *trans*-lycopene	µg/dL	no data	0.8 (< 1%)	no data	0.8 (< 1%)
Serum total lycopene	µg/dL	no data	no data	no data	1.0 (< 1%)
Serum retinyl palmitate	µg/dL	0.2 (16%)	0.2 (2%)	no data	1.3 (22%)
Serum retinyl stearate	µg/dL	0.5 (86%)	0.5 (87%)	no data	0.7 (88%)
Serum 25-hydroxyvitamin D	nmol/L	no data	3.7 (0%)	3.7 (0%)	3.7 (0%)
Fatty Acids - Saturated					
Plasma myristic acid (14:0)	µmol/L	no data	no data	1.6 (0%)	no data
Plasma palmitic acid (16:0)	µmol/L	no data	no data	8.2 (0%)	no data
Plasma stearic acid (18:0)	µmol/L	no data	no data	23.7 (0%)	no data
Plasma arachidic acid (20:0)	µmol/L	no data	no data	0.6 (0%)	no data
Plasma docosanoic acid (22:0)	µmol/L	no data	no data	0.2 (0%)	no data
Plasma lignoceric acid (24:0)	µmol/L	no data	no data	0.1 (0%)	no data

Indicator	Units	1999-2000	2001-2002	2003-2004	2005-2006
Fatty Acids - Monounsaturated					
Plasma myristoleic acid (14:1n-5)	µmol/L	no data	no data	0.1 (0%)	no data
Plasma palmitoleic acid (16:1n-7)	µmol/L	no data	no data	0.6 (0%)	no data
Plasma cis-vaccenic acid (18:1n-7)	µmol/L	no data	no data	0.3 (0%)	no data
Plasm oleic acid (18:1n-9)	µmol/L	no data	no data	5.2 (0%)	no data
Plasma eicosenoic acid (20:1n-9)	µmol/L	no data	no data	0.2 (0%)	no data
Plasma docosenoic acid (22:1n-9)	µmol/L	no data	no data	0.3 (3%)	no data
Plasma nervonic acid (24:1n-9)	µmol/L	no data	no data	0.4 (0%)	no data
Fatty Acids - Polyunsaturated					
Plasma linoleic acid (18:2n-6)	µmol/L	no data	no data	2.2 (0%)	no data
Plasma alpha-linolenic acid (18:3n-3)	µmol/L	no data	no data	0.2 (0%)	no data
Plasma gamma-linolenic acid (18:3n-6)	µmol/L	no data	no data	0.1 (0%)	no data
Plasma eicosadienoic acid (20:2n-6)	µmol/L	no data	no data	0.1 (0%)	no data
Plasma homo-gamma-linolenic acid (20:3n-6)	µmol/L	no data	no data	0.2 (0%)	no data
Plasma arachidonic acid (20:4n-6)	µmol/L	no data	no data	0.3 (0%)	no data
Plasma eicosapentaenoic acid (20:5n-3)	µmol/L	no data	no data	0.1 (0%)	no data
Plasma docosatetraenoic acid (22:4n-6)	µmol/L	no data	no data	0.2 (0%)	no data
Plasma docosapentaenoic acid (22:5n-3)	µmol/L	no data	no data	0.2 (0%)	no data
Plasma docosapentaenoic acid (22:5n-6)	µmol/L	no data	no data	0.1 (0%)	no data
Plasma docosahexaenoic acid (22:6n-3)	µmol/L	no data	no data	0.1 (0%)	no data
Trace Elements					
Iron-Status Indicators					
Serum ferritin	ng/mL	1.1 (0%)	1.1 (0%)	3 (1%)	3 (1%)
Serum soluble transferrin receptor	mg/L	no data	no data	0.5 (0%)	0.5 (0%)
Urinary iodine	ng/mL	no data	1.0 (0%)	1.0 (0%)	1.0 (0%)
Isoflavones and Lignans					
Urinary genistein	µg/L	0.3 (6%)	0.8 (< 1%)	0.3 (< 1%)	1.0 (< 1%)
Urinary daidzein	µg/L	0.5 (1%)	1.6 (7%)	0.3 (< 1%)	0.4 (< 1%)
Urinary equol	µg/L	3 (28%)	3.3 (30%)	0.3 (< 1%)	0.06 (< 1%)
Urinary O-desmethylangolensin	µg/L	0.2 (25%)	0.4 (27%)	0.2 (7%)	0.2 (4%)
Urinary enterodiol	µg/L	0.8 (8%)	1.5 (4%)	0.3 (1%)	0.04 (< 1%)
Urinary enterolactone	µg/L	0.6 (2%)	1.9 (1%)	0.3 (< 1%)	0.1 (0%)
Acrylamide Hemoglobin Adducts					
Acrylamide hemoglobin adduct	pmol/g Hb	no data	no data	3 (< 1%)	no data
Glycidamide hemoglobin adduct	pmol/g Hb	no data	no data	4 (2%)	no data

Reference

Taylor JK. Quality assurance of chemical measurements. Chelsea (MI): Lewis Publishing; 1987.

Appendix G
Selected References of Descriptive NHANES Papers on Diet-and-Nutrition Biochemical Indicators

Water-Soluble Vitamins

Bailey RL, Mills JL, Yetley EA, Gahche JJ, Pfeiffer CM, Dwyer JT, et al. Unmetabolized serum folic acid and its relation to folic acid intake from diet and supplements in a nationally representative sample of adults aged >=60 y in the United States. Am J Clin Nutr. 2010;92:383–389.

Bailey RL, McDowell MA, Dodd KW, Gahche JJ, Dwyer JT, Picciano MF. Total folate and folic acid intake from foods and dietary supplements of US children aged 1–13 y. Am J Clin Nutr. 2010;92:353–358.

Bailey RL, Dodd KW, Gahche JJ, Dwyer JT, McDowell MA, Yetley EA, et al. Total folate and folic acid intake from foods and dietary supplements in the United States: 2003–2006. Am J Clin Nutr. 2010;91:231–237.

Bentley TGK, Willett WC, Weinstein MC, Kuntz KM. Population-level changes in folate intake by age, sex, and race/ethnicity after folic acid fortification. Am J Public Health. 2006;96:2040–2047.

Boulet SL, Yang Q, Mai C, Mulinare J, Pfeiffer CM. Folate status in women of childbearing age by race/ethnicity– United States 1999–2000, 2001–2002, and 2003–2004. Morb Mortal Wkl Rep. 2007;55(51):1377–1380.

Dietrich M, Brown CJP, Block G. The effect of folate fortification of cereal-grain products on blood folate status, dietary folate intake and dietary folate sources among adult non-supplement users in the United States. J Am Coll Nutr. 2005;24:266–274.

Ganji V, Kafai MR. Hemoglobin and hematocrit values are higher and prevalence of anemia is lower in the post-folic acid fortification period than in the pre-folic acid fortification period in US adults. Am J Clin Nutr. 2009;89:363–371.

Ganji V, Kafai MR. Demographic, lifestyle, and health characteristics and serum B vitamin status are determinants of plasma total homocysteine concentrations in the post-folic acid fortification period, 1999–2004. J Nutr. 2009;139:345–352.

Ganji V, Kafai MR. Trends in serum folate, RBC folate, and circulating total homocysteine concentrations in the United States: analysis of data from National Health and Nutrition Examination Surveys, 1988–1994, 1999–2000, and 2001–2002. J Nutr. 2006;136:153–158.

Ganji V, Kafai MR. Population reference values for plasma total homocysteine concentrations in US adults after the fortification of cereals with folic acid. Am J Clin Nutr. 2006;84:989–994.

Ganji V, Kafai MR. Population references for plasma total homocysteine concentrations for US children and adolescents in the post-folic acid fortification era. J Nutr. 2005;135:2253–2256.

Ganji V, Kafai MR. Serum total homocysteine concentration determinants in non-Hispanic white, non-Hispanic black, and Mexican-American populations of the United States. Ethn Dis. 2004;14:476–482.

Ganji V, Kafai MR. Demographic, health, lifestyle, and blood vitamin determinants of serum total homocysteine concentrations in the Third National Health and Nutrition Examination Survey, 1988–1994. Am J Clin Nutr. 2003;77:826–833.

Hamner HC, Mulinare J, Cogswell ME, Flores AL, Boyle CA, Prue CE, et al. Predicted contribution of folic acid fortification of corn masa flour to the usual folic acid intake for the US population: National Health and Nutrition Examination Survey, 2001–2004. Am J Clin Nutr. 2009;89:305–315.

McDowell MA, Lacher DA, Pfeiffer CM, Mulinare J, Picciano MF, Rader JI, et al. Blood folate levels: The latest NHANES results. NCHS data briefs, no 6. Hyattsville, MD: National Center for Health Statistics. 2008.

Morris MS, Jacques PF, Rosenberg IH, Selhub J. Circulating unmetabolized folic acid 5-methyltetrahydrofolate in relation to anemia, macrocytosis, and cognitive test performance in American seniors. Am J Clin Nutr. 2010;91:1733–1744.

Morris MS, Sakakeeny L, Jacques PF, Picciano MF, Selhub J. Vitamin B6 intake is inversely related to, and the requirement is affected by, inflammation status. J Nutr. 2010;140:103–110.

Morris MS, Picciano MF, Jacques PF, Selhub J. Plasma pyridoxal-5'-phosphate in the US population: the National Health and Nutrition Examination Survey, 2003–2004. Am J Clin Nutr. 2008;87:1446–1454.

Morris MS, Jacques PF, Rosenberg IH, Selhub J. Folate and vitamin B12 status in relation to anemia, macrocytosis, and cognitive impairment in older Americans in the age of folic acid fortification. Am J Clin Nutr. 2007;85:193–200.

Morris MS, Jacques PF, Rosenberg IH, Selhub J. Elevated serum methylmalonic acid concentrations are common among elderly Americans. J Nutr. 2002;132:2799–2803.

Must A, Jacques PF, Rogers G, Rosenberg IH, Selhub J. Serum total homocysteine concentrations in children and adolescents: results from the Third National Health and Nutrition Examination Survey (NHANES III). J Nutr. 2003;133:2643–2649.

Pfeiffer CM, Osterloh JD, Kennedy-Stephenson J, Picciano MF, Yetley EA, Rader JI, et al. Trends in circulating concentrations of total homocysteine among US adolescents and adults: findings from the 1991–1994 and 1999–2004 National Health and Nutrition Examination Surveys. Clin Chem. 2008;54:801–813.

Pfeiffer CM, Johnson CL, Jain RB, Yetley EA, Picciano MF, Rader JI, et al. Trends in blood folate and vitamin B12 concentrations in the United States, 1988–2004. Am J Clin Nutr. 2007;86:718–727.

Pfeiffer CM, Caudill SP, Gunter EW, Osterloh J, Sampson EJ. Biochemical indicators of B vitamin status in the U.S. population after folic acid fortification: results from the National Health and Nutrition Examination Survey 1999–2000. Am J Clin Nutr. 2005;82:442–450.

Schleicher RL, Carroll MD, Ford ES, Lacher DA. Serum vitamin C and the prevalence of vitamin C deficiency in the United States: 2003–2004 National Health and Nutrition Examination Survey (NHANES). Am J Clin Nutr. 2009;90:1252–1263.

Selhub J, Jacques PF, Rosenberg IH, Rogers G, Bowman BA, Gunter EW. Serum total homocysteine concentrations in the Third National Health and Nutrition Examination Survey (1991–1994): population reference ranges and contribution of vitamin status to high serum concentrations. Ann Intern Med. 1999;131:331–339.

U.S. Centers for Disease Control and Prevention. Folate status in women of childbearing age, by race/ethnicity—United States, 1999–2000. Morb Mortal Wkl Rep. 2002;51:808–810.

Wright JD, Bialostosky K, Gunter EW, Carroll MD, Najjar MF, Bowman BA, et al. Blood folate and vitamin B12: United States, 1988–1994. National Center for Health Statistics. Vital Health Stat Series No. 11(243), 1998.

Yang Q, Cogswell ME, Hamner HC, Carriquiri A, Bailey LB, Pfeiffer CM, et al. Folic acid source, usual intake, and folate and vitamin B12 status in US adults: National Health and Nutrition Examination Survey (NHANES) 2003–2006. Am J Clin Nutr. 2010;91:64–72.

Yang Q-H, Botto LD, Gallagher M, Friedman JM, Sanders CL, Koontz D, et al. Prevalence and effects of gene-gene and gene-nutrient interactions on serum folate and serum total homocysyteine concentrations in the United States: findings from the third National Health and Nutrition Examination Survey DNA Bank. Am J Clin Nutr. 2008;88:232–246.

Yang Q-H, Carter HK, Mulinare J, Berry RJ, Friedman JM, Erickson JD. Race-ethnicity differences in folic acid intake in women of childbearing age in the United States after folic acid fortification: findings from the National Health and Nutrition Examination Survey, 2001–2002. Am J Clin Nutr. 2007;85:1409–1416.

Yeung LF, Cogswell ME, Carriquiry AL, Bailey LB, Pfeiffer CM, Berry RJ. Contributions of enriched cereal-grain products ready-to-eat cereals and supplements to folic acid and vitamin B-12 usual intake and folate and vitamin B-12 status in US children: National Health and Nutrition Examination Survey (NHANES) 2003–2006. Am J Clin Nutr. 2011;93:172–185.

Yeung L, Yang Q, Berry RJ. Contributions of total daily intake of folic acid to serum folate concentrations. J Am Med Assoc. 2008;300:2486–2487.

Fat-Soluble Vitamins and Nutrients

Bailey RL, Dodd KW, Goldman JA, Gahche JJ, Dwyer JT, Moshfegh AJ, et al. Estimation of total usual calcium and vitamin D intakes in the United States. J Nutr. 2010;140:817–822.

Ford ES, Schleicher RL, Mokdad AH, Ajani UA, Liu S. Distribution of serum concentrations of a-tocopherol and g-tocopherol in the U.S. population. Am J Clin Nutr. 2006;84:375–383.

Ford ES, Ajani UA, Mokdad AH. Brief communication: the prevalence of high intake of vitamin E from the use of supplements among U.S. adults. Ann Intern Med. 2005;143:143–145.

Ford ES, Liu S, Mannino DM, Giles WH, Smith SJ. C-reactive protein concentration and concentrations of blood vitamins, carotenoids, and selenium among United States adults. Eur J Clin Nutr. 2003;57:1157–1163.

Gillespie C, Ballew C, Bowman BA, Donehoo R, Serdula MK. Intraindividual variation in serum retinol concentrations among participants in the third National Health and Nutrition Examination Survey, 1988–1994. Am J Clin Nutr. 2004;79:625–632.

Ginde AA, Liu MC, Camargo CA. Demographic differences and trends of vitamin D insufficiency in the US population, 1988–2004. Arch Intern Med. 2009;169:629–632.

Gruber M, Chappell R, Millen A, LaRowe T, Moeller SM, Iannaccone A, et al. Correlates of serum lutein + zeaxanthin: findings from the Third National Health and Nutrition Examination Survey. J Nutr. 2004;134:2387–2394.

Knutsen SF, Fraser GE, Linsted KD, Beeson WL, Shavlik DJ. Comparing biological measurements of vitamin C, folate, alpha-tocopherol and carotene with 24-hour dietary recall information in nonhispanic blacks and whites. Ann Epidemiol. 2001;11:406–416.

Kumar J, Muntner P, Kaskel FJ, Hailpern SM, Melamed ML. Prevalence and associations of 25-hydroxyvitamin D deficiency in US children: NHANES 2001–2004. Pediatrics 2009;124:e1–9.

Looker AC, Lacher DA, Pfeiffer CM, Schleicher RL, Picciano MF, Yetley EA. Data advisory with regard to NHANES serum 25-hydroxyvitamin D data. Am J Clin Nutr. 2009;90:695.

Looker AC, Pfeiffer CM, Lacher DA, Schleicher RL, Picciano MF, Yetley EA. Serum 25-hydroxyvitamin D status of the US population: 1988–1994 versus 2000–2004. Am J Clin Nutr. 2008;88:1519–1527.

Looker AC, Dawson-Hughes B, Calvo MS, Gunter EW, Sahyoun NR. Serum 25-hydroxyvitamin D status of adolescents and adults in two seasonal subpopulations from NHANES III. Bone. 2002;30:771–777.

Nesby-O'Dell S, Scanlon KS, Cogswell ME, Gillespie C, Hollis BW, Looker AC, et al. Hypovitaminosis D prevalence and determinants among African American and white women of reproductive age: Third National Health and Nutrition Examination Survey, 1988–1994. Am J Clin Nutr. 2002;76:187–192.

Stimpson JP, Urrutia-Rojas X. Acculturation in the United States is associated with lower serum carotenoid levels: Third National Health and Nutrition Examination Survey. J Am Diet Assoc. 2007;107:1218–1223.

Zadshir A, Tareen N, Pan D, Norris K, Martins D. The prevalence of hypovitaminosis D among US adults: data from the NHANES III. Ethn Dis. 2005;15(4 Suppl 5):S5-97–101.

Trace Elements

Iron-Status Indicators

Brotanek JM, Gosz J, Weitzman M, Flores G. Iron deficiency in early childhood in the United States: risk factors and racial/ethnic disparities. Pediatrics. 2007;120:568–575.

Cogswell ME, Looker AC, Pfeiffer CM, Cook JD, Lacher DA, Beard JL, Lynch SR, et al. Assessment of iron deficiency in US preschool children and nonpregnant females of childbearing age: National Health and Nutrition Examination Survey 2003–2006. Am J Clin Nutr. 2009;89:1334–1342.

Looker AC, Cogswell ME, Gunter EW. Iron deficiency—United States, 1999–2000. Morb Mortal Wkly Rep. 2002;51:897–899.

Looker AC, Dallman PR, Carroll M, Gunter EW, Johnson CL. Prevalence of iron deficiency in the United States. J Am Med Assoc. 1997;277:973–975.

Looker AC, Gunter EW, Johnson CL. Methods to assess iron status in various NHANES surveys. Nutr Rev. 1995;53:246–254.

Looker AC, Gunter EW, Cook JD, Green R, Harris JW. Comparing serum ferritin values from different population surveys. National Center for Health Statistics. Vital Health Stat Series No 2(111), 1991.

Mei Z, Cogswell ME, Looker AC, Pfeiffer CM, Cusick SE, Lacher DA, et al. Assessment of iron status in US pregnant women from the National Health and Nutrition Examination Survey 1999–2006. Am J Clin Nutr. 2011; in print.

Michels Blanck H, Cogswell ME, Gillespie C, Reyes M. Iron supplement use and iron status among US adults: results from the Third National Health and Nutrition Examination Survey. Am J Clin Nutr. 2005;82:1024–1031.

Ramakrishnan U, Frith-Terhune A, Cogswell M, Kettel Khan L. Dietary intake does not account for differences in low iron stores among Mexican American and non-Hispanic white women: Third National Health and Nutrition Examination Survey, 1988–1994. J Nutr. 2002;132:996–1001.

Iodine

Caldwell KL, Makhmudov A, Ely E, Jones RL, Wang R. Iodine status of the U.S. population, National Health and Nutrition Examination Survey, 2005–2006 and 2007–2008. Thyroid 2011;21:419–427.

Caldwell KL, Miller GA, Wang RY, Jain RB, Jones RL. Iodine status of the U.S. population, National Health and Nutrition Examination Survey 2003–2004. Thyroid. 2008;18:1207–1214.

Caldwell KL, Jones R, Hollowell JG. Urinary iodine concentration: United States National Health and Nutrition Examination Survey 2001–2002. Thyroid. 2005;15:692–699.

Hollowell JG, Staehling NW, Hannon WH, Flanders DW, Gunter EW, Maberly GF, et al. Iodine nutrition in the United States. Trends and public health implications: iodine excretion data from National Health and Nutrition Examination Surveys I and III (1971–1974 and 1988–1994). J Clin Endocrinol Metab. 1998;83:3401–3408.

Semba RD, Ricks MO, Ferrucci L, Xue QL, Guralnik JM, Fried LP. Low serum selenium is associated with anemia among older adults in the United States. Eur J Clin Nutr. 2009;64:93–99.

Vogt TM, Ziegler RG, Patterson BH, Graubard BI. Racial differences in serum selenium concentrations: analysis of US population data from the Third National Health and Nutrition Examination Survey. Am J Epidemiol. 2007;166:280–288.

Isoflavones and Lignans

U.S. Centers for Disease Control and Prevention. Fourth National Report on Human Exposure to Environmental Chemicals. Atlanta (GA): CDC; 2009. [cited 2011]. Available from: http://www.cdc.gov/exposurereport.

Valentin-Blasini L, Sadowski MA, Walden D, Caltabiano L, Needham LL, Barr DB. Urinary phytoestrogen concentrations in the U.S. population (1999–2000). J Expo Anal Environ Epidemiol. 2005;15:509–523.

Valentin-Blasini L, Blount BC, Caudill SP, Needham LL. Urinary and serum concentrations of seven phytoestrogens in a human reference population subset. J Expo Anal Environ Epidemiol. 2003;13:276–282.

Acrylamide Hemoglobin Adducts

Vesper HW, Caudill SP, Osterloh JD, Meyers T, Scott D, Myers GL. 2009. Exposure of the U.S. population to acrylamide in the National Health and Nutrition Examination Survey 2003–2004. Environ Health Perspect. 2010;118:278–283.

www.ingramcontent.com/pod-product-compliance
Lightning Source LLC
Chambersburg PA
CBHW080227180526

45167CB00006B/2242